Educational Review Manual in Infectious Disease

4th Edition – 2009

Edited by

Burke A. Cunha, MD, MACP
Chief, Infectious Disease Division
Winthrop-University Hospital
Mineola, New York
and
Professor of Medicine
State University of New York School of Medicine
Stony Brook, New York

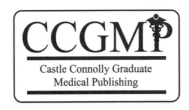

Castle Connolly Graduate Medical Publishing, Ltd.

17 Battery Place, Suite 643 • New York, NY 10004 • Tel: 212.644.9696 • Fax: 646.827.6443 • www.ccgmp.com • e-mail: info@ccgmp.com

Castle Connolly Graduate Medical Publishing, Ltd., publishes review manuals to assist residents and fellows in preparing for board certification exams.

Cover Photo:
This 2005 scanning electron micrograph (SEM) depicted numerous clumps of methicillin-resistant *Staphylococcus aureus* bacteria, commonly referred to by the acronym MRSA; Magnified 9560x. Image ID 10046 CDC-PHIL

Content Provider: CDC/ Janice Haney Carr/ Jeff Hageman, M.H.S.

Photo Credit: Janice Haney Carr, Electron Microscopist

NOTICE

Our thanks to Copy Editor Sarah Herndon

About the Editor-in-Chief

Burke A. Cunha, MD, MACP

Dr. Cunha is Chief, Infectious Disease Division at Winthrop-University Hospital, Mineola, New York, and Professor of Medicine, State University of New York School of Medicine, Stony Brook, New York. He established the first Infectious Disease Fellowship training program on Long Island in 1980.

Dr. Cunha is internationally recognized as a teacher-clinician and he is the recipient of many teaching awards including the prestigious Aesculapius Award, the highest distinction for teaching excellence awarded by the State University from the New York School of Medicine at Stony Brook. He was selected Distinguished Alumni Fellow of the Pennsylvania State University College of Medicine. For years, Dr. Cunha has been listed annually in Castle Connolly Medical's *America's Top Doctors*.

He serves on over two dozen infectious disease journal editorial boards and is a reviewer for over 30 infectious disease/medical journals. Dr. Cunha has written/co-authored 125 abstracts, 1,130 articles, and 180 book chapters. He has edited 27 books on various infectious disease topics including the highly respected *Antibiotic Essentials*, now in its 8th edition, *Pneumonia Essentials*, now in its 3rd edition, and *Infectious Disease in Critical Care Medicine*, also in its 3rd edition. He has served as the Editor-in-Chief of the journals *Infectious Disease Practice* and *Antibiotics for Clinicians*, and is Infectious Disease Editor-in-Chief of the world's first Internet textbook of medicine (*eMedicine*).

Dr. Cunha is a Fellow of the Infectious Disease Society of America, American Academy of Microbiology, American College of Clinical Pharmacology, and American College of Chest Physicians. Dr. Cunha is also a Master of the American College of Physicians, awarded for lifetime achievement as a master clinician and teacher of infectious diseases.

Dedication

This book is dedicated to:

*The great master teacher-clinicians
of the past and present
who taught me the art of the differential
diagnosis using the clinical
syndromic approach.*

Contributors

Burke A. Cunha, MD
Chief, Infectious Disease Division
Winthrop-University Hospital
Mineola, New York
and
Professor of Medicine
State University of New York School of Medicine,
Stony Brook, New York

Marvin J. Bittner, MD, MSc
Attending Physician
Veterans Administration Medical Center
and
Associate Professor of Medicine
Creighton University School of Medicine
Omaha, Nebraska

John L. Brusch, MD
Associate Chief of Medicine
Cambridge Health Alliance
Cambridge, Massachusetts
Medical Director
Somerville Hospital
Somerville, Massachusetts
and
Assistant Professor of Medicine
Harvard Medical School
Boston, Massachusetts

Daniel Caplivski, MD
Attending Physician
Division of Infectious Disease
Director, Travel Medicine Program
and
Assistant Professor of Medicine
Mt. Sinai School of Medicine
New York, New York

Stanley W. Chapman, MD
Director, Division of Infectious Diseases
Vice-Chair Department of Medicine Academic and
Clinical Affairs
University of Mississippi Medical Center
and
Professor of Medicine and Microbiology
University of Mississippi School of Medicine
Jackson, Mississippi

Dennis Cleri, MD
Chairman, Department of Medicine
St. Francis Medical Center
and
Professor of Medicine
Seton Hall University
School of Graduate Medical Education
Trenton, New Jersey

Nancy F. Crum-Cianflone, MD
Clinical Research Physician,
Infectious Disease Section
and
Voluntary Associate Professor
Naval Medical Center San Diego
San Diego, California

Sherwood L. Gorbach, MD
Professor of Public Health and Medicine
Tufts University School of Medicine
Boston, Massachusetts

Braden R. Hale, MD, MPH
Attending Physician,
Infectious Diseases Section
Naval Medical Center San Diego
San Diego, California

Davidson H. Hamer, MD
Director, Travel Clinic of Boston Medical Center
Tufts University Friedman School of Nutrition Science and
Policy
Boston, Massachusetts
and
Associate Professor of Nutrition
Associate Professor of International Health
Boston University School of Public Health
Boston, Massachusetts

Nancy Khardori, MD, PhD
Chief, Infectious Disease Division
Southern Illinois University School of Medicine
and
Professor of Medicine and Microbiology
Southern Illinois University School of Medicine
Springfield , Illinois

Raymond S. Koff, MD
Clinical Professor of Medicine
University of Connecticut School of Medicine
Farmington, Connecticut

Camille Kotton, MD
Clinical Director,
Transplant Infectious Disease and Compromised Host Program
Infectious Diseases Division
Massachusetts General Hospital
and
Assistant Professor
Harvard Medical School
Boston, Massachusetts

Edith Lederman, MD
Director, Travel Clinic of Naval Medical Center
and
Infectious Disease Specialist
Naval Medical Center San Diego
San Diego, California

Fred A. Lopez, MD
Vice Chairman, Department of Medicine
Louisiana State University of Health Sciences Center
and
Associate Professor of Medicine
Louisiana State University School of Medicine
New Orleans, Louisiana

Larry I. Lutwick, MD
Director, Infectious Disease Division
Brooklyn Veterans Administration Medical Center
and
Professor of Medicine
State University of New York at Downstate
Brooklyn, New York

James H. Maguire, MD, MPH
Master Clinician,
Division of Infectious Diseases
Brigham and Women's Hospital
Boston, Massachusetts
and
Professor of Medicine,
Harvard Medical School
Boston, Massachusetts

Brian P. McDermott, DO
Infectious Disease Fellow
Infectious Disease Division
Winthrop-University Hospital
Mineola, New York
and
Instructor in Medicine
SUNY School of Medicine
Stony Brook, New York

Maria D. Mileno, MD
Attending Physician,
Infectious Disease Division
The Miriam Hospital
and
Associate Professor of Medicine,
Brown University School of Medicine
Providence, Rhode Island

Francisco M. Pherez, MD
Infectious Disease Fellow
Infectious Disease Division
Winthrop-University Hospital
Mineola, New York
and
Instructor in Medicine
SUNY School of Medicine
Stony Brook, New York

Nitin Patel, MD
Infectious Disease Fellow
Infectious Disease Division
Southern Illinois University School of Medicine
Springfield , Illinois

Laurel C Preheim, MD
Chief, Department of Medicine
Veterans Administration Nebraska-Western Iowa Care System
and
Professor of Medicine, Medical Microbiology and Immunology
Creighton University School of Medicine and University of
Nebraska School of Medicine
Omaha, Nebraska

Michael F. Rein, MD
Emeritus Professor of Medicine, Division of Infectious Diseases
University of Virginia Health System

William S. Jordan, Jr.
Professor of Medicine
University of Virginia School of Medicine
Charlottesville, Virginia

Anthony J. Ricketti, MD
Chairman, Department of Medicine
and
Head Section of Allergy and Immunology
Associate Program Director, Internal Medicine Residency
St. Francis Medical Center
and
Associate Professor of Medicine
Seton Hall University School of Graduate Medical Education
South Orange, New Jersey

Keith Rodvold, PharmD
Professor of Pharmacy Practice and Medicine
Colleges of Pharmacy and Medicine
University of Illinois at Chicago
Chicago, Illinois

Charles V. Sanders, MD
Chairman, Department of Internal Medicine
Louisiana State University Health Science Center
and
Edgar Hull Professor of Medicine
Professor of Microbiology, Immunology, and Parasitology
Louisiana State University School of Medicine
New Orleans, Louisiana

Paul E. Sax, MD
Clinical Director,
Division of Infectious Diseases & HIV Program
Brigham and Women's Hospital
Boston, Massachusetts
and
Associate Professor of Medicine
Harvard Medical School
Boston, Massachusetts

Leon G. Smith, MD
Chairman, Department of Medicine
St. Michael's Medical Center
and
Professor of Medicine
Seton Hall School of Medicine
Newark, New Jersey

Stephen M. Smith, MD
Chief, Infectious Disease Division
St. Michael's Medical Center
and
Associate Professor of Medicine
Seton Hall School of Medicine
Newark, New Jersey

Donna C. Sullivan, PhD
Attending Physician,
Division of Infectious Diseases
and
Professor of Medicine
University of Mississippi Medical Center
Jackson, Mississippi

John R. Vernaleo, MD
Chief, Division of Infectious Diseases
Wyckoff Heights Medical Center
Brooklyn, New York

Mark R. Wallace, MD
Infectious Disease Specialty Leader
Infectious Disease Section
Naval Medical Center San Diego
and
Clinical Professor of Medicine
University of California, San Diego
San Diego, California

Contents

SECTION 4.
ANTIMICROBIAL THERAPY / PROPHYLAXIS

SECTION 5.
QUESTIONS FOR THE ID BOARDS

Preface

Fourth Edition

We are most pleased to be able to provide you with this *Educational Review Manual in Infectious Disease,* now in its 4th edition, through the generous support of Ortho-McNeil-Janssen Pharmaceuticals, Inc.

This manual was written by a group of distinguished clinicians to provide you with a board-relevant review of key topics in clinical infectious disease that will facilitate your preparation for the infectious disease board examination.

I would like to thank the authors for their excellent contributions. I am particularly indebted to Dr. Michael Wolf, whose editorial expertise and advice were invaluable. His staff at Castle Connolly Graduate Medical Publishing is to be commended for their fine efforts in producing such an excellent and comprehensive board review manual for Infectious Disease fellows.

Special thanks go to Lisa Haave at Winthrop-University Hospital for her assistance.

Building on your Infectious Disease fellowship training and your own reading, this book should be of great value in helping you to review for the Infectious Disease boards.

Burke A. Cunha, MD, MACP
Editor-in-Chief

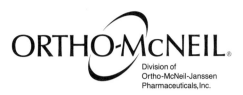

ORTHO-MCNEIL®

Division of
Ortho-McNeil-Janssen
Pharmaceuticals, Inc.

June 19, 2009

Dear Infectious Disease Fellow:

Ortho-McNeil® is proud to sponsor the *Educational Review Manual In Infectious Disease* 2009.

This manual is a tool to assist you through the completion of your fellowship training. It was
prepared under the guidance of editor-in-chief Burke A. Cunha, MD, MACP, Chief, Infectious Disease Division,
Winthrop-University Hospital Mineola, New York, and Professor of Medicine, State University of New York
School of Medicine, Stony Brook, New York. Written by expert educators from medical centers around the US, this
manual will be an invaluable tool for you in the months and years ahead.

As a leader in anti-infectives, Ortho-McNeil® is committed to developing new antimicrobials that will help healthcare
professionals care for their patients.

Ortho-McNeil® is committed to the continued education of healthcare professionals and commends the authors and
the esteemed editor for an outstanding effort in developing this review.

We hope that the wealth of information presented herein will enrich your understanding of Infectious Diseases and
help you during your training.

If you are licensed in any State or other jurisdiction, or an employee or contractor of any organization or
governmental entity, that limits or prohibits any items of value from pharmaceutical companies, your name, the
value, and purpose of this educational gift may be reported as required by state or federal law. Once reported, this
information may be publicly accessible.

Regards,

Susan Nicholson, MD
Therapeutic Area Lead, Anti-Infective Franchise
Ortho-McNeil Janssen Scientific Affairs, LLC

Test Taking Strategies

Burke A. Cunha, MD

- There are now annual in-service examinations for Infectious Disease fellows preparing to take the boards. These exams are helpful in identifying areas of strengths and weakness and to gauge your board review efforts.

- Another important benefit of taking the annual in-service Infectious Disease exams is giving fellows test taking practice and appreciation of topic distribution, the type of test questions, and degree of difficulty.

- Give yourself sufficient time to prepare before the Infectious Disease subspecialty boards. Between 9-12 months is optimal. Starting earlier extends the process over too long a period and you will be unable to remember key points. Less than 6 months of preparation is usually too short and inadequate.

- Be sure to review all infectious diseases, but concentrate particularly on those areas where you have had limited experience, e.g., virology, tropical medicine, parasitology, infections in transplants, zoonoses, or congenital/acquired immune defects, etc. Briefly review your areas of strength, but concentrate on areas of potential weakness.

- The time relegated to review various infectious disease topics should be inversely related to mastery of a topic. The less familiar you are with a topic, the more times the topic should be given in review preparation.

- Board review time is often limited by personal/professional commitments. Use the infectious disease sections of Harrison's Principles of Internal Medicine to quickly overview most infectious disease topics. The infectious diseases section in Harrison's is concise and excellent.

- If needed, additional texts may be used. A tropical medicine text would be useful for certain topics. Strickland's, Manson's, Guerrant, or Weller & Walker's Tropical Infectious Diseases are recommended.

- For infection control and hospital epidemiology, either Mayhall's Hospital Epidemiology and Infection Control or Wenzel's Prevention and Control of Nosocomial Infections provide depth, if needed, on specific topics.

- In-service exam courses and atlases are helpful in infectious disease board review. Atlases of microbiology and parasitology will help you to recall key points of infectious diseases not seen frequently. Atlases also reinforce key points about infections recently reviewed. Color atlases of skin rashes are particularly useful. Color atlases of general infectious diseases, sexually transmitted diseases, and tropical medicine are helpful and should be used in conjunction with your review efforts.

- Infectious Disease fellows preparing for the exam should try to study for at least two hours per night during the week and at least four hours during each weekend. On weekdays, new topics should be covered.

- Weekends should be used for reviewing the information covered during the preceding week and for utilization of color atlases and supplementary materials to solidify and reinforce memory.

- Infectious Disease board review courses also can identify problem areas, and are of most benefit for becoming more familiar with answering board type questions.

- The forte of the Infectious Disease consultant is differential diagnostic skills, and Infectious Disease fellows should concentrate on the syndromic approach to differential diagnosis during the review process.

- Don't learn simply what is "consistent" with the diagnosis but rather concentrate on what is "characteristic" of each infectious disease.

- Keeping differential diagnostic considerations foremost, learn the key differentiating features of clinical syndromes using pertinent history, physical examination, and non-specific laboratory tests.

- Infectious Disease boards are difficult and contain many "red herrings," but sufficient clues are present to select the correct diagnosis/answer.

- Differentiating between non-infectious and infectious diseases is the key in consultative infectious disease practice. Learning to discern the mimics of infectious diseases from their infectious counterparts is essential. Learn to separate the "look-alikes" using the clinical syndromic approach.

- If you don't know the likely differential/diagnostic possibilities, you can't possibly select appropriate correct therapy.

- Concentrate on epidemiology, clinical presentation, differential diagnosis, and complications of infectious diseases. Prognostic factors and therapy are important, but are stressed less.

- The boards are scored on the number of answers that are correct. Therefore, leave no questions unanswered since you cannot be given any credit for questions left blank. Blind guessing should be avoided. However, after narrowing possibilities, intelligent guessing is definitely recommended. Usually, two or three answers can be eliminated for one reason or another and the final selection is between two choices.

- Some questions will seem impossibly difficult, so don't spend too much time answering one difficult test question. Do the best you can and quickly move on so that you complete all sections by the end of the test. Difficult and relatively easy questions have the same value.

- By proceeding in this fashion over the course of the test, if you can limit your selective guessing to one of two possible correct answers, your score will be much better than if you try to blindly guess the correct answer from five possible choices.

- When you read the question, read it over quickly three times before answering. First, quickly read to determine the nature of the question (e.g., this is a question about CNS mass lesions in a renal transplant). Second, re-read for any modifying terms e.g., always, usually, never, double negatives, etc. that may modify the meaning of the question. Third, re-read to determine the point of the question.

- Try to figure out why this question is being asked. What are they trying to test with this question? For example, if a gram-positive bacillus is seen on Gram stain of the CSF patient with meningitis, the differential diagnosis is between a skin organism (e.g., Corynebacterium/Propionibacterium vs. Listeria). The point in asking such a question is related to the microbiologic differentiation between Listeria and gram-positive bacilli from the skin contaminating CSF. Hemolysis on blood agar and "tumbling motility" would clearly differentiate Listeria from gram-positive skin flora. The point of the question is that you should know that Listeria are hemolytic on blood agar and are motile.

- If you cannot figure out the point of the question, you can't possibly select the correct answer. After all, all of the answers are correct for some other question. If you can determine the point of the question, the correct answer should be readily apparent.

- Time may be a factor when taking the test. Look over each test section and gauge approximately how much time you have for each question. Answer the least difficult questions as quickly as you can to possibly gain extra time for those more difficult questions that may be solved with some additional time.

- When reviewing completed questions, do not change an answer unless you are certain it's correct. The initial answer is usually the correct answer.

- When the test is over, you may feel exhausted mentally and emotionally. Remember the most important benefit of taking the Infectious Disease boards is the obligatory review of all Infectious Disease topics during test preparation. Without Infectious Disease boards, few Infectious Disease fellows would spend the time and effort to review the entire discipline with the rigor required for the boards. For many, this is the only time they will review the entire discipline in depth.

- The Infectious Disease boards perform a valuable function in encouraging such a comprehensive review, which subsequently will make the Infectious Disease fellows better Infectious Disease consultants.

- I trust that this manual has been helpful to you in reviewing for the Infectious Disease boards.

- Good luck with the test!

Burke A. Cunha, MD, MACP
Editor-in-Chief
and
Chief, Infectious Disease Division
Winthrop-University Hospital
Mineola, New York
and
Professor of Medicine
State University of New York School of Medicine
Stony Brook, New York

This page was left blank intentionally

Chapter 1:
Fever for the ID Boards

Burke A. Cunha, MD

Contents

1. Fever Patterns

The diagnostic significance of acute fevers depends on their frequency, elevation, pattern and relationship to the pulse.

2. Magnitude of the Fever

General Concepts

- The diagnostic usefulness of fever patterns is most helpful *when there are no other signs suggesting an infectious or noninfectious disorder.*

- *Characteristics of the fever may be the only clue to the diagnosis or* a guide to further diagnostic testing.

Temperatures 100°F
- Patients who are leukopenic-compromised hosts, who are elderly or who have *chronic renal failure* may demonstrate little/no fever in response to an infection.

- Slight elevation of temperatures in leukopenic-compromised hosts often has diagnostic significance.

Temperatures 102°-106°F
- *Most* infectious fevers occur between 102°F-106°F in immunocompetent hosts.

Temperatures <102°F
- Temperatures ≤102°F *may be infectious or noninfectious.*

ID Board Pearls

Hypothermia (≤97°F)
- Usually indicates an inability of the host to mount a febrile response. *Hypothermia is a poor prognostic sign.*

- May be due to overzealous antipyretic therapy.

- May be an indication of infection.

Causes of hypothermia:
- Advanced age

- Uremia

- Cold exposure

- Hypothalamic dysfunction

- Hypothyroidism

- Overwhelming infection

Extreme Hyperpyrexia (>106ºF)
- *Extreme hyperpyrexia* (≥ 106°F) is *not* usually due to infection.

- Malignant hyperthermia

- Central fevers (infection, malignancy,

- Malignant neuroleptic syndrome (usually drug-induced) trauma, hemorrhage, etc.)

- Heat stroke

- Drug fevers

ID Board Pearls

- The only infectious disease that may cause extreme hyperpyrexia is tetanus

3. Diagnostic Significance of 102°F (The 102° Rule)

General Concepts

- *Some* infections have the *potential* for exceeding 102°F while others do not.

- The "102°F" rule is useful in the differential diagnosis of a variety of similar disorders.

ID Board Pearls

- Infectious diseases or disorders that have the potential to *exceed 102°F* do not *always* have temperatures ≥102°F.

4. Frequency of Fever Spikes

General Concepts

- Fevers may be described as *intermittent, continuous, sustained* or *remittent*.

- Relapsing fevers recur in various intervals after the initial febrile episode with or without repetitive pattern.

- *Most* infectious diseases have *no* specific fever patterns.

- Fever patterns based on *frequency* of fever spikes are useful in *selected* diseases, which *are otherwise difficult to diagnose*.

- Single fever spikes commonly occur *after blood or blood product transfusion* (including platelet transfusions) or manipulation or instrumentation of a *colonized* or *infected* mucosal surface/tissue.

- Transfusion-related fevers have a bimodal distribution. The temperatures occurring after blood product transfusion *usually occur within 72 hours. Less commonly,* there may be a febrile reaction 5-7 *days after the initial transfusion*.

- Fever secondary to a transfusion reaction should not be considered for fevers occurring 7 days after transfusion.

ID Board Pearls

- Fevers occurring *more* than 7 days posttransfusion may be related to blood transfusion-related *infection*, but *not* a febrile reaction to blood components per se.

- *Single fever spikes are virtually never due to an infectious cause*.

5. Diagnostic Fever Patterns

General Concepts

Camel-Back Fever Curves

- Refers to 2 febrile episodes separated by a decrease in temperature to normal or near normal *over a 5-7 day period*.

- Differential diagnosis of camel-back fevers:

    * Colorado tick fever (CTF)

    * Ehrlichiosis (rarely)

    * Dengue fever

General Concepts

Double Quotidian Fevers

- Double quotidian fever refers to 2 fever spikes occurring within each 24-hour period (not induced by antipyretics).

ID Board Pearls

    * Differential diagnosis of double quotidian fever:

    * Mixed malarial infections

    * Kala-azar (visceral leishmaniasis)

    * Miliary TB (rarely)

    * Still's disease (adult JRA)

    * Right-sided gonococcal ABE

General Concepts

Morning Temperature

- Typhoid fever spikes

- PAN

- TB

- Whipples's Disease

6. Relapsing Fevers

General Concepts

- Relapsing fevers have a *longer period between febrile episodes* and the temperature *returns to normal* between the febrile episodes.

ID Board Pearls

- *Differential diagnosis of relapsing fevers:*

  * Dengue fever

  * Cholangitis

  * Yellow fever

  * Malaria

  * Brucellosis

  * Rat-bite fever *(S minus* or *S moniliformis)*

  * Relapsing fever *(Borrelia recurrentis)*

- Unlike relapsing fever, remittent fevers have very *short intervals between fever spikes* and the temperature does *not return to normal* between fever spikes.

7. Non-Relapsing Infections Prone to Relapse

- In contrast to relapsing fevers with a biphasic fever pattern usually separated by 1 or more weeks, certain infectious diseases are *prone to relapse without periodicity.*

- *Noninfectious disorders prone to relapse may be confused with infectious diseases.*

ID Board Pearls

- *Differential diagnosis infectious diseases prone to relapse:*

  * Leptospirosis

  * Chronic meningococcemia

  * Bartonella

  * EBV

  * Q fever

  * CMV

  * Melioidosis

  * Babesiosis

  * Lymphocytic choriomeningitis (LCM)

  * Malaria

- *Common causes of noninfectious disorders prone to relapse:*

  * Cyclic neutropenia

  * Familial Mediterranean Fever (FMF)

  * Crohn's disease

  * FAPA syndrome

  * Weber-Christian disease

  * SLE

  * Behçet's disease

* Hyper IgD syndrome

* Sweet's syndrome

* Relapsing polychondritis

8. Fever Defervescence Patterns

General Concepts

- Fever *defervescence* patterns confirm the infection is resolving. *Departure from the usual defervescence pattern may suggest a complication* (eg, myocardial infarction, emboli, etc.).

- Most *viral* infections usually defervesce *gradually* over a week or more.

- Antipyretics and steroids decrease temperatures nonspecifically and are *unhelpful* diagnostically.

- Appropriately treated bacterial infections are manifested by a *rapid* decrease in temperature.

- *Infections due to different organisms defervescence temperature at different rates, which may be used clinically.*

- Temperatures due to febrile *noninfectious* disease disorders do *not decrease* rapidly without antipyretic or specific therapy.

Rapid Fever Defervescence Patterns
- Viridans streptococcal SBE

- *S pneumoniae* CAP

Delayed Defervescence Pattern
- Enterococcal SBE (not as slow as ABE nor as rapid as viridans SBE).

- Defervesce with a "hectic/septic" pattern over 5-7 days.

ID Board Pearls

Reappearance of Fever after an Initial Decrease
- May suggest a *relapse or a complication:*

  * Gout

  * Pulmonary embolus

  * Pancreatitis

  * Drug fever

* Myocardial infarction

- *Rarely due to antibiotic resistance occurring during therapy.*

Pulse-Temperature Relationships (Relative Bradycardia and Relative Tachycardia)

- Elevations in temperature are accompanied by an appropriate increase in pulse rate to deliver increased oxygen to tissues, remove metabolic waste products, and to decrease the temperature of the host.

- In healthy adults, for *every degree of elevation of temperature in degrees Fahrenheit, there is a commensurate increase in the pulse of 10 beats/min* (Table 1).

- If the pulse rate is elevated *above what is appropriate for the temperature, the pulse/temperature* relationship is termed *relative tachycardia.*

9. Relative Tachycardia

General Concepts

- An increase in pulse above that appropriate for the temperature is termed relative tachycardia.

- Differential diagnosis of *relative tachycardia:*

ID Board Pearls

- Anxiety

- Hypoxemia (any cause)

- Hypothyroidism

- Diphtheria

- Arrhythmia

- Gas gangrene

- Pulmonary emboli

10. Relative Bradycardia

General Concepts

- *If the pulse is less than would be appropriate for a given degree of temperature elevation*, the pulse temperature relationship is termed *relative* bradycardia (Figure 1).

- Relative bradycardia should be distinguished from *absolute* bradycardia (a decrease in the pulse to ≤60 bpm in the absence of fever).

- Before a patient with a pulse-temperature deficit is considered to have relative bradycardia (for diagnostic purposes), the *following conditions, which cause pulse temperature deficits, should be excluded:*

- Lev's disease

- Lenègre's disease

- β-blocker medications

- Diltiazem

- Pacemaker rhythms

- Verapamil

- Relative bradycardia may be caused by a *variety of infectious and noninfectious disorders*.

Noninfectious Disorders
- Drug fever

- Central fevers

- Lymphomas

- Factitious fever

Infectious Causes
- Typhoid fever

- Typhus

- Malaria

- Babesiosis

- Rocky Mountain Spotted Fever

- Ehrlichiosis

- Leptospirosis

- Yellow fever

- Dengue fever

- African hemorrhagic fevers

- Psittacosis

- Q fever

- Legionnaires' disease

ID Board Pearls

- Pulse-temperature relationships are *not* affected by the following medications:

  * Digitalis preparations

  * Most calcium channel blockers

  * ACE inhibitors

Reappearance of Fever after an Initial Decrease
- May suggest a *relapse or a complication*:

  * Gout

  * Pulmonary embolus

  * Pancreatitis

  * Drug fever

  * Myocardial infarction

  * Abscess

Figure 1

Relative bradycardia (Pulse-temperature deficit) in a patient with Legionnaires' disease

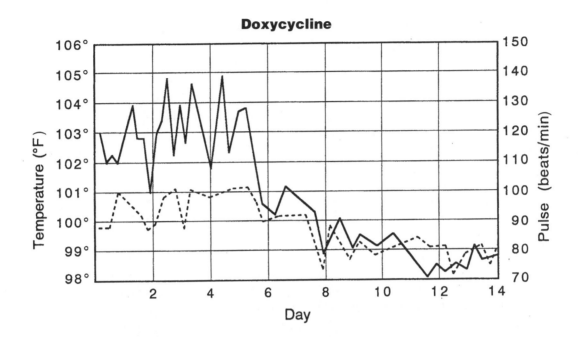

From Cunha BA. The clinical significance of fever patterns. Infect Dis Clin North Am. *1996;10:33-44.*

Table 1

Pulse-Temperature Relationships

Temperature	Appropriate Pulse Response (beats/min)	Relative Bradycardia Pulse (beats/min)
106°F (41.1°C)	150	< 140
105°F (40.6°C)	140	< 130
104°F (40.7°C)	130	< 120
103°F (39.4°C)	120	< 110
102°F (38.9°C)	110	< 100

From Cunha BA. Antibiotic Essentials, *8th ed. Jones & Bartlett, Sudbury, MA, 2009.*

11. Drug Fever

- Drug fevers account for approximately *10% of fevers in hospitalized patients*.

- The mechanism of drug fever is poorly understood but is *probably mediated via the liver*.

- *Drug fever is unaccompanied by rash* and may be the sole manifestation of the hypersensitivity response to a medication.

- *Drug fever is a diagnosis of exclusion*.

- Patients with drug fevers are usually atopic, but need not be.

- Patients with drug fever look *relatively well for the degree of fever (Table 2)*.

- Drug fevers may occur at <102°F or >106°F but *most often occur between 102°F and 104°F*.

- In drug fever, cultures are negative, *excluding* contaminants or in patients without concurrent infection.

- Patients *may have a drug fever with an infectious disease that may occur from either an antibiotic or nonantibiotic medication*.

- Relative bradycardia is the *cardinal* finding in drug fever.

- The type of fever seen following exposure to the medication is variable and may occur after 1 dose or years after the initial sensitizing dose.

- If on only 1 sensitizing medication likely to cause drug fever, the medication should be discontinued.

- If on multiple sensitizing medications, the *non-life supporting sensitizing medications should be discontinued*, which should result in a decrease in temperature over 3 days.

ID Board Pearls

- The *likelihood of the medication causing drug fever increases, not decreases, over time*.

- The longer the patient is on a medication, the *more likely* (*not* less likely) to have a reaction to the medication.

- If a patient develops a drug fever and the offending medication is discontinued, fever decreases to normal/near-normal levels *within 72 hours*.

- Fevers in patients with a drug *rash* may take *days or weeks to resolve*, even after the medication is discontinued.

Table 2

Clinical Features of Drug Fevers

History

Many individuals are atopic
May have been on sensitizing medication for days or years

Physical Examination

Low- to high-grade fevers (102°F - 106°F usual)
Relative bradycardia (with temperature greater than 102°F)
Look "inappropriately well" for degree of fever

Laboratory Tests

Elevated WBC count (usually with left shift)
Atypical lymphocytes (<5%) often present, but atypical lymphocytosis less common
Eosinophils are present, but eosinophilia is uncommon (< 20%)
Elevated erythrocyte sedimentation rate (ESR) in majority of cases (may be very rapid; 60 to ≥100 mm/h)
Mild /transient elevations of serum transaminases (> 90%) is common

Adapted from Cunha BA. Approach to the patient with fever. In: Samiy AH, ed. Textbook of Diagnostic Medicine. *Philadelphia, PA: Lea & Febiger; 1987:154.*

12. Causes of Fever in the ICU

General Concepts

- The *major* diagnostic problem is to differentiate *noninfectious disorders from infectious* disorders. This is done best by history, physical, selected laboratory tests, and taking into account the characteristics of the fever pattern.

- It is important to differentiate sepsis from non-infectious disorders, which may *mimic* sepsis.

- For sepsis to occur, there must be a *gross breach of host defenses to permit a large inoculum of organisms to overwhelm host defenses.*

ID Board Pearls

- *Sepsis does not occur randomly* and requires a *major* disruption of host defenses.

13. Fever in Neurosurgical ICUs

General Concepts

- Fever in neurosurgical patients may be neuro-surgically or *not* neurosurgically related.

- The *major* diagnostic problem is to differentiate *noninfectious from infectious* causes.

- *Infectious* causes are usually related to *open head trauma or AV/VP shunt-related infections.*

- Common *non*-neurosurgically related infections include:

  * Nosocomial pneumonia

  * Central IV line infections

ID Board Pearls

- Common noninfectious causes of fever in the ICU include:

  * Central fever

  * Drug fever

  * Subdural hematoma

  * Phlebitis

  * Intracranial hemorrhage

  * Pulmonary embolus or infarction

  * Posterior fossa syndrome

14. Pseudosepsis

General Concepts

- Pseudosepsis is a term for fever, leukocytosis and hypotension *not* due to infection.

ID Board Pearls

- Differential diagnosis of *pseudosepsis* includes:

  * Acute myocardial infarction

  * Overzealous diuresis

  * Pulmonary embolism or infarction

  * Relative adrenal insufficiency

  * Gastrointestinal hemorrhage

  * Acute pancreatitis

  * Rectus sheath hematoma

- Certain infections *do not* cause sepsis unless there are other extenuating circumstances:

  * Osteomyelitis

  * CAP (*excluding* hyposplenia or asplenia)

  * Septic arthritis (excluding GC arthritis/dermatitis syndrome)

  * Meningitis (*without* meningococcemia)

  * Viridans or enterococcal subacute endocarditis(SBE)

  * Catheter-associated bacteriuria (CAB), pre-existing renal disease/stone disease in normal hosts

15. Further Reading

Cluff LE, Johnson JE. *Clinical Concepts of Infectious Diseases*. 3rd ed. Baltimore, MD: Williams & Wilkins; 1982.

Cohen J, Powderly WG. *Infectious Diseases*. 2nd ed. New York, NY: Mosby; 2004.

Cristie AB. *Infectious Diseases: Epidemiology and Clinical Practice*. 4th ed. Vols. 1 and 2. New York, NY: Churchill Livingstone; 1987.

Cunha BA, ed. *Infectious Diseases in Critical Care Medicine*. 3rd ed. New York, NY: Informa Healthcare; 2009.

Cunha BA. Infectious diseases. In: Samiy AH, Bardoness J, Douglas RG, eds. *Textbook of Diagnostic Medicine*. Philadelphia, PA: Lea & Febiger; 1987.

Isaac B, Kernbaum S, Burke M. *Unexplained Fever*. Boca Raton, FL: CRC Press; 1991.

Gorbach SL, Bartlett JG, Blacklow NR. *Infectious Diseases*. 3rd ed. New York, NY: Lippincott Williams & Wilkins; 2004.

Kluger MJ. *Fever: Its Biology, Evolution, and Function*. Princeton, NJ: Princeton University Press; 1979.

Lawson JH. *A Synopsis of Fevers and Their Treatment*. London, England: Lloyd-Luke Ltd; 1977.

Mackowiak PA. *Fever: Basic Mechanisms and Management*. 2nd ed. New York, NY: Lippincott Williams & Wilkins; 1997.

Mandell GL. *Principles and Practice of Infectious Diseases*. 6th ed. Philadelphia, PA: Churchill Livingstone; 2005.

Root RK. *Clinical Infectious Diseases: A Practical Approach*. 1st ed. New York, NY; Oxford University Press; 1999.

Schlossberg D, Shulman JA, eds. *Differential Diagnosis of Infectious Disease*. Baltimore, MD; Lippincott Williams & Wilkins; 1996.

Woodward TE. The fever pattern as diagnostic aid. In: Mackowiak PA, ed. *Fever: Basic Mechanisms and Management*. 2nd ed. Philadelphia, PA: Lippincott-Raven; 1997.

Chapter 2:
Rash and Fever for the ID Boards

Fred A. Lopez, MD
Charles V. Sanders, MD

Contents

This chapter is designed for educational and informational purposes only. Readers should confirm the information contained herein with other sources, especially when prescribing and dosing medications.

Note: Though many of these organisms can infect multiple organ systems, this review will focus on their cutaneous manifestations.

1. Aeromonas

Synonyms

- Aeromonads

Causative Organisms

- Most common: *A hydrophila; A caviae; A veronii* biovar *sobria*

- Less common: *A veronii* biovar *veronii; A jandaei; A schubertii*

Epidemiology

- Wide distribution including freshwater lakes and rivers, brackish water, and even chlorinated water

- Increased isolation in warm summer months

- Usually community-acquired

- More common in immunocompromised adults and infants
    * Chronic liver disease or cirrhosis
    * Malignancy
    * Diabetes mellitus

Key Clinical Features

Intestinal (Most Due to *A hydrophila; A caviae; A veronii* biovar *sobria*)
Diarrhea and gastroenteritis
- Asymptomatic colonization
    * Usually acute with watery stools
        - Emesis may develop
        - Similar to "traveler's diarrhea"

- Occasional bloody diarrhea
    * Fever
    * Abdominal pain
    * Rarely chronic
    * Similar to dysentery

- Hemolytic uremic syndrome
    * Rarely caused by *Aeromonas*-associated diarrhea
    * Cytotoxin distinct from that associated with *E coli* O157:H7

Figure 1

Aeromonas septicemia

Aeromonas septicemia in a patient with acute leukemia showing a small cutaneous infarct on the hip that resolved

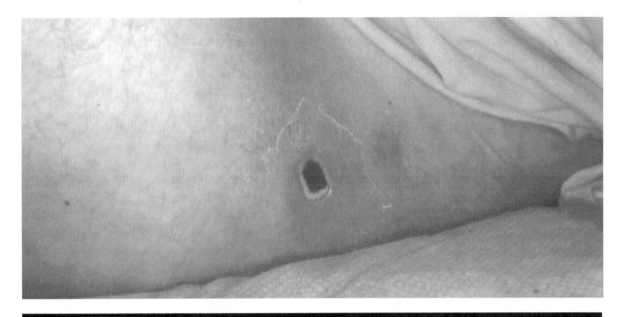

Courtesy of Dr Charles V. Sanders. From Johnson RA, Avram M, Chan E. Skin infections in the immunocompromised host – non-HIV. In: Sanders CV, Nesbitt LT Jr, eds. The Skin and Infection: A Color Atlas and Text. *Baltimore, MD: Williams & Wilkins; 1995:264. Used with permission.*

Extraintestinal
Wound and soft tissue infections (Figure 1)
- Often trauma-associated with aeromonad contaminated aquatic exposure
    * Usually due to abrasion, laceration or puncture injury
        - Typically lower extremities >> upper extremities
        - Cellulitis and abscess most characteristic
    * Crush injuries, severe burns
        - Cellulitis
        - Beware of necrotizing skin, soft tissue, and muscle infections including necrotizing fasciitis, myonecrosis, pyomyositis and gas gangrene
    * Medical procedures including vascular catheterization

- Medicinal leech-associated
    * Aeromonas species inhabit foregut of leech
    * Wound and bloodstream infections

Bloodstream infection
- Typically seeded from GI tract
    * GI symptoms
    * Fever
- Can result in sepsis

Other
- Peritonitis
    * Spontaneous bacterial peritonitis
    * Chronic ambulatory peritoneal dialysis-associated infection
    * Peritonitis secondary to bowel perforation

- Meningitis

- Respiratory tract infections
    * Lung abscess
    * Pneumonia with parapneumonia involvement
        - Secondary to aquatic exposures in immunocompetent individuals
        - Secondary to dissemination from GI tract in immunodeficient individuals

* Ocular infections, infective endocarditis, urinary tract infection and osteomyelitis

Key Laboratory and Radiology Features

Microbiology
- Oxidase-positive

- Gram-negative bacilli with single polar flagellum

- Nonsporulating facultative anaerobe

- Carbohydrate fermentation

- Variable lactose fermentation

- Often beta-hemolytic on blood agar

- Selective media (cefsulodin-Irgasan-novobiocin; media containing ampicillin) can be helpful in isolating from other enteric bacteria

Diagnosis

- Can be isolated from blood, stool, bile fluids and wounds

- Selective media (cefsulodin-Irgasan-novobiocin; media containing ampicillin) can be helpful in isolating from other enteric bacteria

- Automated machines can identify to genus level and at times species level

- Biochemical tests most useful to identify to species level

Differential Diagnosis

Includes other infectious diseases associated with exposure to water. These infections may be difficult to distinguish.

- *Edwardsiella tarda* (Gram-negative bacillus)
    * Gastroenteritis most common manifestation
    * Extra-gastrointestinal disease more common in liver disease and excess iron states
    * Can cause cellulitis, septic arthritis, necrotizing fasciitis and sepsis

- *Streptococcus iniae* (Gram-positive coccus)
    * Infects individuals who incur skin wounds while handling farm-raised fish (particularly tilapia)
    * Short incubation period after exposure
    * Cellulitis, purulent draining ulcers, and lymphangitis
    * Bacteremia with arthritis, endocarditis, and meningitis also reported

- *Erysipelothrix rhusiopathiae* (Gram-positive bacillus)
    * Does not cause gastrointestinal disease
    * Occupational disease of butchers and fish-handlers
    * Manifests as localized skin infection (ie, erysipeloid), diffuse skin involvement, or disseminated disease with infective endocarditis

- *Mycobacterium marinum* (Gram-positive, acid-fast bacillus)
    * Does not cause gastrointestinal disease
    * Typically affects individuals who experience trauma while working with aquariums or engaging in water sports
    * Typically localized skin infection on extremity beginning as papule or plaque; occasionally, sporotrichoid distribution of nodules along lymphatics
    * Extension to tendon and joint can occur but dissemination is rare
    * Usually indolent with absence of systemic signs

- *Vibrio vulnificus* (Gram-negative rod)
    * Found in brackish waters in warmer summer months
    * Short incubation period after exposure
    * Infection of skin due to direct trauma and water exposure or from hematogenous dissemination after ingestion of contaminated shellfish, most commonly oysters
    * More common in immunocompromised host with chronic liver disease (cirrhosis), iron overload states, malignancy or diabetes mellitus
    * Consider in toxic-appearing patient with rapidly progressive cellulites and associated hemorrhagic bullae and necrosis or necrotizing fasciitis

Noninfectious Disease Mimics
- *Contact dermatitis*
  - * History of exposure to irritant with direct skin toxicity (ie, cleansing detergents) or allergen with immunologically-mediated inflammation (ie, poison ivy) most important
  - * Lesion configuration and location dependent on exposure
    - Acute: erythematous patches with vesicles and crusts
    - Longer-standing: erythema, desquamation, lichenification, excoriated papules
    - Lesions typically pruritic
  - * Systemic signs and symptoms absent unless severe
  - * Patch testing for diagnosis of allergen-associated dermatitis; avoidance of suspected precipitant with improvement is often interpreted as diagnostic confirmation of both allergen- and irritant-induced contact dermatitis
  - * Often self-limited unless exposure persists
  - * Avoidance of exposure paramount
    - Short-course topical or systemic steroids, wet-to-dry compresses and antihistamines may be used for management (particularly when allergen-induced)

- *Severe drug-induced cutaneous hypersensitivity drug reactions (Stevens-Johnson syndrome and toxic epidermal necrolysis)*
  - * Usually within 3 weeks of starting medication
    - Can be associated with infections (remember herpes simplex virus) and malignancies
  - * Often associated with history of aminopenicillins, sulfa drugs, NSAIDs, allopurinol or anticonvulsant use
  - * Mucocutaneous involvement
    - \>2 mucosal surfaces involved
    - Initially diffuse erythema or disseminated red macules progressing to desquamation of epidermis
  - * <10% of body surface area consistent with Stevens-Johnson syndrome; >30%, toxic epidermal necrolysis
  - * Histopathology: full-thickness epidermal necrosis
  - * Supportive care with debridement as needed
    - Treat as burn patient

- Insufficient research from well-designed clinical trials to support routine use of prophylactic antibiotics, corticosteroids, intravenous immunoglobulin

- *Neutrophilic dermatosis (Sweet's syndrome)*
  - * Viral-illness typically precedes skin lesions
  - * Suspect in patient with underlying malignancy
  - * Often painful nonpruritic erythematous papules progressing to plaques or pustules
    - Characteristically located on upper body, particularly face, neck, hands and arms
    - Fever, myalgias, arthralgias or conjunctivitis common
  - * Labs may reveal increased acute phase reactants and leukocytosis with peripheral neutrophilia
  - * Histopathology reveals angiocentric neutrophilic infiltrate
  - * Refractory to antibiotics; standard treatment is with prednisone
    - NSAIDs and other anti-inflammatory steroid-sparing agents have been used

Other diagnostic possibilities to consider in the appropriate settings include skin manifestations of collagen vascular diseases, thermal injuries and cutaneous involvement of metastatic malignancy.

Empiric and Definitive Therapy

Skin and Soft Tissue Infection (Length of Therapy Approximately 10-21 days)

Empiric therapy after fresh water exposure
- First, third or 4th generation cephalosporin plus levofloxacin, 500 mg IV daily, or ciprofloxacin, 400 mg IV BID

Advantages
- Broad coverage of fresh water-associated pathogens

Disadvantages
- Decreased activity against *V vulnificus*

Note: Some would recommend gentamicin in lieu of quinolone to provide synergy with a beta-lactam against certain Gram-negative bacilli.

• If marine water exposure, add doxycycline 100 mg IV or PO for better coverage of *V vulnificus*

Definitive Therapy
(Based on Susceptibility Testing)
Preferred
• Levofloxacin 500 mg IV daily or ciprofloxacin 400 mg IV twice daily or daily

Advantages
• Well tolerated

• Oral formulation with excellent bioavailability

Disadvantages and potential adverse effects
• Expensive

• Diarrhea, nausea and vomiting

• Headache and insomnia

• Rash (rare)

Alternative
• Trimethoprim-sulfamethoxazole 10 mg/kg IV daily in 4 divided doses given q6h.

Advantages
• Pathogen-directed therapy

Disadvantages
• Numerous drug interactions and adverse effects (hypersensitivity reactions including rash, GI intolerance, bone marrow suppression)

• Use with caution in patients with renal insufficiency

• In some areas of the world (eg, southeast Asia), resistance to TMP-SMX is increasingly reported

Note: In necrotizing skin infections, early surgical debridement in addition to effective antimicrobials is imperative!

Complications of
***Aeromonas*-associated Skin Infection**
• Localized extension of infection into joints and bones

• Compartment syndromes and skin necrosis resulting in loss of limb (particularly with necrotizing fasciitis)

• Bacteremia with metastatic infections and abscesses

• Sepsis, multi-organ system failure and death

Prognostic Factors

• Crude mortality rates of 25-50%
• Poor prognosis in hospitalized patients with:
    * Renal insufficiency at admission
    * Underlying cirrhosis
    * Multiple blood cultures positive for *Aeromonas*
    * Community-acquired infections
    * Secondary source of bacteremia
    * Increased severity of illness scores

• Prevention by avoiding exposure of skin wound to potentially contaminated water and/or ingesting contaminated water

Infectious Disease Pearls: *Aeromonas*

1. *Aeromonas* is widely distributed and can be found in freshwater lakes and rivers, brackish/estuarine water, and even chlorinated water

2. Though this organism can infect immunocompetent hosts, it more commonly causes severe infections in immunocompromised hosts particularly those with cirrhosis, diabetes mellitus or cancer.

3. *Aeromonas* spp can intestinal and extraintestinal infections. Extraintestinal manifestations more commonly include skin and soft infections and blood stream infections.

4. Fluoroquinolone or trimethoprim-sulfamethoxazole are used for medical management of *Aeromonas* infections.

5. Like Vibrio vulnificus, this organism can cause necrotizing skin and soft tissue infections requiring aggressive surgical therapy in addition to medical management.

2. *Erysipelothrix*

Synonyms

• Erysipeloid; erysipeloid of Rosenbach; whale finger; seal finger; diamond skin disease

Causative Organisms

• *Erysipelothrix rhusiopathiae*

Epidemiology

• Ubiquitous: primarily a pathogen in animals
    * Swine are most important reservoir
    * Occupational risk for fish handlers and butchers

• Organism can survive for long periods in nature

• Most cases occur in summer months

• Infection in males >> females

• Infection initiated by introduction of organism through injured skin

Key Clinical Features (Figure 2)

• Three clinical syndromes: localized cutaneous infection (erysipeloid); generalized cutaneous infection; and systemic infection
    * Cutaneous infections constitute >90% of all infections

Localized Cutaneous Infection

• Most common form of infection

• Incubation period of <7 days

• Occurs at site of inoculation, typically fingers or dorsum of hands

• Pruritic, painful, purplish lesion
    * Well-defined plaque that slowly extends peripherally and clears centrally
    * Suppuration not characteristic
    * Fever, chills, joint pains and lymphadenopathy in less than one-third of all cases

Figure 2

Erysipeloid

Violaceous maculopapular lesions of the fingers that developed after cleaning fish

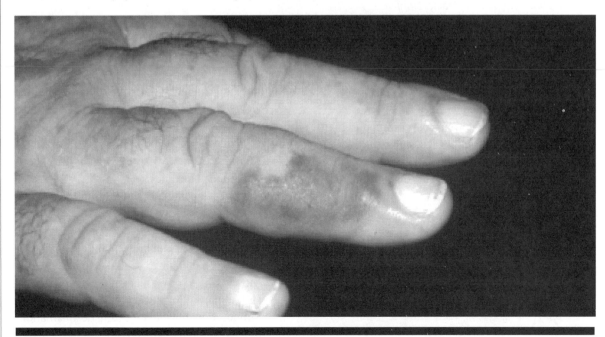

Courtesy Dr Lee T. Nesbitt Jr. From Jester JD. Skin signs of infectious zoonoses. In: Sanders CV, Nesbitt LT Jr, eds. The Skin and Infection: A Color Atlas and Text. *Baltimore, MD: Williams & Wilkins; 1995:89. Used with permission.*

• Usually resolves spontaneously within 2 to 4 weeks

Generalized Cutaneous Infection
• Similar in appearance to localized infection
    * Progressively involves more sites on body
    * Lesions distant from site of inoculation

• Bullous lesions may develop

• Systemic symptoms of fever, chills, joint pains, and lymphadenopathy more common

• Like localized infection, can be self-limited
    * Resolution slower
    * Recurrences more common

• Not associated with bacteremia

Systemic Infection
• Bacteremia uncommon but increasing in incidence

• Immunocompromised patients, particularly those with alcohol-associated liver disease, at increased risk
    * Systemic symptoms of fever and malaise common

• About 30%-40% of patients will have a characteristic skin lesion
    * Consumption of contaminated food also associated with primary bacteremia

• Infective endocarditis very common association (approximately 90% of cases)
    * Aortic valve involved in two-thirds of cases
        • 40% of cases with prior valvular disease
        • Usually native valves
    * Sub acute presentation most common
    * Can cause significant valvular destruction
    * Risk factors include alcohol abuse and occupations associated with farming and animal, fish and water exposure
    * Mortality rate 30%-40%

• Less common manifestations include septic arthritis, cerebritis, osteomyelitis and pleural disease

Key Laboratory, Microbiology and Radiology Features

• Gram-positive bacillus
    * Nonspore forming, nonmotile
    * Facultative anaerobe

• No standard serologic testing

• Culture and Gram stain of skin lesion associated material, usually unrevealing organism deep in dermis
    * Full-thickness skin biopsy at leading edge of lesion recommended

• Blood cultures useful in bacteremic patients

• Microbiology lab essential
    * Gram stain, colony morphology, vancomycin resistance and negative catalase properties may cause confusion with *Lactobacillus* and *Enterococcus* spp.
    * Hydrogen sulfide production essential in differentiation
    * Isolation by initial inoculation in brain-heart infusion enrichment both followed by *Erysipelothrix*-selective broth (ESB) consisting of vancomycin, kanamycin, neomycin, serum and tryptose

Differential Diagnosis

Infectious Diseases
Erysipelas
• Major etiologic agent: Group A *Streptococcus* (*S pyogenes*)

• Infection of superficial layer of skin
    * Manifests as rapidly spreading, erythematous, indurated painful lesion
    * Well-demarcated margins

• In contrast to erysipeloid:
    * Incubation period shorter (acute vs. within one week)
    * More likely to be on face
    * Erythematous rather than violaceous
    * Suppuration, vesiculation, and desquamation of lesions more characteristic

* Fever and other constitutional symptoms
  more common

• Treated with penicillin or cefazolin

Anthrax
• Caused by Gram-positive rod, *Bacillus anthracis*

• Like *E rhusiopathiae, B anthracis* primarily an
  occupational-associated pathogen
    * Consider in individuals who work with poten-
      tially infected animals and their carcasses or
      hair from swine, goats, sheep, cattle, or deer
    * Consider postal workers or others who come into
      contact with anthrax contaminated materials
    * Inoculated through skin, by ingestion or
      inhalation

• Primarily causes cutaneous infections
    * Incubation period up to 1 week
    * Lesions most common on hands, arms and face
    * Low-grade fever may be present
    * Unlike *E rhusiopathiae,* skin lesions initially
      papular before progressing to vesicle that
      ulcerates with a central black, necrotic eschar
    * Treated with penicillin G, ciprofloxacin or
      doxycycline
    * Other forms of infection include inhalational,
      meningeal and gastrointestinal

Herpetic whitlow
• Infection of finger after inoculation of herpes simplex virus type 1 or 2

• Characterized initially by acute swelling, pain and
  erythema; vesiculopustular lesions are classic

• Fever with associated lymphadenopathy more
  common than erysipeloid

• Acyclovir-based therapy

Erythema migrans (EM)
• Etiologic agent is spirochete, *Borrelia burgdorferi*

• Transmitted and inoculated through skin by tick bite

• Epidemiology important
    * More common in northeastern, western and
      midwestern United States

• Incubation period variable, from several days to 1
  month

• Expanding red annular plaque with central clearing
  known as erythema migrans
    * Unlike erysipeloid, skin lesions usually
      asymptomatic

• Constitutional symptoms of fever, headache,
  malaise and myalgia more common than
  erysipeloid
    * Approximately 50% of patients have EM

• Treated with oral doxycycline, amoxicillin or
  cefuroxime

Noninfectious Disease Mimics
Contact dermatitis
• History of exposure to irritant with direct skin toxicity (ie, cleansing detergents) or allergen with
  immunologically-mediated inflammation (ie, poison
  ivy) most important

• Lesion configuration and location dependent on
  exposure
    * Acute: erythematous patches with vesicles
      and crusts
    * Longer-standing: erythema, desquamation,
      lichenification, excoriated papules
    * Lesions typically pruritic

• Systemic signs and symptoms absent unless severe

• Patch testing is done for diagnosis of allergen-
  associated dermatitis; avoidance of suspected precipitant with improvement is often interpreted as
  diagnostic confirmation of both allergen- and irritant-induced contact dermatitis

• Often self-limited unless exposure persists

• Avoidance of exposure paramount
    * Short-course topical or systemic steroids,
      wet-to-dry compresses and antihistamines
      may be used for management (particularly
      when allergen induced)

Severe drug-induced cutaneous hypersensitivity drug reactions (Stevens-Johnson syndrome and toxic epidermal necrolysis)
• Usually within 3 weeks of starting medication
  * Can be associated with infections (remember herpes simplex virus) and malignancies

• Often associated with history of aminopenicillins, sulfa drugs, NSAIDs, allopurinol, or anticonvulsant use

• Mucocutaneous involvement
  * >2 mucosal surfaces involved
  * Initially diffuse erythema or disseminated red macules, progressing to desquamation of epidermis

• <10% of body surface area consistent with Stevens-Johnson syndrome; >30%, toxic epidermal necrolysis

• Histopathology: full-thickness epidermal necrosis

• Supportive care with debridement as needed
  * Treat as you would a burn patient
  * Insufficient research from well-designed clinical trials to support routine use of prophylactic antibiotics, corticosteroids, or intravenous immunoglobulin

Neutrophilic dermatosis (Sweet's syndrome)
• Viral illness typically precedes skin lesions

• Suspect in patient with underlying malignancy

• Often painful nonpruritic erythematous papules progressing to plaques or pustules
  * Characteristically located on upper body, particularly face, neck, hands and arms
  * Fever, myalgias, arthralgias or conjunctivitis common

• Labs may reveal increased acute phase reactants and leukocytosis with peripheral neutrophilia

• Histopathology reveals angiocentric neutrophilic infiltrate

• Refractory to antibiotics; standard treatment is with prednisone
  * NSAIDs and other anti-inflammatory, steroid-sparing agents have been used

Other diagnostic possibilities to consider in the appropriate settings include skin manifestations of collagen vascular diseases, thermal injuries, and cutaneous involvement of metastatic malignancy.

Empiric Therapy

Parenteral Therapy
(For nonspecific cellulitis of unknown cause requiring hospitalization)
• Nafcillin, 2 g IV q4h, or cefazolin, 1 g IV TID, for 10-14 days

Advantages
• Organism typically sensitive to beta-lactam antibiotics

Disadvantages
• Needs to be administered every 4 hours

• Vancomycin, 1 g IV BID for 10-14 days

Advantages
• Excellent Gram-positive coverage including methicillin-resistant *S aureus* (MRSA)

Disadvantages
• *Erysipelothrix rhusiopathiae* is **resistant to vancomycin**

• Increased risk for VRE

• Neutropenia: dose- and duration-dependent; reversible

Definitive Therapy

Cutaneous Disease
(Usually self-limited, but therapy for 7-14 days will expedite symptomatic improvement and decrease risk for progression or relapses)

Preferred
• Penicillin VK, 500 mg PO q6h (aminopenicillin can be used)

Advantages
- Narrow spectrum of activity and its acceptance as a drug of choice based on antimicrobial susceptibility

Disadvantages
- Adverse effects
    * Hypersensitivity reactions, GI intolerance and rash more common than bone marrow suppression, interstitial nephritis and CNS effects including seizures

Alternative
- Ciprofloxacin, 250-500 mg PO BID or levofloxacin 500-750 mg PO daily

Advantages
- Excellent bioavailability and well tolerated

- Once- or twice-daily administration

Disadvantages and adverse effects
- More expensive than penicillin

- Diarrhea, nausea, vomiting

- Headache, insomnia

- Rash (rare)

Systemic Disease or Infective Endocarditis (Treatment Duration: 4-6 weeks)
Preferred
- Penicillin G, 2 to 4 million units IV q4h

Alternative
- Ciprofloxacin, 400 mg IV or levofloxacin, 500 mg IV daily OR Ceftriaxone, 2 g IV daily (if no IgE-mediated immediate hypersensitivity to penicillin)

Advantages and disadvantages
- See above

Note: Historically, valve replacement surgery is required in approximately one third of patients with infective endocarditis due to *E rhusiopathiae*.

Complications

- Progression to diffuse cutaneous disease or systemic disease with bacteremia and infective endocarditis

- Destruction of heart valve and/or metastatic abscesses due to septic emboli
    * Glomerulonephritis as complication of infective endocarditis

- Mortality rate of almost 40% for endocarditis; almost double the rate for other causes of infective endocarditis

Prognostic Factors

- Delay in recognition of infection
    * May allow progression to generalized cutaneous infection and/or bacteremia with infective endocarditis

- Endocarditis accounts for >90% of deaths due to *E rhusiopathiae*

- Abuse of alcohol and other immunosuppressive medical conditions may increase risk for systemic infections and infective endocarditis

Infectious Disease Pearls: Erysipelothrix rhusiopathiae

1. Fish handlers, slaughterhouse workers, veterinarians, butchers and farmers are most classically at risk for infection with this organism.

2. Infection is initiated by introduction of organism through injured skin.

3. Cutaneous infections constitute more than 90% of all infections, classically involving the dorsum of the hand and fingers.

4. Bloodstream infections are more commonly seen in immunocompromised hosts and often are complicated by infective endocarditis.

5. *Erysipelothrix is intrinsically resistant to vancomycin.* Penicillin is a drug of choice based on antimicrobial susceptibility.

3. Eikenella

Synonym

- Formerly *Bacteroides corrodens; Bacteroides ureolyticus*

Causative Organism

- *Eikenella corrodens*

Epidemiology

- Normal flora of oral cavity, upper respiratory tract, GI tract and GU tract
  * Skin and soft tissue infections often secondary to closed-fist injuries or human bites
  * Increased incidence in intravenous drug users
    - Oral secretions contaminating needles
    - Nonsterile preparation of injectable materials
  * Infections more common in the immunocompromised (particularly those with head and neck cancers) and elderly patients
  * Can be sole pathogen, but often part of polymicrobial infection
    - Streptococci often co-isolated

Key Clinical Features

- Sites of infection most commonly include skin and soft tissue, oropharynx, lung and heart valves

Skin and Soft Tissue Infection
- Often involves hand
  * Oral secretions inoculated through traumatized skin

- Look for erythematous, swollen, skin lesions including abscesses
  * Marked tenderness frequently present
  * Local lymphadenopathy
  * Foul-smelling purulent drainage

Key Laboratory and Radiology Features

Laboratory Features
- Elevated ESR

- Leukocytosis (although WBC can be normal)

- Gram-negative bacillus

- Can be cultivated in standard blood cultures

- Grows slowly on chocolate or blood agar incubated with 5%-10% CO_2
  * Characteristic pinpoint colonies often described as "pitting" into agar and surrounded by green discoloration
  * May require up to 1 week to grow
  * Produces odor reminiscent of bleach

Plain Radiographs of Injured Area
- Assess for foreign bodies including tooth particles

- Assess for presence of gas

- Assess for deep infections of the bone or even fractures

Differential Diagnosis

Infectious Diseases
Cellulitis or cutaneous abscesses secondary to other causes
- Distinguishing features dictated by exposure history (ie, human bite vs. animal bite vs. trauma vs. chronic skin abnormalities)

- Usually due to *S aureus* or *S pyogenes*

- Necrotizing fasciitis
  * Spreads rapidly
  * Initially very painful
  * More likely to be associated with sepsis

Noninfectious Disease Mimics
Contact dermatitis
- History of exposure to irritant with direct skin toxicity (ie, cleansing detergents) or allergen with immunologically-mediated inflammation (ie, poison ivy) most important

- Lesion configuration and location dependent on exposure
  * Acute: erythematous patches with vesicles and crusts
  * Longer-standing: erythema, desquamation, lichenification, excoriated papules
  * Lesions typically pruritic

- Systemic signs and symptoms absent unless severe

- Patch testing for diagnosis of allergen associated dermatitis; improvement with avoidance of suspected precipitant is often interpreted as diagnostic confirmation of both allergen- and irritant-induced contact dermatitis

- Often self-limited unless exposure persists

- Avoidance of exposure paramount
    * Short-course topical or systemic steroids, wet-to-dry compresses and antihistamines may be used for management (particularly when allergen induced)

Empiric Therapy

- Irrigation of skin wound with saline

- Debridement of necrotic tissue

- Elevation of injured limb

- Tetanus assessment and immunization as indicated

- Do not suture human bite-associated wounds if:
    * Frank infection present
    * More than 24 hours post-injury
    * Often avoided when hands involved (concern over closed-space infection)

- Prophylactic antibiotics for human bite wounds:
    * Amoxicillin-clavulanic acid, 875/125 mg PO BID (if parenteral, choose ampicillin-sulbactam, cefoxitin or ertapenem)
    * Oral medication alternatives for penicillin-allergic patients: clindamycin, 300-450 mg PO, plus ciprofloxacin, 500 mg PO BID (or other flouroquinolones such as levofloxacin)

Note: Eikenella corrodens is **resistant to clindamycin.**

Empiric Parenteral Therapy
(Duration of treatment is 14 days if adequate debridement and drainage are attained)

Preferred
- Ampicillin-sulbactam, 3 g IV q6h (other beta-lactam or beta-lactamase inhibitors also acceptable)

Advantages
- Broad spectrum of activity against mixed aerobes and anaerobes associated with human bites

Disadvantages
- Expensive

- Diarrhea

- Pain at injection site

Alternative
- Other acceptable parenteral agents include cefoxitin, 1g (IV) q 6-8 h or ertapenem, 1g (IV) q 24 h

- Levofloxacin, 500 mg IV daily or ciprofloxacin, 400 mg IV BID plus clindamycin, 600 mg IV q8h (particularly for penicillin-allergic patient)

Advantages
- Provides coverage of mixed anaerobes and aerobes associated with human bites

- Can be given to individuals with IgE mediated hypersensitivity reaction to penicillin

Disadvantages
- *C difficile*-associated colitis

Definitive Therapy for *Eikenella* monomicrobial skin/soft tissue infection with documented susceptibility

- Duration of therapy for skin wound infection is 14 days if adequate debridement and drainage are obtained

Preferred
- Penicillin G, 2 million units IV q4h (or ampicillin)

Advantages
- Pathogen-directed

- Inexpensive

Disadvantages
- Adverse effects
    * Hypersensitivity reactions and rash.

Alternative
- Levofloxacin, 500-750 mg IV daily (see previous section for advantages and disadvantages)

Complications of Skin and Soft Tissue Infection

- Tenosynovitis

- Septic arthritis

- Osteomyelitis

- Bacteremia and sepsis

- Infective endocarditis
    * Usually due to poor dentition or intravenous drug use

- Tetanus infection

Prognostic Factors

- Delays in diagnosis due to failure to present promptly after injury

- Delay in appropriate treatment (ie, antibiotics and/or surgical debridement and drainage)

- Adult bites more likely to become infected (bites by children not as deep)

Infectious Disease Pearls: *Eikenella*

1. Eikenella is part of the normal flora of the oral cavity, upper respiratory tract, GI tract and GU tract.

2. Skin and soft tissue infections are often secondary to closed-fist injuries or human bites.

3. Though it can cause a monomicrobial infection, it often is part of a polymicrobial infection.

4. If infection secondary to Eikenella alone, then penicillin often a drug of choice based on susceptibility. If part of a poly- microbial bite-wound infection then a beta lactam/beta-lactamase inhibitor combination such as ampicillin-sulbactam or amoxicillin-clavulanic acid should be used.

5. Tenosynovitis, septic arthritis and osteomyelitis are local complications of infection that can warrant more aggressive therapy.

4. Group A Streptococci

Synonyms

• *Streptococcus pyogenes;* "flesh-eating bacteria"

Causative Organism

• *Streptococcus pyogenes* (Figure 3)

Epidemiology

• *S pyogenes* colonizes the skin and oropharynx
  * Transmitted by aerosolization and skin contact

• Impetigo is usually seen in young children in warm, humid summer months after minor trauma

• Increased risk for cellulitis with trauma, venous insufficiency, lower extremity edema, obesity and lymphedema

• Bacteremia most common in very young and elderly
  * Risk factors: varicella infection, burns, peripheral vascular disease, immunosuppressed conditions including malignancy, diabetes and corticosteroid administration

• Necrotizing fasciitis
  * Usually community-acquired without sex or age predilection
  * Age distribution usually 20-60 years of age
  * Can affect healthy hosts
  * Risk factors include varicella infection, minor trauma, surgical procedures, burns, childbirth, IVDU and possibly NSAIDs
  * Seen in approximately 50% of patients with streptococcal toxic shock syndrome

Key Clinical Features of Selected Skin Infections Due to *S pyogenes*

Impetigo
• Vesicle or pustule that evolves to thick, honey-crusted plaque
  * Often on arms, legs and face
  * Localized adenopathy often seen
  * Minimal generalized symptoms

• Ecthyma extends deeper into epidermis with resultant crater-like ulcers and eventual scarring

Figure 3

Streptococci

Gram stain appearance of *Streptococcus pyogenes*

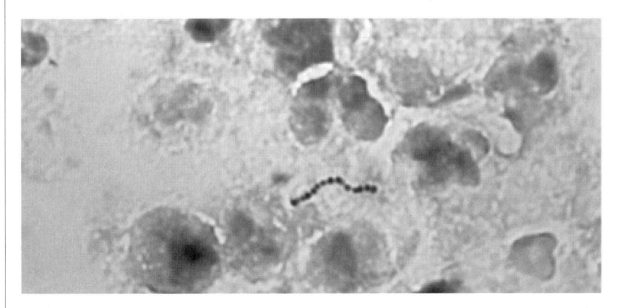

Courtesy of Charles V. Sanders, MD

Figure 4

Streptococci

Early cellulitis on an adult's leg. Note the hemorrhagic nature of the lesion.

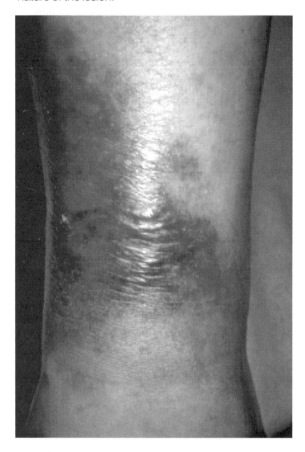

Courtesy Dr Lee T. Nesbitt Jr. From Leyden JJ, Gately LE. Staphylococcal and streptococcal infections. In: Sanders CV, Nesbitt LT Jr, eds. The Skin and Infection: A Color Atlas and Text. *Baltimore, MD: Williams & Wilkins; 1995:36. Used with permission.*

Cellulitis (Figure 4)

• Deeper infection involving epidermis, dermis, and subcutaneous fat
  * More superficial infection of lower extremities or face that does not involve subcutaneous tissues and is characterized by palpable serpiginous and well-demarcated borders progressing to erysipelas

• Manifests as confluent macular erythema with tenderness, warmth and edema

  * Regional lymphadenopathy and lymphangitis, fever and myalgias possibly associated

Necrotizing Fasciitis

(Also known as beta-hemolytic streptococcal gangrene or type II necrotizing fasciitis when due to *S pyogenes)*

• Entry site may not be obvious

• Initially appears like cellulitis (see above)

• Rapidly extends from original site of involvement over 1-2 days

• Change in color of skin from red to purplish-blue

• Bullae develop before obvious skin necrosis becomes apparent

• Prominent feature includes severe localized pain
  * Later localized anesthesia as soft tissue-associated nerves are destroyed

• Fever

• GI complaints in approximately 50% of cases

• No gas typically appreciated in soft tissue

• Progression to shock with multiple organ system dysfunction including mental status changes

Key Laboratory and Radiology Features

Impetigo
• Diagnosis usually made on clinical basis

• Gram stain and culture of infected material diagnostic

Cellulitis
• Diagnosis usually made on clinical basis

• Culture of aspirate of leading edge of lesion positive in less than 20% of cases
  * Most helpful in patients with underlying disease (liver disease, cardiovascular disease, diabetes mellitus) or no fever response to skin infection at admission

- Punch biopsy cultures positive in approximately 20% of patients

- Blood cultures positive in <5% of patients

- Lab findings nonspecific

- Plain films to assess for presence of gas, foreign bodies or osteomyelitis

Necrotizing Fasciitis
(Classified as type II when caused by *S pyogenes*)

- Clinical suspicion paramount

- Labs nonspecific
  * Elevated creatinine kinase may suggest necrotizing infection with muscle involvement
  * Blood cultures should be obtained
  * Laboratory Risk Indicator for Necrotizing Fasciitis (LRINEC) uses total white cell count, hemoglobin, sodium, glucose, serum creatinine and C-reactive protein to generate a score that assists in predicting presence of necrotizing fasciitis.

- Full-thickness frozen-section soft tissue biopsy can provide early diagnosis
  * Histopathology: intact epidermis and superficial dermis with necrosis, neutrophil infiltration and vessel thrombosis involving deeper dermis, subcutaneous fat and fascia

- Surgical exploration with biopsy for histopathologic and microbiologic work-up

- Plain films uncommonly reveal gas in soft tissue

- MRI appears best for evaluating the location and extent of the necrotizing process

Differential Diagnosis

Infectious Diseases
- Impetigo needs to be differentiated from:
  * Herpes simplex virus infection

- Herpes labialis affecting area around mouth

- Initially vesicles that ulcerate

- Characterized by recurrences

- Diagnosis often made on clinical grounds

- Tzanck smear will show multinucleated giant cells

- Acyclovir-like agent used for treatment

Cellulitis
- See differential for *Aeromonas* and *Erysipelothrix* (exposure history important)

Necrotizing fasciitis
- Differentiation from other necrotizing skin infections can be difficult

Bacterial synergistic gangrene
- Involves epifascial soft tissue

- Mixed infection including streptococci, staphylococci, anaerobes, and aerobic Gram-negative rods

- More chronic and indolent than necrotizing fasciitis

- Manifests as tender ulcer with surrounding gangrenous skin

- Usually associated with surgery including bowel diversion procedures

- Diagnosis made at time of surgical intervention

Clostridial cellulitis
- Involves epifascial soft tissue

- Caused by *Clostridium perfringens*

- Usually associated with surgery wound or traumatic wound

- Lesions appear clean or with minimal exudates

- Minimal systemic toxicity and mild localized pain

- Gas in tissues may be felt on physical exam or visualized in radiographs

- Debridement and antibiotic therapy consisting of penicillin or metronidazole or clindamycin

Nonclostridial cellulitis
- Similar clinical presentation to clostridial cellulitis
- Increased risk with diabetes mellitus

- Caused by non-spore forming anaerobes and facultative aerobes such as staphylococci, streptococci and Gram-negative bacilli

Gas gangrene
- Also known as clostridial myonecrosis

- Rapidly progressive infection involving deep muscle compartments

- Predisposing factors typically include trauma and surgery; cancer of colon associated with spontaneous nontraumatic gas gangrene

- Caused by clostridial species; *C septicum* typically associated with spontaneous nontraumatic gas gangrene

- Incubation period of 2-3 days on average

- Characterized by severe muscle pain with eventual "bronze" discoloration of overlying skin and bullous skin lesions

- "Dirty brown" discharge often noted

- Systemic toxicity prominent, including fever and delirium

- Gas formation in tissue

- Diagnosis confirmed with surgical exploration

- Treatment includes aggressive debridement and anticlostridial antibiotics

Noninfectious Disease Mimics
Contact dermatitis
- History of exposure to irritant with direct skin toxicity (ie, cleansing detergents) or allergen with immunologic-mediated inflammation (ie, poison ivy) most important

- Lesion configuration and location dependent on exposure

- * Acute: erythematous patches with vesicles and crusts
  * Longer-standing: erythema, desquamation, lichenification, excoriated papules
  * Lesions typically pruritic

- Systemic signs and symptoms absent unless severe

- Patch testing for diagnosis of allergen associated dermatitis; avoidance of suspected precipitant with improvement is often interpreted as diagnostic confirmation of both allergen- and irritant-induced contact dermatitis

- Often self-limited unless exposure persists

- Avoidance of exposure paramount
  * Short-course topical or systemic steroids, wet-to-dry compresses and antihistamines may be used for management (particularly when allergen-induced)

Severe drug-induced cutaneous hypersensitivity drug reactions (Stevens-Johnson syndrome and toxic epidermal necrolysis)
- Usually within 3 weeks of starting medication
  * Can be associated with infections (remember herpes simplex virus) and malignancies

- Often associated with history of aminopenicillins, sulfa drugs, NSAIDs, allopurinol or anticonvulsant use

- Mucocutaneous involvement
  * >2 mucosal surfaces involved
  * Initially diffuse erythema or disseminated red macules progressing to desquamation of epidermis

- <10% of body surface area consistent with Stevens-Johnson syndrome; >30%, toxic epidermal necrolysis

- Histopathology: full thickness epidermal necrosis

- Supportive care with debridement as needed
  * Treat as burn patient
  * Insufficient research from well-designed clinical trials to support routine use of prophylactic antibiotics, corticosteroids, intravenous immunoglobulin

Neutrophilic dermatosis (Sweet's syndrome)
• Viral-illness typically precedes skin lesions

• Suspect in patient with underlying malignancy

• Often painful nonpruritic erythematous papules
  progressing to plaques or pustules
      * Characteristically located on upper body,
        particularly face, neck, hands and arms
      * Fever, myalgias, arthralgias, or conjunctivitis
        common

• Labs may reveal increased acute phase reactants
  and leukocytosis with peripheral neutrophilia

• Histopathology reveals angiocentric neutrophilic
  infiltrate

• Refractory to antibiotics; standard treatment is
  with prednisone
      * NSAIDs and other anti-inflammatory,
        steroid-sparing agents have been used

Other diagnostic possibilities to consider in the
appropriate settings include skin manifestations of
collagen vascular diseases, thermal injuries and
cutaneous involvement of metastatic malignancy.

Therapy

Impetigo
(Usually caused by *S pyogenes* or *S aureus*)

Empiric
• Preferred: dicloxacillin, 250-500 mg PO q6h, *or*
  cephalexin, 500 mg PO q6h, for approximately 10
  days

Advantages
• Both active against *S aureus* and *S pyogenes*

Disadvantages
• Dicloxacillin not as effective against *S pyogenes* as
  penicillin G or cephalexin

• Most common adverse effects: GI disturbances
  including diarrhea, rash, hypersensitivity reactions

• Dicloxacillin has improved absorption if given 1
  hour before or 2 hours after meals

• Neither effective against methicillin-resistant
  staphylococci (MRSA)

Alternative for penicillin-allergic patient
• Erythromycin, 500 mg PO q6h, for approximately
  10 days

Advantage(s)
• Active against *S aureus* and *S pyogenes*

Disadvantages
• Not reliably effective against *S aureus*
  (clindamycin an acceptable alternative)

• Gastrointestinal intolerance, particularly abdominal pain, diarrhea (including C *difficile*-associated)
  and nausea

Topical
• Mupirocin ointment (2%), topically 3-4 times
  daily for 5 days, for milder cases
      * Alternative includes retapamulin ointment
        applied to affected area for 5 days

Advantages
• Topical administration

Disadvantages
• Not indicated for diffusely distributed lesions

• Not to be used for patients with systemic
  symptoms

• Major adverse effect is local irritation

• Prolonged use can result in high-level resistance in
  S aureus

Definitive Therapy for Impetigo Due to *S pyogenes*
Preferred
• Penicillin VK, 500 mg PO q6h, for approximately
  10 days

Advantages
• Drug of choice for *S pyogenes* infections

• *S pyogenes* uniformly susceptible to penicillin

Disadvantages
• Adverse effects
   * Hypersensitivity reactions

Or for milder cases, Mupirocin ointment TID x 5 days (see above for advantages and disadvantages)

Alternative
• Clindamycin, 300 mg PO TID, for approximately 10 days (increasing resistance being reported)

• Erythromycin, 500 mg PO q6h, for approximately 10 days

Advantages
• Active against *S aureus* and *S pyogenes*

• Not beta-lactam agents

Disadvantages
• Gastrointestinal intolerance, particularly abdominal pain, diarrhea and nausea

Cellulitis
(Usually caused by *S pyogenes* or *S aureus*)

Empiric
• Preferred: cefazolin, 1g IV TID, for 10 to 14 days (milder cases: cephalexin, 500mg PO q6h)

Advantages
• Generally well tolerated

• Beta-lactam agent with good activity against *S aureus* and *S pyogenes*

Disadvantages
• Can cause diarrhea

• Not effective against methicillin-resistant staphylococci (MRSA)

• Like other beta-lactams, may be less effective against higher concentrations of slow-growing organisms

• Not recommended for patients with IgE mediated

hypersensitivity reactions to penicillin

Alternative for penicillin-allergic patients
• Vancomycin, 15 mg/kg IV BID, for 10-14 days (milder cases: clindamycin, 300-450 mg PO q6h; IV form can be administered for more severe forms of cellulitis)

Advantages
• Active against most gram-positive organisms including *S pyogenes* and *S aureus* (both methicillin-sensitive and methicillin-resistant)

Disadvantages
• Needs to be dosed based on renal function

• "Red neck syndrome"
   * Pruritus, flushing, erythematous rash of chest and neck and sometimes hypotension associated with rapid infusion
• Inferior methicillin-sensitive antistaphylococcal activity when compared to betalactams like nafcillin or oxacillin

• Overuse will result in increased Gram-positive resistance to this agent

Clindamycin or linezolid are additional alternative agents if oral administration is preferred

Definitive Therapy for *S pyogenes*
Preferred
• Penicillin G, 2-4 million units IV q 4-6h, for 10-14 days (mild disease: penicillin VK, 500 mg PO q6h, for approximately 10-14 days)

Advantages
• Drug of choice for *S pyogenes* infections

• *S pyogenes* remains susceptible to penicillin

Disadvantages
• Adverse effects
   * Anaphylactic hypersensitivity reactions

Alternative
• Cefazolin, 1 g IV TID, for 10-14 days (milder cases: cephalexin, 500 mg PO q6h)

Advantages
• Generally well-tolerated

• Beta-lactam agent with good activity against
  S aureus and *S pyogenes*

Disadvantages
• Can cause diarrhea

• Not effective against methicillin-resistant
  staphylococci (MRSA)

• Like other beta-lactams, may be less effective
  against higher concentrations of slow-growing
  organisms

• Not recommended for patients with IgE mediated
  hypersensitivity reactions to penicillin

Necrotizing Fasciitis
(Type I caused by mixed aerobic and anaerobic bacteria; type II caused by *S pyogenes)*

• The cornerstone of therapy for necrotizing fasciitis
  is surgical debridement. Duration of antimicrobial
  therapy is approximately 14 days provided definitive debridement is attained.

• Community-associated MRSA reported as cause
  of necrotizing fasciitis
    * If considered, vancomycin IV should be
      added

Type I necrotizing fasciitis
• Preferred: imipenem, 500 mg IV q6h or
  meropenem 1 g (IV) TID

Advantages
• Broad spectrum of activity against aerobic and
  anaerobic bacteria

Disadvantages
• Imipenem risk for seizure activity with increased
  doses, renal insufficiency or previous central nervous system abnormality

• C difficile colitis

Alternative
• Piperacillin-tazobactam, 4.5 grams IV TID,
  Clindamycin, 600-900 mg/rs 12

Advantages
• Broad spectrum of activity against aerobic and
  anaerobic bacteria (broadest spectrum of coverage
  of the penicillin and beta-lactamase inhibitor combinations)

Disadvantages
• Not active against methicillin-resistant
  staphylococci

• Adverse reactions most commonly include gastrointestinal disturbances (diarrhea, nausea, constipation), headache and insomnia

• If penicillin-allergic, consider clindamycin IV plus
  aminoglycoside or fluoroquinolone like
  ciprofloxacin or levofloxacin for Type I necrotizing skin infection.

Type II necrotizing fasciitis
(See streptococcal toxic shock-like syndrome in
next section for other possible therapeutic interventions)

• Preferred: penicillin G, 4 million units q4h, *plus*
  clindamycin, 900 mg IV TID

Advantages
Penicillin G
• Drug of choice for *S pyogenes* infections

• *S pyogenes* remains susceptible to penicillin

Clindamycin
• Suppresses synthesis of toxic shock-associated
  toxin and organism-associated penicillin-binding
  proteins by inhibiting protein production

• Post-antibiotic effect longer than that of beta-lactams

• Not affected by growth phase or inoculum size of
  bacteria

Disadvantages

Penicillin G
- May be less effective against infections with high inoculum of slow-growing organisms (ie, necrotizing fasciitis/toxic shock syndrome)
    * Known as "Eagle effect"

- Adverse effects
    * Hypersensitivity reactions

Clindamycin
- *C difficile*-associated diarrhea/colitis

Alternative
- Clindamycin (alone), 900 mg IV TID, if history of IgE-mediated type I hypersensitivity to penicillin

- Though usually due to S pyogenes, type II necrotizing fasciitis can be caused by MRSA. When considered due to increased prevalence of MRSA in the community, anti-MRSA therapy with an agent such as vancomycin should be empirically included.

Complications

Impetigo
- Cellulitis (approximately 10% of cases)

- Poststreptococcal glomerulonephritis: antibiotic treatment not effective in prevention

- Rarely, osteomyelitis, septic arthritis, lymphangitis, sepsis

Cellulitis
- Abscess(es)

- Thrombophlebitis

- Localized extension of infection into joints and bones

- Bacteremia with metastatic infections

- Toxic shock-like syndrome

- Resultant lymphedema may increase risk for recurrent episodes

- Necrotizing fasciitis

- Compartment syndromes and skin necrosis resulting in loss of limb

- Toxic shock-like syndrome with hypotension, renal failure, shock, multisystem organ failure

- Death

Prognostic Factors

- Delay in diagnosis resulting in less than optimal antibiotic selection and/or surgical management results in poorer outcomes

    * Rapid progression of hemodynamic instability and toxicity may rule out surgical options

- Admission levels of serum sodium and lactate may be useful in predicting mortality secondary to necrotizing soft-tissue infections
    * Increased mortality when lactate level >54.1 mg/dL; sodium < 135 mEq/L

- Use of NSAIDs may delay diagnosis and worsen outcome of necrotizing fasciitis by masking the inflammatory response and impairing immune responses

- Other factors potentially worsening outcome in necrotizing infection include older age, malnutrition, peripheral vascular disease and diabetes mellitus

- Mortality rate of approximately 30% with necrotizing fasciitis

- Outcome for cases of impetigo and cellulitis generally good

Infectious Disease Pearls: Group A Streptococci

1. Group A streptococci cause skin and soft-tissue infections that include impetigo, erysipelas, cellulitis and necrotizing fasciitis.

2. Impetigo is usually seen in young children in warm, humid summer months after minor trauma.

Figure 5

Staphylococci

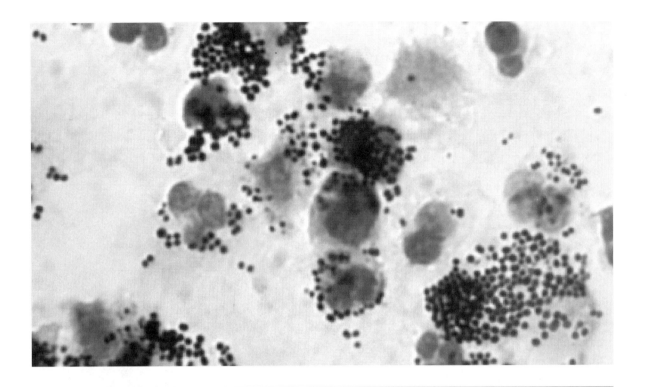

Courtesy of Charles V. Sanders, MD

3. In cellulitis, culture of aspirate obtained from the leading edge of the lesion is positive in less than 20% of cases.

4. A prominent feature of necrotizing fasciitis includes initial severe localized pain with later evolution to localized anesthesia when soft tissue-associated nerves are destroyed.

5. The drug of choice for Group A streptococci infections remains penicillin. Clindamycin should be added in Group A streptococcus-associated necrotizing fasciitis and toxic shock syndrome for killing of organism as well as suppressing production of the toxic shock-associated toxin.

Figure 6

Staphylococcal toxic shock syndrome

Petechial hemorrhages on the oral mucosa

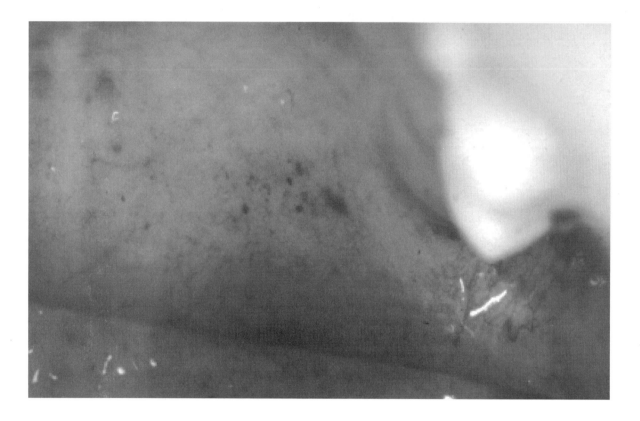

Courtesy of Dr Charles V. Sanders. From Leyden JJ, Gately LE. Staphylococcal and streptococcal infections. In: Sanders CV, Nesbitt LT Jr, eds. The Skin and Infection: A Color Atlas and Text. *Baltimore, MD: Williams & Wilkins: 1995: 34. Used with permission.*

5. Toxic Shock Syndrome

Synonyms

- Staphylococcal toxic shock syndrome; streptococcal toxic shock syndrome; streptococcal toxic shock-like syndrome

Causative Organisms

- *Staphylococcus aureus; Streptococcus pyogenes* (see Figures 3 and 5)

- Group B and Group C streptococci reported to cause TSS-line syndrome

Epidemiology

Staphylococcal Toxic Shock Syndrome (TSS)
- Menses associated with tampon use (50% of cases)
    * Increased risk with extended use of same tampon, particularly if high absorbency type

- Nonmenstrual-associated (50% of cases)
    * Associated with surgical wound infection (most common), obstetric wound infection, sinus infection, bone infection, burns, HIV infection, intravenous drug use

- Approximately 75% of cases diagnosed in women

- Primarily reported in 15- to 35-year-old age group

Streptococcal TSS
- Infections sporadic, ie, not outbreak-associated

- Primarily reported in the 20- to 50-year-old age group

- Classically, most individuals not immunosuppressed
    * At least one study revealed increased risk for streptococcal TSS in the elderly and those with underlying medical conditions, including heart disease, lung disease and alcohol abuse

- No predilection for either sex

- Predisposing factors
    * Preceding viral infection (ie, influenza)
    * Trauma with disruption of skin and mucous membranes

    * Primary varicella zoster infections
        • Wounds associated with surgery, burns, bites, minor trauma including cuts, intravenous drug use
        • Vaginal delivery
    * Blunt trauma with ecchymoses and hematoma development
    * NSAID use
    * In up to 50% of cases, no entry site identified
    * Very rarely associated with streptococcal pharyngitis

Key Clinical Features

Staphylococcal TSS
Symptoms
- Prodrome of chills and general malaise
- Fatigue, confusion, lightheadedness, and fever after several days
- Diarrhea common

Signs
- Fever
- Hypotension
- Diffuse erythematous rash ("erythroderma") with subsequent desquamation 1-2 weeks later
    * Conjunctival suffusion, "strawberry tongue," and petechiae in oropharynx may also be present (Figure 6)
    * Desquamation typically includes palms and soles
- Multi-organ-system involvement (>3)
    * Gastrointestinal, muscular, mucous membranes, kidney, liver, brain, hematologic

Streptococcal TSS
Symptoms
- Initially nonspecific
- 1 out of every 5 patients will have flu-like syndrome with fever, chills and gastrointestinal disturbances
- Most common complaint is pain
    * Severe
    * Sudden onset
    * Usually involves an extremity

Signs
- More than 50% of patients with:
    * Fever
    * Confusion

* Tachycardia
* Hypotension
* Skin or soft tissue infection seen in 80% of patients with streptococcal TSS
* Edema and erythema most common cutaneous manifestations
* Bullae 10% of patients; desquamation, 20%

Key Laboratory and Radiology Features

• Elevated creatinine with renal insufficiency

• Urine hemoglobinuria

• Hypoalbuminemia

• Hypocalcemia

• Creatinine phosphokinase (CPK) level in serum increased when deeper skin, soft tissue, fascia and/or muscles involved
    * Tissue necrosis more common in streptococcal TSS

• Mildly increased white blood cell count with increased immature granulocytes

• Thrombocytopenia

• Bacteremia
    * Reported in approximately 60% of patients with streptococcal TSS
    * Uncommon in staphylococcal TSS (approximately 5% of cases)
• Isolation of *S pyogenes* from infected sites in approximately 95% of cases; *S aureus* isolated from infected sites in approximately 50% of individuals with nonmenstrual-associated TSS and 85% of individuals with menstrual-associated disease
    * Isolation of organism included in case definition for streptococcal TSS, not staphylococcal TSS

• Negative work-up for other clinical mimics including RMSF, measles and leptospirosis

Differential Diagnosis

Infectious Diseases
Leptospirosis
• Caused by a spirochete

• Associated with bathing or swimming in water contaminated with urine from livestock, dogs, or rats

• Clinical presentations:
    * Milder anicteric form is biphasic
        • Initial septic phase with abrupt presentation of fever, GI disturbances, headache, conjunctival injection and myalgias (up to 7-day duration); then fever abates for 2 days before second phase of disease begins
        • Immune phase characterized by fever, headache, spleen and liver enlargement, uveitis, rash, adenopathy, and lung abnormalities
    * Severe icteric form (Weil's syndrome):
        • Characterized by liver insufficiency with jaundice, renal insufficiency, mental status changes and pulmonary hemorrhage.

• Abnormal labs include peripheral neutrophilia, thrombocytopenia, increased liver function studies, increased CPK, azotemia, abnormal urine sediment and increased white blood cells in cerebrospinal fluid

Diagnosis
• Microscopic dark-field examination

• Isolation from blood or CSF in first 10 days

• Isolation from urine after first 10 days

• Serologic testing for antibodies against

Leptospira

• Treatment usually penicillin or doxycycline

• Mortality rate of 5%-35% for icteric form of disease

Typhoid fever
- Etiologic agent: *Salmonella enterica* (serotype *typhi)*

- Transmitted with ingestion of contaminated consumables

- Incubation period of 1-2 weeks

- Three phases of infection:
  * Beginning of symptoms including headache, cough, sore throat, disturbance in stool patterns (increased or decreased frequency), and gradual stepwise increase in fever
  * Period of greatest severity often accompanied by pulse-temperature discordance, altered mental status, and cutaneous manifestation of "rose spots"
    - Blanching macules approximately 2 mm in size that are pink-brown in color, found on the trunk and resolving slowly over 4 days
  * Slow resolution of symptoms followed by possible relapse or carriage

- Leukopenia characteristic

- Can culture organism from blood (usually in first week) and stool (usually after first week); bone marrow cultures can be helpful early in the course
  * Rose spot-associated skin biopsy specimens can be culture-positive >50% of time

- Organism may be susceptible to trimethoprim-sulfamethoxazole, ampicillin, ceftriaxone or fluoroquinolones

Meningococcemia
- Etiologic agent: Gram-negative diplococcus, *Neisseria meningitidis*

- Skin lesions develop sooner than in RMSF, in which rash typically appears on third to fourth day
  * Petechial lesions most common; macular, maculopapular and, in severe cases, purpuric and ecchymotic skin lesions may also be seen
  * Rash can involve palms and soles
  * Skin lesions may be tender

- Pharyngitis and hypotension can develop

- Diagnosis usually confirmed by isolation from blood, cerebrospinal fluid, or aspirate from skin lesion

- Treatment: Penicillin or ceftriaxone

Rubeola (Measles)
- Vaccine-preventable disease caused by rubeola virus belonging to genus *Morbillivirus*

- Seen in winter and spring most commonly

- Clinical features include fever, cough, conjunctivitis, coryza, photophobia and rash

- Enanthem (ie, Koplik's spots): buccal mucosa-associated erythematous macules with central white focus that appear about 2 days before rash are pathognomonic

- Prominent red-brown maculopapular rash typically originates on face before involving trunk and upper extremities

- No specific antiviral therapy; supportive care

Rocky Mountain Spotted Fever
- See section below

Noninfectious Disease Mimics
Heatstroke
- Clinical presentation includes dehydration, altered consciousness, high fever, hypotension, renal dysfunction (sometimes liver and cardiac dysfunction) and lack of sweating

- Predisposing factors include:
  * Exertion in setting of high ambient temperatures
  * Compromised temperature homeostasis induced by medications including phenothiazene antipsychotics and anticholinergics
  * Treatment includes supportive care, discontinuation of precipitants, and quick reduction of core temperature

Empiric Therapy

• Duration of therapy approximately 14 days provided all foci of infection are removed

Preferred Treatment for Serious Gram-positive Cocci Infections

• Vancomycin, 15 mg/kg IV BID (Add clindamycin, 600 mg -900 mg IV q8h if symptoms consistent with toxic shock are present)

Advantages
• Active against most Gram-positive cocci including *S pyogenes* and *S aureus* (both methicillin-sensitive and methicillin-resistant strains)

Disadvantages
• Needs to be dosed based on renal function

• "Red neck syndrome"
    * Pruritus, flushing, erythematous rash of chest or neck and (sometimes) hypotension associated with rapid infusion

• Overuse will result in increased VRE

• Inferior methicillin-sensitive anti-staphylococcal activity when compared to beta-lactams like nafcillin or oxacillin

Note: MRSA strains associated with TSS warrant consideration of non-beta lactam agents such as vancomycin

Alternative
• Cefazolin, 1-2 g IV TID, or nafcillin *or* oxacillin, 2 g IV q4h

Advantages
Cefazolin
• Generally well-tolerated

• Beta-lactam agent with good activity against *S aureus* and *S pyogenes*

Nafcillin or oxacillin
• Active against *S pyogenes* and *S aureus*

• Improved activity against methicillin-sensitive *S aureus* (MSSA) when compared to vancomycin

• No need to dose-adjust for renal insufficiency (nafcillin)

Disadvantages
Cefazolin
• Can cause diarrhea

• Not effective against methicillin-resistant staphylococci

• Like other beta-lactams, may be less effective against higher concentrations of slow-growing organisms

• Not recommended for patients with IgE mediated hypersensitivity reactions to penicillin

Nafcillin or oxacillin
• Not effective against methicillin-resistant staphylococci (MRSA)

• Frequent dosing

• Extended course of high-dose nafcillin associated with leukopenia

• Oxacillin associated with hepatic dysfunction

Definitive Therapy (based on susceptibilities and presence of syndromes)

Staphylococcal TSS
• Preferred: Nafcillin or oxacillin, 2 g IV q4h, *plus* clindamycin, 600-900 mg IV TID

Advantages
Nafcillin or oxacillin
• Improved activity against methicillin-sensitive *S aureus* (MSSA) when compared to vancomycin

• No need to dose-adjust for renal insufficiency

Clindamycin
• Suppresses synthesis of toxic shock-associated toxin and organism-associated penicillin-binding proteins by inhibiting protein production

• Post-antibiotic effect longer than that of beta-lactams

• Not affected by growth phase or inoculum size of bacteria

Disadvantages
Nafcillin or oxacillin
• Frequent dosing

• Can cause transaminitis and thrombophlebitis

• Extended course of high-dose nafcillin associated with leukopenia

• Oxacillin associated with hepatic dysfunction

• Not effective against methicillin-resistant staphylococci (MRSA)

Clindamycin
• *C difficile*-associated colitis

Alternative
• Cefazolin plus clindamycin (see above for doses and advantages and disadvantages)

Note: MRSA strains associated with TSS warrant consideration of non-beta-lactam agents. Therefore, empiric therapy for staphylococcal TSS should include vancomycin plus clindamycin. If MSSA, then change to nafcillin/oxacillin plus clindamycin.

Streptococcal TSS
• Preferred: Penicillin G, 4 million units IV q4h, *plus* clindamycin, 600-900 mg IV TID

Figure 7

Vibrio vulnificus

Hemorrhagic and bullous skin lesions of the feet and lower legs, also showing hemorrhagic necrosis of the dorsum of the left foot

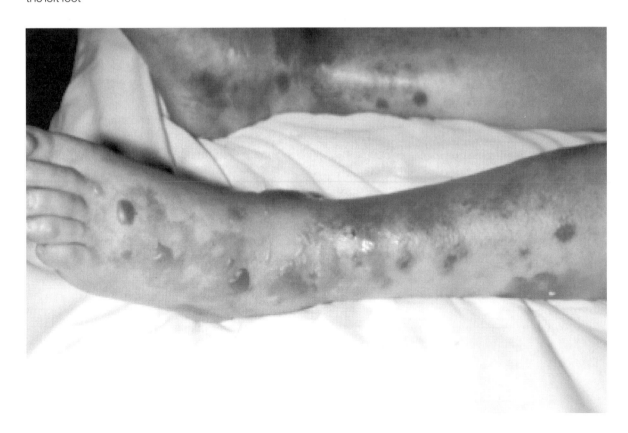

Courtesy of Dr Charles V. Sanders. From Septimus EJ, Musher DM. Other bacterial infections. In: Sanders CV, Nesbitt LT Jr, eds. The Skin and Infection: A Color Atlas and Text. *Baltimore, MD: Williams & Wilkins; 1995:57. Used with permission.*

Advantages
Penicillin G
• *S pyogenes* remains susceptible to penicillin

• Drug of choice for *S pyogenes* infections

Clindamycin (see above)

Disadvantages
Penicillin G
• May be less effective against infections with high inoculum of slow-growing organisms (ie, toxic shock syndrome)

• Adverse effects:
　* Hypersensitivity reactions, GI intolerance, and rash more common than bone marrow suppression, interstitial nephritis and CNS effects (including seizures)

Clindamycin (see above)

Alternative
• Clindamycin, 600-900 mg IV TID (see above for advantages and disadvantages)

Other therapeutic modalities for management of toxic shock syndrome include:
• Hemodynamic monitoring with intravenous fluids and vasopressor support as needed

• Prompt surgical intervention including removal of nidus of infection and aggressive exploration, irrigation, and debridement of all associated infected necrotic material

• Intravenous immune gamma-globulin
　* Antibodies neutralize toxic shock syndrome-associated toxin

• Hyperbaric oxygen
　* No data to recommend its standard use

• Corticosteroids
　* No effect on mortality when used in treatment of staphylococcal TSS

Complications

• Deep-seated tissue involvement (particularly in streptococcal TSS) can lead to necrotizing fasciitis and myositis

• Bacteremia
　* More common in streptococcal TSS (approximately 60% of cases) than staphylococcal TSS (approximately 5% of cases)

• Hypotension and septic shock

• Renal dysfunction, acute respiratory distress syndrome, and additional manifestations of multiorgan system involvement
　* Renal impairment usually reversible

• Morbidity from surgical procedures
　* Incision and debridement procedures
　* Amputation

• Mortality rate of approximately 50% for streptococcal TSS; approximately 5% for staphylococcal TSS

• Recurrences can occur
　* Particularly well-described in staphylococcal TSS (one-third of cases)

• Residual neuropsychiatric impairment

Prognostic Factors

• Mortality rates significantly higher in streptococcal TSS vs. staphylococcal TSS

• Mortality rates higher in nonmenstrual-associated staphylococcal TSS vs. menstrual-associated

• Delay in diagnosis resulting in less than optimal antibiotic selection and/or timing of surgical interventions can result in poorer outcomes
　* Rapid progression of hemodynamic instability and toxicity may rule out surgical options

• Greater number of dysfunctional organ systems results in higher mortality rates

Infectious Disease Pearls: Toxic Shock Syndrome

1. *Staphylococcus aureus* and *Streptococcus pyogenes* are the organisms primarily associated with toxic shock syndrome(s).

2. TSS should be considered when a patient presents with a multi-organ syndrome manifesting clinical signs and symptoms such as fever, confusion, tachycardia, hypotension and skin/soft tissue involvement.

3. Bacteremia is reported in approximately 60% of patients with streptococcal TSS, but is uncommon in staphylococcal TSS (approximately 5% of cases).

4. Clindamycin is added to specific staphylococcal and/or streptococcal targeted therapy in order to suppress protein synthesis particularly targeting toxic shock-associated toxin(s).

5. The mortality rate is approximately 50% for streptococcal TSS and 5% for staphylococcal TSS.

6. *Vibrio vulnificus*

Synonyms

• None

Causative Organism

• *Vibrio vulnificus*

Epidemiology

• Infections most common in warmer months between April and October
    * Requires temperatures >18°C and briny or marine water environment with approximately 1% salt concentration
    * In the United States, highest prevalence of infections originate from southeastern Gulf Coast waters

• Much more common in men >40 years of age

• Immunocompromised hosts most susceptible
    * Liver disease, iron-excess states, malignancy, diabetes, renal disease, HIV-infection

• Leading cause of seafood-related deaths in the U.S.

Key Clinical Features (Figure 7)

• 3 clinical syndromes: septicemia, wound infection and gastroenteritis

Septicemia
• Onset after ingestion of *V vulnificus*-contaminated shellfish, primarily oysters

• Fever and chills (>90%) >> nausea, vomiting, diarrhea (approximately 50%)
    * Hypotension at admission portends poor prognosis (~ 90% mortality rate)

• Skin lesions (50%-75% of patients with septicemia)
    * Commonly on lower extremities
    * Cellulitis with hemorrhagic bullae progressing to necrotizing fasciitis and necrosis
    * Secondary to hematogenous dissemination

Wound Infection

- Develops in wounds exposed to seawater or shellfish

- May manifest as mild cellulitis or progress rapidly to invasive necrotic disease involving fascia and muscle

- Secondary bacteremia in one-third of cases

- Hypotension in approximately 25% of cases

- Fever present in about three-quarters of wound infections

Gastroenteritis

- Least common clinical syndrome

- Abdominal pain, emesis and/or diarrhea

- *V vulnificus* typically isolated from stool alone

- Can be morbid but unlikely to be fatal

Laboratory Features

- Leukopenia more common than leukocytosis

- Thrombocytopenia

- Look for evidence of disseminated intravascular coagulation

- Blood cultures
  - Positive in 70%-100% of patients with septicemia
  - Positive in 30% of wound infections
- Gram stain of bullous skin lesion
  - Curved Gram-negative rod

- Culture of infected material
  - Grows on sodium chloride-containing media
  - Selective media: thiosulfate, citrate, bile salts, sucrose (TCBS) media

- Nucleic acid-based testing of blood samples available in research setting

Differential Diagnosis

Infectious Diseases
Group A streptococcal necrotizing fasciitis
- Rapidly spreading and initially very painful

- Approximately 50% of patients with toxic shock-like syndrome will develop necrotizing fasciitis

- Can occur in young, healthy individuals
  - Predisposing factor usually minor trauma that leads to varicella infection (eg, abrasions, lacerations, burns, intravenous drug use)
  - Unlike *V vulnificus*, seawater exposure not a classic association

- Gram stain of aspirate from bullous lesion or blood cultures can be diagnostic
  - Gram-positive cocci in short chains
  - Bacteremia in >50% of patients with streptococcal toxic shock-like syndrome

- Treatment: early surgical debridement and antibiotics (penicillin plus clindamycin)

Aeromonas (Gram-negative bacillus)
- Usually community-acquired after exposure to soil or contaminated fresh water (versus brackish or seawater association with *V vulnificus*)

- Like *V vulnificus*, increased isolation in warm summer months

- Like *V vulnificus*, more common in males and immunocompromised hosts (including adults and infants)
  - Chronic liver disease or cirrhosis
  - Malignancy
  - Diabetes mellitus

- Like *V vulnificus*, can cause soft-tissue infection and bacteremia with sepsis

- Microbiology lab essential in distinguishing *V vulnificus* from *Aeromonas*

Edwardsiella tarda (Gram-negative bacillus)
• Gastroenteritis most common manifestation

• Extra-gastrointestinal disease more common in liver disease and excess iron states

• Can cause cellulitis, septic arthritis, necrotizing fasciitis and sepsis

Streptococcus iniae (Gram-positive coccus)
• Infects individuals who incur skin wounds while handling farm-raised fish (particularly tilapia)

• Short incubation period after exposure

• Cellulitis, purulent draining ulcers and lymphangitis

• Bacteremia with arthritis, endocarditis and meningitis reported

Erysipelothrix rhusiopathiae (Gram-positive bacillus)
• Does not cause gastrointestinal disease

• Occupational disease of butchers and fish handlers

• Manifests as localized skin infection (ie, erysipeloid); diffuse skin involvement; or disseminated disease with infective endocarditis

Mycobacterium marinum (Gram-positive, acid-fast bacillus)
• Does not cause gastrointestinal disease

• Typically affects individuals who experience trauma while working with aquariums or engaging in water sports

• Typically localized skin infection on extremity beginning as papule or plaque; occasionally, sporotrichin distribution of nodules along lymphatics

• Extension to joint can occur but dissemination rare

• Usually indolent and without systemic signs

Noninfectious Disease Mimics
Contact dermatitis
• History of exposure to irritant with direct skin toxicity (ie, cleansing detergents) or allergen with immunologic-mediated inflammation (ie, poison ivy) most important

• Lesion configuration and location dependent on exposure
    * Acute: erythematous patches with vesicles and crusts
    * Longer-standing: erythema, desquamation, lichenification, excoriated papules
    * Lesions typically pruritic

• Systemic signs and symptoms absent unless severe

• Patch testing for diagnosis of allergen-associated dermatitis; avoidance of suspected precipitant with improvement is often interpreted as diagnostic confirmation of both allergen- and irritant-induced contact dermatitis

• Often self-limited unless exposure persists

• Avoidance of exposure paramount
    * Short-course topical or systemic steroids, wet-to-dry compresses and antihistamines may be used for management (particularly when allergen induced)

Severe drug-induced cutaneous hypersensitivity drug reactions (Stevens-Johnson syndrome and toxic epidermal necrolysis)
• Usually within 3 weeks of starting medication
    * Can be associated with infections (remember herpes simplex virus) and malignancies

• Often associated with history of aminopenicillin, sulfa drug, NSAID, allopurinol, or anticonvulsant use

• Mucocutaneous involvement
    * >2 mucosal surfaces involved
    * Initially diffuse erythema or disseminated red macules progressing to desquamation of epidermis

• <10% of body surface area consistent with Stevens-Johnson syndrome; >30%, toxic epidermal necrolysis

- Histopathology: full-thickness epidermal necrosis

- Supportive care with debridement as needed
    * Treat as burn patient
    * Insufficient research from well-designed clinical trials to support routine use of prophylactic antibiotics, corticosteroids, intravenous immunoglobulin

Neutrophilic dermatosis (Sweet's syndrome)
- Viral-illness typically precedes skin lesions

- Suspect in patient with underlying malignancy

- Often painful nonpruritic erythematous papules progressing to plaques or pustules
    * Characteristically located on upper body, particularly face, neck, hands and arms
    * Fever, myalgias, arthralgias or conjunctivitis common

- Labs may reveal increased acute phase reactants and leukocytosis with peripheral neutrophilia

- Histopathology reveals angiocentric neutrophilic infiltrate

- Refractory to antibiotics; standard treatment is with prednisone
    * NSAIDs and other anti-inflammatory steroid-sparing agents have been used

Other diagnostic possibilities to consider in the appropriate settings include skin manifestations of collagen vascular diseases, thermal injuries and cutaneous involvement of metastatic malignancy.

Empiric Therapy

Skin and Soft Tissue Infection
(Length of Therapy Approximately 10-21 days)
Empiric therapy after freshwater exposure
- Ceftazidime, 1-2 g IV TID, plus levofloxacin, 500 mg IV daily or ciprofloxacin, 400 mg IV BID

Advantages
- Broad coverage of organisms associated with water exposure

Disadvantages
- Decreased activity against *V vulnificus*

Note: Some would recommend gentamicin in lieu of quinolone, providing synergy with beta-lactam against certain Gram-negative bacilli.

- If marine water exposure, add doxycycline 100 mg IV bid daily for better coverage of *V vulnificus*

Definitive Therapy

- Doxycycline, 100 mg IV or PO BID, plus ceftazidime, 2 g IV TID

- An aminoglycoside (gentamicin, 5 mg/kg IV QD) may be added to above regimen by some authorities

Advantages
- Effective anti-*Vibrio vulnificus* activity

Disadvantages
- Effective antibiotic delivery may be difficult to attain in necrotic, devitalized tissue

Alternative
- Ciprofloxacin, 400 mg IV BID or levofloxacin, 500 mg IV daily

Advantages
- Effective pathogen-directed therapy based on susceptibilities

Disadvantages
- Effective antibiotic delivery may be difficult to attain in necrotic devitalized tissue

- Early surgical debridement imperative in rapidly progressing necrotic skin infections.

Complications

- Compartment syndromes and skin necrosis and gangrene resulting in loss of limb (particularly with necrotizing fasciitis)

- Bacteremia with metastatic infections and abscesses

- Sepsis, disseminated intravascular coagulation, multiorgan system failure and death

Prognostic Factors

• Hypotension at presentation (~ 90% mortality rate)

• Septicemia (mortality rate of 60%); wound infection (mortality rate of 30%)
  * Increased when diagnosis is delayed, surgical intervention is delayed, or in patients with underlying disease (particularly liver disease)

• Prevention in immunocompromised hosts imperative
  * Avoid consumption of raw shellfish
  * Avoid exposure of skin wound to potentially contaminated water

• Post-harvest processing of oysters (ie, quick freezing, pasteurization, and high hydrostatic pressure) can reduce inoculum of *V vulnificus*
  * May decrease risk for infection

Infectious Disease Pearls: *Vibrio vulnificus*

1. Infections with *Vibrio vulnificus* are most common in warmer months between April and October because the organism requires temperatures >18°C in addition to a briny or marine water environment with approximately 1% salt concentration.

2. Infections are much more common in men greater than 40 years of age. Immunocompromised hosts are most susceptible particularly those with liver disease, iron-excess states, malignancy, diabetes, renal disease and HIV-infection.

3. *Vibrio vulnificus* is the leading cause of seafood-related deaths in the United States.

4. The 3 clinical syndromes associated with *V vulnificus* infection include septicemia, wound infection and gastroenteritis. These infections are caused by ingestion of undercooked shellfish (particularly oysters) or when pre-existing wounds are exposed to or wounds occur in water contaminated with *V vulnificus*.

5. Hemorrhagic bullous lesions are the classical cutaneous manifestations of infection with *V vulnificus*.

7. *Mycobacterium chelonae* and *M fortuitum*

Synonyms

• *Mycobacterium fortuitum* complex; Runyon group IV rapid growers

Causative Organisms

• *Mycobaterium fortuitum; M chelonae*

Epidemiology

• Ubiquitous organisms found in soil, dust and water; also isolated from contaminated hospital materials

• Common nontuberculous mycobacterial causes of nosocomial infection

• Cutaneous infections observed in the settings of:
  * Surgery
  * Trauma secondary to abrasion, post-needle injection, peritoneal or vascular catheters
  * Disseminated disease in immunocompromised patients (end-stage renal disease, organ transplantation, collagen vascular diseases, hematologic malignancies and use of corticosteroids or cytotoxic chemotherapy)
  * Nail salon whirlpool footbaths

Key Clinical Features

• Lesions or drainage often located at site of trauma both in the environmentally or nosocomially

• Incubation period of approximately 4-6 weeks

• Primary cutaneous disease: minimally tender nodules, cellulitis, abscesses, draining fistulas, ulcers, sporotrichoid lesion

• Disseminated disease-associated skin lesions: nodules, multiple abscesses, uniform morbilliform eruption, draining nodular subcutaneous erythematous lesions

• Noncutaneous disease manifestations can include osteomyelitis, meningitis, endocarditis, pericarditis, keratitis, and hepatitis

Figure 8

Mycobacterium marinum infection

Nodular plaques on the elbow

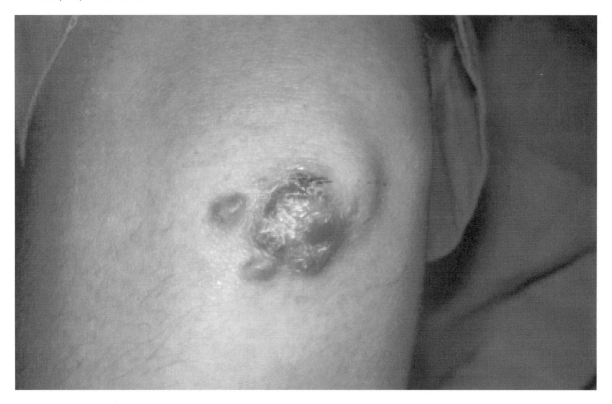

Courtesy of Dr Lee T. Nesbitt Jr. From Lee BD, Greer DL. Cutaneous signs of nontuberculosis mycobacteria. In: Sanders CV, Nesbitt LT Jr, eds. The Skin and Infection: A Color Atlas and Text. Baltimore, MD: Williams & Wilkins; 1995: 145. Used with permission.

- Infections usually chronic and indolent

- *M. chelonae* more likely to present as multiple lesions vs. single lesions in *M fortuitum*

Key Laboratory and Radiology Features

- *M fortuitum* grows best at 28°-37°C; *M chelonae*, 28°C

- Rapid growers: colonies grow within 1 week on mycobacterial culture media

- Colonies not pigmented

- Identification of these two rapid growers (as well as the other clinically significant rapid grower, *M abscessus*) relies on biochemical and drug susceptibility testing
  * Susceptibility panel consists of sulfonamide, imipenem, doxycycline, clarithromycin, amikacin, fluoroquinolone and cefoxitin
  * Both *M fortuitum* and *M chelonae* are resistant to the drugs usually used to treat tuberculosis

Differential Diagnosis

- Same as other atypical mycobacteria reviewed in this section (see *M marinum* and *M ulcerans* sections that follow)

Antimicrobial Therapy

Severe skin and soft-tissue infection including osteomyelitis

M fortuitum
• Initially, amikacin, 10-15 mg/kg IV in 2 divided doses (target level of approximately 20 mcg/mL) plus cefoxitin, 12 g daily in 4 divided doses, for at least 2 weeks and until clinical improvement noted in patients with serious cutaneous infections

M chelonae
• IV tobramycin more active than amikacin

Note: Imipenem is an alternative to cefoxitin for either *M fortuitum* or *M chelonae*.

If susceptible to oral antimicrobials, consider change to regimen consisting of combination of 2 of the following oral agents after initial parenteral therapy in more extensive disease or as therapy for limited skin/soft tissue infection:
• Sulfonamides (ie, trimethoprim-sulfamethoxazole)
• Doxycycline

Note: Linezolid has excellent potential for treatment of *M fortuitum* and *M chelonae*.

• *Macrolide such as clarithromycin or azithromycin*

• *Levofloxacin*

Figure 9

Mycobacterium marinum infection

Ulcerative nodules on the arm

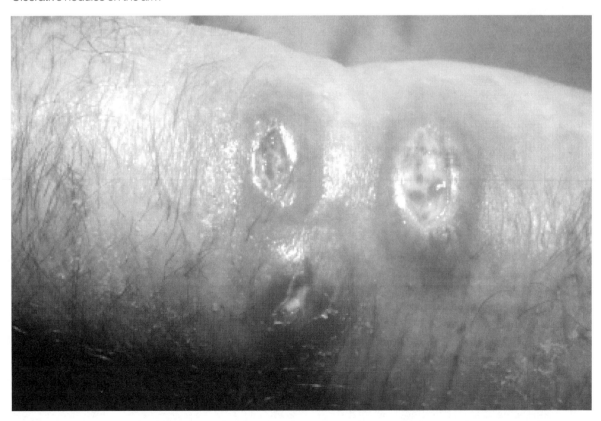

Courtesy of Dr Charles V. Sanders. From Lee BD, Greer DL. Cutaneous signs of no-tuberculosis mycobacteria. In: Sanders CV, Nesbitt LT Jr, eds. The Skin and Infection: A Color Atlas and Text. *Baltimore, MD: Williams & Wilkins; 1995: 145. Used with permission.*

Figure 10

Mycobacterium marinum infection

Large, ill-defined erythematous plaques on the arm

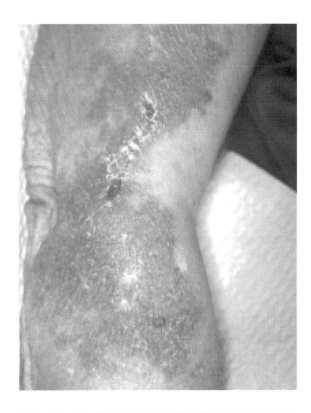

Courtesy of Dr Lee T. Nesbitt, Jr. From Lee BD, Greer DL. Cutaneous signs of nontuberculosis mycobacteria. In: Sanders CV, Nesbitt LT Jr, eds. The Skin and Infection: A Color Atlas and Text. *Baltimore, MD: Williams & Wilkins; 1995: 144. Used with permission.*

Definitive Therapy

• Guided by susceptibility testing
  * Duration: Approximately 4 months for severe cutaneous disease; 6 months for bony involvement

Adverse Effects

• Amikacin and tobramycin: auditory vestibular toxicity manifesting as ataxia, vertigo, hearing difficulty, tinnitus

• Clarithromycin: diarrhea; nausea; vomiting; headache; hearing difficulty; liver function abnormalities; elevated BUN; cytochrome P450-associated drug interactions

• Cefoxitin: bone marrow suppression; diarrhea; hypersensitivity reaction consisting of rash, fever, and increased eosinophils

• Imipenem: risk for seizure activity with increased doses, renal insufficiency, or previous central nervous system abnormality

• Sulfonamides: hypersensitivity reactions including Stevens-Johnson syndrome and toxic epidermal necrolysis; bone marrow suppression; aseptic meningitis; hepatitis and pancreatitis; hyperkalemia

• Tetracyclines: diarrhea, nausea, vomiting; photosensitivity; hepatotoxicity; dizziness

• Ciprofloxacin: diarrhea, nausea, vomiting; CNS effects including headache, restlessness, insomnia

• Linezolid: diarrhea, nausea, and vomiting; headache; bone marrow depression

• Indications for surgery include:
  * Extensive disease
  * Multinodular or localized abscess formation
  * Difficulty administering drug or ineffective drug options
  * Removal of necrotic tissue and infected foreign material

Complications

• Extension to bone with development of osteomyelitis

• Multiple organ involvement with disseminated disease

Prognostic Factors

• Outcome affected by timely diagnosis, antibiotic susceptibility-driven therapy, and surgery when indicated

• Immune status of individual also important, particularly in individuals whose infection appears secondary to immunosuppressive effects of agents such as corticosteroids and cytotoxic chemotherapy
    * Reduce immunosuppressive therapy as tolerated
    * Role of cytokine immune modulation being investigated

Infectious Disease Pearls: *M fortuitum* and *M chelonae*

1. *M fortuitum* and *M chelonae* are ubiquitous organisms found in soil, dust, water and contaminated hospital materials.

2. Lesions or drainage from wound infections secondary to these organisms are often located at the site of trauma.

3. These organisms are known as rapid growers because colonies grow within 1 week on mycobacterial culture media.

4. Both *M fortuitum* and *M chelonae* are resistant to the drugs usually used to treat tuberculosis.

5. Duration of therapy is approximately 4 months for localized skin disease and at least 6-12 months for more severe disease including bony involvement and disseminated disease.

8. *Mycobacterium marinum*

Synonyms

• Fish tank granuloma

• Swimming pool granuloma

• Previously *Mycobacterium balnei* and *M platypoecilus*

• Runyon group I photochromogen

Causative Organisms

• *Mycobacterium marinum*

Epidemiology

• Worldwide distribution

• Infection after exposure to contaminated water including salt water, fresh water, brackish water, stagnant water
    * Classically develops after handling water from aquariums and domestic fish tanks
    * Organism inoculated through skin
    * Vectors include fish and shellfish
    * Unlikely to be found in swimming pool water with chlorine concentrations >0.6 mg/L

Key Clinical Features

• Cutaneous disease in immunocompetent patients

• Dissemination rare and almost always in immuno-compromised hosts

Cutaneous Infection (Figures 8, 9 and 10)
• Occurs at site of inoculation
    * Hands, fingers, elbows and knees most commonly

• Incubation period approximately 2-6 weeks

• Manifests as:
    * Violaceous papule
    * Verrucous, ulcerated, or scaly plaque
    * Suppurating nodules in sporotrichoid pattern spreading along lymphatics

- Systemic symptoms rare

- Regional lymphadenopathy uncommon

- Usually follows indolent course

- Deeper penetration can result in arthritis, bursitis, osteomyelitis and tenosynovitis

Key Laboratory and Radiology Features

- Biopsy from margin or leading edge of skin lesion
    * Histopathology

- Acute lesions with inflammation, possible suppuration

- Later, granulomas with or without caseation
    * Acid-fast bacilli more likely present in acute suppurative lesion; atypical mycobacteria usually larger than tuberculous mycobacteria
    * Culture
        - Gold standard
        - *M marinum* grows best at 28°-32°C
        - Photochromogenic (appear yellow under light) on Lowenstein-Jensen or Middlebrook solid media
        * May take up to 3-4 weeks to grow (ask lab to hold for 6 weeks)

Differential Diagnosis

Infectious Diseases
Sporotrichosis
- Infection caused by dimorphic fungus: *Sporothrix schenckii*

- Worldwide distribution in warmer, humid climates

- Inhabitant of vegetation (soil, plants)
    * Inoculation through skin of individuals engaged in gardening

- Cutaneous sporotrichosis is the most common infectious manifestation, presenting as lymphocutaneous disease (75%) or "fixed" form (25%)

Lymphocutaneous sporotrichosis
- Most common cutaneous manifestation

- Incubation period of weeks to months

- Typically on extremity

- Erythematous painless papule enlarges before ulcerating

- Nodules develop along lymphatics
    * Can ulcerate and drain pus

- Systemic symptoms absent

"Fixed" form
- Plaque-like lesions
    * May also present as nodular, ulcerative or verrucous lesion(s)

- Do not spread along lymphatics

- Facial involvement as likely as extremity involvement

- Diagnosis by biopsy
    * Histopathology reveals characteristic asteroid body or cigar-shaped yeast forms
    * Culture on Sabouraud's dextrose agar

- Cutaneous disease treated with itraconazole

Leishmaniasis
- Vector: sandfly

- Associated with travel to or residence in endemic areas such as South America, Central America, Asia, Africa and southern part of Europe

- Clinical syndromes include cutaneous leishmaniasis, mucocutaneous leishmaniasis and visceral leishmaniasis

- *Cutaneous leishmaniasis*
    * Incubation period 2-8 weeks
    * Initial erythematous papule, plaques or crusty ulcerative lesions form later
    * Look for palpable borders and base with granulation tissue
    * Can see sporotrichoid distribution of nodules along lymphatics

- *Mucocutaneous leishmaniasis*
    * Mucosal involvement of mouth, lips, nose, pharynx
    * Initially, tender papulonodular lesion on skin, which ulcerates and later forms scar

Diagnosis
- Scrapings, aspiration or punch biopsy of involved skin tissue

- Look for amastigote form of parasite with Wright-Giemsa smear

- Kinetoplasts seen on culture or tissue smears are characteristic

- Can culture with specific media

- Nucleic acid-based testing can be helpful

- Medical treatment of cutaneous disease
    * Meglumine antimonate, stibogluconate or pentamidine

- Medical treatment of mucocutaneous disease
    * Stibogluconate
    * Amphotericin B for refractory cases

- Some lesions will heal spontaneously

Nocardia
- Ubiquitous in soil and water

- Cutaneous infection typically caused by traumatic inoculation through skin
    * Cellulitis in immunocompetent hosts usually due to *N brasiliensis*
    * Systemic infection(s) usually due to *N asteroides* in immunocompromised hosts

- Incubation period of 1-6 weeks

- Initially, painful nodule or abscess on extremity, then later, lymphangitic spread with suppuration of lesions

- Beaded, branching, filamentous Gram-positive, weakly acid-fast organisms in biopsy specimen or aspirate

- Culture diagnostic
    * Need to hold for longer period in microbiology laboratory because growth may be slow
    * Enhanced growth in CO_2-enhanced environment at 32°-35°C

- Sulfonamides are drugs of choice

The differential diagnosis is lengthy and may also include tularemia, other mycobacterial species, treponemal infections including yaws and syphilis, and endemic fungal infections such as histoplasmosis, coccidioidomycosis and blastomycosis.

Noninfectious Disease Mimics
Gout
- Acute in onset (not indolent as in *M marinum* infections)

- History of recurrences

- Look for chronic tophaceous deposits on ears, hands, olecranon and feet

- Intra articular infection usually involving first metatarsophalangeal joint
    * Sodium urate crystals in joint fluid diagnostic
    * Evaluate joint fluid for microbial infection

- Fever more common than with *M marinum* infections

- Acute attacks responsive to anti-inflammatory agents

Sarcoid
- Myriad skin manifestations in one-quarter of cases, including erythema nodosum; nodular lesions; plaques; maculopapular eruption; ulcerative lesions

- Histopathology may be similar (ie, non-caseating granulomas) to *M marinum* infections

- Major differences:
    * Sarcoid: systemic multi-organ disease with lung involvement in 90% of cases
    * *M marinum* infections: typically localized without extracutaneous manifestations

Empiric Therapy

Empiric Therapy After Fresh Water Exposure
- Ceftazidime, 2 g IV TID, *plus*
  levofloxacin, 500 mg IV daily *or*
  ciprofloxacin, 400 mg IV BID

Advantages
- Broad spectrum of activity against many water-associated organisms

Disadvantages
- None of these drugs is first-line therapy against *M marinum*

Note: If marine water exposure, add doxycycline 100 mg IV or PO BID.

Advantages
- Doxycycline effective against *M marinum*

Disadvantage(s)
- Need to identify *M marinum*
  * Cutaneous disease secondary to *M marinum* requires >3 months duration of therapy

Definitive Therapy

Susceptibility testing not indicated unless treatment failure. Organism susceptible to clarithromycin, rifampin, rifabutin, ethambutol, sulfonamides (including trimeoprim-sulfamethoxazole); susceptible or intermediately susceptible to doxycycline/minocycline

- Use two active agents for 1-2 months after symptoms resolve (ie, 3-4 months total duration)
  * Effective combinations reported include clarithromycin and ethambutol, clarithromycin and rifampin, ethambutol and rifampin

    - Clarithromycin, 500 mg PO BID

    - Doxycycline or minocycline, 100 mg PO BID

    - Rifampin 600 mg PO QD

    - Ethambutol (15 mg/kg) PO QD

- Trimethoprim-sulfamethoxazole (160/800 mg) PO BID

Advantages
- All recommended because of their efficacy against *M marinum*

Disadvantages
- See previous section on *M fortuitum* and *M chelonae*

- Surgical debridement may be required for necrosis, deep infections in closed spaces or infections refractory to antimicrobials

Complications

- Deeper penetration can result in arthritis, bursitis, osteomyelitis and tenosynovitis
  * Consider clarithromycin, ethambutol and rifampin combination therapy when deep structure infections including bone

- Hematogenous dissemination in immunosuppressed hosts

Prognostic Factors

- Poorer prognosis associated with:
  * Unremitting pain
  * Intralesional corticosteroid administration
  * Sinus tract with drainage despite extended course of antimicrobial treatment
  * Lack of surgical debridement in cases of deep infection

Infectious Disease Pearls: *M marinum*

1. Infection with this organism occurs after exposure to contaminated water including salt water, fresh water, brackish water and stagnant water.

2. Infection classically develops after soft tissue injury while handling water from aquariums and domestic fish tanks since the organism is inoculated through skin.

3. *M marinum* grows best In the microbiology lab at 28°-32°C and may take up to 3-4 weeks to grow.

4. Antimicrobial agents with reported efficacy include clarithromycin, doxycycline or minocycline, rifampin, ethambutol and trimethoprim-sulfamethoxazole.

5. Susceptibility testing for anti-*M marinum* agents is not indicated unless there is suspected treatment failure.

9. *Mycobacterium ulcerans*

Synonyms

• Buruli ulcer disease; "Bairnsdale ulcer"; Runyon group III nonchromogens

Causative Organism

• *Mycobacterium ulcerans*

Epidemiology

• Endemic foci primarily in rural tropical Africa including West Africa
    * Other areas include Australia, Papua New Guinea, Mexico, Malaysia, and scattered areas of Latin America including French Guyana and Bolivia
    * Not endemic in the United States

• Risk factors include living in tropical regions and skin trauma
    * Hypothesized that minor penetrating injury associated with contaminated water, soil, or vegetation results in inoculation of this environmental mycobacterium

• Number of infections greater in children than adults

• Causes disease in immunocompetent individuals

Key Clinical Features

• Incubation period approximately 3 months

• 4 stages of skin infection:
    * Stage 0: latency period between inoculation and clinical manifestations
    * Stage 1: pre-ulcerative stage initially consisting of pruritic intra- or subcutaneous papule evolving to nodule and plaque
    * Stage 2: Necrotic painless ulcer with undermined borders
    * Stage 3: granulomatous healing
    * Stage 4: fibrosis and scarring

• Skin lesions usually on extremities

• Fever and lymphadenitis absent

Key Laboratory and Radiology Features

• Often a clinical diagnosis in endemic areas

• Tissue-associated aspirate and biopsy material may reveal acid-fast bacilli
    * Positive in roughly one-third to two-thirds of cases
    * More likely positive in earlier necrotic lesions than in healing lesions

• Histopathology reveals "ghost" outlines of tissue among areas of subcutaneous necrosis

• Cultivation of organism on Lowenstein-Jensen or Middlebrook solid media
    * Grows best at 30°-33°C
    * Incubation at 37°C may not allow growth
    * Long incubation period required (1-3 months)
    * Non-pigmented colonies (nonchromogen like *M avium-intracellulare* and *M haemophilum*)

• PCR testing of biopsy or ulcer swab

Differential Diagnosis

Infectious Diseases
Cellulitis
• Typically manifests as warm, erythematous, spreading and swollen infection of skin
    * Not as papule, nodule or ulcer

• Lymphangitis common

• Constitutional symptoms may be present

• Leukocytosis usually present in serious infections

• *S pyogenes* and *S aureus* most common etiologic agents

Deep fungal infection with endemic mycoses (Coccidioides, Histoplasma, Blastomyces)
• Often manifest as multiple scattered (not solitary as in *M ulcerans*) nodules, plaques and ulcers due to hematogenous dissemination

• Typically associated with immunosuppressed hosts who are systemically ill

Sporotrichosis
• Infection caused by dimorphic fungus: *Sporothrix schenckii*

• Worldwide distribution in warmer, humid climates

• Inhabitant of vegetation (soil, plants)
    * Inoculation through skin of individuals engaged in gardening

• Cutaneous sporotrichosis is most common infectious manifestation presenting as lymphocutaneous disease (75%) or "fixed" form (25%)

Figure 11

Rocky Mountain spotted fever

Petechial and reticular rash on the dorsum of the foot

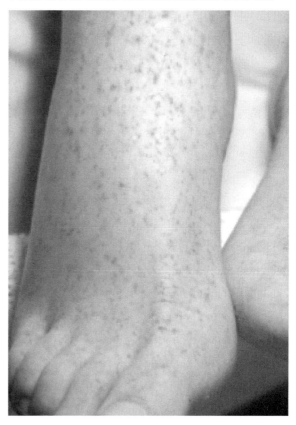

Courtesy of Dr Gene Beyt. From Fine DP. The rickettsioses. In: Sanders CV, Nesbit LT Jr, eds. The Skin and Infection: A Color Atlas and Text. *Baltimore, MD: Williams & Wilkins; 1995: 127. Used with permission.*

Lymphocutaneous sporotrichosis
- Most common cutaneous manifestation

- Incubation period weeks to months

- Typically on extremity

- Erythematous painless papule enlarges before ulcerating

- Nodules develop along lymphatics
    * Can ulcerate and drain pus

- Systemic symptoms absent

"Fixed" form
- Plaque-like lesions
    * May also present as nodular, ulcerative, or verrucous lesion(s)

- Do not spread along lymphatics

- Facial involvement as likely as extremity involvement

- Diagnosis by biopsy
    * Histopathology reveals characteristic asteroid body or cigar-shaped yeast forms
    * Culture on Sabouraud's dextrose agar

- Cutaneous disease treated with itraconazole

Leishmaniasis
- Vector: sandfly

- Associated with travel to or residence in endemic areas such as South America, Central America, Asia, Africa and southern part of Europe

- Clinical syndromes include cutaneous leishmaniasis, mucocutaneous leishmaniasis and visceral leishmaniasis

Cutaneous leishmaniasis
- Incubation period 2-8 weeks

- Initial erythematous papule, then later, plaques or crusty ulcerative lesions

- Look for palpable borders and base with granulation tissue

- Can see sporotrichoid distribution of nodules along lymphatics

Mucocutaneous leishmaniasis
- Mucosal involvement of mouth, lips, nose, pharynx

- Initially, tender papulonodular lesion on skin, which ulcerates and later forms scar

Diagnosis
- Scrapings, aspiration, or punch biopsy of involved skin tissue

- Look for amastigote form of parasite with Wright-Giemsa smear

- Kinetoplasts seen on culture or tissue smears are characteristic

- Can culture with specific media

- Nucleic acid-based testing can be helpful
    * Medical treatment of cutaneous disease
    * Meglumine antimonate, stibogluconate or pentamidine
    * Medical treatment of mucocutaneous disease

- Stibogluconate

- Amphotericin B for refractory cases
    * Some lesions will heal spontaneously

Nocardia
- Ubiquitous in soil and water

- Cutaneous infection typically caused by traumatic inoculation through skin
    * Cellulitis in immunocompetent hosts is usually due to *N brasiliensis*
    * Systemic infections are usually due to

***N asteroides* in immunocompromised hosts**

- Incubation period of 1-6 weeks

- Initially, painful nodule or abscess on extremity, then later, lymphangitic spread with suppuration of lesions

- Beaded, branching filamentous gram-positive, weakly acid-fast organisms in biopsy specimen or aspirate

- Culture diagnostic
    * Need to hold for longer period in microbiology laboratory because growth may be slow
    * Enhanced growth in CO_2-enhanced environment at 32°-35°C

- Sulfonamides are drugs of choice

The differential diagnosis is lengthy and may also include tularemia, other mycobacterial species and treponemal infections, including yaws and syphilis.

Noninfectious Disease Mimics
Pyoderma gangrenosum
- Extraintestinal manifestation of inflammatory bowel disease

- Usually presents as ulcer with necrotic base on lower extremity

- Control of inflammatory bowel disease results in improvement of lesion

Squamous cell carcinoma
- Predisposition typically includes sun exposure

- Presents initially as red indurated nodule
    * Can ulcerate

- Diagnosis with biopsy

- Treatment requires excision

Also consider foreign body granuloma, epidermal cyst, panniculitis and vasculitis.

Empiric Therapy

- Short course of antistaphylococcal and antistreptococcal antibiotics such as cefazolin may be administered until diagnosis is made. This agent has no activity against *M ulcerans*.

Definitive Therapy

- Debridement and wide surgical excision generally recommended
    * Skin grafting often required

- No definitive recommendations regarding combination anti-mycobacterial therapy
    * Usually sensitive in vitro to clarithromycin, ethambutol, some aminoglycosides, some quinolones and rifampin
    * Sulfonamides, clofazimine, dapsone, ciprofloxacin, moxifloxacin and minocycline have also been used
    * 1 consensus group recommends rifampicin plus clarithromycin or ciproflaxin or moxofloxacin when oral regimen indicated
        - Also makes recommendations for use of intravenous amikacin plus oral rifampicin in certain situations such as major relapse, severe/extensive disease, bone involvement, not fully resectable lesions, involvement of deep structures such as major vessels, tendons, nerves, etc.

- Heat treatment and hyperbaric oxygen have been tried
    * No large, well-controlled studies exist to recommend their routine use

Complications

- Small percentage extend to bone resulting in osteomyelitis

- Extensive scarring with decreased function of affected area (eg, contractures of limbs)

- Bacterial superinfection of ulcers

Prognostic Factors

- Early recognition of infection with surgical intervention can be curative
    * Prevents opportunity for secondary bacterial infections of large ulcers and extension of infection to bone

    * Prevents progression of disease and resultant extensive scarring and potential functional disabilities

Infectious Disease Pearls: *Mycobacterium ulcerans*

1. Risk factors for cutaneous infection include living in tropical regions and skin trauma.
2. Skin lesions are usually on extremities and fever and lymphadenitis are classically absent.

3. Diagnosis of Buruli ulcer disease secondary to Mycobacterium ulcerans in endemic areas is often a clinical one.

4. This organism grows best at 30°-33°C. Colonies are non-pigmented.

5. Debridement and wide surgical excision are generally recommended as medical therapy is generally disappointing.

10. Rocky Mountain Spotted Fever (RMSF)

Causative Organism

- *Rickettsia rickettsii*
    * Gram-negative, obligate, intracellular bacteria

Epidemiology

- Tick vectors in the United States include *Dermacentor variabilis* and *Rhipicephalus sanguineas*

- Wide distribution of cases across U.S.
    * Incidence greatest in southeastern, south Atlantic and south central areas of U.S.
    * Highest annual incidence in North Carolina

- Also found in Canada, Mexico, Central America and parts of South America including Bolivia, Brazil and Columbia

- Highest incidence of infection in children 5-9 years of age

- Males more likely to be infected than females

- >90% of cases occur from April to September

- Other reported risks for infection include living in wooded areas and exposure to dogs

- 30%-50% of case patients do not recall a tick bite

Key Clinical Features

- Incubation period of 3-12 days (average 7 days)

- Classic triad of tick bite, rash and fever
    * Seen in up to 70% of illnesses by second week after exposure to tick vendor

- May include sudden onset of:
    * Fever, chills, myalgias (typically calf-associated)
    * Nausea, vomiting, abdominal pain, diarrhea
    * Frontal headache, photophobia, mental status changes, conjunctival suffusion
    * Cough; cardiac arrhythmia (secondary to myocarditis)

- Rash appears after 2-6 days of illness (Figure 11)
  * Blanching erythematous macular rash initially on ankles, palms, wrists and soles with centripetal spread to arms, legs, neck, trunk and face
  * Evolution of lesions to petechiae
  * Eschar at site of inoculation (rare)
  * Reflects a vasculitic process

Key Laboratory and Radiology Features

- General laboratory findings nonspecific but suggestive

- Thrombocytopenia characteristic

- Peripheral white blood cell count may be depressed or normal
  * Over two-thirds of cases with increased band counts

- Usually normal hemoglobin

- Look for elevated CPK

- Elevated serum transaminases and bilirubin

- Hyponatremia

- Cerebrospinal fluid profile:
  * Cell count normal or with minimal lymphocytic pleocytosis
  * Glucose normal
  * Protein normal to elevated

- Chest x-ray:
  * Infiltrates consistent with pneumonitis, pulmonary edema, or ARDS may be seen

- Electrocardiogram:
  * Arrhythmia with myocardial or conduction tissue involvement

Diagnostic Tests

- Serologic antibody tests (immunofluorescent, latex agglutination, complement fixation)
  * Usually requires acute and convalescent specimens

- * Weil-Felix test for cross-reacting antibodies against Proteus vulgaris antigens not recommended

- PCR of whole blood available through health departments

- Cell culture isolation

- Skin biopsy/immunochemistry of organism from clinical specimen
  * Direct immunofluorescent staining of tissue
    • Helpful for diagnosis in early stage of infection
    • Sensitivity. 70%; specificity, 100%
- Clinical suspicion important in appropriate epidemiologic setting

Differential Diagnosis

Infectious Diseases
Meningococcemia
- Etiologic agent: Gram-negative diplococcus, *Neisseria meningitidis*

- Skin lesions develop sooner than in RMSF, in which rash typically appears on third to fourth day
  * Petechial lesions most common; macular, maculopapular and, in severe cases, purpuric and ecchymotic skin lesions may develop
  * Rash can involve palms and soles in both diseases
  * Rash more likely to be tender in meningococcal infection than in RMSF

- Pharyngitis and hypotension more likely with *N meningitidis* infection than RMSF

- Nausea, vomiting, diarrhea, pulse-temperature disparity, edema of distal extremities and around orbit, conjunctival injection, hepatosplenomegaly, and increased serum transaminases more likely in RMSF

- Diagnosis usually by isolation from blood, cerebrospinal fluid or aspirate from skin lesion

- Treatment: Penicillin or ceftriaxone

Typhoid fever
- Etiologic agent: *Salmonella enterica* (serotype typhi)

- Transmitted with ingestion of contaminated consumables

- Incubation period of 1-2 weeks

- 3 phases of infection:
  * Beginning of symptoms include headache (like RMSF), cough, sore throat (unlike RMSF), disturbance in stool patterns (increased or decreased frequency), and gradual stepwise increase in fever
  * Period of greatest severity often accompanied by pulse-temperature discordance, altered mental status, and cutaneous manifestation known as "rose spots"

- Blanching macules approximately 2 mm in size that are pink-brown in color, located on the trunk and resolving slowly over 4 days
  * Slow resolution of symptoms followed by possible relapse or carriage

- Leukopenia more characteristic than in RMSF; thrombocytopenia and lymphocytic pleocytosis of CSF more likely in RMSF; increased serum transaminases in both

- Can culture organism from blood (usually in first week) and stool (usually after first week); bone marrow cultures can be helpful early in course
  * Rose spot-associated skin biopsy specimens can be culture-positive >50% of time

- Organism may be susceptible to trimethoprim-sulfamethoxazole, ampicillin, ceftriaxone or fluoroquinolones

Rubeola (measles)
- Vaccine-preventable disease caused by *Morbillivirus* virus

- Winter and spring most common time for infection vs. summer months when RMSF more common

- Clinical features characteristically include fever, cough, conjunctivitis, coryza, photophobia and rash

- Enanthem is pathognomonic (ie, Koplik's spots), buccal mucosa-associated erythematous macules with central white focus that appear approximately 2 days before rash

- Prominent red-brown maculopapular rash that typically originates on face before involving trunk and upper extremities

- No specific antiviral therapy available; supportive care only

Rubella (German measles)
- Vaccine-preventable disease caused by *Rubivirus*

- Pink papular rash that begins on face before spreading to trunk

- Lesions remain distinct, particularly on extremities

- Look for palatal petechiae known as Forchheimer's sign

- Tender postauricular, posterior cervical and suboccipital nodes characteristic

Murine typhus
- Etiologic agent: *Rickettsia typhi*

- Vector: rat flea

- Transmission abetted by poor living conditions

- Clinical symptoms similar to RMSF, albeit milder

- Rash typically present
  * Can be subtle
  * Blanching macular rash, usually on trunk
  * Nonpruritic

Epidemic louse-borne typhus
- Etiologic agent: *Rickettsia prowazekii*

- Vector: human body louse

- Epidemiologically associated with poor hygiene and crowded living conditions

- Clinical presentation similar to RMSF

- Rash begins centrally (axilla and trunk) before spreading centrifugally (different than RMSF)
    * Initially blanching erythematous maculopapular rash which can become petechial
    * Palms, soles, and face are spared (palm and sole involvement more typical of RMSF)

Ehrlichiosis/Anaplasmosis
- Tick-borne disease

- 3 types: human monocytic ehrlichiosis (HME), human granulocytic anaplasmosis (HGA) and human granulocytic ehrlichiosis (HGE)

- Clinically similar to RMSF except rash much less common, ie, "spotless RMSF"
    * 36% of patients with HME
    * 2% of patients with HGA

- Rash typically maculopapular, not petechial

- Rash most prominent on trunk

- Rash spares the soles and palms (unlike RMSF)

- Laboratory abnormalities include elevated liver transaminases, thrombocytopenia and leukopenia

Other infectious diseases to consider include leptospirosis, tularemia, scrub typhus, rickettsialpox, viral hepatitis, and enteroviral infections. Noninfectious disease mimics would include collagen vascular diseases like systemic lupus erythematosus.

Empiric Therapy

Due to relative lack of universally available expedient testing for diagnosis of acute disease, begin empiric therapy if diagnosis suspected.

Preferred
Doxycycline, 100 mg PO/IV BID, *plus* ceftriaxone, 1-2 g IV BID

- Doxycycline for coverage of tick-borne diseases and ceftriaxone for coverage of *N meningitidis*

Advantages
Doxycycline
- Oral and intravenous formulations

- No need for dosage adjustment in renal failure

- Good activity against rickettsial diseases

Chloramphenicol
- May be preferable if central nervous system (CNS) involvement prominent
    * Effective against CNS infections due to meningococci, pneumococci, *H influenzae* and RMSF

- Not contraindicated in pregnancy

Disadvantages
Doxycycline
- Risk of irreversible tooth staining in children less than 8 years of age

- Contraindicated in pregnancy

- Potential adverse effects include nausea and diarrhea.

Chloramphenicol
- Inferior anti-RMSF (*R rickettsii*) activity

- Not effective against Ehrlichia, a potential clinical mimic of RMSF

- Toxicity profile:
    * Dose-related suppression of bone marrow, particularly red blood cells
    * Aplastic anemia
        - Not dose-associated
        - Rare (approximately 1 episode per 30,000 treatment courses)

Alternative
Chloramphenicol, 50-75 mg/kg/d PO/IV in 4 divided doses daily, *plus* ceftriaxone, 1 to 2 g IV BID

Definitive Therapy

Preferred
Doxycycline, 100 mg PO/IV BID

Alternative
Chloramphenicol, 50-75 mg/kg/d PO/IV in 4
divided doses daily

Note: Typically, defervescence noted within 48-72
hours of initiating appropriate antibiotics (exception
with gangrene or multiple organ involvement)

• Duration of therapy: Approximately 5-10 days
  with patient afebrile for at least 48-72 hours

Complications

• Death usually secondary to shock and multiple organ
  system failure including pneumonitis, myocarditis
  and disseminated intravascular coagulation

• Neurologic sequelae include seizure, neuropathy
  and paresis
      * More likely in individuals with extended
        hospital courses

Prognostic Factors
• With advent of effective antibiotics, case fatality
  rate of approximately 3%-5%
      * 20% mortality rate in absence of treatment

• Mortality rate highest in patients >70 years of age
  and lowest in those less than 4 years of age

• Delay in initiation of effective antibiotics, liver
  insufficiency, and G6PD deficiency in African
  American males associated with poorer outcomes

• No vaccine currently available
      * Prevention against possibility of tick bite with
        protective clothing

• Doxycycline prophylaxis against RMSF not recommended after tick bite in endemic area

**Infectious Disease Pearls: Rocky Mountain
Spotted Fever**

1. Incidence of the tick-borne associated RMSF is
   greatest in the southeastern, south Atlantic and
   south central areas of United States.

2. The incubation period is 3-12 days (average 7
   days).

3. RMSF is characterized by the classic tick bite-
   associated triad of headache, rash and fever.

4. A blanching erythematous macular rash initially
   (rapidly progresses to petechial rash) on ankles,
   palms, wrists and soles with centripetal spread to
   arms, legs, neck, trunk and face is characteristic
   of RMSF. Rash appears 2-6 days after the illness
   begins.

5. Doxycycline is the drug of choice for this infection.

11. Dengue Fever

Synonyms

• Dengue; dengue fever; dengue hemorrhagic fever; dengue shock syndrome

Causative Organisms

• Belongs to family of flavivirus

• 4 serotypes of dengue virus, serotypes (ie, DEN-1, DEN-2, DEN-3, or DEN-4)

Epidemiology

• Reservoir: humans, monkeys

• Vector: *Aedes* mosquitoes (primarily *A aegypti* and *A albopictus*)
  * Transmission usually from bites of female *A aegypti* mosquito

• Occurs in tropical and subtropical areas
  * Endemic in Americas, Africa, western Pacific, southeast Asia, eastern part of Mediterranean

• Warmer weather favorable for mosquito life cycle

• In the United States, cases primarily travel-associated
  * Indigenous infections have been reported in Texas and Hawaii

• Approximately 50 to 100 million people infected annually

• Hawaiian outbreak transmitted by inefficient vector of A albopictus

Key Clinical Features

• Incubation period of 3-14 days (usually 4-6 days)

• Clinical manifestations range from asymptomatic to dengue fever to more severe forms of disease such as dengue hemorrhagic fever and dengue shock syndrome (DHF/DHS)

Dengue Fever
• Biphasic fever curve: initial abrupt onset of fever

• Retro-orbital headache

• Severe bone and muscle pain (ie, "breakbone fever")

• Rash initially macular, erythematous and blanching

• Respiratory and gastrointestinal symptoms in some cases

• Conjunctival injection, lymphadenopathy, posterior oropharyngeal erythema and enlarged liver may be appreciated

• Fever subsides after several days, then recurs 1-3 days later (ie, "saddleback" pattern)
  * Diffuse maculopapular rash that spares soles and palms temporally associated with defervescence

• Resolution of illness within 2 weeks

Dengue Hemorrhagic Fever (DHF)
• Occurs after rechallenge with dengue virus
  * DHF/DHS can be seen with primary infection in infants secondary to presence of maternal dengue-associated antibodies

• Initial systemic symptoms of fever, headache, vomiting, then condition deteriorates after approximately 4 days

• Bleeding, bruising, petechiae and plasma leakage (ie, ascites, pleural effusion)

• Encephalopathy observed less commonly

• Lab abnormalities include low platelets, hemoconcentration, prolonged bleeding time, hypoproteinemia, elevated liver function tests

• Rapid recovery after 1-2 days of clinical deterioration

Dengue Shock Syndrome (DSS)
• Essentially DHF + circulatory collapse
  * Hypotension; shock; narrow pulse pressure
  * Mental status changes

Key Laboratory and Radiology Features

Laboratory Features
• Leukopenia

• Thrombocytopenia

• Elevated hematocrit

• Prolonged bleeding time

• Elevated serum aspartate transaminase

• Hypoproteinemia

Diagnostic Tests

(Usually performed by Centers for Disease Control and Prevention)

* Dengue antigen capture ELISA

• **Serologic Testing**
  * Hemagglutination inhibition assay (paired acute and convalescent specimens)
  * IgG (paired acute and convalescent specimens) or IgM enzyme immunoassays

• Virus isolation in tissue or mosquito culture

• PCR most expeditious but not universally accessible

Differential Diagnosis

Infectious Diseases
Yellow fever
• Like dengue virus, a flavivirus

• Vector: *Aedes mosquito*

• Outbreaks primarily in South America and Africa

• Incubation period of 3-6 days

• Range of clinical presentations
  * Subclinical
  * Milder form that includes nonspecific fever, retro-orbital headache, gastrointestinal symptoms
  * Severe form initially resembles milder form, then short remission followed by severe systemic process
    • Insufficiency of multiple organs (including liver, ie, "yellow fever") and bleeding tendencies
    • Fever-pulse disparity characteristic, ie, "Faget's sign"
  * Lab abnormalities: leukopenia and elevated serum transaminases (AST >ALT); more severe infections with azotemia, nephrotic-range proteinuria, thrombocytopenia, liver function abnormalities, prolonged PT, hypoglycemia, hyperkalemia
  * Diagnostic aids include virus isolation in culture or serologic antibody testing (ELISA IgM capture assay; paired acute and convalescent antibody titers)
  * No specific antiviral agent available
  * Mortality rate approximately 10%

Leptospirosis
• Caused by a spirochete

• Associated with bathing or swimming in water contaminated with urine from livestock, dogs or rats

• Clinical presentations
  * Milder anicteric form is biphasic
    • Initial septic phase with abrupt presentation of fever, gastrointestinal disturbances, headache, conjunctival injection and myalgias (up to 7-day duration), then fever abates for 2 days before second phase of disease begins.
    • Immune phase characterized by fever, headache, spleen and liver enlargement, uveitis, rash, adenopathy and lung abnormalities
  * Severe icteric form (Weil's syndrome)
    • Characterized by liver insufficiency with jaundice, renal insufficiency, mental status changes and pulmonary hemorrhage

- Abnormal labs include peripheral neutrophilia, thrombocytopenia, increased liver function studies, increased CPK, azotemia, abnormal urine sediment and increased white blood cells in cerebrospinal fluid

- Diagnosis
  * Microscopic dark field examination
  * Isolation from blood or CSF in first 10 days
  * Isolation from urine after first 10 days
  * Serologic testing for antibodies against *Leptospira*

- Treatment usually penicillin or doxycycline

- Mortality rate of 5%-35% for icteric form of disease

Typhoid fever
- Etiologic agent: *Salmonella enterica* (serotype typhi)

- Transmitted with ingestion of contaminated consumables

- Incubation period of 1-2 weeks

- 3 phases of infection:
  * Beginning of symptoms including headache, cough, sore throat, disturbance in stool patterns (increased or decreased frequency), and gradual stepwise increase in fever
  * Period of greatest severity often accompanied by pulse-temperature discordance, altered mental status, and cutaneous manifestation of "rose spots"
    - Blanching macules approximately 2 mm in size that are pink-brown in color, found on the trunk and resolving slowly over 4 days
  * Slow resolution of symptoms followed by possible relapse or carriage

- Leukopenia characteristic

- Can culture organism from blood (usually in first week) and stool (usually after first week); bone marrow cultures can be helpful
  * Rose spot-associated skin biopsy specimens can be culture positive >50% of time

- Organism may be susceptible to trimethoprim-sulfamethoxazole, ampicillin, ceftriaxone or fluoroquinolones

Malaria
- Vector is female *Anopheles* mosquito

- Clinical triad of high fever, rigors and chills

- Symptoms can be similar to dengue but cutaneous manifestations are rare
  * Urticaria, petechiae, purpura, and mucous membrane bleeding uncommon

- Anemia (not hemoconcentration as in dengue virus infections) is common
- Evaluation of red blood cells in peripheral smear for diagnosis

- Antimicrobials available for treatment

Noninfectious Disease Mimics
Heatstroke
- Clinical presentation includes dehydration, altered consciousness, high fever, hypotension, renal dysfunction (sometimes liver and cardiac dysfunction) and lack of sweating

- Not dependent on exposure to mosquito vector

- Predisposing factors include:
  * Exertion in setting of high ambient temperatures
  * Compromised temperature homeostasis induced by medications including phenothiazene antipsychotics and anticholinergics
  * Treatment includes supportive care, discontinuation of precipitants and quick reduction of core temperature

Therapy

- No specific anti-dengue viral agents available

- Supportive care recommended
  * Fluids and blood products as needed

- Avoid potential antiplatelet agents such as aspirin and NSAIDs (bleeding complications)

- Prevention is key
  * Mosquito control
  * No effective commercial vaccine

Complications

- Bleeding, bruising, petechiae and plasma leakage (ie, ascites, pleural effusion)

- Encephalopathy and liver insufficiency

- Shock

- Death

Prognostic Factors

- With development of DHF, case fatality rate of 1%-5%

- With development of DSS, case fatality rate of about 10%

- Development of encephalopathy and liver failure associated with increased mortality

Prevention

- Avoid exposure to mosquitoes

  *Insect repellent, screened quarters, protective clothing

Infectious Disease Pearls: Dengue Fever

1. The vector for infection is the *Aedes* mosquito (primarily *A aegypti* and *A albopictus*).

2. Infections are primarily seen in tropical and subtropical areas as this infection is endemic in Americas, Africa, western Pacific, southeast Asia and eastern part of the Mediterranean.

3. Clinical manifestations range from asymptomatic to dengue fever to more severe forms of disease such as dengue hemorrhagic fever/dengue shock syndrome (DHF/DHS).

4. Laboratories obtained in patients with dengue fever infections typically reveal leukopenia, thrombocytopenia, elevated hematocrit, a prolonged bleeding time, an elevated serum aspartate transaminase and hypoproteinemia.

5. No specific anti-dengue viral agents are available and supportive care is recommended. Antiplatelet agents such as aspirin and NSAIDs should be avoided to reduce potential bleeding complications.

12. Further Reading

Books

Cunha BA, ed. *Tickborne Infectious Diseases: Diagnosis and Management.* New York, NY: Marcel Dekker; 2000.

Gorbach SL, Bartlett JG, Blacklow NR. Infectious Diseases. 3rd ed. New York, NY: Lippincott Williams & Wilkins; 2004.

Guerrant RL, Walker DH, Weller PF. *Tropical Infectious Diseases: Principles, Pathogens, & Practice.* Vol 1. Philadelphia, PA: Churchill Livingstone; 1999.

Mandell GL. *Principles and Practice of Infectious Diseases.* 6th ed. Philadelphia, PA: Churchill Livingstone; 2005.

Slaven EM, Stone SC, Lopez FA, eds. *Infectious Diseases: Emergency Department Diagnosis and Management.* 1st ed. New York, NY: McGraw Hill; 2007.

Strickland GT, ed. *Hunter's Tropical Medicine and Emerging Infectious Diseases.* 8th ed. Philadelphia, PA: WB Saunders; 2000.

Tan JS, File TM, Salata RA, Tan M, eds. *Expert Guide to Infectious Diseases.* 2nd ed. Philadelphia, PA: ACP Press; 2008.

Journal Articles

Anaya DA, Patchen Dellinger E. Necrotizing soft tissue infection: Diagnosis and management. *Clin Infect Dis.* 2007; 44: 705-710.

Bisno AL, Stevens DL. Streptococcal infections of skin and soft tissues. *N Engl J Med.* 1996;334:240-245.

Chen LF, Sexton DJ. What's new in Rocky Mountain Spotted Fever? *Infect Dis Clin North Am.* 2008; 22:415-432.

Chuang YC, Yuan CY, Liu CY, et al. Vibrio vulnificus infection in Taiwan: report of 28 cases and review of clinical manifestations and treatment. *Clin Infect Dis.* 1992;15:271-276.

Davies HD, McGreer A, Schwartz B, et al. Invasive group A streptococcal infections in Ontario, Canada. *N Engl J Med.* 1996;335:547-554.

Dechet AM, Yu PA, Koram N, Painter J. Nonfoodborne Vibrio infections: An important cause of morbidity and mortality in the United States, 1997-2006. *Clin Infect Dis.* 2008; 46:970-976.

Dunbar SA, Clarridge JE III. Potential errors in recognition of Erysipelothrix rhusiopathiae. *J Clin Microbiol.* 2000;38:1302-1304.

Eagle H. Experimental approach to the problem of treatment failure with penicillin. I. Group A streptococcal infection in mice. *Am J Med.*1952;13:389-399.

Edelstein H. Mycobacterium marinum skin infections: report of 31 cases and review of the literature. *Arch Intern Med.* 1994;154:1359-1364.

Evans MRW, Thangaraj HS, Warnsbrough-Jones MH. Buruli ulcer. *Cur Opin Infect Dis.* 2000;13:109-112.

Ghenghesh KS, Ahmed SF, El-Khalek RA, Al-Gendy A, Klena J. Aeromonas-associated infections in developing countries. *J Infect Developing Countries* 2008; 2(2):81-98.

Gold WL, Salit IE. Aeromonas hydrophila infections of the skin and soft tissue: report of 11 cases and review. *Clin Infect Dis.* 1993;16:69-74.

Gorby GL, Peacock JE Jr. Erysipelothrix rhusiopathiae endocarditis: microbiologic, epidemiologic, and clinical features of an occupational disease. *Rev Infect Dis.*1988;10:317-325.

Halstead SB. Dengue. *Lancet.* 2007; 370:1644-1652.

Hook EW III, Hooton TM, Horton CA, et al. Microbiologic evaluation of cutaneous cellulitis in adults. *Arch Intern Med.*1986;146:295-297.

Jernigan JA, Farr BM. Incubation period and sources of exposure for Mycobacterium marinum infection: case report and review of the literature. *Clin Infect Dis*. 2000;31:439-443.

Johnson PD, Hayman JA, Quek TY, et al for the *Mycobacterial ulcerans* Study Team. Consensus recommendations for the diagnosis, treatment and control of Mycobacterium ulcerans infection (Bairnsdale or Buruli ulcer) in Victoria, Australia. *Med J Aust*. 2007;186:64-68.

Jorgensen JH, Hindler JF. New consensus guidelines from the Clinical and Laboratory Standards Institute for antimicrobial susceptibility testing of infrequently isolated or fastidious bacteria. *Clin Infect Dis*. 2007;44:280-286.

Klontz KC, Lieb S, Schreiber M, et al. Syndromes of Vibrio vulnificus infections: clinical and epidemiologic features in Florida cases, 1981-1987. *Ann Intern Med*.1988;109:318-323.

Lee CC, Chi CH, Lee NY, et al. Necrotizing fasciitis in patients with liver cirrhosis: predominance of monomicrobial Gram-negative bacillary infections. *Diagn Microbiol Infect Dis*. 2008;62:219-225.

Lillis RA, Dugan V, Mills T, et al. A fish hook and liver disease: revisiting an old enemy. *J LA State Med Soc*. 2002;154:20-25.

Lopez FA, Lartchen KS. Skin and soft tissue infections. *Infect Dis Clin North Am*. 2006;20:759-772, v-vi.

Myers SA, Sexton DJ. Dermatologic manifestations of arthropod-borne diseases. *Infect Dis Clin North Am*. 1994;8:689-712.

Paul K, Patel SS. Eikenella corrodens infections in children and adolescents: case reports and review of the literature. *Clin Infect Dis*.2001;33:54-61.

Ramos E, Silva M, Pereira AL. Life threatening eruptions due to infectious agents. *Clin Dermatol*. 2005;23:148-156.

Sheng WS, Hsueh PR, Hung CC, et al. Clinical features of patients with invasive Eikenella corrodens infections and microbiological characteristics of the causative isolates. *Eur J Clin Microbiol Infect Dis*. 2001;20:231-236.

Stevens DL, Bisno AL, Chambers HF, et al. Practice guidelines for the diagnosis and management of skin and soft-tissue infections. *Clin Infect Dis*. 2005;41:1373-1406.

Stevens DL. The toxic shock syndromes. *Infect Dis Clin North Am*.1996;10:727-746.

The Working Group on Severe Streptococcal Infections. Defining the group A streptococcal toxic shock syndrome. *J Am Med Assoc*.1993;269: 390-391.

Thorner AR, Walker DH, Petri WA Jr. Rocky Mountain spotted fever. *Clin Infect Dis*. 1998;27:1353-1359.

Todd J, Fishaut M, Kapral F, Welch T. Toxic-shock syndrome associated with phage-group-I staphylococci. *Lancet*. 1978;2:1116-1118.

Usian DZ, Kowalski TJ, Wengenack NL, Virk A, Wilson JW. Skin and soft tissue infections due to rapidly growing mycobacteria: comparison of clinical features, treatment and susceptibility. *Arch Dermatol*. 2006;142:1287-1292.

Wallace RJ Jr. The clinical presentation, diagnosis, and therapy of cutaneous and pulmonary infections due to the rapidly growing mycobacteria, *M fortuitum* and *M chelonae*. *Clin Chest Med*. 1989;10:419-429.

Woodward TE, Cunha BA. Rocky Mountain spotted fever. *Infect Dis Pract*. 1999;23:73-80.

Chapter 3: Fever in Returning Travelers for the ID Boards

Nancy F. Crum-Cianflone, MD, MPH
Edith R. Lederman, MD, MPH
Braden R. Hale, MD, MPH
Mark R. Wallace, MD

Contents

The views expressed in this chapter are those of the authors and do not reflect the official policy of the Department of the Navy, Department of Defense or the United States government.

Introduction

Returning travelers have different risks for various disease entities depending upon their 1.) itinerary; 2.) length of stay; 3.) known exposures; 4.) underlying immune status (both underlying conditions and vaccination status); and 5.) type of traveler (eg, an individual visiting friends and relatives vs. a cruise ship patron). Furthermore, although the list of pathogens seems vast, for practical purposes, the majority of identifiable causes of fever in the returned traveler are: 1.) malaria; 2.) dysentery; 3.) typhoid fever; 4.) rickettsial infections; and 5.) hemorrhagic fever viruses, namely dengue. Dysentery will not be specifically discussed in this chapter (see Chapter 22). In addition to tropical diseases as a cause of fever in returning travelers, common infections such as upper respiratory infections, streptococcal infections, urinary tract infections and common viral illnesses, as well as non-infectious causes such as deep venous thrombosis (DVT) may occur.

1. Malaria

Causative Organisms

Malaria is caused by protozoa carried by anopheline mosquitoes. There are 4 main human pathogens: Plasmodium falciparum, *P vivax, P malariae and P ovale.* Recently "monkey malaria" (*P knowlesi*) has been found to be a human pathogen in certain areas of Southeast Asia, especially Borneo. The geographic distribution of malaria is shown in Figure 1.

Epidemiology

The WHO estimates that 2.4 billion people live in malaria-endemic areas, 500 million fall ill each year and about 2 million die annually. More deaths occur today than 30 years ago. Over 90% of the malaria deaths occur in sub-Saharan Africa, caused by *P falciparum.* Some generalities can be useful in considering the epidemiology of malaria:

• Nearly all deaths are in children.

• *P falciparum* tends to have more stable transmission, predominating in areas with efficient anthropophagic vectors and less climatic variation.

• *P vivax* may predominate in more temperate climates with less efficient vectors. The scope of morbidity and mortality secondary to P vivax has been traditionally underestimated, and recent publications have highlighted serious manifestations especially among children and pregnant females.

• Chloroquine-resistant *P falciparum* (CRPF) is present throughout most of the malaria endemic world.

• Epidemics of malaria may occur in areas of political instability (loss of vector control/public health infrastructure) or when the ecosystem is altered (eg, introduction of new vector, increase in number of susceptible persons).

Key Clinical Features

The severity of the malaria infection depends on a variety of factors: host immunity and age, the parasite strain and the parasite species (Table 1). Much has been written about the periodicity of the fever, which is often not a practical historical feature in ill patients. However, there are a few key common, yet nonspecific, symptoms and signs:

Figure 1

Global distribution of malaria

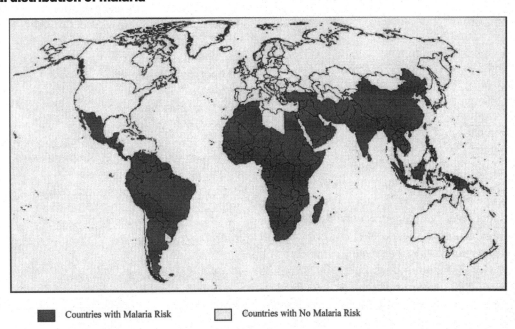

■ Countries with Malaria Risk   ☐ Countries with No Malaria Risk

From: CDC. Health Information for International Travel. *2001-2003*

Table 1

Epidemiology of Malaria Parasites

	P falciparum	*P vivax*	*P malariae*	*P ovale*
Incubation period, days (range)	12 (9-14)	13 (12-17+)	28 (18-40+)	17 (16-18+)
RBCs parasitized	All	Young (large)	Old (small)	Young
Average parasitemia	20,000+	10,000	6000	9000
Periodicity	48 hours	48 hours	48 hours	72 hours
Distribution	Worldwide	Worldwide	Africa, Asia, scattered others	Africa, Haiti, Oceania
Severity	Severe	Mild to moderate	Mild	Mild

• Fever

• Headache

• Chills

• Myalgias

• Splenomegaly

• Hepatomegaly

• A variety of other symptoms (diarrhea, nonproductive cough, jaundice, vomiting) may be present

No constellation of symptoms has proven predictive of malaria infection. Clinical suspicion is critical. Complicated malaria or severe malaria is a multisystem illness with mortality approaching 25% in the untreated nonimmune host (Table 2). In endemic areas, severe malaria is a disease of children. Generally, severe malaria presents with severe anemia, respiratory distress, or mental status changes (coma, seizures). However, in the non-immune adult traveler, severe malaria is a real and potentially fatal entity.

Key Laboratory/Radiologic Features

• Anemia

• Thrombocytopenia

• Hypoglycemia

• Metabolic acidosis: an important factor in respiratory distress (Kussmaul breathing) and changes in mental status

• Elevated transaminases

• Hyperbilirubinemia

• Prolonged PT

• Elevated serum creatinine, BUN

• Hemoglobinuria

Radiology

• The chest radiograph may show pulmonary edema which may develop during or after successful treatment of parasitemia. Superinfection with bacterial pneumonia may also occur.

Differential Diagnosis

Infectious Diseases
• Sepsis, bacterial

• Gastroenteritis (if diarrhea is prominent)

• Meningitis (if seizures and altered mental status are prominent)

• Rickettsial disease

• Pneumonia (if cough is prominent)

• Tropical viral diseases (hemorrhagic fevers)

• Other arboviruses

• Leptospirosis

• Influenza

• Meningococcemia

• Typhoid fever

• Relapsing fever

• Viral hepatitis

Malaria can often be distinguished from at least some of the above by a careful history, examination and assessment of the constellation of signs and symptoms. Obtaining the gold standard test, the thick/thin smear, confirms the diagnosis of malaria. It is important to remember that the semi-immune patient from an endemic area may have incidental parasitemia with illness from other etiologies, which must be separately addressed. It is also important to remember that non-immune travelers may have a low parasitemia which may be difficult to detect on thin smears (many US laboratories cannot reliably perform and interpret thick smears). Therefore, serial thin smears (every 8 hours) should be per-

Table 2

Severe Malaria

Defining criteria for severe malaria (may be revised soon)	Other manifestations (not part of definition but frequently present in severe disease)
• Cerebral malaria with unable to rouse coma	• Impaired consciousness but able to rouse
• Severe normocytic anemia	• Prostration,extreme weakness
• Renal failure	• Hyperparasitemia
• Pulmonary edema	• Jaundice
• Hypoglycemia	• Hyperpyrexia
• Shock or circulatory collapse	
• Disseminated intravascular coagulation (DIC)/ spontaneous bleeding	
• Repeated generalized convulsions	
• Acidemia/acidosis	
• Macroscopic hemoglobinuria	

formed if you are entertaining the diagnosis of malaria.

Empiric Therapy

Empiric therapy should not be performed, with the possible exception of personnel in remote field conditions, without any diagnostic or therapeutic alternatives (such as Peace Corps volunteers). In remote settings, the following are acceptable options:

• Atovaquone-proguanil (Malarone) 2 tablets PO BID for 3 days

• Mefloquine 750 mg followed by 500 mg 6 hours later

• Chloroquine 1000 mg PO followed by 500 mg at 6, 24 and 48 hours if in a location with CSPF

• Artemether-lumefantrine fixed dose combination (FDA-approval anticipated later in 2009)

[a]Mefloquine has a high incidence of adverse effects at this dose level and should generally not be distributed for emergency self-treatment.

Definitive Therapy
(please consult current resistance maps prior to prescribing malaria treatment, as drug resistance continues to emerge)

• For uncomplicated CSPF and *P malariae:*
  * Chloroquine 1000 mg PO (600 g base) followed by 500 mg (300 mg base) at 6, 24 and 48 hours

• For chloroquine-susceptible *P vivax* (CSPV) and *P ovale*:
  * Chloroquine 1000 mg PO followed by 500 mg at 6, 24, and 48 hours, followed by primaquine 30 mg PO QD for 14 days (check G6PD status first)

• For chloroquine-resistant *P vivax* (CRPV):
  * Mefloquine 750 mg followed by 500 mg 6 hours later
  * Quinine sulfate 650 mg PO TID for 7 days, *plus* doxycycline 100 mg PO BID for 7 days
  * Atovaquone-proguanil (Malarone) 2 tablets PO BID for 3 days (less published data, but appears effective)
    • Also followed by primaquine as noted above

- For uncomplicated CRPF:
  - * Artemether-lumefantrine 4 tablets PO now and 4 tablets PO 8 hours later; then 4 tab PO BID for 2 more days (when available)
  - * Quinine sulfate 650 mg PO TID for 7 days, *plus* doxycycline 100 mg PO BID for 7 days *or* clindamycin 900 PO TID for 5 days (in pregnancy, not severe)
  - * Atovaquone-proguanil (Malarone) 2 tablets PO BID for 3 days
  - * Mefloquine 750 mg followed by 500 mg 6 hours later

- If the identity of the parasite is unclear, but is likely to be due to *P vivax* or *ovale* based on the location of travel, radical cure with primaquine 15 mg (or 30 mg if from a primaquine-tolerant *P vivax* [PTPV] area) daily for 14 days. You may also opt to do this if the individual has been in an area with significant rates of *P vivax* or *P ovale* to presumptively treat the liver stage of the parasite and prevent relapse (known as PART (presumptive anti-relapse treatment). Check G6PD status first.

Advantages/Disadvantages

Artemesinin compounds have supplanted quinine-based therapy as the standard of care for severe malaria in the developing world as they have superior parasite clearance and treatment outcomes. Although not currently available in the United States, artemether+lumefantrine is under FDA processing for approval. Quinine is clearly effective, although it has troublesome, but generally not serious side effects, most commonly cinchonism. Mefloquine induces nausea and emesis in a significant number of people at treatment doses, even when given in divided doses, and cannot be administered to those with cardiac conduction abnormalities, seizure disorders and psychiatric disorders. It can be given to those on beta-blockers. Malarone is expensive, but has few side effects. Halofantrine has been used in the past, but associated cardiac toxicity limits its use today given the availability of other treatment options.

- Severe *P falciparum*:
  - * Artesunate (if available) 2.4 mg/kg IV per day in four divided doses for 3 days followed by malarone, doxycycline, mefloquine or clindamycin, given the short half life of artesunate.
  - * Quinine IV 20 mg/kg loading dose over 4 hours followed by 10 mg/kg TID (not generally available)
  - * Quinidine IV 10 mg/kg loading dose (max: 600 mg) over 2 hours followed by continuous infusion of 0.02 mg/kg/min—follow QT interval closely. Skip loading dose if mefloquine was already administered.
  - * For quinine or quinidine regimens, continue until parasite density is <1% and patient is able to take oral medications, then switch to oral quinine for 3 days (use 7 days for SE Asia). Also give doxycycline 100mg IV BID or clindamycin (10mg/kg load, then 5 mg/kg IV TID) with quinine/quinidine regimens.
  - * Adjunctive measure—consider exchange transfusion if patient meets criteria for severe malaria (controversial)
  - * Consider broad-spectrum antibiotic coverage of bacterial sepsis (especially Gram-negative rods) and/or bacterial pneumonia, commonly coexisting with severe malaria.

Complications

- *P falciparum* –severe malaria (see above); black-water fever; superinfection with bacterial sepsis, pneumonia and death

- *P malariae* – nephrotic syndrome

- *P vivax* and *P ovale* – splenic rupture

ID Board Pearls

- The diagnosis of malaria should be entertained in any febrile traveler returning from a malaria-endemic area.

- The most important considerations in choosing the appropriate therapy are the *Plasmodium* species causing the infection, the severity of illness and the geographic location where the infection was acquired. In addition, if the infection involves a relapsing form (*P ovale* or *vivax*), then primaquine for terminal cure is advised.

- The two most common causes of sudden deterioration in patients with severe malaria are bacterial infection/sepsis and hypoglycemia (due to *Plasmodium*-infected RBCs utilizing glucose, the effect of quinine/quinidine and impaired hepatic gluconeogenesis).

- Non-immune travelers may present with low parasitemia despite prominent clinical symptoms. This may lead to increased difficulty of diagnosis in these cases; therefore, serial thin smears (every 8 hours) as well as thick smears must be performed to rule out malaria.

- When available in the U.S., artemesinin compounds will be the preferred treatment for *P falciparum* malaria. In the meantime, quinine/quinidine plus doxycycline or clindamycin is the treatment for severe cases.

2. Typhoid Fever

Synonyms

Enteric fever

Causative Organisms

Salmonella typhi is the cause of typhoid fever; enteric fever refers to both typhoid and paratyphoid fever, which is caused by paratyphoid A, B, and C.

Epidemiology

- A human pathogen; all cases can be traced to an infected human.

- Usually spread through infected food or water.

- Occasionally acquired in laboratory accidents.

- Primarily a pathogen of the developing world, with 8 million cases per year in Asia, 5 million in Africa and 500,000 in South America.

- 25,000 cases annually in the developed world.

- 1%-3% of typhoid patients become asymptomatic fecal or urinary carriers.

Key Clinical Features

- Incubation period 10-14 days.

- Insidious onset: malaise, chills, dull headache, myalgias, arthralgias, night sweats and fever.

- Stool symptoms not helpful; some patients have loose stools, others constipation, many with neither.

- Fever always present in early stages: "stair step" pattern may be helpful in diagnosis.

- Second week of untreated illness: patients may have GI hemorrhage or perforation (1-5% risk). Fevers continue, and physical findings such as rose spots, splenomegaly and abdominal tenderness become more apparent.

- Third week: treated patients are now well; untreated patients are in the typhoidal state (disoriented, toxic, waxy appearance; weak, profoundly lethargic). A slow recovery begins during the third and fourth weeks (in survivors).

- Unusual presentations of typhoid fever:
    * Neuropsychiatric
    * Pneumonia

Key Laboratory Features

Definitive Diagnosis
- Positive cultures of blood, bone marrow (highest yield), or rose spot biopsy for S typhi.

Helpful, But Not Definitive
- Rapid tests for typhoid have improved sensitivity and specificity and are helpful, but not conclusive evidence of recent infection.

- Positive stool culture (could be a carrier with another cause of fever).

- Positive urine culture (same as above).

- Mild hyponatremia, proteinuria, hematuria and/or elevated transaminases.

Not Helpful
- Widal test (a nonspecific serology).

Differential Diagnosis

Infectious Diseases
- Tuberculosis: Usually CXR/sputum studies help in differential, but abdominal TB can mimic typhoid.

- Brucellosis: Symptoms similar, but cultures and serology readily differentiate.

- Intraabdominal abscess: CT scan differentiates.

- Amebic liver abscess: In developing world, this is often confused with typhoid. Use ultrasound/CT of abdomen for diagnosis.

- Endocarditis: Typhoid can cause a mild myocarditis, but doesn't cause murmurs or peripheral stigmata.

- HIV seroconversion: May be a tough call; presence of GI symptoms more consistent with typhoid.

- Malaria

- SLE

- Vasculitic syndromes

- IBD

Therapy for Typhoid Fever (Table 3)

- All patients require careful attention to fluid status, early ambulation to avoid DVT, and supplemental nutrition (for advanced cases).

- Empiric therapy (Table 3) involves a quinolone or third-generation cephalosporin. Increasing resistance to quinolones is being reported, so avoid use in cases from areas of known resistance.

- High-dose dexamethasone useful in *severe* typhoid.

Therapy for Carrier State

- Quinolones (ciprofloxacin, norfloxacin, ofloxacin, levofloxacin) orally for 28 days clears 90%.

- Oral ampicillin and TMP-SMX clear about 60% (if sensitive).

- Chloramphenicol is not useful.

- Cholecystectomy occasionally required to resolve carrier state, especially if gallstones present.

Complications

- The "typhoidal state" occurs in the third to fourth week of untreated (or improperly treated) typhoid. During this period of waxy, wasting immobility, patients may develop secondary infections, aspiration pneumonia, DVT, decubitus ulcers, etc.

Table 3

Antibiotic Therapy for Typhoid Fever

Antibiotic	Dose	Duration	Problems
Ceftriaxone	2 g IV QD	7-14 days	2009 drug of choice as empiric
Ciprofloxacin	500 mg PO BID	7-10 days	Steadily increasing resistance; quinolones no longer drug of first choice[a]
Ofloxacin	400 mg PO BID	7-10 days	Avoid in children[a]
Levofloxacin	500 mg PO QD	7-10 days	Avoid in pregnancy[a]
Azithromycin	1 g PO QD	5-10 days	Occasional failure
Chloramphenicol	500 mg PO QID	14 days	Resistance, increased carriage[b]
TMP-SMX	1 DS tab PO BID	14 days	Resistance
Ampicillin	1 g PO QID	14 days	Resistance, slow response[b]

[a] Applies to all quinolones.

[b] Rarely used in clinical setting any longer due to high levels of resistance.

- Bowel perforation occurs in 1%-5%; suspect if there is a sudden deterioration in condition with peritoneal signs; treat with surgery plus antibiotics (ceftriaxone/metronidazole).

- GI hemorrhage in 1%-8%; much less common/severe if timely antibiotic therapy is used.

- Pneumonia can be due to *S typhi* itself or aspiration of oral organisms.

- Relapse in 10% occurs 2-10 weeks after apparent recovery.

- Long-term gallbladder *S typhi* carriers may develop cancer.

Prognostic Factors

- Untreated mortality 10%-30%.

- Treated has mortality rate of only 1%.

- U.S. mortality higher than necessary (5%-10%) as diagnosis is often delayed or missed.

- Poor premorbid health status and advanced age associated with higher mortality.

ID Board Pearls

- *S typhi* is restricted to humans and all cases can be traced to an infected human.

- Transmission usually occurs through ingestion of contaminated food or water.

- Diagnosis is established by positive cultures of blood, bone marrow, or rose spot biopsy for *S typhi*.

- Suspected typhoid fever should be treated empirically pending diagnostic confirmation.

- Treatment of typhoid since about 1990 has usually started with a quinolone; given increasing rates of quinolone-resistance from Asia and other parts of the world, an alternate agent (eg, ceftriaxone) should be first-line therapy in cases from these areas.

3. Leptospirosis

Synonyms

- Canicola fever; hemorrhagic jaundice; mud fever; Swineherd disease; Fort Bragg fever

Causative Organism

- The spirochete Leptospira interrogans, a thin, coiled, Gram-negative bacteria with characteristic hooks on both ends.

- L interrogans has at least 218 serovars.

- Leptospires are obligate aerobes that are motile (visualize with darkfield microscopy) and slow growing (use long-chain fatty acids in culture media).

Epidemiology

- Zoonosis with a worldwide distribution; may be the most common zoonotic disease in the world.

- Most cases occur in the tropics, especially Latin America and Southeast Asia.

- The exact number of infections is unknown since manifestations are nonspecific; some states report cases, but this is not universal.

- Up to 80% of residents in highly endemic areas are seropositive for leptospirosis.

- Approximately 100 cases/year occur in the United States, most in Hawaii.

- Seasonal variation with highest incidence in July-October in the U.S.

- Leptospires infect wild and domestic animals that excrete the causative organism in their urine or tissues of parturition propagating the infection to other animals and to humans.

- Common animals that become infected include rodents, dogs and livestock.

- Animals may serve as reservoirs with leptospires persisting in the renal tubules.

- Human infection occurs through direct contact with infected urine, most commonly while swimming in contaminated water or via soil contact.

- The causative organism may remain viable in the environment for months.

- Leptospires enter via abrasions of the skin, mucous membranes or conjunctivae.

- Rare cases of transmission occur via breast milk and sexual intercourse.

- Peak occurrence of human infections occurs after heavy rains (epidemics after flooding).

- Humans are accidental hosts.

- Highest incidence is in animal workers such as hunters, farmers, veterinarians and military personnel. Overall, males are infected more often than females.

- Swimming, rafting and water contact activities are also risk factors for infection. Outbreaks have been associated with ecotourism.

Key Clinical Features

- Incubation period is generally 5-14 days, but may range up to 30 days.

- The severity of infection ranges from subclinical to life threatening.

- Clinically recognizable disease manifests either as:

    * A self-limited, influenza-like illness (90%); or

    * A potentially fatal illness with renal failure, hepatic dysfunction with jaundice, pneumonitis, meningitis, myocarditis and/or bleeding.

- The combination of renal and hepatic failure defines Weil's syndrome.

- Clinical disease has 2 phases: an acute septicemic phase followed by an immune phase.

- The *acute phase* has symptoms including fevers, headache, myalgias of the lumbar area and calves, chills, conjunctival suffusion without purulent discharge, nausea/vomiting, abdominal pain and pretibial maculopapular rash.

- Myalgias may involve the abdominal musculature and may mimic a surgical abdomen.

- Acute symptoms generally last from 3-7 days.

- The most specific signs and symptoms of leptospirosis are the conjunctival suffusion and the myalgias of the calves.

- Examination may also show hepatomegaly.

- The *immune phase* is heralded by defervescence.

- During this phase, a serologic response develops, and the blood/CSF becomes culture negative while the urine becomes culture positive.

- The second phase of the disease may include aseptic meningitis (80%), pretibial palpable purpura, uveitis or chorioretinitis, which are typically due to the immune response.

- Severe disease usually occurs during the second week of illness.

- Weil's syndrome (icteric leptospirosis with renal and hepatic dysfunction), myocarditis, hemorrhagic pneumonitis and/or ARDS may occur with the recurrence of high fevers in a minority of patients.

Key Laboratory/Radiology Features

- Routine laboratory values are nonspecific.

- The WBC count may be low, normal or high in the acute phase.

- Regardless of the WBC count, neutrophilia is usually present.

- The WBC count is typically elevated in Weil's syndrome.

- The erythrocyte sedimentation rate is elevated.

- Urinalysis may show proteinuria, pyuria, and in some cases, hematuria.

- Elevated creatinine phosphokinase (MM) and aldolase with myalgias.

- Lung involvement in 20% of cases.

  * Chest radiograph findings are nonspecific; most common pattern is small, patchy infiltrates in the lung periphery.

- Aseptic meningitis: lymphocyte pleocytosis, elevated protein and normal glucose.

- Severe disease:

  * Hepatic dysfunction: elevated bilirubin (may be >80 mg/dL) with only modest elevations of alkaline phosphatase, ALT or AST.

  * Prolonged PT that corrects with vitamin K.

  * Renal failure with elevated BUN and creatinine.

- Diagnosis can be established by cultures of the blood, CSF and urine.

  * Gold standard diagnostic tool is isolation of leptospires using a culture medium such as Fletcher's; may take 4-8 weeks for growth.

- Blood and CSF cultures positive during the first week; urine cultures positive during the second week (after 5-7 days of illness).

- Serologies: obtain acute 1-2 weeks after symptoms appear and convalescent studies 2-3 weeks later.

  * Standard serology is the micro-agglutination test (MAT); alternatives are ELISA, CF, or IHA.

  * Confirmed with a four-fold rise or a single titer of at least 1:800.

  * Serology may cross-react with Lyme, syphilis or relapsing fever.

- Antigen detection "dipsticks" are rapid means for diagnosis.

- Silver stain showing organisms in tissue is diagnostic.

Differential Diagnosis

Infectious Diseases
- Viral hepatitis (leptospirosis mainly affects the bilirubin which is usually much higher than ALT)

- Viral aseptic meningitis

- Appendicitis with significant abdominal muscle cramps

- Rocky Mountain Spotted Fever

- Influenza

Tropical Infectious Diseases
- Malaria (negative malaria smear and marked leukocytosis in leptospirosis)

- Typhoid fever (unusual to have leukocytosis and renal failure)

- Scrub typhus (splenomegaly and lymphadenopathy usually absent in leptospirosis)

- Hantaan virus infection (typically liver disease is not a manifestation of Korean hemorrhagic fever; co-infections with both Hantaan virus and leptospirosis have been reported).

Noninfectious Diseases
- Pediatric leptospirosis may resemble Kawasaki's disease.

Empiric Therapy

- Penicillin G 1.5 mU IV q6 for spirochete illnesses.

- Leptospirosis should always be suspected if there

is a history of water/animal contact with severe myalgias and/or conjunctival suffusion is present.

Definitive Therapy

• Supportive care with meticulous fluid and electrolyte management.

• Treatment of severe and late disease: penicillin G 1.5 million units IV QID hours. Ceftriaxone (1 g IV daily) has been shown to be equally effective. The treatment course is 7 days.

• Infections requiring hospitalization are generally treated with IV penicillin.

• For early, mild disease: doxycycline 100 mg PO BID or amoxicillin or cefuroxime for 1 week.

• Treatment most beneficial if given early in the disease process; however, all cases should be treated.

Prevention

• Prevention via avoidance of contaminated water/soil and/or use of doxycycline 200 mg once weekly.

Complications

• Development of severe disease including Weil's syndrome as noted above; however, there is no residual liver dysfunction after recovery.

• Infection during pregnancy may cause abortion and intrauterine death.

• Treatment may be complicated by a Jarisch-Herxheimer reaction with penicillin therapy.

Prognostic Factors

• Death is extremely rare in the acute phase of illness except for the possibility of a spontaneous abortion in a pregnant female.

• Fatality of severe disease is 5%-40%.

ID Board Pearls

• Leptospirosis has a worldwide distribution and may be the most common zoonosis in the world.

• Human infection occurs through direct contact with infected urine, most commonly while swimming in contaminated water or via soil contact.

• Classic symptoms include conjunctival suffusion and calf myalgias.

• Weil's syndrome is a complicated form of leptospirosis involving both renal and hepatic failure.

• The diagnosis is usually established by serology, specifically the micro-agglutination test (MAT).

• Treatment is with penicillin or ceftriaxone; mild disease may be treated with doxycycline.

4. Rickettsial Diseases

Causative Organisms

- Rickettsioses are zoonotic diseases caused by rickettsiae, which are obligate intracellular Gram-negative bacteria.

- Organisms enter via an arthropod bite (eg, ticks, fleas, mites and lice) and have a propensity for invading endothelial cells as well as inducing endovascular lesions.

- Rickettsial diseases are usually divided into 3 main groups:

    *1) the spotted fever group (ie, Rocky Mountain Spotted Fever [*R rickettsii*], Mediterranean spotted fever [*R conorii*], and African tick bite fever [*R africae*]);

    *2) the typhus group including murine typhus (*R typhii*); and

    *3) scrub typhus (*Orientia tsutsugamushi*).

- Infections in returning travelers are usually due to the latter four organisms, the most common being African tick bite fever. Rocky Mountain Spotted Fever most commonly occurs in the continental United States (especially the mid-Atlantic states), but has been reported in southern Canada, Central America, Mexico and parts of South America.

- Several other rickettsioses exist (eg, epidemic typhus [*R prowazekii*]; North Asian tick typhus [*R sibirica*] and Queensland tick typhus [*R australis*]), but are uncommon causes of disease among travelers, and are reported mainly in case reports.

Epidemiology

- *R africae* is found in sub-Saharan and South Africa as well as the eastern Caribbean area. Transmission to humans occurs via the bite of an *Amblyomma* cattle tick. Most cases to date have been found among tourists and game hunters to South Africa. Outbreaks have been reported in safari tourists, military personnel and hunters.

- Mediterranean spotted fever [*R conorii*] along with the related agents of Astrakhan fever, Israeli tick typhus and Indian tick typhus are acquired in the Mediterranean basin of Europe and Africa as well as in the Middle East, South Asia and the Caspian area of Russia. Dog ticks are responsible for human infections, and many cases report contact with local dogs.

- *R typhi* is transmitted via a rat flea (*Xenopsylla cheopsis*) by inoculation of the flea feces into the bite wound. It is found predominantly in tropical and subtropical areas, but may occur worldwide. Port cities and costal regions, where there are large numbers of rodents, are common locations. *R felis*, transmitted by cat fleas, was recently found to cause a murine-like disease.

- *O tsutsugamushi*, the cause of scrub typhus, is transmitted by the trombiculid mite (chiggers) and is most commonly found in rural Asia, Japan and Oceania. Imported cases from Europe, North America and other locations are described, but are uncommon. Travel to rural areas and engaging in camping or trekking places travelers at highest risk.

Key Clinical Features

- African tick bite fever presents as fever, flu-like illness and rash (usually maculopapular or vesicular). A characteristic finding is inoculation eschars and local adenopathy. Of note, eschars are often multiple unlike other rickettsial infections. In addition, mouth ulcerations may also be seen. Symptoms typically begin 5-10 days after tick bite. Most cases are self-limited, but neuropathy (central or peripheral) has been reported. There have been no fatalities reported to date.

- Mediterranean spotted fever is typically a mild infection presenting with an inoculation eschar (tache noire) at the inoculation site as well as rash and fever. Complications have been described such as acute respiratory distress syndrome and neurologic findings.

- Murine typhus typically presents with fever, headache, myalgias, gastrointestinal symptoms and a poorly visualized rash (predominantly on the trunk). Meningitis, deafness and renal failure may occur in severe cases.

- The most common symptoms of scrub typhus are fever, rash, eschar, malaise, headache, myalgias and generalized lymphadenopathy. Complications include acute respiratory distress syndrome, disseminated intravascular coagulation, renal dysfunction and neurological involvement, such as meningoencephalitis.

Key Laboratory/Radiology Features

- Infections are often accompanied by leucopenia, thrombocytopenia and elevated transaminases.

- Rickettsial infections are often clinically diagnosed. Serologic testing by immunofluorescence assay (IFA) can be performed with the best sensitivity using paired serum samples one month apart. Cross reactivity is noted among the rickettsial species within their respective serologic groups.

- Biopsy of the eschar can be performed applying polymerase chain reaction or immunohistochemistry for diagnosis.

- Culture is rarely used since it is difficult and potentially hazardous.

Differential Diagnosis

Infectious Diseases
- Ehrlichioses

- Meningococcemia

- Measles

- Secondary syphilis

- Toxic Shock

Noninfectious Diseases
- Kawasaki syndrome

Therapy
- Therapy for a suspected rickettsial infection should be immediately initiated based on clinical and epidemiologic diagnosis, as confirmation is often difficult and requires several days to weeks. Treatment is with doxycycline 100 mg PO/IV twice daily for 7 days. Doxycycline resistance in scrub typhus cases from Thailand has been described. Studies have shown that azithromycin or telithromycin were as effective doxycycline for scrub typhus.

Prevention
- Prevention is via avoidance of arthropod bites. Use of protective clothing (impregnated with permethrin) and topical repellents are recommended. Daily self-checking and removal of arthropods is indicated.

- Weekly doxycycline (200 mg) was protective for scrub typhus in a military study. The effect of such prophylactic strategies for other rickettsial infections is unknown.

- No vaccines are currently available.

Complications
- See Clinical Features section.

Prognostic Factors
- Early management and antibiotic therapy are important in optimizing patient outcomes.

- Outcome is also related to both the organism as well as host factors. For example, the highest mortality rates are with *R rickettsii* and *R prowazekii* (Louse-borne [epidemic] typhus); other rickettsial infections which are more likely to be seen in the returning traveler typically have a more benign and self-limited course. Host factors such as age, male gender and other underlying diseases are also important prognostic factors.

ID Board Pearls

- Rickettsioses are transmitted to humans by arthropod bites.

- Rickettsial diseases are divided into 3 groups: the spotted fever group, the typhus group and scrub typhus.

- The most common rickettsioses in the returning traveler is African tick bite fever (*R africae*) caused by bite of an Amblyomma cattle tick.

- The diagnosis of rickettsioses is usually established by immunofluorescence assay (IFA), however cross reactivity among the rickettsial species within their respective serologic groups may occur.

- Empiric therapy with doxycycline should be immediately initiated for a suspected rickettsial infection.

5. Yellow Fever

Synonyms

Mosquito-borne viral hemorrhagic fever

Causative Organism

- A virus in the genus *Flavivirus*, family Flaviviridae

Epidemiology

- 2 transmission cycles exist in nature: a sylvatic (jungle) cycle involving primates and an urban cycle involving humans.

- Transmission through bites of *Aedes aegypti* (Africa) and the *Haemagogus* species complex (South America) mosquitoes.

- Disease reservoir in the sylvatic cycle is mosquitoes, monkeys, marsupials; in the urban cycle it is humans and mosquitoes.

- Eradication of the disease is not feasible, making prevention by mosquito control and vaccination essential.

- Disease limited to South America and Africa (between 15°N and 10°S latitude).

- Up to 5000 cases in Africa and 300 in South America are reported annually, but the true incidence is likely up to 50-fold higher.

- Incidence in South America is lower than in Africa because most transmission occurs in forest canopies (highest risk with logging).

- Mosquito breeding is augmented in the presence of containers that hold rainwater; these should be discarded to reduce the number of infections.

- After the bite of an infected mosquito, the human becomes viremic and may serve as a source of infection for other mosquitoes.

- There is no human-to-human transmission (unlike most other viral hemorrhagic fevers).

- Risks to a traveler for acquiring YF are based on immunization status, geographic location, season, duration of exposure and activities.

- The overall risk of YF for an average 2-week trip to an endemic area is estimated at 1:267.

Key Clinical Features

- Incubation 3-6 days.

- Viremia leads to seeding of the lymph nodes, liver, spleen, and bone marrow.

- Mild unapparent infections are common in endemic areas (5%-50% of cases).

- Classic triad of clinical illness is hepatitis, hemorrhagic diathesis, and proteinuria.

- Clinical symptoms during the *period of infection* include the sudden onset of fever, chills, headache, backache, myalgias, nausea, vomiting and prostration.

- Examination may reveal:

    * Bradycardia and a weak pulse with fever (Faget's sign).

    * Conjunctival injection and facial flushing.

- Patient's blood is infective for mosquitoes during the first 3-5 days of illness.

- Most infections resolve by the fifth day (*period of remission*).

- In 15%-25% of cases, after a brief remission of symptoms near day 5, a *period of intoxication* occurs with recurrence of fevers, myalgias, and abdominal pain.

- Hemorrhagic symptoms (epistaxis, hematemesis, melena), liver dysfunction with jaundice and kidney failure may occur.

- Encephalopathy and coma may develop due to cerebral edema and metabolic acidosis.

- Shock and death may follow, usually occurring within 7-10 days of symptom onset.

- For those who recover, prolonged weakness and fatigue for several months is characteristic.

Key Laboratory/Radiology Features

- Leucopenia and neutropenia early in the disease course (nadir at approximately day 5 of illness).

- Albuminuria (proteinuria of 3-20 g/L), renal dysfunction and anuria may occur.

- Elevations of transaminases (AST >ALT).

- Elevated direct bilirubin to 5-10 mg/dL, whereas alkaline phosphatase is only slightly elevated.

- With disease progression, thrombocytopenia, prolonged PT and PTT, and fibrin-split products develop.

- Cerebrospinal fluid may reveal an elevated opening pressure and elevated protein without pleocytosis, consistent with cerebral edema.

- With the onset of myocarditis, ST-T wave changes and arrhythmias may appear on the electrocardiogram.

- Diagnosis is established by viral isolation from the serum by inoculation of suckling mice, mosquitoes or cell cultures.

- Diagnosis also achieved by demonstration of viral antigen, detection of an antibody response (IgM), or by PCR of the blood or liver tissue.

Differential Diagnosis

Infectious Diseases
- Other viral hemorrhagic fevers in Africa and South America:

    * These are definitively differentiated by laboratory confirmation.

* YF stands apart from other viral hemorrhagic fevers by its universal appearance of jaundice, severity of liver dysfunction and lack of a rash.

* Clues such as secondary transmission suggests that the disease is not YF (consider a filovirus or Crimean-Congo), and the presence of rash also suggests an alternative diagnosis (Ebola, dengue).

• Viral hepatitis, especially hepatitis E (YF is suggested by the albuminuria/proteinuria and bleeding diathesis)

• Leptospirosis

• Malaria

• Typhoid fever

• Typhus

• Relapsing fever

Noninfectious Diseases
• Toxin-related hepatitis

• Acute fatty liver of pregnancy

Therapy

• Supportive therapy is the mainstay.

• Hospitalization

• Fluids and vasopressors to maintain blood pressure.

• Correction of electrolyte disturbances.

• Consider an H2-receptor antagonist or sucralfate to reduce GI bleeding.

• Fresh frozen plasma and vitamin K as needed to replenish clotting factors.

• Antibacterial agents for secondary bacterial infections.

• No clinical data in primates or humans to support ribavirin or other antivirals.

Prevention

• Use of the live, attenuated YF 17D vaccine as a single dose.

• Revaccination every 10 years.

• Avoid vaccine in those with egg allergy.

• Postvaccinal encephalitis is an issue for infants <7 months of age and rarely in elderly patients.

• YF 17D is a live viral vaccine, so it is generally avoided in the immunocompromised (HIV infected persons with a CD4 count >200 cells/mm3 have been vaccinated successfully but all data is retrospective).

• Avoidance of mosquito bites and mosquito control

Complications

• Secondary bacterial infections may occur, especially during the second week of illness, resulting in sepsis or pneumonia.

• If recovery occurs, chronic hepatitis does not develop.

Prognostic Factors

• Mortality is 5% among indigenous populations in endemic areas, but may reach 20%-50% in outbreaks and among travelers.

• Progression into the period of intoxication is associated with a poor prognosis.

ID Board Pearls

• Yellow fever is acquired via the bite of *Aedes aegypti* (Africa) and the *Haemagogus* species complex (South America).

• Yellow fever exists only in South America and Africa (between 15°N and 10°S latitude).

- Unlike most other viral hemorrhagic fevers, there is no human-to-human transmission.

- The classic triad of Yellow fever is hepatitis, hemorrhagic diathesis and proteinuria.

- Prevention of Yellow fever among travelers involves the use of the live, attenuated YF 17D vaccine and avoidance of mosquito bites.

6. Other Hemorrhagic Fever Viruses including Dengue Fever

Causative Organisms

Hemorrhagic fever viruses (HFVs) are a loosely defined group of viruses of various classes that can cause bleeding. This relatively large group can be divided into New World and Old World viruses, with some having worldwide distribution.

- New World hemorrhagic fever viruses

    * Junin virus (Argentinean hemorrhagic fever [AHF])

    * Machupo virus (Bolivian hemorrhagic fever)

    * Guanarito virus (Venezuelan hemorrhagic fever [VHF])

    * Sabia virus (Brazilian hemorrhagic fever)

- Old World hemorrhagic fever viruses

    * Crimean-Congo hemorrhagic fever virus (CCHF)

    * Rift Valley fever virus (RVF)

    * Hantaan (hemorrhagic fever with renal syndrome [HFRS])

    * Lassa fever virus

    * Ebola virus

    * Marburg virus

    * Omsk hemorrhagic fever virus

    * Kyasanur fever virus

- Worldwide hemorrhagic fever viruses

    * Dengue

    * Yellow Fever (discussed above)

Epidemiology

These pathogens are a mix of flavivirus, arenavirus and bunyavirus, among others. The epidemiology varies widely, but a few generalities can be drawn:

- The South American HFVs are all arenaviruses. The viruses are thought to be transmitted to people by inhalation of rodent excreta. Generally, the viruses affect rural agricultural populations and have fairly focal distribution. Sabia virus has an unknown epidemiology as there has only been one naturally occurring case, and the reservoir is unknown (although a rodent host has been implicated similar to other arenaviruses). Person-to-person transmission is possible in AHF and well-documented in Bolivian hemorrhagic fever (nosocomial and familial). Epidemics have occurred with Bolivian hemorrhagic fever in association with rodent migration into populated areas.

- Rift Valley fever (bunyavirus) is spread by a variety of mosquitoes, infecting livestock and humans in Africa and more recently, the Arabian peninsula. Given its jump to Arabia, there are increasing concerns that climate change and other factors could eventually results in its introduction to Europe or additional areas of Asia. Handling or consumption of infected body fluids or raw milk is a major mode of transmission to humans. Aerosol transmission occurs as well, and accidental transmission in the laboratory has occurred by this route. Those with extensive contact with domestic animals are at increased risk of infection (veterinarians, abattoir workers, farmers, etc.), particularly during epizootics. The virus may be transmitted by mosquitoes as well, and this has been a significant mode of transmission in some epidemics. An epizootic with significant animal mortality may be the first evidence of an impending RVF epidemic in humans.

- CCHF (bunyavirus) is transmitted principally by *Hyalomma* ticks in Africa, Asia and Eastern Europe, with seasonal variation. Many animal species are potential reservoirs (including rodents), and domesticated animals are important reservoirs. Handling or consumption of infected body fluids or raw milk is a major mode of transmission. Those with extensive contact with

domestic animals are at increased risk of infection (veterinarians, abattoir workers, farmers, etc.). Nosocomial transmission is well documented.

- Lassa fever (arenavirus) is transmitted by contact or inhalation of rodent excreta, and is widely distributed in West Africa. Nosocomial and intrafamilial transmission is well documented.

- Ebola and Marburg are filoviruses with unclear epidemiology. The reservoirs remain undefined despite extensive investigation, but these viruses have been responsible for outbreaks in central Africa notable for high case fatality rates. Multiple Ebola outbreaks have occurred in the Democratic Republic of the Congo (DRC), Gabon, Ivory Coast and Sudan, while the first outbreak of Marburg occurred in the DRC in May 1999. Marburg and Ebola are morphologically indistinguishable. It is generally thought that cases occur after contact with infected body fluids. Large droplet transmission does not seem to occur, but the large numbers of cases occurring in medical personnel (after institution of contact precautions) in the Uganda outbreak in 2000 have fueled speculation of possible airborne transmission. A strain of Ebola was identified in monkeys originating from the Philippines, and very recently, one from swine was also identified in the Philippines.

- HFRS was first well characterized during the Korean War and is still primarily a concern in East Asia, although the causative agents are more widely distributed. The Puumala virus is associated with the red bank vole. The Hantaan and Seoul viruses are associated with *Apodemus* mice and *Rattus norvegicus*, respectively. Seoul virus has been linked to urban outbreaks of HFRS, particularly in Asia but also worldwide. Hantaan virus is predominantly rural. These agents are transmitted to humans through inhalation of rodent excreta.

- Dengue (flavivirus) is transmitted by mosquitoes, and has a complex worldwide cycle. Dengue has no other reservoir except for humans, and is transmitted in many areas by *Aedes aegypti*. This mosquito has adapted to man-made conditions, making urban transmission frequent. The dengue virus has 4 serotypes, each with a number of genotypes.

- Omsk hemorrhagic fever and Kyasanur Forest disease are exotic fevers unlikely to be encountered on a board exam and will not be further discussed (see Further Reading).

- Chikungunya (Alphavirus) is transmitted to humans by virus-carrying *Aedes* mosquitoes. There have been several recent outbreaks in Africa, Asia and Europe. Illness resembles dengue fever (fevers followed by prolonged arthralgias), but is not typically hemorrhagic in nature and will not be further discussed.

Key Clinical Features

Most hemorrhagic fevers share many clinical features: fever, chills, headache, myalgia, arthralgias, nausea and vomiting, conjunctival injection, meningismus, relative bradycardia and changes in mental status are common. Clearly, hemorrhagic features define the condition and include petechial/purpuric rash, mucosal bleeding, epistaxis, bloody diarrhea, hematemesis and bleeding from puncture sites. Particular features are noted below.

- South American arenaviruses share many clinical features: insidious onset of symptoms, early facial flushing, periorbital edema, cervical lymphadenopathy, palatal vesicles, axillary petechiae, fine tremor, decreased deep tendon reflexes and ataxia. Patients generally improve within a week or two, but about 20% will develop severe hemorrhage with or without neurologic signs. Convalescence may be prolonged (1-3 months).

- Rift Valley fever (RVF) is usually asymptomatic or a relatively mild flu-like illness. A small percentage may develop hemorrhagic features or meningoencephalitis. Ocular (retinal) injury may result from even mild cases and result in significant permanent visual deficits.

- Lassa fever has a gradual onset, with fever, chills, nonproductive cough, severe headache, retrosternal chest pain and sore throat. Exudative pharyngitis may be seen on examination. Hemorrhagic signs are less frequent (15%-20%) and generally limited to mucosal surfaces. However, patients demonstrating CNS involvement or facial edema have a poorer prognosis. Hearing loss is a common consequence of infection. Like RVF, most cases are not fatal.

- Ebola and Marburg virus cause rapid onset of severe hemorrhagic fever syndrome, with prominent gastrointestinal manifestations. Rash may be prominent in some, occasionally desquamating later.

- CCHF is a severe illness with the abrupt onset of fever, chills and severe body aches. Ecchymoses may be prominent. Mental status changes such as mood changes (irritability) are common.

- The classic HFRS syndrome occurs in 5 stages: febrile, hypotensive, oliguric, diuretic and convalescent, beginning suddenly with fever, chills, headache, increased thirst, anorexia and diffuse abdominal pain. In practice, the presentation is variable and diagnosis is difficult. Physical clues to the diagnosis are conjunctival injection, pharyngeal erythema, palatal petechiae, periorbital edema and petechial rash.

- Dengue is generally subdivided into 4 clinical syndromes: a mild flu-like illness, classic dengue, dengue hemorrhagic fever and dengue shock syndrome (Table 4). DHF/Dengue Shock Syndrome (DSS) may manifest after a few days of typical dengue symptoms, classically starting as the temperature normalizes.

Key Laboratory/Radiology Features

The various viruses included in this section have obviously varied manifestations in the human host, but common features include:

- Thrombocytopenia

- Elevated transaminases

- Leucopenia

- Hematuria

- Proteinuria

Table 4

Grades of Dengue Fever

Grade	Definition
Grade I	Dengue + positive tourniquet test
Grade II	Grade I + spontaneous bleeding (usually skin)
Grade III	Circulatory failure (weak, rapid pulse; narrowed pulse pressure [<20]; hypotension with cold, clammy skin and restlessness/agitation)
Grade IV	Profound shock with undetectable BP or pulse

Grades III and IV are considered DSS

• Neutrophilia may occur late in CCHF and Ebola infection

Differential Diagnosis

Infectious Diseases
• Malaria

• Rickettsial diseases

• Typhoid fever

• Meningococcemia

• Infectious mononucleosis

• Other bacterial sepsis

• Leptospirosis

• Relapsing fever

• Viral hepatitis

• Acute African trypanosomiasis

• Measles in a compromised host (malnourished)

• Other arboviruses

• Influenza

Noninfectious Diseases
• Hemolytic-uremic syndrome

• Thrombotic thrombocytopenic purpura (TTP)

• Acute rheumatologic syndromes (SLE)

• Ergot intoxication, other intoxications

The hemorrhagic fevers have no prominent examination or laboratory findings to alert the clinician. In some cases, the prevalence of bleeding tendency is low (Lassa, Rift Valley). The constellation of historical and examination findings, plus laboratory data, should help to eliminate or confirm other possible etiologies.

Empiric Therapy

If a specific viral hemorrhagic disease is suspected, and other obvious possible causes have been excluded, treatment should be initiated as appropriate. The therapy for each is listed under **Definitive Therapy**. Intravenous fluid support and, often, vasopressors are part of therapy. Intramuscular injections are obviously inappropriate in patients with suspected hemorrhagic fevers.

Definitive Therapy

• Arenaviruses (Lassa, CCHF, Junin, Machupo, Guanarito, Sabia, HFRS): Ribavirin is effective therapy. A loading dose of 30 mg/kg (max: 2 g) is given, followed by 15 mg/kg (max: 1 g) QID for 4 days, followed by 7.5 mg/kg (max: 500 mg) TID for 6 days.

• Supportive therapy is also given (for all, especially filovirus, DHF/DSS, CCHF, arenaviruses and HFRS).

- Immune serum is a well-proven therapy for AHF, but must be given within 8 days of illness for efficacy and is associated with a late-onset neurologic syndrome in 10% of treated cases. Immune serum is generally not available for the other viruses.

Complications

Generally, severe hemorrhagic symptoms portend a poor prognosis. Multiple organ systems can be involved in these viral infections, but neurologic sequelae are possible in most, and renal injury may occur. Recovery is generally complete in those surviving dengue.

Prevention

Vaccination for AHF is safe and effective, and cross-immunity to BHF has been documented. RVF vaccine is available on an IND basis and has been used for decades in lab workers and outbreak control. Research efforts into vaccines are ongoing for many HFVs.

ID Board Pearls

- Dengue is the most common hemorrhagic fever virus diagnosed in the returning traveler.

- Most hemorrhagic fevers share many clinical features including systemic complaints such as fever, chills, headache and myalgias as well as hemorrhagic complications including petechial/purpuric rash and bleeding from mucosal and puncture sites.

- Rift Valley fever (bunyavirus) is spread by mosquitoes in Africa and the Arabian peninsula, and may result in retinal damage.

- Dengue is subdivided into 4 clinical syndromes: a mild flu-like illness, classic dengue, dengue hemorrhagic fever and dengue shock syndrome.

- Therapy is largely supportive for most hemorrhagic fever viruses including dengue; however, arenaviruses (Lassa, CCHF, Junin, Machupo, Guanarito, HFRS) can be treated with ribavirin and AHF with immune serum.

7. Leishmaniasis

Synonyms

- Visceral leishmaniasis: kala azar

- Mucosal leishmaniasis: espundia

- Cutaneous leishmaniasis: Oriental sore, Baghdad boil, many others.

Causative Organisms

Leishmania are protozoa which cause a spectrum of human disease. The major species are shown in Table 5. Of note, some *Leishmania* sp. cause more than one type of these syndromes.

Key Clinical Features

- Spread by the bite of sand flies (*Lutzomyia* in the Americas and *Phlebotomus* elsewhere).

- A broad spectrum of pathology. As in leprosy, the clinical manifestations depend considerably on the vigor of the host response.

Table 5

Leishmania That Cause Human Disease

	New World	Old World
Visceral	L chagasi[a]	L donovani
		L infantum
Cutaneous	L mexicana	L aethiopica
	L guyanensis	L tropica (urban)[b]
	L amazonensis	L major (rural)
	L peruviana	
	L venezuelensis	
	L braziliensis	
	L panamensis	
	L chagasi	
Mucosal	L braziliensis	L aethiopica (rare)

[a] L chagasi *is the same as* L infantum
[b] L tropica *may also cause viserotropic disease as seen among US military troops stationed in central Asia.*

- Visceral leishmaniasis is characterized by an indolent course with months of fever, wasting, hepatosplenomegaly, lymphadenopathy, hypergammaglobulinemia and pancytopenia. Most commonly found in India, Brazil, Sudan and Bangladesh.

- Cutaneous leishmaniasis typically evolves over several weeks (incubation from 2 weeks to a few years) from a nodule to ulcers and resolves with a scar. Usually 1 or 2 lesions are present on an exposed area (head, hand, wrist, lower extremity); multiple lesions may occur (sometimes in sporotrichoid fashion).

- Mucosal leishmaniasis is rarely seen in the Old World. New World mucosal disease occurs following cutaneous disease in 1%-5% of patients after the cutaneous lesions have apparently healed. Initial symptoms may include nasal stuffiness or discharge. The organisms progressively damage nasopharyngeal structures and may be extremely deforming or life threatening. Most commonly found in Brazil, Peru and Bolivia.

- Diffuse cutaneous leishmaniasis occurs in both the New and Old World in a small subset of patients who lack CMI to *Leishmania*. Diffuse nodular lesions occur, often on the face and extremities. As in mucosal leishmaniasis, it is often disfiguring.

Key Diagnostic Features

- Visceral leishmaniasis may be suspected if imaging reveals hepatosplenomegaly in a compatible clinical setting, but definite diagnosis requires the demonstration of amastigotes on Giemsa-stained aspirates of spleen, marrow, liver, nodes (in the order of the most sensitive biopsy site) or a positive culture in NNN media. Many serologic assays are available for visceral disease (IFA, ELISA and others are sometimes helpful), but these are not well-standardized.

- Cutaneous and mucosal disease is diagnosed through microscopic examination and culture (NNN media) of tissue obtained through needle aspirates, punch biopsies and smears of lesions. Mucosal disease and more chronic cutaneous lesions tend to have fewer amastigotes and are harder to diagnose. Serology is of limited value in cutaneous disease.

- PCR is becoming the best technology for the diagnosis of cutaneous and mucosal leishmaniasis. Available through some reference laboratories, it offers enhanced sensitivity and specificity.

Differential Diagnoses

Visceral Leishmaniasis

Infectious diseases

- Malaria (check blood smears)

- Disseminated (miliary) TB: distinguish by biopsy, AFB stains and cultures

- Typhoid fever

- Schistosomiasis (stool O & P; rectal or liver biopsy; pipestem fibrosis on liver imaging)

- Trypanosomiasis (blood smears)

- Brucellosis (culture, serology)

- Disseminated histoplasmosis (urine antigen, culture)

- Tropical splenomegaly syndrome (a tough differential; liver biopsy often helpful)

- Endocarditis (echocardiogram, blood cultures)

Noninfectious diseases

- Cirrhosis (any cause) with splenomegaly

- Lymphoma (biopsy of marrow, liver)

- Leukemia (blood smears, marrow biopsy)

- Disseminated malignancy

- Sarcoid

Cutaneous Leishmaniasis

Infectious diseases
- Bacterial, fungal (such as sporotrichosis), and mycobacterial infections (distinguished by biopsy, cultures)

- Diphtheria

- Tertiary syphilis (gummas): check serology

- Blastomycosis, chromomycosis

Noninfectious diseases
- Trauma (history helpful)

- Insect bites (rapid onset)

- Foreign body reactions

- Skin cancers

Mucosal Leishmaniasis

Infectious diseases
- Fungal infections (histoplasmosis, paracoccidioidomycosis, blastomycosis)

- Syphilis

- Leprosy

Noninfectious disease differential
- Sarcoidosis

- Various malignancies

Diffuse Cutaneous Disease

- Looks much like lepromatous leprosy. Lesions of diffuse cutaneous leishmaniasis are soft as opposed to the indurated lesions of leprosy.

Empiric Therapy

- Visceral leishmaniasis: amphotericin lipid formulations (AmBisome® or Abelcet®), amphotericin B or antimonials (sodium stibogluconate or meglumine antimonate). Amphotericin lipid formulations preferred due to better toxicity profile and potential superior efficacy (see Table 6 for dosages). In India, antimonials are no longer utilized due to high rates of resistance; most cases are treated with amphotericin or miltefosine, an oral agent not yet available in the U.S.

- Cutaneous/mucosal leishmaniasis: often hold off on therapy pending diagnosis unless rapidly progressive disease. In areas where there are no mucosal forms of the disease and the cutaneous lesion is healing, follow expectantly. In cases where the species may cause mucosal disease or the lesion is associated with a mucosal surface, a joint or the lesion is cosmetically disfiguring, treatment should be utilized, most commonly with pentavalent antimonials. Lipid formulations of amphotericin for cutaneous disease should be avoided as these concentrate in the reticuloendothelial system rather than the skin. Most experts would favor an antimonial over amphotericin B, as there is more experience with these agents. Other options for only cutaneous disease include oral azoles, topical paromomycin, miltefosine, heat or cryotherapies (Table 6).

Complications

- Visceral leishmaniasis will progress to severe pancytopenia and is often fatal without appropriate therapy.

- Cutaneous leishmaniasis is usually uncomplicated and scars uneventfully over a period of months. Therapy should be directed to those with larger, multiple, function-limiting or cosmetically unacceptable lesions. Superinfection is a possibility with all cutaneous lesions.

- Mucosal disease (espundia) many cause horrific destruction of the nasal, pharyngeal or buccal mucosa. Mucosal disease occurs months to years after apparent resolution of the cutaneous disease caused by some New World species. Disfigurement or death often occurs due to espundia or its sequelae.

Prognostic Factors

Leishmaniasis is a complex illness. Outcome is critically dependent on multiple factors, including:

Table 6

Definitive Therapy for Leishmaniasis

Type of disease	Preferred drug	Alternatives	Dosing	Comments
Visceral	Lipid amphotericin B agents: AmBisome® IV, Abelcet® IV		2-4 mg/kg/d; dose and duration depend on region, host	Well-tolerated, expensive
		Amphotericin B IV	1 mg/kg/d x 3 wk	Effective; usual amphotericin B toxicity
		Sodium stibogluconate IV[a]/IM	20 mg/kg/d x 28 d	Toxic; obtain from CDC
		Meglumine antimonate IV[b]/IM	20 mg/kg/d x 28 d	Not available in U.S.
		Pentamidine IV/IM	4 mg/kg qod x 30+ d	A last resort
		Miltefosine PO	100 mg/d for 28 d	GI toxicity; promising new therapy
Cutaneous (limited to moderate disease)	No therapy			Small; inconspicuous lesions
		Itraconazole PO	200 mg bid x 28 d	Well tolerated
		Fluconazole PO	200 mg qd x 42 d	Nontoxic
		Ketoconazole PO	600 mg qd x 28 d	Other azoles preferred
		Topical paromomycin	Apply BID for 2 weeks	Limited data; promising
		Intralesional antimonials	Weekly injections	Quite painful
		Miltefosine PO	100 mg/d x 28 d	Little data
		Imiquimod cream	Apply QOD for 20 d	Promising
		Sodium stibogluconate IV[a]	20 mg/kg QD x 20 d	Toxic; from CDC
		Meglumine antimonate [b] IV	20 mg/kg QD x 20 d	Toxic
Mucosal or extensive cutaneous disease	Sodium stibogluconate IV[a]		20 mg/kg/d x 28 d	Toxic, but drug of choice
	Meglumine antimonate[b]		20 mg/kg/d x 28 d	Not available in U.S.
		Amphotericin B IV	1 mg/kg/d x 3 wk	Usual amphotericin B toxicity
		Pentamidine IV/IM	4 mg/kg QOD x 30+ d	Toxic; risk of diabetes

a Sodium stibogluconate is known as Pentostam®, available from CDC
b Meglumine antimonate sold as Glucantine® not available in U.S.

- Infecting species

- Location of infection

- Timing and intensity of therapy

- Immune status of the host (HIV, nutritional status, comorbid illness)

General Advice

The diagnosis and treatment of leishmaniasis is often extremely difficult for physicians who do not routinely deal with this infection. Fortunately, a dedicated group of leishmania experts ("leishmaniacs") exists. All of them welcome calls and are eager to offer advice, and often diagnostic assistance. Sodium stibogluconate (Pentostam®) is available from the CDC and certain military facilities.

ID Board Pearls

- Leishmaniasis may be visceral (kala azar), mucosal (espundia) or cutaneous.

- Spread is by the bite of sand flies (*Lutzomyia* in the Americas and *Phlebotomus* elsewhere).

- Visceral leishmaniasis presents with fevers, hepatosplenomegaly, adenopathy, wasting, pancytopenia and increased gamma globulin.

- Diagnosis is made by microscopic examination and culture (NNN media) of infected tissues; PCR is also useful and available through some reference laboratories.

- The cornerstone of therapy for visceral, mucosal or severe cutaneous leishmaniasis is antimonial agents (sodium stibogluconate or meglumine antimonate)

8. Fever and Eosinophilia in the Returning Traveler (Southeast Asia, Latin America, Africa)

Causative Organisms

- Most common infectious cause is helminthic, although eosinophilia is not a universal finding in helminthic infections. Eosinophilia is usually most prominent during tissue invasion.

- The only protozoa commonly associated with eosinophilia are *Isospora belli* and *Dientamoeba fragilis* (both rare pathogens in the returning traveler and eosinophilia is mild if present).

- *Ascaris lumbricoides* larval forms produce eosinophilia, but adult, established infections do not. Suspect concurrent Toxocara, Schistosomiasis or Strongyloidiasis if an adult Ascaris infection is associated with a notable eosinophilia.

- Schistosomiasis

- Fascioliasis/fasciolopsiasis

- Filariasis (*Brugia malayi*, *Wuchereria bancrofti*, *Loa loa*, *Mansonella* spp.)

- Onchocerciasis

- Hookworm (*Ancylostoma duodenale* and *Necator americanus*), *Ancylostoma braziliense* and *caninum* (causes of cutaneous larva migrans); typically produce eosinophilia without fever.

- Cysticercosis (*T solium*)

- *Clonorchis sinensis/Opisthorchis viverrini*

- Strongyloides stercoralis

- Angiostrongylus cantonensis/costaricensis

- Trichinella spiralis

- Toxocariasis

- Paragonimiasis

- Echinococcosis

- Gnathostomiasis

- Tuberculosis

- HIV (eosinophilia extremely common and does not necessarily imply a parasitic process)

- Coccidioidomycosis (the only fungus commonly associated with eosinophilia)

Epidemiology

- Southeast Asia: ascariasis, hookworm, clonorchiasis/opisthorchiasis, schistosomiasis, fasciolopsiasis, gnathostomiasis (predominantly Thailand), paragonimiasis, angiostrongyliasis, HIV, filariasis and strongyloidiasis.

- Latin America: ascariasis, hookworm, echinococcosis, taeniasis/cysticercosis, angiostronglyiasis, onchocerciasis (Guatemala and Mexico), fascioliasis (Cuba), filariasis (Caribbean), schistosomiasis (Brazil), strongyloidiasis, HIV and coccidioidomycosis (Mexico, Central America, Columbia, Venezuela, Paraguay and Argentina).

- Africa: ascariasis, hookworm, echinococcus, fascioliasis, schistosomiasis, dracunculiasis (very rare in returning travelers), onchocerciasis, loiasis, strongyloidiasis and HIV.

Key Clinical Features

- Important historical points include the exact dates and locations of travel, the kind of accommodations, unusual activities, sexual contacts, animal contacts and sources of food. In particular, raw or undercooked food, or food from an unusual source should be noted.

- The physical examination should be comprehensive. Special note should be made of conjunctivitis or conjunctival suffusion, jaundice, organomegaly or lymphadenopathy. Appropriate initial laboratory studies include a complete blood count with differential, electrolytes and liver function tests. Stool ova and parasites (3 tests). Serum IgE quantitation may help distinguish infectious and allergic causes of eosinophilia from other causes (eg, malignancy). The term "eosinophilia" is variably defined, but most authorities consider

numbers greater than 500 per microliter to be clinically significant.

Ascariasis

Children are particularly at risk for high worm burdens. Peak eosinophilia occurs during the migratory phase (first 10-12 weeks after ingestion of eggs), and may be associated with pulmonary hypersensitivity (wheezing, Charcot-Leyden crystals in sputum) and chest x-ray infiltrates (Loeffler's syndrome). Worms may also obstruct the pancreatic duct or biliary tree. Heavy worm burden may cause intestinal obstruction. Mature infections not associated with eosinophilia.

Schistosomiasis

5 main species cause human disease (*S haematobium*, *mansoni*, *japonicum*, *mekongi*, and *intercalatum*). *S haematobium* worms reside in the urinary bladder venous plexus, whereas the other species migrate to the venous plexus of the large or small intestine. Snails are essential to the reproductive cycle; fresh water contact with exposed skin is a key historical point. Dermatitis may occur shortly after exposure to cercariae. Katayama fever (fever, chills, abdominal pain, eosinophilia, hepatosplenomegaly, nausea/vomiting, lymphadenopathy) may occur 5-7 weeks after acute infection and can be fatal. Chronic schistosomiasis is mostly characterized by fibrotic or granulomatous reactions to deposited eggs, and thus is rarely a febrile illness.

Fasciola hepatica and *gigantica/ Fasciolopsis buski*

Historical association with sheep or domestic livestock. Snails are the intermediate host. Human infection usually occurs after eating freshwater vegetation (such as watercress) contaminated by metacercariae. *Fasciola hepatica* and *gigantica* are pathogens of the biliary tree, whereas *Fasciolopsis buski* infects the small bowel. Signs and symptoms of acute fascioliasis (fever, eosinophilia, hepatomegaly, urticaria, nausea/vomiting, abdominal pain) usually occur in the first few weeks after infection. Chronic infection may result in persistent abdominal discomfort and abnormal liver function tests. Fasciolopsiasis, in contrast, presents with symptoms of small bowel pathology: malabsorption, diarrhea and anemia.

Filariasis

Usually only seen in indigenous populations or long-term expatriates. All cases are spread through biting insects. Fevers, chills and malaise, with pain and swelling in the associated lymph nodes and distal extremities, characterize acute attacks. Asymptomatic filaremia may be present for years prior to the first attack. Eosinophilia is prominent during acute episodes. Whereas *W bancrofti* is often an indolent cause of elephantiasis, *B malayi* infection is usually more abrupt. Both are associated with tropical pulmonary eosinophilia, a form of allergic hypersensitivity to worms entrapped in the pulmonary vasculature. *Loa loa* is associated with painless angioedema of the subcutaneous tissues (Calabar swellings); occasionally patients will report worms migrating across the surface of the eye ("eyeworm").

Onchocerciasis

Also known as river blindness, caused by *Onchocerca volvulus*; rarely a cause of fever and eosinophilia in the returning traveler. Disease may take the form of pruritic skin lesions (papules or vesicles) caused by the inflammatory reaction evoked by an adult worm. Skin nodules containing adult worms may be palpable over bony prominences. More devastating are the corneal lesions caused by chronic inflammation in the eye, which after repeated cycles of infection may lead to permanent blindness. Risk of disease increases with duration of stay.

Hookworm

Worldwide distribution. Localized dermatitis may occur as the larvae penetrate the skin; *cutaneous larva migrans* and eosinophilia may develop. Loeffler's syndrome may also develop as the larvae enter the alveoli. Epigastric pain, nausea, and diarrhea may occur as the larvae invade the small bowel. Severe iron deficiency anemia may result in chronic cases (*N americanus* and *A duodenale*). Mature infections rarely febrile, eosinophilia variable.

Cysticercosis

Caused by the pork tapeworm, *Taenia solium*. Principal cause of infection is ingestion of food contaminated by viable eggs, not by consumption of larvae (which leads to a purely luminal infection). However, poor hygiene can lead to autoinfection. The most common form of disease is neurocysticercosis, which generally manifests as epilepsy. Elevated intracranial pressure may cause headache, nausea and vomiting. Chronic meningitis can also result, causing cranial nerve deficits. Noncommunicating hydrocephalus may occur if cysts occlude the cerebral aqueduct. Cysticerci can also present in subcutaneous tissue, which may be an important physical exam finding, and in many other organs as well.

Clonorchis sinensis/Opisthorchis viverrini/Opisthorchis felineus

Principal risk factor is consumption of infected undercooked fish. Snails are the intermediate hosts. Patients may have fever, lymph node enlargement, rash and eosinophilia 1-3 weeks after acute infection. Most infections, however, are asymptomatic. Additionally, patients may complain of abdominal tenderness (right upper quadrant), anorexia, flatulence, loose stool and malnutrition. The liver may enlarge and become cirrhotic; cholangiocarcinoma has been associated with chronic infection.

Strongyloidiasis

Spread by dermal penetration after contact with contaminated soil. *S stercoralis* is the *par excellence* example of autoinfection; continuous replicative cycles (hyperinfection) are possible within the human host, particularly in the context of immune suppression (steroid use, HTLV-1, but not HIV). *Larva currens* may be apparent: serpiginous tracks around the perianal skin as the larvae develop in the colorectal area and infiltrate the buttocks. Likewise, Loeffler's syndrome may develop during the period of worm migration through the lung. Chronic infection may persist for decades, manifesting as recurring episodes of abdominal pain, urticaria and diarrhea. In hyper infected patients, sepsis from intraabdominal pathogens may occur.

Angiostrongylus cantonensis

It is the most common cause of eosinophilic meningitis. The principal risk factor is the consumption of undercooked snails, seafood, or contaminated water plants. Symptoms usually begin 2 weeks after infection: severe headache, nausea, vomiting, stiff neck and occasionally altered mental status. Cranial nerves may be affected. Peripheral eosinophilia is common; the CSF opening pressure is generally elevated with a high white count and increased eosinophil count (25%-75%). *Angiostrongylus costaricensis* (a pathogen of South America and the Caribbean) has a predilection for invading the intestinal wall, particularly in the ileocecal region. Thrombosis and necrosis of affected tissue is common. Metastatic disease to the liver and testes can also occur.

Trichinosis

Multiple species, of which *T spiralis* is the most significant. Strong association with undercooked pork, as well as more exotic meats (eg, cougar, walrus, bear). After ingestion of the larva and incubation, the acute infection period begins; early on, intestinal symptoms (nausea, abdominal pain, diarrhea) may predominate, followed by fever, eosinophilia, myalgia and periorbital and other soft tissue edema. Acute infection lasts 1-8 weeks. Mental status changes and myocarditis may result from larvae migrating through CNS and cardiac tissue.

Toxocariasis

Two species, *T canis* (dogs) and *T cati* (cats). Infection occurs through ingestion of foodstuffs contaminated with eggs; after excystation, the larvae migrate throughout the body. Both *ocular larva migrans* (OLM) and *visceral larva migrans* (VLM) may result. OLM may cause granulomatous scarring of the retina with vision loss; the lesion may be confused with a retinoblastoma. VLM is characterized by eosinophilia, fever, hepatomegaly and occasional pulmonary (asthma-like) or neurological involvement.

Paragonimiasis

Most common species is *P westermani*. Unlike other flukes, the primary site of infection is the lung. Eggs are expectorated (and sometimes aspirated and passed out in the feces), whereupon they hatch in water and infect the snail (first intermediate host). Infected snails then produce cercariae that infect crustaceans, which if eaten uncooked can then retransmit disease to humans. Thus, the principal risk factor is consumption of raw seafood such as "drunken crab." Prominent clinical features include pneumonia (variable presentations) and pleural effusion, with macroscopically visible lung cysts. Lesions may occur elsewhere in the body as well, including the CNS. During the migratory phase (from intestine to lung), the patient may experience fever, abdominal pain and eosinophilia. Pulmonary symptoms follow: cough, sputum production and shortness of breath. Hemoptysis may occur. Ring-shaped opacities may appear on chest x-ray.

Echinococcosis

In the tropics, the principal pathogen is *E granulosus*, the agent of cystic *hydatid* disease (*E multilocularis* is primarily a pathogen of the temperate Northern Hemisphere). A key historical point is association with livestock, especially in settings with working dogs who are fed with raw slaughtered animals. The most common sites for cyst formation are liver and lung, but any organ can be involved. Rupture of a cyst may cause fever, pain and eosinophilia; rupture of a lung cyst may cause a pneumonia-like syndrome. Anaphylaxis due to release of cyst contents may occur.

Gnathostomiasis

Caused by a nematode of cats and dogs. Humans are infected by ingestion of larva from flesh of contaminated hosts (freshwater fish), occasionally from contaminated water. 2 clinical diseases exist: larval gnathostomiasis and myeloencephalitis. Larval gnathostomiasis is characterized by fever, eosinophilia, hepatomegaly, pneumonitis, creeping eruptions caused by the migrating worm and painless subacute swellings not unlike the Calabar swellings of *Loa loa*. Eyelids are commonly involved, and chemosis and conjunctival edema are frequent findings. Eosinophilic myeloencephalitis occurs when the worm migrates up a nerve trunk into the CNS, causing nerve root pain, paresis and urinary retention. Meningitis is classically eosinophilic as well. CNS disease is associated with a high mortality rate.

Tuberculosis

Generally does not cause a high-grade eosinophilia, but due to its extremely high prevalence throughout the developing world, it should always be considered as a possible cause of fever.

HIV

Commonly associated with mild-moderate eosinophilia. Due to its increasing prevalence and implications for diagnosis of other infectious conditions, it should be considered as a cause of fever in the returning traveler.

Key Laboratory/Radiology Features

• *Ascariasis* is usually diagnosed on the basis of stool ova and parasites (submit on alternate days for maximum sensitivity). Endoscopic evaluation of the biliary tree can be diagnostic in cases of obstruction.

• *Schistosomiasis* may be diagnosed by stool examination, but in the acutely ill returning traveler, serological methods are preferable (assuming the traveler comes from a low-incidence population), as stools will be negative.

• *Fascioliasis/fasciolopsiasis* in later stages can be diagnosed on the basis of O & P or serology; biliary imaging can also be diagnostic in the case of fascioliasis.

• *Filariasis:* The principal method of making the diagnosis relies on demonstrating nematodes in the bloodstream. Diagnosis complicated by the periodicity of filaremia (nocturnal for W bancrofti and B. malayi, diurnal for L loa). Specialized laboratories offer serologic testing for antifilarial antibodies. Lymphoscintigraphy may help demonstrate obstructed flow.

• *Onchocerciasis:* Eosinophilia and skin nodules in a longtime resident from an endemic area are the keys to the diagnosis. Diagnosis is confirmed by skin snip biopsies or aspiration of skin nodules. Slit lamp examination of affected eyes may demonstrate the microfilariae. The Mazzotti test (giving the patient a provocative dose of DEC, 25-50 mg) may help in patients with low filarial burdens, although there is a risk of provoking a severe inflammatory reaction in patients with heavy burdens.

• *Hookworm:* Diagnosis primarily made by stool ova and parasite exam. It should be noted that the O & P may not be positive during the period of acute gastrointestinal symptoms, cutaneous larva migrans, or eosinophilia.

• *Cysticercosis:* Many diagnoses are made incidentally, on CNS or other imaging obtained for some other purpose. The classic radiologic appearance is of a cystic lesion with a hyperdense center (the scolex). Degenerating cysticerci may have surrounding tissue enhancement. Nonviable cysts are generally calcified. The diagnosis can be confirmed serologically.

• *Clonorchis and Opisthorchis* infections can sometimes be diagnosed on the basis of cholangiograms or ultrasound exam of the liver.

• *Strongyloidiasis* is difficult to diagnose on routine stool O & P; the laboratory should be notified if this is in the differential. Serum serology is useful if done by a qualified laboratory. Eosinophilia is common but not universal, and is less common in immune-suppressed patients. This diagnosis must always be considered before giving immunosuppressive therapy to a person who has lived in an endemic area.

• *Angiostrongylus* is typically diagnosed based on clinical presentation and a compatible history of exposure, together with the presence of pronounced eosinophilic meningitis (A cantonensis) or ileocecal inflammation (A costaricensis). Peripheral eosinophilia is usually present. Serologic tests are useful when available. In cases of A. costaricensis, diagnosis can be made by examination of the excised specimen.

- *Trichinosis* may be recognized by the history of ingestion of relevant meat products, the constellation of fever, eosinophilia and edema, and an elevated creatine kinase. Diagnosis is confirmed by muscle biopsy (deltoid or gastrocnemius) and/or circulating antibody.

- *Toxocariasis* is diagnosed on the basis of consistent physical exam findings (especially in the case of OLM) and serological studies.

- Sputum samples may be useful in diagnosing *paragonimiasis*. However, serology is required in most cases.

- *Echinococcal disease* may be diagnosed based on the appearance of a cyst on ultrasound of the liver or CT scan of a pulmonary cyst. Diagnosis should be confirmed with serologic assay.

- *Gnathostomiasis* is difficult to diagnose except by history and physical examination; the nerve root pain of myeloencephalitis gnathostomiasis helps differentiate it from the eosinophilic meningitis of *Angiostrongylus*. Serologic testing may be useful, but often not available in non-endemic areas.

Differential Diagnosis

Noninfectious Disease Mimics
- Drug allergy (statistically most likely cause of eosinophilia)

- Malignancy (leukemia, lymphoma, adenocarcinoma)

- Collagen vascular disease

- Atopic dermatitis

- Allergic bronchopulmonary aspergillosis

- Allergic asthma

- Episodic angioedema

- Idiopathic hypereosinophilic syndrome

Empiric Therapy

- A broad generalization is virtually impossible, but albendazole 400 mg x 1 dose is generally very well-tolerated and has broad activity against nematodes. In refugee settings, mass prophylaxis using albendazole is a common strategy. Caution should be exercised if there is any concern for neurocysticercosis or eosinophilic meningitis due to *Angiostrongylus cantonensis*; CNS symptoms may acutely worsen.

- Praziquantel is useful for a wide variety of trematode infections as well as many cestode infections.

Definitive Therapy

- *Ascariasis:* albendazole 400 mg dose for mebendazole 500 mg for 1 dose.

- *Schistosomiasis:* praziquantel 40-60 mg/kg for 1 dose (higher dose in S japonicum). Egg excretion may occur for months after successful treatment. A mild Loeffler's-like syndrome may occur as the dying worms are expelled.

- *Fascioliasis/fasciolopsiasis:* praziquantel 25/kg mg TID for 2 days.

- *Filariasis* is generally treated with diethylcarbamazine (DEC), but doxycycline directed against the Wolbachia endosymbionts is increasingly used. Marked inflammatory reactions provoked by the dying worms may cause severe tissue destruction and systemic reactions, especially with L loa. Cytapheresis or albendazole may help reduce worm burden prior to treatment. Ivermectin is an alternative for L loa. Repeated cycles of therapy are usually needed.

- *Onchocerciasis* is best treated with ivermectin 150 mcg/kg, repeated semi-annually for 2 years. A mild Mazzotti-type reaction may occur.

- *Hookworm:* albendazole 400 mg PO x 1 dose (mebendazole 500 mg for 1 is an alternative).

- *Cysticercosis:* Stable lesions (especially those discovered on incidental radiology studies) in asymptomatic patients do not necessarily require therapy.

Symptomatology (usually seizures) usually denotes degeneration of the cyst, and anti-seizure medications are indicated. If a decision is made to eradicate living cysticerci, the preferred drug is albendazole, 15 mg/kg/d (max 800 mg/d) x 1-2 weeks, with concomitant steroids to reduce CNS inflammation.

- *Clonorchis/Opisthorchis:* praziquantel 25 mg/kg TID x 3 days.

- *Strongyloidiasis:* ivermectin 200 mcg/kg/day x 2 days; repeated doses may be needed. Alternative is albendazole, but it has a comparatively inferior response rate.

- *Angiostrongylus infection* is best treated with serial lumbar punctures and/or corticosteroids to relieve headache. Disease is usually self-limiting. Treatment with anthelmintics is contraindicated, as inflammation from the dying parasites may cause symptoms to worsen.

- *Trichinosis:* Gastrointestinal symptoms are treated with albendazole 400 mg/d x 3 days (alternatives are pyrantel pamoate 10 mg/kg QD or mebendazole 200 mg/d, both for 5 days). In the presence of acute severe infection, the goal is diminution of muscle damage; therefore prednisolone 40-60 mg/d is added to the anthelmintic. There is no treatment for chronic sequelae of infection.

- *Toxocariasis:* Treatment has not been shown consistently to be of benefit. Albendazole 400 mg PO BID x 5 days or mebendazole 100-200 mg BID x 5 days are preferred. OLM is treated primarily with steroids (systemic and intraocular); anthelmintics have no established role.

- *Paragonimiasis:* praziquantel 25 mg/kg TID x 2 days.

- *Cystic hydatid disease:* Calcified cysts require no treatment. Percutaneous aspiration with instillation of hypertonic saline is the preferred method of draining cysts; surgical removal has a higher complication rate. Anaphylactic complications and dissemination of cyst contents with risk of subsequent cyst formation, may occur during either procedure; perioperative and postoperative (28 days) albendazole 400 mg PO BID is usually used to prevent complications.

- *Gnathostomiasis* is treated by surgical removal of the worm. Albendazole 400 mg daily for 3 weeks or ivermectin 200 mcg/kg daily for 2 days has been effective for isolated cutaneous disease.

ID Board Pearls

- Eosinophilia and fever in the returning traveler is usually due to a helminthic infections, HIV, tuberculosis, coccidioidomycosis and rarely a protozoa (*Isospora belli* and *Dientamoeba fragilis*), depending on the area of travel and types of exposures.

- Important historical points include the exact dates and locations of travel, the kind of accommodations, unusual activities, sexual contacts, animal contacts, and sources and types of food (in particular, ingestion of raw or undercooked food items).

- Exposure to freshwater in an endemic area with the development of fever, chills, abdominal pain, eosinophilia, hepatosplenomegaly and/or lymphadenopathy within approximately 6 weeks should prompt an evaluation for acute schistosomiasis (Katayama fever).

- *Angiostrongylus cantonensis* is the most common cause of eosinophilic meningitis and is related to the consumption of undercooked snails, seafood or contaminated water plants.

- Strongyloidiasis should always be considered before giving immunosuppressive therapy to a person who has lived in an endemic area. Eosinophilia is variably present; diagnosis is by serology.

9. Pneumonia in the Returning Traveler (Southeast Asia, Latin America, Africa)

Causative Organisms

• Most likely causes of pneumonia are no different than in temperate North America.

• Southeast Asia: tuberculosis, melioidosis, histoplasmosis, Penicillium marneffei and paragonimiasis.

• Latin America: tuberculosis, coccidioidomycosis, paracoccidioidomycosis, paragonimiasis and histoplasmosis.

• Africa: tuberculosis and paragonimiasis.

Epidemiology

• Melioidosis is reported throughout Southeast Asia, particularly in association with exposure to standing water. Occasional cases occur elsewhere, including in Florida.

• The endemic dimorphic fungi of Latin America have restricted geographical distributions. Coccidioidomycosis is common only in the lower Sonoran life zone, ie, Mexico, the pampas of Argentina, and isolated areas of Venezuela and Colombia. Paracoccidioidomycosis (AKA South American blastomycosis) is seen in Brazil, Colombia, Venezuela, Argentina, and Paraguay. It is thought to favor moist soil with lush vegetation. Histoplasmosis is found worldwide, but in the tropics is found throughout Latin America and Southeast Asia, in association with river valleys and bird guano. All the dimorphic fungi are spread through inhalation of airborne conidia.

• Paragonimiasis may be a cause of fever and pulmonary infiltrates in persons who have consumed undercooked crustaceans (eg, "drunken crab").

• Tuberculosis is common throughout the developing world; drug resistance is on the rise worldwide.

• *Penicillium marneffei* is found in Southeast Asia or southern China. Most commonly it occurs among immunocompromised persons residing or visiting endemic areas, but has been described in normal hosts.

• Although influenza is a seasonal disease, it should be kept in mind that the seasons in the Southern Hemisphere are the reverse of those in the Northern Hemisphere, and thus travelers going from one hemisphere to the other may be at risk. Furthermore, influenza can be transmitted year-round in the tropics. Travel to bird markets in Asia should raise clinical suspicion for avian influenza although this infection has yet to be diagnosed in a returned traveler.

Key Clinical Features

• The prevalence of drug-resistant *S pneumoniae* is increasing in most areas of the world.

• Melioidosis: caused by *Burkholderia pseudomallei*, a common environmental organism isolated from wet soil in Southeast Asia. Patients are generally infected by inhalation of aerosolized organisms; the latency period has been known to last decades. Most patients with severe disease have comorbid conditions (diabetes, renal failure, malignancy, alcoholism). Patients frequently present with diffuse pneumonia and septicemia. Metastatic abscesses may occur in lung, liver, spleen, the musculoskeletal system and the CNS.

• Coccidioidomycosis (caused by *Coccidioides immitis* or *posadasii*) may present with fever, cough and weight loss (in the pulmonary form), or as osteomyelitis, skin/soft tissue abscess or meningitis in the disseminated form. Frequently, the diagnosis is only made after failure of treatment of community acquired pneumonia, or a diagnosis of flu-like illness which fails to improve. Africans, Filipinos and probably Hispanics are at increased risk for disseminated disease, as is anyone in an immune-compromised state. Persons with disseminated disease may not report a history of pneumonia or flu-like illness.

• Histoplasmosis may present as an acute pulmonary or disseminated disease, the latter being especially common in immune-suppressed patients. In the pulmonary form, patients may present with fever, night sweats, severe cough and weight loss; patients with disseminated disease may have cutaneous lesions of histoplasmosis and bone marrow infiltration. Reactivation disease may occur years after acute infection, especially in the elderly or immune suppressed, and generally takes the form of disseminated disease. Occasional patients will have chronically progressive histoplasmosis: fever, cough, weight loss and chronic chest x-ray infiltrates. In the disseminated form of chronic histoplasmosis, oral ulcers are frequently noted. Mediastinal fibrosis may cause symptoms related to compression of the bronchi, esophagus and great vessels.

- Paracoccidioidomycosis (*Paracoccidioides brasiliensis*) rarely presents as an acute infection; most patients who are infected have self-limited disease and may not present for treatment. However, a sub acute form of disease is reported among children and adolescents: this is described as presenting with fever, anorexia, weight loss, subcutaneous abscesses, hepatosplenomegaly and lymphadenopathy. The prognosis is poor. For unclear reasons, in adults there is a large preponderance of male patients. Pulmonary disease may cause fever, cough and shortness of breath, sometimes with productive sputum. Weight loss is common. Painful mucosal lesions may be noted on the nose, lips or tongue; laryngeal lesions may cause dysphonia. Skin lesions may be apparent around the mouth, anus and genitalia. Adenopathy and adrenal involvement are occasionally noted.

- Paragonimiasis usually presents about 6 months after exposure, but presentation can be up to years later. Patients complain of cough, sputum production and shortness of breath. Physical examination may demonstrate a mild fever and wheezing. In endemic populations, cerebral metastatic lesions may cause focal neurologic deficits, seizures or an encephalitic syndrome. Abdominal and subcutaneous nodules may arise; if biopsied, these contain adult flukes.

- *P marneffei* infections typically present with a chronic illness of fever, cough, weight loss, and/or skin lesions. Skin lesions are variable, but may resemble molluscum contagiosum. Other sites of infection have been described including adenopathy, hepatosplenomegaly, colonic lesions, bony disease and pericarditis. Disease is most commonly noted in the immunocompromised (eg,

AIDS patients) and may occur several years after the exposure in an endemic area.

- Influenza presents with fever, chills, myalgia and malaise. Pulmonary symptoms may be caused either by primary influenza pneumonia or by secondary bacterial superinfection (eg, *S pneumoniae* and *S aureus*); the latter may have more purulent sputum and positive sputum or blood cultures. Cases of community-acquired MRSA complicating influenza cases are well documented.

Key Laboratory/Radiology Features

- *B pseudomallei* readily grow on routine media. You should alert the laboratory staff if you suspect this diagnosis as cultures are infective and should be handled in a BSL-2 facility. Chest x-ray may show diffuse pneumonia or embolus-like abscesses.

- Coccidioidomycosis is generally diagnosed by ELISA, although the traditional complement fixation (CF) test is still required to monitor the course of disease (and response to treatment). CF titers greater than 1:16 predict a higher risk of dissemination and mandate a bone scan to look for bony disease. If the patient has any CNS complaints (including headache) a lumbar puncture to rule out meningitis is mandatory: ELISA and CF antibodies can make the diagnosis on CSF. Diagnosis also can be made by culture and histopathology with pathonomonic spherules. If biopsy material or sputum is submitted for culture, the laboratory should be warned that coccidioidomycosis is in the differential, and the mycelial form is highly infectious (patients themselves are not transmission risks). On chest x-ray, pulmonary disease can appear either alveolar or interstitial; hilar lymphadenopathy is common. Over time, nodular densities and cavitary lesions may appear in the lungs.

- Histoplasmosis is most commonly diagnosed by detecting urine histoplasma antigen, which should turn negative as the disease resolves. Histoplasmosis antibodies are less useful as they may be positive in any person who resided in an endemic area. The detection of fungal elements is straightforward on tissue biopsy; preferred sites in disseminated disease include buffy coat smears and, in particular, bone marrow biopsy.

- Paracoccidioidomycosis is diagnosed by culture of biopsy specimens. Serologic testing is available and may be helpful in the traveler returning from a low endemicity population. Chest x-ray findings are described as perihilar, frequently bilateral and symmetric, with a nodular pattern; adenopathy is relatively rare.

- Eosinophilia is common in paragonimiasis. The chest x-ray may show ill-defined opacities, lobar pneumonia, pleural effusion, calcified nodules or cysts. Antibody testing is helpful in confirming the diagnosis. Ova of P westermani may be visualized in the sputum or bronchoscopy washings of infected patients.

- *P marneffei* is usually diagnosed by identifying the organism by smear, culture or histopathologic examination. Most often the organism is found in biopsies of skin lesions, sputum, bone marrow or lymph node biopsies. Chest radiography may show nodular, reticulonodular, diffuse infiltrates or cavitary lesions.

- Influenza may be diagnosed in the office by a variety of commercial rapid detection methods. Direct fluorescent antibody screening of nasopharyngeal swabs is the most widely available laboratory confirmatory method. The chest x-ray appearance may be variable; diffuse interstitial infiltrates are classically seen with primary influenza pneumonia, whereas bacterial superinfection is associated with a lobar/airspace pattern.

Differential Diagnosis

Infectious Diseases
- Malaria can occasionally present with pulmonary infiltrates (due to capillary leak syndrome); a generally accepted rule is that any febrile traveler returning from a malaria zone must be evaluated for malaria, regardless of competing diagnoses.

- Typhoid fever can present with pneumonitis and cough, and with minimal abdominal symptomatology.

- Loeffler's syndrome (pneumonitis due to migration of helminths through lung parenchyma) can cause pulmonary infiltrates that mimic pneumonia.

- Tropical pulmonary eosinophilia due to filariasis. Likewise, acute schistosomiasis may be associated with cough and pulmonary infiltrates.

- Severe acute respiratory syndrome (SARS) is caused by the SARS coronavirus and may present with fever and respiratory distress, especially in the setting of travel to an area with an ongoing outbreak of disease.

Noninfectious Disease Mimics
- Churg-Strauss syndrome

- Wegener's granulomatosis

- Acute eosinophilic pneumonia - associated with dust exposure and seen in US troops deployed to Iraq

Empiric Therapy

- Treatment of pneumonia in the returning traveler should in general adhere to the commonly accepted principles of treating community acquired pneumonia in the United States, with exceptions made for patients at special risk (recently hospitalized, immune compromised, etc). Tuberculosis can present either as a *de novo* infection or as reactivation.

- For most patients, appropriate empiric therapy can follow either American Thoracic Society or Infectious Disease Society of America guidelines for community acquired pneumonia. Amphotericin B is considered first line treatment for all severely ill patients with dimorphic fungal infections; the exception is coccidioidal meningitis, for which fluconazole is the preferred choice.

- In patients who are suspected of having influenza, treatment with neuraminidase inhibitors (zanamavir may be preferred due to reports of increasing oseltamivir resistance); the combination of rimantidine-oseltamivir reasonable if zanamavir not available or contraindicated. Most beneficial if started within the first 36 hours of symptoms.

- In patients with suspected tuberculosis, a determined effort to obtain diagnostic cultures before starting therapy is imperative, as the rising prevalence of multidrug resistance in the developing world makes empiric therapy difficult.

Definitive Therapy

- Melioidosis is usually treated with ceftazidime 120 mg/kg/d in divided doses. Carbapenem therapy is an alternative, and there is some evidence that carbapenems may be superior, but a prospective study is not yet available. Once patients are clearly improving, the usual practice is to continue oral antibiotics (trimethoprim- sulfamethoxazole, doxycycline, chloramphenicol or a combination of two of the above) to complete a 20-week treatment course. *B pseudomallei* are intrinsically resistant to all aminoglycosides. The overall mortality despite therapy remains high at 50%.

- Coccidioidomycosis need not be treated in all cases, although most authorities would treat anyone at high risk for dissemination (Africans, Filipinos, Hispanics, the immunocompromised), or with a high complement fixation titer (>1:16). Most authorities would treat uncomplicated cases with fluconazole 400 mg/d or itraconazole 200 mg BID (the latter is favored in soft tissue or bony disease). Amphotericin B is indicated in severe cases (coccidioidal meningitis should not be treated with intravenous amphotericin: the preferred drug is fluconazole, usually at 800 mg or more a day). Treatment, once begun, is usually continued for at least 6-12 months, or longer, depending on how quickly symptoms resolve and the complement fixation titer drops (ideally 4-fold or more). The exception is coccidioidal meningitis; these patients generally receive treatment for life. Newer azoles (posaconazole, voriconazole) are active against Coccidioides, but their role has not been defined by clinical trials or guidelines.

- Histoplasmosis is usually self-limiting in immunocompetent patients. For the severely symptomatic or immune suppressed, the preferred choice of therapy is amphotericin until symptoms resolve;

therapy is generally continued with itraconazole (200 mg twice a day) for 4-6 weeks or longer.

- Paracoccidioidomycosis is optimally treated with itraconazole 200 mg daily for 6 months. An induction course of amphotericin may be used in severe cases. Sulfonamindes are an alternate treatment option. Treatment frequently continues for 2-3 years.

- Paragonimiasis is optimally treated by praziquantel 25 mg/kg TID x 2 days. Side effects are generally minimal and symptoms resolve within several months.

- *Penicillium* is usually treated with amphotericin B. After 2 weeks of therapy, often therapy is switched to itraconazole 200 mg BID. Fluconazole is inferior to itraconazole for this disease.

Complications

- Melioidosis is prone to recrudescence if antibiotic therapy is not continued for a sufficient length of time.

- Disseminated coccidioidomycosis can relapse years after apparently successful initial therapy. Meningitis should be treated for life. Cavitary disease may cause spontaneous hemoptysis and may be colonized by aspergillus (aspergilloma); surgical resection may be needed.

- Resolved histoplasmosis will frequently cause chronic splenic or pulmonary calcifications and stable hilar lymphadenopathy. Chronic progressive fibrosis may cause obstruction of airways or major vessels; surgery may be necessary, but the disease often recurs. Histoplasmomas may form in the lung; these do not usually require treatment unless they impinge on a vital structure, but may be confused with malignancy. Cavitary pulmonary disease may occur, particularly in patients with preexisting emphysema. If the patient has a thick-walled cavity (associated with worse prognosis), progressive pulmonary decline, or persistent infiltrates, treatment with itraconazole or amphotericin is indicated. Ocular histoplasmosis may result in posterior uveitis and choroiditis.

This appears to be an immune-mediated phenomenon and generally occurs years after acute infection.

- Paracoccidioidomycosis can relapse even after prolonged effective therapy. Retreatment with standard regimens is indicated.

- Relapses of *Penicillium* are well described among HIV-infected persons; secondary prevention with itraconazole is often utilized.

Prognostic Factors

- In general, extremes of age, comorbid medical conditions, and immune-compromised states are associated with worse prognosis.

ID Board Pearls

- Usual respiratory pathogens (eg, *S pneumoniae*) are the most likely causes of pneumonia in the returning traveler.

- Influenza can be transmitted year-round in the tropics; as such, it should be considered during pre-travel counseling and in the returning traveler with respiratory symptoms.

- Malaria can occasionally present with pulmonary infiltrates (due to capillary leak syndrome); any febrile traveler returning from a malaria zone must be evaluated for malaria, regardless of competing diagnoses.

- The dimorphic fungi coccidioidomycosis, paracoccidioidomycosis (AKA South American blastomycosis), and histoplasmosis may be acquired during travel to various parts of Latin America.

- Treatment of pneumonia in the returning traveler should in general adhere to the commonly accepted principles of treating community-acquired pneumonia in the United States, with exceptions made for patients at special risk (recently hospitalized, immune compromised, exposure during an outbreak, high-risk of tuberculosis, etc).

10. Further Reading

Books

Christie AB, ed. *Infectious Diseases: Epidemiology and Practice*. 4th ed. New York, NY: Churchill-Livingstone; 1987.

Cook GC, Zumla A. *Manson's Tropical Diseases*. 22nd ed. United Kingdom: WB Saunders; 2008.

Deepe GS. Histoplasma capsulatum. In: Mandell GL, Bennet JE, Dolin R, ed. *Principles and Practice of Infectious Diseases*. 2nd ed. Philadelphia, PA: Churchill Livingstone; 2005:506-516.

Guerrant RL, Walker DH, Weller PD. *Tropical Infectious Diseases*. Vol I. 2nd ed. Philadelphia, PA: Churchill Livingstone; 1999.

Strickland GT, ed. *Hunter's Tropical Medicine and Emerging Infectious Diseases*. 8th ed. Philadelphia, PA: WB Saunders; 2000.

DuPont HL, Steffen R, eds. *Textbook of Travel Medicine and International Health*. 3rd ed. Hamilton, Ontario, Canada: BC Decker; 1997.

Richman DD, Whitley RJ, Hayden FG, eds. *Clinical Virology*. 3rd Ed. Washington, DC: ASM Press; 2001.

Magill AJ. Leishmaniasis. In: Strickland GT, ed. *Tropical Medicine Emerging Infectious Diseases*. 8th ed. New York, NY: WB Saunders; 2002: 665-687.

Warrell DA, Gilles HM, ed. *Essential Malariology*. London, England: Arnold Publishers; 2002.

Wilson ME. *A World Guide to Infections*. New York, NY: Oxford University Press; 1991.

Journal Articles

Fatal yellow fever in a traveler returning from Amazonas, Brazil, 2002. *JAMA*. 2002;287:2499-2500.

Update on management of patients with suspected viral hemorrhagic fever—United States. *MMWR*. 1995;44:475-479.

Antony SJ. Leptospirosis— An emerging pathogen in travel medicine: A review of its clinical manifestations and management. *J Travel Med*. 1963;3:113-118.

Arevalo I, Ward B, Miller R, et al. Successful treatment of drug-resistant cutaneous leishmaniasis in humans by use of imiquimod, an immunomodulator. *Clin Infect Dis*. 2001;33:1847-1851.

Aronson NE, Wortmann GW, Johnson SC, et al. Safety and efficacy of intravenous sodium stibogluconate in the treatment of leishmaniasis: Recent U.S. military experience. *Clin Infect Dis*. 1998;27:1457-1464.

Baird JK, Hoffman SL. Progress in prevention and treatment of malaria. *Curr Opin Infect Dis*. 1996;9:319-329.

Berman JD. Editorial response: US Food and Drug Administration approval of AmBisome (liposomal amphotericin B) for treatment of visceral leishmaniasis. *Clin Infect Dis*. 1999;28:9-51.

Boria L, Inglesby T, Peters CJ, et al. Hemorrhagic viruses as biological weapons. *JAMA*. 2002;287: 2391-2405.

Bruno P, Hassell LH, Brown J, Tanner W, Lau A. The protean manifestations of hemorrhagic fever with renal syndrome. *Ann Intern Med*. 1990;113:385-391.

Colebunders R, Borchert M. Ebola hemorrhagic fever–A review. *J Infect Dis*. 2000;40:16-20.

Cunha BA. Diagnosis of imported malaria in returning travelers. *Arch Intern Med*. 2001;161:1926-1928.

Cunha BA. Osler on typhoid fever: Differentiation of typhoid from typhus and malaria. *Infect Dis Clin North Am*. 2004;18:111-126.

Cunha BA. The importance of non-specific laboratory tests in suspecting malaria in returning travelers. *Ann Intern Med*. 2004;14:e141/7/547.

Cunha BA. The microscopic mimics of malaria. *Infect Dis Pract*. 2002;26:89-90.

Cunha BA, Bonoan JT, Schlossberg D. Atypical lymphocytes in acute malaria. *Arch Intern Med*. 1997;157:1140-1141.

Currie BJ, Fisher DA, Howard DM, et al. Endemic melioidosis in tropical northern Australia: a 10 year perspective and review of the literature. *Clin Infect Dis*. 2002;31:981-986.

Enria DA, Pinheiro F. Rodent-borne emerging viral zoonosis. *Infect Dis Clin North Am*. 2000;14: 167-184.

Farr RW. Leptospirosis. *Clin Infect Dis*.1995;21:1996.

Fisher-Hoch SP, Khan JA, Rehman S, et al. Crimean congo hemorrhagic fever treated with oral ribavirin. *Lancet*. 1995;346:472-475.

Gajdusek DC. Virus hemorrhagic fevers. *J Pediatr*. 1962;60:841-857.

Galgiani JN, Ampel NM, Catanzaro A, et al. Practice guidelines for the treatment of coccidioidomycosis. *Clin Infect Dis*. 2000;30:658-661.

Griffith ME, Hospental DR, Murray CK. Antimicrobial therapy of leptospirosis. *Curr Opin Infect Dis*. 2006;19:533-537.

Herwaldt BL. Leishmaniasis. *Lancet*. 1999;354:1191-1199.

Hoerauf A. Filariasis: new drugs and opportunities for lymphatic filariasis and onchocerciasis. *Curr Opin Infect Dis*. 2008;21:673-681.

Hoffman SL. Diagnosis, treatment and prevention of malaria. *Med Clin North Am*. 1992;76:1327-1355.

Hoffman SL, Punjabi NH, Kumala S, et al. Reduction of mortality in chloramphenicol treated severe typhoid fever by high-dose dexamethasone. *N Engl J Med*. 1984;310:82-88.

Isaacson M. Viral hemorrhagic fever hazards for travelers in Africa. *Clin Infect Dis*. 2001;33:1707-1712.

Jha TK, Sundar S, Thaku CP, et al. Miltefosine, an oral agent, for the treatment of Indian visceral leishmaniasis. *N Engl J Med*. 1999;341:1795-1800.

Jensenius M, Fournier PE, Raoult D. Rickettsioses and the international traveler. *Clin Infect Dis*. 2004;39:1493-1499.

Karunajeewa HA, Mueller I, Senn M, et al. A trial o f combination antimalarial therapies in children from Papua New Guinea. *N Engl J Med*. 2008;359:2601-2603.

Kim YS, Yun HJ, Shim SK, Koo SH, Kim SY, Kim S. A comparative trial of a single dose of azithromycin versus doxycycline for the treatment of mild scrub typhus. *Clin Infect Dis*. 2004;39:1329-1335.

Lee HW. Hemorrhagic fever with renal syndrome in Korea. *Rev Infect Dis*. 1989;11(suppl 4):S864-S876.

Levett PN. Leptospirosis. *Clin Microbiol Rev*. 2001;14:296-326.

Lomar AV, Diamant D, Torres JR. Leptospirosis in Latin America. *Infect Dis Clin North Am*. 2000;14:23-39.

Magill AJ, Grogl M, Gasser RA, et al. Visceral infection caused by Leishmania tropica in veterans of Operation Desert Storm. *N Engl J Med*. 1993;328:1383-1387.

Manns BJ, Baylis BW, Urbanski SJ, Gibb AP, Rabin HR. Paracoccidioidomycosis: case report and review. *Clin Infect Dis*. 1996;23:1026-1032.
Marianneau P, Georges-Courbot M, Deubel V. Rarity of adverse effects after 17D yellow fever vaccination. *Lancet*. 2001;358:84-85.

McClain JBL, Ballou WR, Harrison SH, et al. Doxycycline therapy of leptospirosis. *Ann Intern Med*. 1984;100:696.

McDonald JC, MacLean JD, McDade JE. Imported rickettsial disease: clinical and epidemiologic features. *Am J Med*. 1988;85:799-805.

Miller KD, Greenberg AE, Campbell CC. Treatment of severe malaria in the United States with a continuous infusion of quinidine gluconate and exchange transfusion. *N Engl J Med*. 1989;321:65-70.

Monath TP. Yellow fever: An update. *Lancet Infect Dis*. 2002;1:11-20.

Monath TP, Cetron MS. Prevention of yellow fever in persons traveling to the tropics. *Clin Infect Dis*. 2001;34:1369-1378.

Moore TA, Nutman TB. Eosinophilia in the returning traveler. *Infect Dis Clin North Am*. 1998;12:503-521.

Murphy GS, Oldfield EC. Falciparum malaria. *Infect Dis Clin North Am*. 1996;10:747-775.

Murray HW, Berman JD, Davies CR, Saravia NG. Advances in leishmaniasis. *Lancet*. 2005;366:1561-1577.

Nutman TB, Kradin RL. A 24-year-old woman with paresthesias and muscle cramps after a stay in Africa. *N Engl J Med*. 2002;346:115-122.

Olson JG, Bourgeois AL, Fang RC, Coolbaugh JC, Dennis DT. Prevention of scrub typhus. Prophylactic administration of doxycycline in a randomized double blind trial. *Am J Trop Med Hyg*. 1980;29:989-997.

Panaphut T, Domrongkitchaiporn S, Vibhagool A, et al. Ceftriaxone compared with sodium penicillin G for treatment of severe leptospirosis. *Clin Infect Dis*. 2003;36:1507-1513.

Phillips P, Nantel S, Benny WB. Exchange transfusion as an adjunct to the treatment of severe malaria: case report and review. *Rev Infect Dis*. 1990;12:1100-1108.

Phuong CXT, Bethell DB, Phuong PT, et al. Comparison of artemisinin suppositories, intramuscular artesunate and intravenous quinine for the treatment of severe childhood malaria. *Trans R Soc Trop Med Hyg*. 1997;91:335-342.

Ratcliff A, Siswantoro H, Kenangalem E, et al. Two fixed-dose artemisinin combinations for drug-resistant falciparum and vivax malaria in Papua, Indonesia: an open-label randomised comparison. *Lancet*. 2007;369:757-765.

Robertson SE, Hull BP, Tomori O, et al. Yellow fever: A decade of reemergence. *JAMA*. 1996;276:1157-1162.

Rothenburg ME. Eosinophilia. *N Engl J Med*. 1998;338:1592-1599.

Rowe B, Ward LR, Threlfall J. Multi-drug resistant Salmonella typhi: A worldwide epidemic. *Clin Infect Dis*. 1997;24(suppl 1):S106-S109.

Schoch PE, Iancu D, Lobato M, Cunha BA. Mixed malarial infections: P falciparum and P vivax. *Dis Pract*. 1998;22:61-63.

Schulte C, Krebs B, Jelinek T, et al. Diagnostic significance of blood eosinophilia in returning travelers. *Clin Infect Di*s. 2002;34:407-411.

Sejvar J, Bancroft E, Winthrop K, et al. Leptospirosis in "Eco- Challenge" athletes, Malaysian Borneo. *Emerg Infect Dis*. 2000;9:702-707.

Shorr AF, Scoville SL, Cersovsky SB, et al. Acute eosinophilic pneumonia among US Military personnel deployed in or near Iraq. *JAMA*. 2004;292:2997-3005.

Sideridis AK, Canario D, Cunha BA. Dengue fever A: diagnostic importance of a camelback fever pattern. *Heart Lung*. 2003;32:414-418.

Solomon T, Mallewa M. Dengue and other emerging flaviviruses. *J Infect*. 2001;42:104-115.
Speil C, Mushtaq A, Adamski A, Khardori N. Fever of unknown origin in the returning traveler. *Infect Dis Clin North Am*. 2007;21:1091-1113.

Strickland GT. Fever in the returned traveler. *Med Clin North Am*. 1992;76:1375- 1392.

Swanepoel R, Gill DE, Shepherd AJ, et al. The clinical pathology of Crimean-Congo hemorrhagic fever. *Rev Infect Dis*. 1989;11(suppl 4):S794-S800.

Takafuji ET, Kirkpatrick JW, Miller RN, et al. An efficacy trial of doxycycline chemoprophylaxis against leptospirosis. *N Engl J Med*. 1984;310:497-500.

Vinetz JM. Leptospirosis. *Curr Opin Infect Dis*. 2001;14:527-538.

Wallace MR, Sharp TW, Smoak B, et al. Malaria among US troops in Somali. *Am J Med*. 1996;100:49-55.

Wallace MR, Yousif AA, Mahroos GA, et al. Ciprofloxacin versus ceftriaxone in the treatment of multiresistant typhoid fever. *Eur J Clin Microbiol Infect Dis*. 1993;12:907-910.

Watt G, Warrell DW. Leptospirosis and the Jarisch-Herxheimer reaction. *Clin Infect Dis*. 1995;20:1437-1438.

Wilson ME, Weld LH, Boggild A, et al. Fever in returned travelers: results from the GeoSentinel Surveillance Network. *Clin Infect Dis*. 2007;44:1560-1568.

World Health Organization. Severe and complicated malaria. *Trans Roy Soc Trop Med Hyg*. 1980;84(suppl 2):1-65.

World Health Organization. Yellow Fever, 1996–1997. Part 1. Weekly Epidemiology Record. 1984;46:354-357.

Chapter 4:
Fever of Unknown Origin (FUO) for the ID Boards

Burke A. Cunha, MD

Contents

1. Fever of Unknown Origin (FUO)

Definition

Classic
• Fever of unknown origin (FUO) is defined as prolonged febrile illness lasting 3 weeks, with temperature ≥101° F (38.3° C) that defies diagnosis after 1 week of in-hospital evaluation.

Current
• Undiagnosed fever after 3 days of hospitalization or 3 outpatient visits or 1 week of intensive outpatient investigations.

Fever of Unknown Origin in Adults

• Traditionally, *infections* were the commonest cause of FUO followed by collagen vascular diseases and malignancies.

• Currently, *malignancies and infectious diseases remain the most common causes of FUO in adults* (Table 1).

• *SBE is still an important FUO cause.*

• Rheumatologic diseases, particularly rheumatoid arthritis and systemic lupus erythematosus (SLE) are now *rare* causes of FUO.

• Adult Still's disease and temporal arteritis remain important rheumatic causes of FUO.

• Tuberculosis (TB) and subacute bacterial endocarditis (SBE) are *less common* causes of FUO.

• Intraabdominal abscesses *still* are important causes of FUO.

ID Board Pearls

• *The more prolonged the period of undiagnosed fever in a patient with FUO, the more likely it is due to a noninfectious etiology.*

Fever of Unknown Origin in Children

• FUO etiology varies with age.

• Infections in children are a more common cause of FUO than neoplasms.

• Viral illnesses are common causes of FUO in children.

• Common FUO in the pediatric age group include cat-scratch disease (Bartonella), while others are rare, eg, SBE.

• FUO due to regional arteritis, SLE, cytomegalovirus (CMV) and lymphomas are common in young children/adults.

Table 1

Diseases Causing Fever of Unknown Origin

	Common	Uncommon	Rare
Malignancy	Lymphomas Metastases (liver or CNS) Hypernephromas	Hepatomas Preleukemias	Atrial myxomas CNS tumors Myeloproliferative disorders Pancreatic carcinomas Colon carcinomas

Infections	Renal TB
	TB meningitis
	Miliary TB
	Intra-abdominal abscesses
	Subdiaphragmatic
	   abscesses
	     Periappendiceal
	     Pericolonic
	     Hepatic
	Pelvic abscesses
		Subacute bacterial
		   endocarditis (SBE)
		Cytomegalovirus (CMV)
		Toxoplasmosis
		Salmonella sp. enteric fevers
		Intra- and perinephric
		   abscesses
		Splenic abscesses
			Small brain abscesses
			Chronic sinusitis
			Subacute vertebral
			   osteomyelitis
			Chronic meningitis or
			   encephalitis
			Listeria
			Yersinia
			Brucellosis
			Relapsing fever
			Rat-bite fever
			Chronic Q fever
			Cat-scratch disease (CSD)
			HIV
			Epstein-Barr virus (EBV)
			   mononucleosis (elderly)
			Leptospirosis
			Blastomycosis
			Histoplasmosis
			Coccidioidomycosis
			Cryptococcosis
			Infected aortic aneurysm
			Infected vascular grafts
			Leishmaniasis
			Trypanosomiasis
			Trichinosis
			Lymphogranuloma venereum
			   (LGV)
			Relapsing mastoiditis
			Septic jugular
			   thrombophlebitis
			Whipple's disease

Rheumatologic	Still's disease
	   (adult juvenile
	   rheumatoid arthritis)
	Temporal arteritis (TA)
		Periarteritis nodosa (PAN)
		Late onset rheumatoid
		   arthritis (LORA)
			Systemic lupus
			   erythematosus (SLE)
			Vasculitis (eg, Takayasu's
			   arteritis, hypersensitivity
			   vasculitis)
			Felty's syndrome
			Pseudogout
			Behçet's disease
			Familial Mediterranean fever
			   (FMF)

(continued)

Table 1

Diseases Causing Fever of Unknown Origin *(continued)*

	Common	**Uncommon**	**Rare**

Miscellaneous causes	Drug fever
	Cirrhosis
	Alcoholic
	   hepatitis
		Granulomatous
		   hepatitis
			Regional enteritis (RE)
			Fabry's disease
			Hyperthyroidism
			Addison's disease
			Subacute thyroiditis
			Cyclic neutropenia
			Polymyositis
			Weber-Christian disease
			Occult hematomas
			Subacute dissecting aortic
			   aneurysm
			Wegener's granulomatosis
			Sarcoidosis (eg, basilar
			   meningitis, hepatic
			   granulomas)
			Pulmonary emboli (multiple,
			   recurrent)
			Hypothalamic dysfunction
			Giant hepatic hemangiomas
			Pseudolymphomas
			Kikuchi's disease
			Takayasu's arteritis
			Malakoplakia
			Hyper IgD syndrome
			Habitual hyperthermia
			Factitious fever

Adapted from Cunha BA. Fever of unknown origin (FUO). In: Gorbach SL, Bartlett JB, Blacklow NR, eds. Infectious Diseases. *3rd ed. Philadelphia, PA: Lippincott Williams & Wilkins; 2004 and Cunha Ba, ed.* Fever of the Unknown Origin. *New York, NY: Informa Healthcare: 2007.*

2. Causes of Fever of Unknown Origin

Malignancies

Lymphomas

- Retroperitoneal lymphomas are a common cause of FUOs.

- Retroperitoneal lymphomas are common in the elderly.

ID Board Pearls

- Retroperitoneal lymphomas may be associated with systemic symptoms, eg, weight loss, decreased appetite and malaise, *but often have no symptoms except fever.*

Metastatic Malignancies

- Fever *may be the only sign of metastatic disease* of the liver or central nervous system (CNS).

- Physical findings are usually absent.

Hypernephromas

- Renal cell carcinoma commonly presents as FUO.

- Hypernephromas, *"the internist's tumor,"* often presents with multisystem involvement when metastatic.

ID Board Pearls

- Most patients with hypernephroma do not have hematuria.

- *Left* varicocele in an *adult* should suggest hyper-nephroma.

Colon Carcinoma

- *Right*-sided colon carcinomas may present as FUO.

- Colon cancer may be *missed* by colonoscopy and CT scanning.

Hepatic and Pancreatic Carcinomas

- Hepatomas often present with hepatomegaly, hepatic bruit or rub.

- Multifocal hepatomas mimic metastatic liver disease.

- Symptoms of pancreatic carcinoma include *vague changes in mental status, hyperglycemia* and abdominal discomfort.

Preleukemias

- *Preleukemic monocytic leukemia is a frequent cause of FUO.*

ID Board Pearls

- Sternal tenderness may be the *only sign.*

- *Blasts* are *not* present in the *peripheral* blood smear.

Atrial Myxomas

- Atrial myxomas mimic SBE.

- Atrial myxomas may present with fever, emboli or a heart murmur.

ID Board Pearls

- *FUO with a heart murmur and polyclonal gammopathy on SPEP suggests atrial myxoma (vs. SBE).*

Infectious Diseases

Extrapulmonary Tuberculosis
Renal tuberculosis

- Renal tuberculosis presents with *sterile pyuria, microscopic hematuria or slowly progressive renal failure.*

- Renal tuberculosis is one of the few diseases that *simultaneously affects the upper and lower urinary tracts*.

Tuberculous meningitis

- Early TB meningitis may present with intermittent low-grade fevers, cognitive difficulties, mild headaches or difficulties in concentration.

- *Serial* lumbar punctures may be necessary to make the diagnosis of TB meningitis to demonstrate the "*protein-glucose dissociation.*"

- Chest x-ray may be *normal* in TB meningitis.

ID Board Pearls

- In TB basilar meningitis, cranial nerve abnormalities and *unilateral or bilateral abducens nerve palsies are late findings*.

- With TB meningitis, the *CSF glucose falls as the CSF protein rises*.

Miliary tuberculosis

- Miliary tuberculosis has *no localizing signs*.

- Elderly patients and those on *corticosteroids* may have disseminated disease.

- The diagnosis may be made by *biopsy of the liver or bone marrow*.

- An *empiric trial* of anti-tuberculous agents in a *rapidly deteriorating patient with suspected miliary TB is reasonable*.

Intraabdominal or Pelvic Abscesses

- Periappendiceal or pericolonic collections are common causes of FUO.

- Subdiaphragmatic collections and intrahepatic abscesses are common causes of FUO in the *elderly*.

- *Splenic* abscesses should suggest SBE, typhoid fever or brucellosis.

- Perinephric abscesses from chronic pyelonephritis may present as FUO.

Enteric Fevers (Salmonella)

- Usually there are *no* localizing signs with typhoid fever.

- Typhoid fever often presents with *splenomegaly* or *spinal* tenderness.

Toxoplasmosis

- Toxoplasmosis FUO in *immunocompetent* adults may present as *prolonged infectious mononucleosis-like illness*, or as isolated regional lymphadenopathy.

- Few physical findings with *atypical lymphocytosis* and *mild liver abnormalities* are clues to acquired toxoplasmosis in normal adults.

ID Board Pearls

- Onion skin appearance on biopsy of the affected node is *characteristic*.

Epstein-Barr Virus (EBV)

- Elderly patients with EBV present without posterior cervical adenopathy or pharyngitis.

ID Board Pearls

- In an elderly patient, mild hepatitis with FUO *with atypical lymphocytosis should suggest EBV*.

Subacute Bacterial Endocarditis (SBE)

- SBE is less common cause of FUO because of early blood cultures and echocardiographic studies.

ID Board Pearls

- The most common FUO causes of true *culture negative endocarditis are brucellosis* or Q fever.

Cat-scratch disease (CSD)

• Cat-scratch disease (*Bartonella*) primarily occurs in children but may occur in adults, and is frequently manifested by *fever and regional adenopathy*.

Brucellosis

• Often there are no *localizing signs* in *chronic* brucellosis.

• Unexplained headache, *unusual affect, or cognitive difficulties* may be the *only* findings.

• Renal and genitourinary involvement is uncommon.

• Arthritis of the knee, sacro-iliac or vertebral is t*ypical* of brucellosis.

Rheumatologic/Inflammatory Causes

Still's Disease (Adult JRA)

• Juvenile rheumatoid arthritis (adult Still's disease) is an important rheumatic cause of FUO in adults.

ID Board Pearls

• *Double quotidian fever* with hepatosplenomegaly and evanescent truncal salmon-colored rash and some joint/eye findings should suggest the diagnosis.

• *ANA and rheumatoid factor are negative*.

Temporal Arteritis (TA)

• Granulomatous arteritis of the temporal arteritis is a common cause of FUO in the elderly.

• Patients may complain of *vague headache or visual disturbances*.

• Tenderness over the temporal arteries *is not* always present.

Periarteritis Nodosa (PAN)

• Periarteritis nodosa is a midsize vasculitis characterized by multi-system involvement.

ID Board Pearls

• Abdominal pain or headache is common in PAN.

• *PAN may be suggested by otherwise unexplained hypertension, peripheral eosinophilia, acalculous cholecystitis, or epididymo-orchitis*.

• Pain over the angle of the jaw may be present.

Kikuchi's Disease

• Kikuchi's disease is *necrotizing adenitis with leukopenia* that usually occurs in young women.

• *Necrotizing mediastinal or retroperitoneal adenopathy* with or without splenomegaly are characteristic.

Miscellaneous Causes

Drug Fever

• FUO is an important manifestation of drug fever.

• Fever may be the *sole* manifestation of a hypersensitivity reaction.

• Most drugs are potentially sensitizing.

• Important causes of drug fever include cardiac medications, anti-arrhythmics, pain medications, sulfacontaining diuretics, sulfa-containing stool softeners, sleep medications and tranquilizers.

• Serum transaminases are *mildly* and transiently elevated *early*.

• Patients are often on medications *for years* before drug fever occurs.

ID Board Pearls

• Eosinophils are *commonly* present in the CBC, but *eosinophilia is infrequent*.

- *Don't assume that because the patient has been on a medication chronically it is not the cause of drug fever.*

Alcoholic Liver Disease

- Alcoholic liver disease is a common cause of FUO.

- Cirrhosis and alcoholic hepatitis are *frequently* missed causes of FUO.

Sarcoidosis

- Sarcoidosis is an *afebrile* disorder.

- Sarcoidosis may be associated with fever *if* there is bilateral hilar adenopathy with or without erythema nodosum, uveal tract/parotid involvement (Heerfordt's syndrome) or massive hepatic granulomas.

ID Board Pearls

- Sarcoidosis with *fever* should suggest coexisting TB or an alternate diagnosis (eg, lymphoma).

Familial Mediterranean Fever (FMF)

- FMF is characterized by intermittent pleuritic or abdominal pain and *joint pain*.

- Otherwise unexplained intermittent abdominal pain with fever in individuals of western European Mediterranean ancestry should suggest the diagnosis.

Whipple's Disease

- The combination of *mental status changes and arthritic symptom* should suggest Whipple's disease.

- Skin *hyperpigmentation* and adenopathy are variably present.

- Diagnosis is by *PAS-positive* material on small intestine biopsy.

- Most patients have *low carotene serum levels*.

Hypergammaglobulinemia IgD Syndrome

- Hypergammaglobulinemia IgD syndrome presents as periodic prolonged fever with *abdominal pain, arthralgias and cervical adenopathy*.

- Large joints are usually affected and some patients have an erythematous extremity rash.

- There is an increased risk of malignancy, particularly lymphomas.

ID Board Pearls

- Serum IgD levels are elevated in sarcoidosis, Hodgkin's lymphoma, HIV and TB, *but are very highly elevated in the hyper IgD syndrome* (>100 U/mL).

Factitious Fever

- Patients with factitious fevers are *usually young females in the medical field*.

- Factitious fevers are usually high and are *not accompanied by an appropriate pulse response*.

- With a suspected factitious fever, *measure the temperature of a recently voided urine sample*, which closely approximates core temperature.

3. Diagnostic Approach

History

- The *history is usually more important than the physical* examination in providing clues.

- Features that limit diagnostic possibilities are the most useful diagnostically (Table 2).

Physical Examination

General Concepts

- The eye, cardiac, lymph node and abdominal exam of the patient with FUO are particularly important.

- A heart murmur may suggest subacute endocarditis or an atrial myxoma.

- Hepatomegaly may point to lymphoma, metastatic carcinoma or alcoholic liver disease.

- Adenopathy is an important finding in FUO patients with lymphomas, rheumatoid arthritis, SLE, disseminated tuberculosis, EBV infectious mononucleosis, CMV, toxoplasmosis or human immunodeficiency virus (HIV) (Table 3).

ID Board Pearls

- *Trapezial* tenderness may be the *only* subtle expression of an occult subdiaphragmatic abscess.

- *Epididymal or testicular tenderness* may be the only clue to renal tuberculosis, blastomycosis, lymphoma, brucellosis, leptospirosis, periarteritis nodosa (PAN) or EBV infectious mononucleosis.

Diagnostic Approach

- Use clues from the patient's history and physical examination to guide the workup.

- Do *not* include every conceivable cause of FUO. The *work-up should be directed by the clinical presentation* and *pattern of organ involvement*.

- A previous intraabdominal or pelvic infection or surgery would suggest the possibility of an abscess if an infectious etiology is likely.

- In adults, *don't overlook malignancy* as a cause of FUO.

ID Board Pearls

- Drug fevers *should always be considered* in FUO patients *without localizing signs*.

- In adults, *don't overlook malignancy* as a cause of FUO.

Fever Patterns

General Concepts

- Fever patterns in the FUO patient with no localizing signs may provide the only clue to the diagnosis.

- Drug fevers presenting as FUOs *usually* have low grade temperatures (<102° F).

- Fevers ≥102° F suggest an *infectious* etiology, lymphoma or vasculitis.

- *Relative bradycardia* is an important diagnostic clue suggesting typhoid fever, psittacosis, leptospirosis, lymphoma or drug fever.

- *Double quotidian fever* may be the only clue to Still's disease (adult juvenile rheumatoid arthritis), visceral leishmaniasis (kala-azar), malaria or miliary tuberculosis.

- *Periodic or relapsing fevers* point to cyclic neutropenia, malaria, lymphoma, or one of the relapsing fevers due to *Borrelia, Spirillum or Streptobacillus*.

- *Intermittent hectic/septic fevers* suggest abscess, miliary tuberculosis or lymphoma.

ID Board Pearls

- In FUO patients, *reversal of diurnal temperature rhythm* with a *morning* temperature spike may suggest periarteritis nodosa, tuberculosis or factitious fever.

Table 2

Historic Clues to Fever of Unknown Origin

Medication or toxic substances
Drug fever
Fume fever

Tick exposure
Relapsing fever

Animal contact
Psittacosis
Leptospirosis
Brucellosis
Toxoplasmosis
Cat-scratch disease (CSD)
Q fever
Rat-bite fever

Myalgias
Trichinosis
SBE
PAN
Late onset rheumatoid arthritis (LORA)
FMF
Polymyositis
Whipple's disease

Cerebrovascular accident (CVA)
SBE
Takayasu's arteritis
PAN

Nonproductive cough
TB
Q fever
Psittacosis
Typhoid fever
Pulmonary neoplasms
RMSF
Temporal arteritis (TA)

Vision disorders or eye pain
Temporal arteritis (emboli)
SBE
Relapsing fever
Takayasu's arteritis (TA)

Angle of Jaw pain
PAN
TA

Neck pain
Subacute thyroiditis
Still's disease (adult JRA)
Temporal arteritis (TA)
Relapsing mastoiditis
Septic jugular phlebitis

Headache
Relapsing fever
Rat-bite fever
Brucellosis
CNS neoplasms
Whipple's Disease

Abdominal pain
RE
PAN
FMF
Relapsing fever

Back pain
Brucellosis
SBE

Fatigue
Carcinomas
Lymphomas
EBV/CMV mononucleosis
Enteric fevers
SLE
Late onset rheumatoid arthritis
    (LORA)
Toxoplasmosis

Mental confusion
Sarcoid meningitis
TB meningitis
Carcinomatous meningitis
CNS neoplasms
Brucellosis
Typhoid fever
Whipple's Disease

Adapted from Cunha BA. Fever of unknown origin (FUO). In: Gorbach SL, Bartlett JB, Blacklow NR, eds. Infectious Diseases. *3rd ed. Philadelphia, PA: Lippincott Williams & Wilkins; 2004.*

Table 3

Physical Clues to Fever of Unknown Origin

Skin hyperpigmentation
Whipple's disease
Histoplasmosis
Kala-azar

Band keratopathy
Still's disease (adult JRA)

Dry eyes
SLE
LORA
Sarcoidosis

Epistaxis
Relapsing fever
Psittacosis
Acute leukemias

Conjunctivitis
TB
Cat-scratch disease (CSD)
Brucellosis
SBE
CMV
LGV
Still's disease (adult JRA)

Conjunctival suffusion
Leptospirosis
Relapsing fever
Trichinosis

Subconjunctival hemorrhage
SBE
Trichinosis
Leptospirosis

Uveitis
TB
Still's disease (adult JRA)
SLE
Histoplasmosis
Brucellosis
LGV
CSD
Leptospirosis

Cytoid Bodies
SBE
CSD
PAN
SLE
TA
Atrial myxoma
Still's disease (adult JRA)

Tongue tenderness
Relapsing fever

Lymphadenopathy
Lymphomas
Cat-scratch disease (CSD)
TB
LGV
EBV infectious mononucleosis
CMV infectious mononucleosis
Toxoplasmosis
HIV
Still's disease (adult JRA)
Brucellosis
Whipple's disease
Pseudolymphoma
Kikuchi's disease
Kimura's disease

Sternal tenderness
Metastatic carcinoma
Preleukemias

Heart murmur
SBE
Atrial myxoma

Watery eyes
PAN
Histoplasmosis
Kala-azar

Hepatomegaly
Hepatoma
Relapsing fever
Lymphomas
Metastatic carcinoma
Alcoholic liver disease
Brucellosis
Q fever
Typhoid fever
Malaria
Kala-azar
Bartonella

Splenomegaly
Leukemia
Lymphomas
TB
Brucellosis
SBE
EBV infectious mononucleosis
CMV
Psittacosis
Q fever
Kikcuhi's disease
Kala-azar
Malaria

Relative bradycardia
Enteric fever
Leptospirosis
Psittacosis
Q fever
Central fever
Drug fever

Splenic abscess
SBE
Brucellosis
Enteric fevers
Still's disease (adult JRA)

Epididymo-orchitis
Tuberculosis
Lymphoma
Brucellosis
Leptospirosis
PAN
EBV infectious mononucleosis

Spinal tenderness
Subacute vertebral
    osteomyelitis
SBE
Brucellosis
Typhoid fever

Trapezius tenderness
Subdiaphragmatic abscess
Polymyositis

Arthritis & joint pain
FMF
Pseudogout
Rat-bite fever
LORA
SLE
LGV
Whipple's Disease
Brucellosis
Hyper IgD syndrome

Thrombophlebitis
Psittacosis

Thigh tenderness
Brucellosis
Polymyositis

Adapted from Cunha CB. Infectious Disease Differential Diagnosis. In: Cunha BA, (Editor): Antibiotic Essentials, (8th ed).
Jones & Bartlett, Sudbury, Massachusetts, 2009.

Table 4

Laboratory Clues to Fever of Unknown Origin

Monocytosis
Whipple's disease
Histoplasmosis
TB
PAN
Temporal arteritis (TA)
CMV
Histoplasmosis
Kala-azar
Malaria
Brucellosis
SBE
SLE
Lymphomas
Carcinomas
Regional enteritis (RE)
Myeloproliferative disorders

Leukopenia
Miliary TB
Brucellosis
SLE
Lymphomas
Preleukemias
Enteric fevers
Kikuchi's disease
Kala-azar
Psitticosis
EBV infectious mononucleosis
CMV infectious mononucleosis
Histoplasmosis
Cyclic neutropenia

Abnormal renal tests
SBE
Renal TB
PAN
Fabry's disease
Leptospirosis
Brucellosis
Lymphomas
SLE
Myeloproliferative disorders

Lymphocytosis
TB
EBV infectious mononucleosis
CMV infectious mononucleosis
Toxoplasmosis
Lymphomas
Histoplasmosis
Kala-azar
Whipple's disease

Basophilia
Carcinomas
Lymphomas
Preleukemias
Myeloproliferative disorders

Eosinophilia
Trichinosis
Lymphomas
Drug fever
Addison's disease
PAN
RE
Histoplasmosis
Hypernephroma
Myeloproliferative disorders

Lymphopenia
HIV
Whipple's disease
Histoplasmosis
Miliary TB
Malaria
SLE
Lymphomas
CMV
Typhoid fever
Whipple's Disease

Atypical lymphocytosis
EBV infectious mononucleosis
CMV infectious mononucleosis
Brucellosis
Malaria
Toxoplasmosis
Drug fever

Thrombocytosis
Myeloproliferative disorders
TB
Carcinomas
Lymphomas
PAN
Temporal arteritis (TA)
Subacute osteomyelitis
SBE
Q fever

Thrombocytopenia
Leukemias
Lymphomas
Myeloproliferative disorders
Relapsing fever
EBV infectious mononucleosis
Vasculitis
SLE
HIV
Malaria
Kala-azar
Miliary TB
Histoplasmosis

SPEP (polyclonal gammopathy)
Atrial myxomas
Alcoholic cirrhosis
Lymphomas
PAN
HIV
Takayasu's arteritis

↑Rheumatoid IgM factors
SBE
Chronic active hepatitis
Late onset rheumatoid arthritis
Hypersensitivity vasculitis

↑IgD immunoglobulins
Hyper IgD syndrome

ESR (>100 mm/h)
Still's disease (adult JRA)
Temporal arteritis
Hypernephroma
SBE
Drug fever
Carcinomas
Lymphomas
Myeloproliferative disorders
Abscesses
Subacute osteomyelitis
Polymyositis
Hyper IgD syndrome

↑Alkaline phosphatase
Hepatoma
Miliary TB
Histoplasmosis
Lymphomas
Still's disease (Adult JRA)
Subacute thyroiditis
Temporal arteritis
PAN
Liver metastases

↑Serum transaminases
EBV infectious mononucleosis
CMV
Q fever
Psittacosis
Drug fever
Leptosriopsis
Toxoplasmosis
Brucellosis
Relapsing fever
Kikuchi's disease

Adapted from Cunha CB. Infectious Disease Differential Diagnosis. In: Cunha BA, (Editor): Antibiotic Essentials, (8th ed). Jones & Bartlett, Sudbury, Massachusetts, 2009.

Laboratory Tests

CBC

• Routine laboratory tests may provide important clues about FUO (Table 4).

• *Leukopenia* may suggest *miliary TB, brucellosis, SLE or lymphoma*.

• *Monocytosis* may be the initial clue to *CMV, tuberculosis, brucellosis, lymphoma, regional enteritis (RE) or carcinoma*.

• *Eosinophilia* suggests *lymphoma, trichinosis, drug fever or periarteritis nodosa (PAN)*.

• *Basophilia* suggests *carcinoma* or *lymphoma*.

• *Chronic* lymphocytosis suggests CMV, *mononucleosis, TB, toxoplasmosis or CLL*.

ESR

• ESR is a sensitive but nonspecific test and is most useful when combined with other clinical and laboratory abnormalities.

> * *ESR >100 mm/h in a patient with FUO suggests drug fever, adult Still's disease, TA, LORA, FMF, PAN, SLE, subacute endocarditis, abscess, osteomyelitis, carcinoma and/or lymphoma*.

> * The *absence* of an elevated ESR *does not* rule out infectious, rheumatic or neoplastic causes of FUO.

LFTs

• Many of the diseases causing FUO have **hepatic** involvement.

• Elevations of *alkaline phosphatase* out of proportion to serum transaminases suggests an infiltrative or obstructive process, eg, *adult Still's disease*, subacute thyroiditis, TA or periarteritis nodosa (PAN).

• Elevations of the *serum transaminases*, with minimal or no elevations of the serum alkaline phosphatase, suggests infection of the liver, particularly CMV, EBV, Q fever, psittacosis or drug fever.

Serum protein electrophoresis (SPEP)

• SPEP may provide a clue to lymphoma with an *isolated elevation of the alpha 1/2 globulins*.

• *Polyclonal gammopathy* in a patient with an FUO suggests atrial myxoma, sarcoidosis, malaria, kala-azar, lymphoma or HIV.

Imaging Tests

• CT and MRI are useful in detecting intrahepatic, intrasplenic and intra-perinephric mass lesions.

• *Ultrasound of the abdomen often misses pathology*.

• Transthoracic (TTE) or transesophageal echocardiography (TEE) has been useful in detecting vegetations in SBE and cardiac myxomas.

• CT and MRI scans have been useful in detecting intracranial, intraabdominal and pelvic pathology.

• CT and MRI scans are the *best* way to detect *retroperitoneal lymphomas or subacute vertebral osteomyelitis*.

• *Gallium or indium scans* are useful in detecting abscesses or malignancies.

Invasive Diagnostic Procedures

• Liver biopsy and bone marrow biopsies are important diagnostic procedures *if clinical or laboratory clues point to these organ systems*.

• Liver biopsy may be the *only* way to make a diagnosis of miliary TB, or metastatic carcinoma, if infiltrate lesions are small and below the resolution of gallium or indium scanning.

• *Bone marrow biopsy* may provide the diagnosis in patients with enteric fevers, histoplasmosis or kala-azar.

- *Small bowel biopsy* is indicated in patients with the possibility of small intestinal lymphoma or Whipple's disease.

- CSF may provide clues to the presence of *meningeal carcinomatosis, LCM, CNS lymphoma, or basilar meningitis due to TB or sarcoidosis*.

- If temporal arteritis is a diagnostic possibility, then biopsy of the affected segments of the artery is usually diagnostic.

Problem Solving Approach

- Use the combined clinical clues from the history, physical examination, and laboratory tests to localize the process to an organ or organ system (Table 5).

- The *pattern of organ system involvement determines the differential diagnosis* and guides the FUO work-up. (Table 6-9)

Table 5

Recurrent Fever of Unknown Origin

Infectious Causes

Common
- Chronic prostatitis
- Subacute cholangitis

Uncommon
- FAPA syndrome
- Dental abscesses
- Malaria

Noninfectious Causes

Common
- Still's disease (adult JRA)
- Familial Mediterranean Fever (FMF)
- Regional enteritis (RE)
- SLE
- Drug fever
- Lymphomas
- Hyper IgD syndrome

(continued)

Table 5 *(continued)*

Uncommon
- Factitious fever
- Cyclic neutropenia
- Adrenal insufficiency
- Atrial myomas
- Beçet's disease
- Fabry's disease
- Gaucher's disease
- Fume fever
- Mastocytosis
- Habitual hyperthermia
- Ankylosing spondylitis
- Pseudolymphomas
- Rosai-Dorfman disease
- Kikuchi's disease
- Castleman's disease
- Hemophagocytic syndrome
- Familial Hibernian fever (TRAPS)
- Erdheim-Chester disease
- Muckle-Wells syndrome

Adapted from Cunha BA. Fever of unknown origin (FUO). In: Gorbach SL, Bartlett JB, Blacklow NR, eds. Infectious Diseases. 3rd ed. Philadelphia, PA: Lippincott Williams & Wilkins; 2004.

Adapted from Cunha BA, ed. Fever of Unknown Origin. New York, NY: Informa Healthcare: 2007.

Table 6

FUO Panels and Testing

FUO Infectious Panel	FUO Neoplastic Panel	FUO Rheumatic/Inflammatory Panel

Blood Tests
Special blood cultures
  (CO_2/6 weeks)
Q fever serology
Brucella serology
Bartonella serology
Salmonella serology
Viral serologies
  EBV
  CMV
  HHV-6
	Blood Tests
	Ferritin
	SPEP
		Blood Tests
		DS DNA
		SPEP
		Ferritin
		CPK
		ACE

Radiologic Tests
CT/MRI abdomen/pelvis[a]
Gallium scan
Panorex film of jaws (if all else negative)
	Radiologic Tests
	CT/MRI abdomen/pelvis
	Gallium scan
	BM biopsy (if myelophthistic anemia
	  abnormal RBCs/WBCs)
	TTE (if heart murmur with negative
	  blood cultures)
	PET scan
		Radiologic Tests
		Head/chest CT/MRI
		Temporal artery biopsy
		  (if ESR >100 without
		  alternate diagnosis)
		Low dose steroids
		  (Prednisone 10 mg/day
		  if PMR likely)
		PET scan

Other Tests Naprosyn test Anergy panel/PPD	**Other Tests** Naprosyn test	

[a] *Chest/head CT/MRI (if infectious etiology suspected in head/chest)*
Adapted from Cunha BA. Fever of Unknown Origin (FUO). *New York, NY: Informa Healthcare; 2007.*

Table 7

Focused Diagnostic Approach to FUO: Clues to Malignant Disorders

History

Fatigue (any neoplastic disorder)

Decreased appetite/weight loss (any neoplastic disorder)

Headache (primary/metastatic CNS neoplasms)

Cough (pulmonary neoplasms)

Night sweats (any neoplastic disorder)

Physical Findings

Relative bradycardia (lymphomas)

Sternal tenderness (preleukemias, myeloproliferative disorders, lymphoreticular malignancies)

Pleural effusion (lymphomas, pulmonary neoplasms, metastases)

Heart murmur (atrial myoma)

Hepatomegaly (hematoma, metastases, lymphomas)

Splenomegaly (leukemias, lymphomas)

Ascites (peritoneal/omental metastases)

Lymphadenopathy (lymphomas, CLL)

Epididymoorchitis (lymphoma)

Nonspecific Laboratory Tests

CBC

Leukocytosis (MPD, CLL)

Leukopenia (lymphoreticular malignancies)

Anemia (any malignancy)

Myocytes/metamyelocytes/nucleated RBCs/ "teardrop RBCs" (neoplastic bone marrow involvement)

Atypical (small/uniform) lymphocytes (CLL)

Eosinophilia (MPD, leukemias, lymphomas)

Basophilia (MPD, leukemias, lymphomas)

Thrombocytopenia (any malignancy with bone marrow involvement)

Thrombocytosis (any malignancy)

ESR

Highly elevated ESR >100 mm/hr (any neoplastic disorder)

LFTS

Increased alkaline phosphatase (hepatomas, lymphomas, liver metastases)

SPEP

Increased monoclonal gammopathy (multiple myeloma)

Increased α_1/α_2 globulins (lymphomas)

Serum Ferritin

Increased ferritin levels (MPD, any malignancy)

CNS = central nervous system; CLL = chronic lymphocytic lymphoma; ESR = erythrocyte sedimentation rate; SPEP = serum protein electrophoresis; MPD = myeloproliferative disorder
Adapted from Cunha BA. Fever of Unknown Origin (FUO). New York, NY: Informa Healthcare; 2007.

Table 8

Focused Diagnostic Approach to FUO: Clues to Rheumatic/Inflammatory Disorders

History

Dry eyes (LORA, SLE)

Watery eyes (PAN)

Vision disorders/eye pain (Takayasu's arteritis, TA)

Headache (temporal pain, TA)

Neck pain (jaw pain, adult JRA)

Dry cough (TA)

Abdominal pain (PAN, SLE)

Myalgias/arthralgias (PAN, adult JRA, FMF, LORA, SLE)
    generalized
    localized

Physical Findings
Eyes

Band keratopathy (adult JRA)

Conjunctivitis (SLE)

Uveitis (adult JRA, sarcoidosis, SLE)

Dry eyes (LORA, SLE)

Watery eyes (PAN)

Fundi [("cytoid bodies" (SLE), "candlewax drippings" (sarcoidosis)]

Lymphadenopathy (Kikuchi's disease, adult JRA)

Splenomegaly (SLE, LORA, sarcoidosis, Kikuchi's disease)

Epididymoorchitis (PAN)

(continued)

Table 8 *(continued)*

___

Focused Diagnostic Approach to FUO: Clues to Rheumatic/Inflammatory Disorders

Nonspecific Laboratory Tests
Blood Tests (all rheumatic disorders)

CBC

___

Leukopenia (SLE)

___

Lymphopenia (sarcoidosis/lymphoma syndrome)

___

Eosinophilia (sarcoidosis, PAN)

___

Thrombocytopenia (SLE)

ESR

___

Highly elevated ESR >100 mm/hr (all rheumatic disorders)

LFTs

___

Increased SGOT/SGPT (Kikuchi's disease, adult JRA)

___

Increased alkaline phosphatase (PAN)

SPEP

___

Polyclonal gammopathy (SLE, PAN, Takayasu's arteritis, Rosai-Dorfman disease)

___

Increased α_1/α_2 globulins (SLE)

Ferritin

___

Increased ferritin levels (adult JRA, SLE, TA, Rosai-Dorfman disease, LORA)

___

ESR = erythrocyte sedimentation rate; JRA = juvenile rheumatoid arthritis; LFTs = liver function tests
LORA = late onset rheumatoid arthritis; SPEP = serum protein electrophoresis; PAN = periarteritis nodosa
TA = temporal arteritis; FMF = familial Mediterranean fever
Adapted from Cunha BA. Fever of Unknown Origin (FUO). *New York, NY: Informa Healthcare; 2007.*

Table 9

Causes of FUO in the Elderly

Malignancies	Lymphomas
	Preleukemias
	Carcinomas
	Metastases
	MPDs
Infections	Subacute bacterial endocarditis (SBE)
	Abscesses
	Intra abdominal and subdiaphragmatic
	Periappendiceal
	Pericolonic
	Hepatic
	Intra- and perinephric
	Periapical dental
	Infected aortic aneurysm
	Infected vascular grafts
	Extrapulmonary tuberculosis
	Renal tuberculosis
	TB meningitis
	Miliary tuberculosis
	EBV infectious mononucleosis (elderly)
Rheumatologic	TA
	Still's disease (adult JRA)
	Late onset rheumatoid arthritis (LORA)
Other Causes	Drug fever
	Cirrhosis
	Vasculitis

Adapted from Cunha BA. Fever of unknown origin (FUO). In: Gorbach SL, Bartlett JB, Blacklow NR, eds. Infectious Diseases.
3rd ed. Philadelphia, PA: Lippincott Williams & Wilkins; 2004.

4. Fever of Unknown Origin in Special Populations

- FUO in *special* populations, eg, the elderly, pediatric patients, neutropenic patients, hospitalized patients and HIV patients.

- The causes of FUO in these subgroups are *largely the same diseases that cause FUOs in the general population*.

- Classifying FUO by specific subgroup population offers *no diagnostic advantage*.

FUO in the Ambulatory Setting

- FUO work-up usually diagnostic unless invasive procedures needed.

FUO in the Elderly

- Malignancy is *common*.

- Among infectious common causes are SBE, abscesses and TB. (Table 10)

FUO in HIV Patients

- Reflects the usual HIV pathogens.

- *Geographical* factors affect pathogen distribution, eg, leishmaniasis (Table 10)

Table 10

Fever of Unknown Origin in Human Immunodeficiency Virus (HIV)

Infectious Causes

Common[a]

HIV

Mycobacterium tuberculosis

Mycobacterium avium-intracellular (MAI)

CMV

Pneumocystis (carinii) jiroveci pneumonia (PCP)

Uncommon

Sinusitis

Toxoplasmosis

non-M tuberculosis/MAI mycobacteria

Noninfectious Causes

Drug fever

[a]*Leishmaniasis and histoplasmosis in patients from endemic areas.*
Adapted from Cunha BA. Fever of unknown origin (FUO). In: Gorbach SL, Bartlett JB, Blacklow NR, eds. Infectious Diseases. *3rd ed. Philadelphia, PA: Lippincott Williams & Wilkins; 2004.*

5. Recurrent Fever of Unknown Origin

- Few infectious diseases present as *recurrent* FUO.

- Usually noninfectious diseases cause recurrent FUOs.

- Some FUOs have no etiologic diagnosis (Table 6).

6. Therapy

Empiric therapy of FUOs

General Concepts

- There are only a few situations where empiric therapy of an FUO is clinically reasonable.

- Treat the *underlying cause* of the fever, *not* the fever itself.

Miliary TB

- In FUO patients when miliary TB is suspected/likely, empiric TB therapy is reasonable for presumed miliary TB in a rapidly deteriorating patient.

Culture Negative Endocarditis

- Patients with a heart murmur, cardiac vegetation, peripheral manifestations or SBE, and negative blood cultures.

Temporal Arteritis (TA)

- Empiric high dose (≥60 mg of prednisone daily) may be sight saving in FUOs when TA is the likely diagnosis.

7. Further Reading

Books

Cunha BA, ed. *Fever of Unknown Origin*. New York, NY: Informa Healthcare; 2007.

Keefer CS, Leard SE. *Prolonged and Perplexing Fevers*. Boston, MA: Little Brown; 1955:1248.

Murray HW, ed. FUO: *Fever of Undetermined Origin*. Mount Kisco, NY: Futura Publishing; 1983.

Journal Articles

Brusch JL, Weinstein L. Fever of unknown origin. *Med Clin North Am*. 1988;72:1247-1261.

Calabro JJ, Marchesano JM. Juvenile rheumatoid arthritis. *N Engl J Med*.1967;277:746-749.

Cunha BA. Fever of unknown origin. *Infect Dis Clin North Am*. 2007; 21:857-1220.

Esposito AL, Gleckman R. Fever of unknown origin in the elderly. *J Am Geriatr Soc*. 1978;26:498-505.

Johnson DH, Cunha BA. Drug fever. *Infect Dis Clin North Am*. 1996;10:85-91.

Kauffman CA, Jones PG. Diagnosing fever of unknown origin in older patients. *Geriatrics*. 1984;39:46-51.

Kazanjian PH. Fever of unknown origin. Review of 86 patients treated in community hospitals. *Clin Infect Dis*. 1992;15:968-973.

Louria DB. Fever of unknown etiology. *Del Med J*. 1971;43:343-348.

Petersdorf RG, Beeson PB. Fever of unexplained origin: report on 100 cases. *Medicine (Baltimore)*. 1961;40:1-30.

Petersdorf RG, Bennett IL. Factitious fever. *Ann Intern Med*. 1957;46:1039-1062.

Weinstein L. Clinically benign fever of unknown origin: a personal retrospective. *Rev Infect Dis*. 1985;7:692-699.

Wolf SM, Fauci SS, Dale DC. Unusual etiologies of fever and their evaluation. *Ann Rev Med*. 1975;26:277-279.

Chapter 5: Microbiology for the ID Boards

Daniel Caplivski, MD

Contents

Microbiology Overview

The infectious diseases board exam includes many images of pathogens that must be identified in order to answer the question correctly. The images in this chapter highlight some important characteristic morphologic findings that can be essential to making the correct diagnosis. Try to identify each of the organisms without looking at the names, and then review the key facts in the figure legend.

1. Acinetobacter

Acinetobacter baumanii is a good example of the challenges that exist in identifying certain bacteria by microscopy. It is described as a Gram-variable cocco-bacillus because as shown it can be either Gram-positive or Gram-negative and some of its forms will be round cocci and others will be short bacilli. It is an important pathogen in nosocomial infections because many isolates have extensive resistance to antimicrobials. (Figure 1)

ID Board Pearls

• *Acinetobacter* may stain Gram-positive or Gram-negative.

• Organisms may appear as cocci or bacilli.

• Despite extensive resistance to antimicrobials may still be susceptible to ampicillin/sulbactam.

2. Actinomyces

Actinomycetes are members of a group of higher order bacteria. This low power view of biopsy of a neck mass shows a characteristic sulfur granule: an actual colony of the organism within the tissue. The organism stains Gram-positive and has a branching, filamentous appearance. Differentiating the organism from *Nocardia, Rhodococcus* and some rapidly-growing *Mycobacteria* can be challenging. *Actinomyces* species replicate under anaerobic or microaerophilic conditions and do not retain acid-fast or modified acid-fast stains. (Figure 2)

ID Board Pearls

• Anaerobic or microaerophilic.

• Sulfur granules may be discharged from infection.

• Gram-positive branching rods that are negative on acid-fast or modified acid-fast stain.

3. Ascaris lumbricoides

Ascaris lumbricoides is the largest of the human nematodes and is readily identifiable with the naked eye. Most patients are asymptomatic, but children are more likely to present with intestinal obstruction in heavy infections because of the smaller diameter of the lumen of their GI tract. (Figure 3)

ID Board Pearls

• One quarter of the world's population is estimated to be infected.

• Can migrate to biliary tree and mimic cholecystitis or cholangitis.

• Usually treated with benzimidazole class (albendazole, mebendazole).

• Migratory path through lungs can cause fleeting infiltrates and eosinophilia (Loeffler's syndrome).

4. Aspergillus

Aspergillus species have a "fruiting head" appearance when grown in culture. This form can also be seen in tissue in patients with aspergilloma. The *aspergillum* is the hollow tube used in the Catholic mass to spread holy water among the pews. This image should help you remember the elemental structure of this mold in culture.

Aspergillus in histopathologic section has thin, septate hyphae with acute angle branching. In this example the organism can be seen traversing the blood vessel wall. This will cause local ischemia and the necrotic destruction of surrounding tissue, especially in immunocompromised hosts. (Figures 4,5)

ID Board Pearls

• May present as non-invasive aspergilloma or allergic bronchopulmonary aspergillosis.

• Duration of neutropenia is an important risk factor for invasive aspergillosis.

• Thin, septate hyphae with acute angle branching (compare to zygomycetes).

5. Babesia

Babesia species in a peripheral blood smear can be difficult to distinguish from *Plasmodium* species when only the ring forms are seen. In this example a tetrad of intraerythrocytic organism is also found. The "Maltese cross" describes this finding when the four merozoites are dividing in a cross formation. Extracellular merozoites are also much more common in *Babesia* infections. (Figure 6)

ID Board Pearls

• Maltese cross formation, extracellular merozoites, smaller rings than *Plasmodium*.

• *Babesia microti* is the most common species transmitted in the United States.

• *Babesia divergens* (found more commonly in Europe) causes more severe disease, especially in asplenic patients.

6. *Bacillus cereus*

Bacillus cereus is a Gram-positive rod that will form short chains. While Gram-positive rods in blood cultures may be inadvertently discounted as contaminants, it is important to be vigilant for invasive Gram-positive rods such as *Bacillus cereus*, *Bacillus anthracis*, *Clostridium perfringens*, *Listeria monocytogenes*, *Corynebacterium jekeium* and *Erysipelothrix* species. (Figure 7)

ID Board Pearls

• May cause infectious gastroenteritis from reheated rice.

• Heat stable toxin produces emetic form of disease.

• Heat labile toxin produces diarrheal form of disease.

7. *Campylobacter*

Campylobacter species appear on Gram stain as curved or spriochetal-like Gram-negative rods. This auramine-rhodamine stain emphasizes the spiral nature of the organism in culture. They have darting motility in wet preps and are a major cause of diarrhea in rural areas of the world where animal contamination of the water supply occurs. (Figure 8)

ID Board Pearls

• Associated with post-infectious Guillain-Barré Syndrome.

• Zoonotic infection sometimes acquired from improperly prepared poultry.

8. Candida

Candida albicans filamentous projections can be visible emanating from the circular colonies.

Candida species on Gram stain may appear as large Gram-positive oval cells that divide via budding. Pseudohyphae are the tubular structures that represent elongation of a new bud from a parent cell. Germ tubes are short, hyphal extensions from yeast cells incubated in human or sheep serum, and the presence of germ tubes is a rapid diagnostic test for *Candida albicans*. (Figures 9,10)

ID Board Pearls

- Candidemia often associated with broad spectrum antibiotics, central venous catheters and total parenteral nutrition.

- Non-*albicans* species may have variable susceptibility to fluconazole.

- *C albicans* is germ tube positive when incubated with human or sheep serum.

9. Clostridium perfringens

Clostridium perfringens in a blood culture Gram stain. These anaerobic Gram-positive rods will often have rounded to square ends. When viewed in India ink preparations, an area of clearing will highlight the capsule that surrounds it. The organism is nonmotile. Isolates of *Listeria* by contrast will have a tumbling, end-over-end motility when incubated at room temperature and have a pleomorphic appearance ranging from short rods to coccobacillary forms. (Figure 11)

ID Board Pearls

- Enterotoxin is heat-labile and may cause gastroenteritis.

- Irregular staining may cause a gram variable appearance.

- Clostridial myonecrosis is signaled by rapidly spreading infection and gas in tissue.

10. Cytomegalovirus

Cytomegalovirus inclusion bodies are seen in this histologic section in a patient with CMV colitis. Intranuclear inclusions are sometimes kidney bean-shaped, and retraction of the nuclear membrane can have the appearance of an owl's eye.
(Figures 35, 36)

ID Board Pearls

• Enlarged infected cell.

• Owl's eye basophilic intranuclear inclusion body.

• Primary infection associated with mononucleosis-like syndrome in older adults.

11. Cryptococcus neoformans

Cryptococcus neoformans from a cerebrospinal fluid stained with India ink. The clear area surrounding the budding yeast cell represents the polysaccharide capsule. The capsule is an important virulence factor and serves as the basis for serum and CSF Cryptococcal antigen testing. On Gram stain the organism can sometimes have a stippled appearance as the crystal violet is unable to fully penetrate the capsule. (Figure 12)

ID Board Pearls

• The only encapsulated yeast in the CSF is *Cryptococcus neoformans*.

• Non-viable *Cryptococcus neoformans* may be seen on CSF India ink stains for years after the infection.

• *Cryptococcus* meningitis is not accompanied by an intense CSF pleocytosis.

12. *Diphyllobothrium latum*

Diphyllobothrium latum egg in stool preparations stained with iodine. The eggs of the fish tapeworm have a lid-like structure called an operculum (barely visible on the bottom of this image). On the opposite (abopercular) end a small knob is visible. Several other members of the flatworm group have opercular structures; in particular the *flukes Fasciola, Paragonimus* and *Opistorchis*.

Diphyllobothrium latum—the fish tapeworm can be acquired by eating undercooked fish. The scolex attaches to the human intestine with two ventral grooves known as bothria. The organism then elongates via strobilization, a gradual addition of segments called proglottids. Eggs are passed in the feces and undergo further maturation in the water where the lifecycle is completed via infection of copepods and eventually fish. (Figures 13,15)

ID Board Pearls

• Scolex with ventral bothria.

• Can cause B12 deficiency.

• Abopercular knob on egg.

13. CA-MRSA

The D-Test is a test of inducible clindamycin resistance that is especially important to request in patients with community-acquired(CA- MRSA) infection. The "D" shape is seen when antibiotic-impregnated discs for erythromycin and clindamycin are placed in adjacent areas on a lawn of freshly prepared medium with CA-MRSA. Notice that there is an indentation in the zone of inhibition in the areas where erythromycin has diffused towards the clindamycin disc. This indicates the presence of the *erm* gene product, which mediates resistance to clindamycin and may predict clinical failure with this antibiotic. (Figure 14)

ID Board Pearls

• D-test predicts clindamycin failure based on inducible resistance.

• Trimethoprim-sulfamethoxazole susceptibility often maintained.

• Abscesses often require drainage for cure.

14. *Exophiala jeanselmei*

Giemsa stain of material expressed from a nodule in a case of cutaneous phaeohyphomycosis. This pigmented fungus can have both yeast cells as well as hyphal elements in tissue and grows as a black mold in culture. These dematiaceous fungi can cause painless subcutaneous nodules when introduced into the tissue from the environment by minor trauma. (Figure 17)

ID Board Pearls

• Phaeohyphomycosis: a group of infections caused by fungi with dark cell walls

• Both yeast cells as well as hyphal elements may be seen in tissue.

• Can cause cutaneous and subcutaneous infections as well as brain abscess and sinusitis

15. *Enterobius vermicularis*

Enterobius vermicularis female gravid with thousands of eggs. The female pinworm has lateral alae that allow her to migrate to the perianal skin and deposit eggs. The eggs produce a perianal inflammatory reaction and children will often scratch the area and end up with eggs under their nails. The autoinoculation cycle is completed when children put their fingers in their mouths. (Figure 16)

ID Board Pearls

• Pinworm eggs are identifiable on "Scotch-tape" test.

• Adequate decontamination of bedclothes required for cure.

• Eggs are thin-walled, ovoid and flattened on one side.

16. Fusarium

Fusarium species in culture have banana-shaped conidia. *Fusarium* is one of the few molds that can routinely be recovered in blood culture—particularly in neutropenic patients with skin lesions. *Fusarium* keratitis outbreaks have occurred as the result of contaminated contact lens care systems. (Figure 18)

ID Board Pearls

• Banana-shaped conidia.

• *Fusarium* keratitis associated with contact lens care systems.

• One of the few molds to be recovered in routine blood culture.

17. Fusobacterium

Fusobacterium species are anaerobic pleomorphic organism that may have a beaded spindle-like appearance. *Fusobacterium necrophorum* is the causative organism of Lemierre's syndrome: septic thrombophlebitis of the internal jugular vein, often accompanied by emboli to the lungs. (Figure 19)

ID Board Pearls

• *Fusobacterium necrophorum* causes Lemierre's syndrome.

• May present initially as sore throat and progress to internal jugular thrombosis and septic pulmonary emboli.

18. *Histoplasma capsulatum*

Histoplasma capsulatum stained with lactophenol blue after culture at 24° C. The filamentous form of this dimorphic fungus is the environmental mold phase. The tuberculate macroconidia at the end of the stalks are morphologically important in identifying the organism, and can be confused with the environmental saprophyte, *Sepodonium*. In the body at 37° C, the organism exists as a yeast cell that divides by budding.

Histoplasma capsulatum seen in its yeast phase on the peripheral blood smear of a patient with disseminated histoplasmosis. The small ovoid cells do not have a true capsule, but an artifact of staining causes a clearing around them that gives the organism its species name. They will be seen replicating within macrophages and granulomas in biopsies of tissues. (Figure 20)

ID Board Pearls

• Dimorphic fungus found in the warm, moist soil of riverbanks in the Midwestern United States, but also distributed globally.

• Yeast phase is morphologically similar to *Leishmania*—distinguished by absence of kinetoplast.

• Mold phase may be inhaled by spelunkers as the organism is found in heavy concentrations in bat guano.

19. *Leishmania*

Leishmania amastigotes are seen here in a Giemsa-stained smear of a scraping from an ulcerative lesion on the skin of a traveler who had spent 6 months in Sicily. The organisms are both intracellular and extracellular in this preparation. The kinetoplast is the small bar-like structure adjacent to the amastigote nucleus. It is important to identify this body, as it distinguishes the amastigote from the yeast phase of *Histoplasma capsulatum*. (Figure 21)

ID Board Pearls

• Transmitted by the sandfly vector.

• May cause cutaneous, mucocutaneous or visceral disease depending on species.

• Amastigotes distinguished from *Histoplasma capsulatum* by the presence of a kinetoplast.

20. *Mycobacterium tuberculosis*

Mycobacterium tuberculosis is shown here in the fluorescent auramine-rhodamine stain after growth in liquid culture. This stain has made screening of sputum specimens more effective, but finding the organism before culture confirmation remains a challenge when there is a paucity of organisms. The beaded, slightly curved shape of the bacilli can be appreciated.

Mycobacterium tuberculosis on Kinyoun (acid-fast) staining after culture in liquid media. The cording phenomenon is seen because the mycolic acid in the cell wall bestows hydrophobicity on the bacterium, which results in water exclusion and coalescing of the cells into serpentine cords. (Figure 22)

ID Board Pearls

• Dry colonies on Lowenstein Jensen Media.

• On microscopy of acid-fast stained smears have a curved, beaded appearance and may exhibit cording.

• MDR strains are resistant to isoniazid and rifampin.

• XDR strains are resistant to isoniazid, rifampin, fluoroquinolones and at least one of the second-line drugs.

21. *Neisseria meningitides*

Neisseria meningitidis in a Gram-stained smear of CSF from a patient with meningitis. The Gram-negative intracellular diplococci may have a kidney bean appearance. The organisms are typed into serogroups based on the polysaccharide capsule antigens. This capsule is also the basis for the quadrivalent conjugated vaccine that is protective against serogroups A, C, Y and W-135. (Figure 23)

ID Board Pearls

• Gram-negative diplococci often intracellular with kidney bean shape

• May cause fulminant meningococcemia with bilateral destruction of adrenal glands (Waterhouse-Friderichsen syndrome).

• Serogroups A, C, Y and W-135 are the capsular strains that are included in conjugate vaccine.

22. Nocardia

Nocardia species have a delicately beaded, branching, filamentous appearance on Gram stain. They can be difficult to distinguish from other Gram-positive organisms that have a tendency to become filamentous (*Actinomyces, Gordona, Rhodococcus*). *Nocardia* will also be identifiable by the modified acid-fast stain. (Figure 24)

ID Board Pearls

• Gram-positive finely-beaded, branching filamentous rods.

• Partial acid-fast staining will retain modified acid-fast stain.

• May cause disseminated disease in immunocompromised hosts, including pulmonary and central nervous system infection.

23. Paracoccidioides brasiliensis

Paracoccidioides brasiliensis is seen here after culture and stained with lactophenol blue. The typical "mariner's wheel" results from multiple budding from the mother cell. This dimorphic fungus can cause invasive pulmonary and gingival infection in patients from South America. There is a strong male predominance that is thought to be related to estrogen inhibition of the organism's conversion from the mold to the yeast phase. (Figure 25)

ID Board Pearls

• "Mariner's wheel" appearance of mother cell budding in multiple directions.

• Endemic in rural South America.

• Prominent male:female ratio possibly related to protective effect of estrogen.

24. Plasmodium falciparum

Plasmodium falciparum malaria can be recognized on peripheral blood smear because of its tendency towards heavy parasitemia and multiply-infected erythrocytes with relatively normal size compared to non-infected cells. Appliqué forms are merozoites that are abutting the inner aspect of the erythrocyte membrane. A banana or sausage-shaped gametocyte is pathognomonic for *falciparum* malaria. The schizonts of *Plasmodium falciparum* are generally not visible in the peripheral blood smear because the infected schizonts express adhesive projections that mediate attachment to endothelial tissue. (Figure 26)

ID Board Pearls

• Heavy parasitemia, fatal disease, infected cells are the same size as non-infected cells.

• Multiply-infected erytherocytes, accole forms, schizonts generally not seen on peripheral blood smear, only ring forms.

• Banana-shaped gametocytes sometimes seen.

25. Proprionibacterium acnes

Proprionibacterium acnes infections of ventricular-peritoneal shunts are important to recognize. *Proprionibacterium acnes* in a single blood culture may be discarded as a contaminant, but this anaerobic bacterium with rudimentary branching may cause true infection in patients with ventricular-peritoneal shunts. (Figure 27)

ID Board Pearls

• Anaerobic Gram-positive branching bacillus.

• May cause ventriculoperitoneal shunt infections.

• May cause acne vulgaris in teenagers and young adults.

26. Zygomycetes

Rhizomucor is shown here on solid media. This opportunistic mold is one of the zygomycetes that causes rhinocerebral mucormycosis. Invasive infection is most often seen in patients with conditions such as neutropenia, organ transplantation and diabetes. Diabetic ketoacidosis and iron chelation therapy with desfuroxime make more iron (a growth factor) available to the organism, and patients with these conditions are also at increased risk for mucormycosis.

Rhizomucor in histologic section stained with methenamine-silver. The histologic appearance is characterized by broad, ribbon-like non-septate hyphae that branch at right angles. As seen here, the organism is capable of penetrating blood vessels and other structures in immunocompromised hosts. (Figure 28, 29)

ID Board Pearls

• Ribbon-like hyphae branching at right angles. No septations.

• Risk factors include diabetic ketoacidosis, neutropenia, organ transplant and desfuroxime iron chelation therapy.

• In culture, root-like structures can be seen.

27. Salmonella typhi

Salmonella typhi seen as Gram-negative rods recovered in the blood culture of a patient with typhoid fever. The organism survives intracellularly and is passed from human to human via contaminated food, water or direct fecal-oral spread. The elongation of some of the bacilli seen in this specimen is likely due to incomplete cell wall synthesis because of inhibition by beta-lactam antibiotics given prior to the blood culture. (Figure 30)

ID Board Pearls

• Gram-negative rods that produce black pigment, triple sugar iron slant.

• Replicate intracellularly and accumulate in Peyer's patches, leading in some cases to intestinal perforation.

• Non-typhoidal strains are also associated with endovascular infection in association with damaged endothelial tissue.

28. Veridans streptococcus

Streptococcus mitis on blood agar plate showing incomplete or alpha hemolysis. Alpha hemolytic streptococci are further divided by their susceptibility to optochin. *Veridans streptococcus* is resistant to optochin, while *Streptococcus pneumoniae* is susceptible. The *veridans* group of streptococci is often associated with subacute presentations of infectious endocarditis.

Streptococcus mitis seen on Gram stain. The organism is seen here as Gram-positive cocci in long chains. When clumps of chains are superimposed they may be confused with the clusters of *Staphylococcus* species. (Figure 31,32)

ID Board Pearls

• *Veridans streptococcus* group is Gram-positive cocci in chains with alpha hemolysis.

• Optochin antibiotic disc: *veridans streptococcus* is optochin-resistant, while *Streptococcus pneumoniae* is optochin-susceptible.

29. Streptococcus pneumoniae

Streptococcus pneumoniae on Gram stain of CSF in a patient with severe pneumococcal meningitis. The Gram-positive cocci will appear as lancet-shaped diplococci. The capsule is at times visible as a clearing of background stain around the organism. The polysaccharide capsule is an important virulence factor and a target of the polyvalent vaccines. (Figure 33)

ID Board Pearls

• Gram-positive lancet-shaped diplococci may appear in short chains.

• Capsular polysaccharide is basis for polyvalent vaccines.

• Higher risk for severe diseases in patients with asplenia and terminal complement deficiencies.

30. *Strongyloides stercoralis*

Strongyloides stercoralis larvae found in the stool of a patient with ulcerative colitis whose diarrhea was worsening with corticosteroid treatment. This nematode maintains a chronic autoinfection cycle over many years as some of the larvae passed in the stool re-enter the body via the perianal skin. Immunosuppression can lead to a hyperinfection syndrome with overwhelming dissemination of the filariform larvae. This syndrome can be accompanied by polymicrobial sepsis from enteric organisms traveling with the larvae. This carries a high mortality when it is not recognized early in the course of the illness. (Figure 34)

ID Board Pearls

• Infective filariform larvae penetrate intact skin. Penetration of perianal skin can lead to cycle of autoinfection for many years.

• Immunosuppression with corticosteroids or other medications may lead to hyperinfection syndrome, possibly presenting with polymicrobial bacterial sepsis with diffuse pulmonary infiltrates.

• Associated with recurrent infections despite treatment in patients infected with HTLV-1.

31. Photomicrographs

Figure 1

Acinetobacter baumanii gram variable

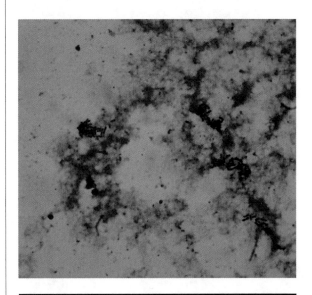

Figure 2

Actinomyces sulfur granule

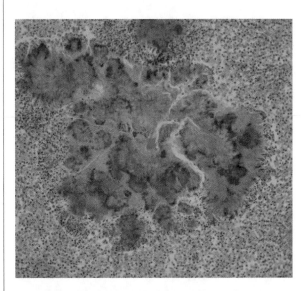

Figure 3

Ascaris lumbricoides

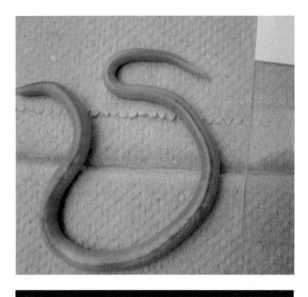

Figure 5

Aspergillus in tissue biopsy

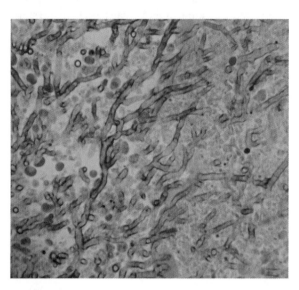

Figure 4

Aspergillus in culture

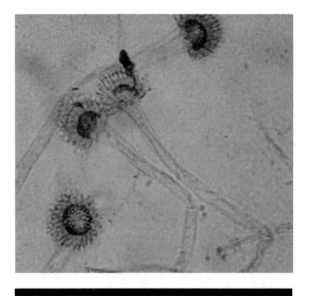

Figure 6

Babesia microti

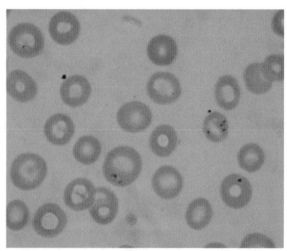

Figure 7

***Bacillus cereus* in blood culture**

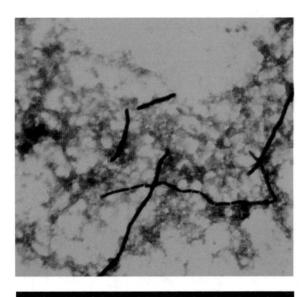

Figure 8

***Campylobacter* on auramine rotamine stain**

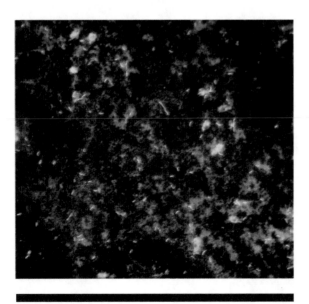

Figure 9

***Candida albicans* foot processes**

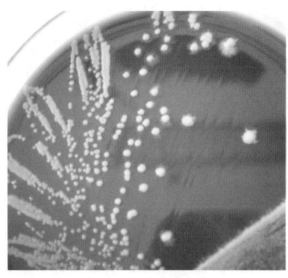

Figure 10

***Candida* with pseduohyphae**

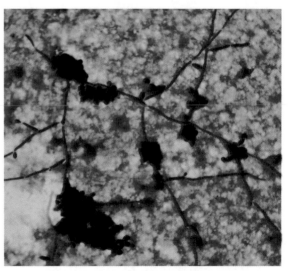

Figure 11

Clostridium perfringens in blood culture

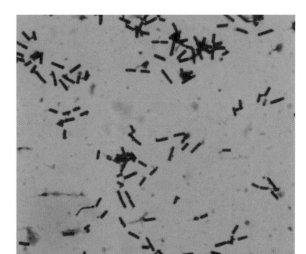

Figure 12

Cryptococcus neoformans India ink stain

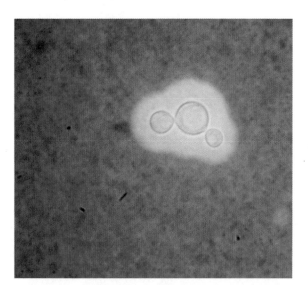

Figure 13

D latum egg with knob on abopercular end

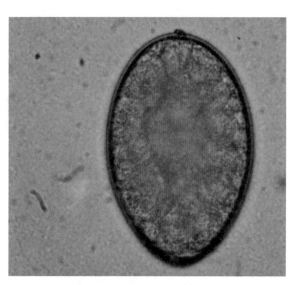

Figure 14

D test for inducible clindamycin resistance

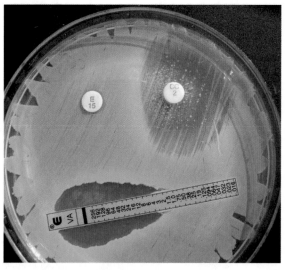

Figure 15

Diphyllobothrium latum

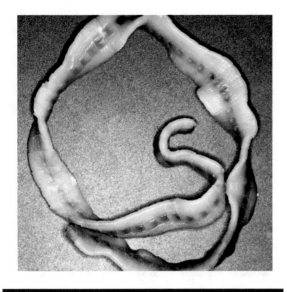

Figure 16

Enterobius gravid female with eggs

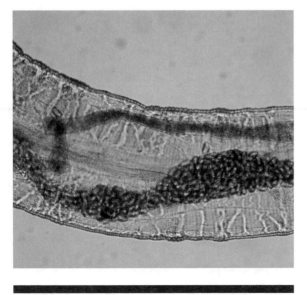

Figure 17

Exophiala jeanselmei on Giemsa stain

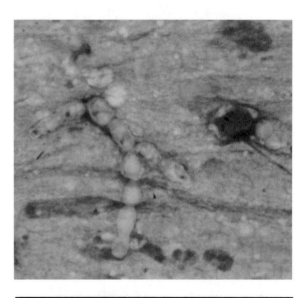

Figure 18

Fusarium banana-shaped conidia

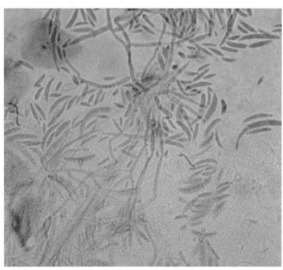

Figure 19

***Fusobacterium* in culture**

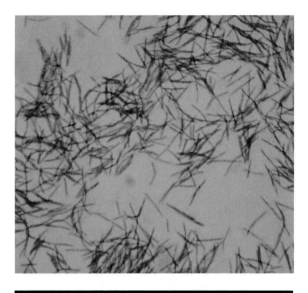

Figure 20

***Histoplasma capsulatum* in culture**

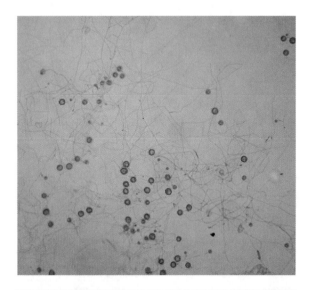

Figure 21

***Leishmania* parasites with prominent kinetoplasts**

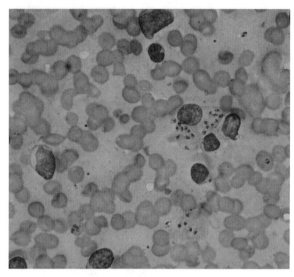

Figure 22

***Mycobacterium tuberculosis* auramine rotamine stain**

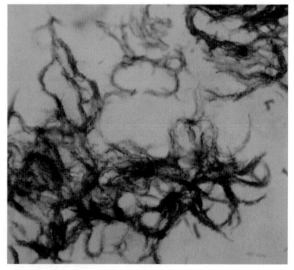

Figure 23

Neisseria meningitidis CSF gram stain

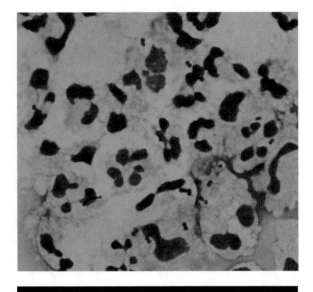

Figure 24

Nocardia Gram stain

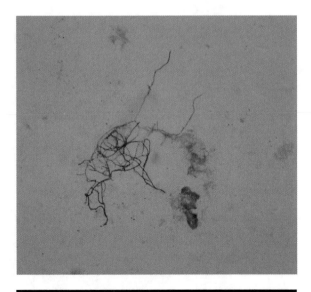

Figure 25

Paracoccidioides brasiliensis in culture with mariner's whee

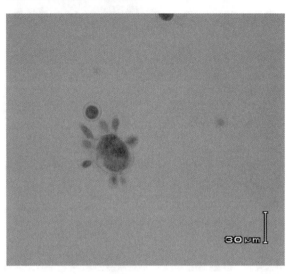

Figure 26

Plasmodium falciparum

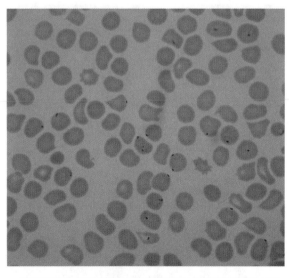

Figure 27

Proprionibacterium acnes CSF shunt infection

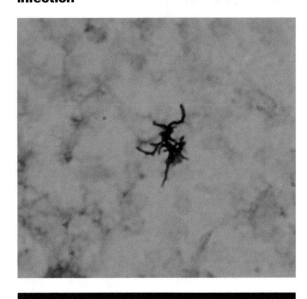

Figure 28

Rhizopus in culture

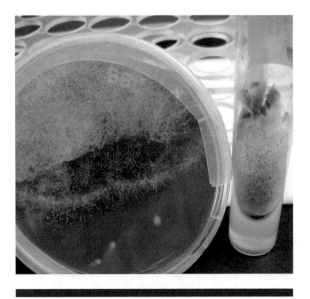

Figure 29

Rhizopus silver stain

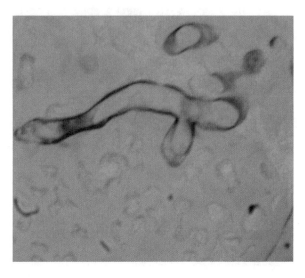

Figure 30

Salmonella typhi Gram stain

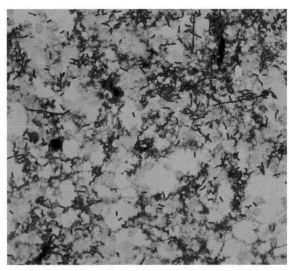

Figure 31

Streptococcus mitis alpha hemolysis

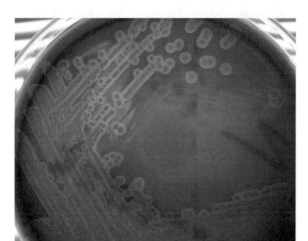

Figure 32

Streptococcus mitis

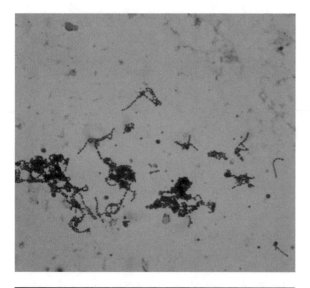

Figure 33

Streptococcus pneumoniae CSF gram stain

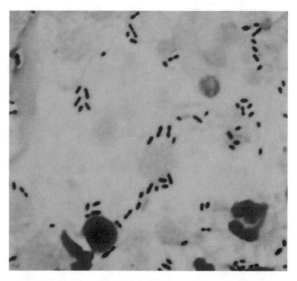

Figure 34

Strongyloides stercoralis larvae in stool specimen

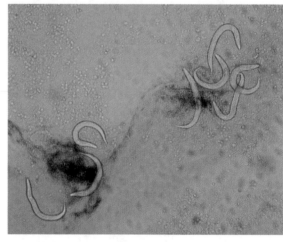

Figure 35

Cytomegalovirus

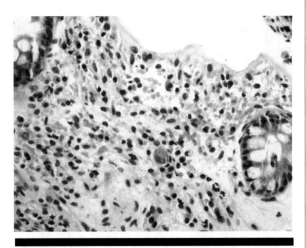

Image courtesy of Alexandros D. Polydorides, M.D., Ph.D.

Figure 36

Immunohistochemical stain specific to CMV antigens

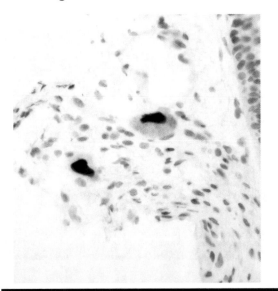

Image courtesy of Alexandros D. Polydorides, M.D., Ph.D.

32. Further Reading

Ash L, Orihel T. *Atlas of Human Parasitology*. 3rd ed. Chicago, IL: ASCP Press; 1990.

Bottone E. *An Atlas of the Clinical Microbiology of Infectious Diseases, Volume 1: Bacterial Agents*. New York, NY: Parthenon Publishing; 2004.

Bottone E. *An Atlas of the Clinical Microbiology of Infectious Diseases, Volume 2*: Viral, Fungal, and Parasitic Agents. Boca Raton, FL: Taylor and Francis; 2006.

Mandell G, Bennett J, Dolin R. *Mandell, Douglas, and Bennett's Principles and Practice of Infectious Diseases*. 6th ed. Philadelphia, PA: Elsevier

Chapter 6: Human Immunodeficiency Virus (HIV) Infection for the ID Boards

Paul E. Sax, MD

Contents

1. Introduction

- Infection with human immunodeficiency virus type-1 (HIV-1) leads to a chronic and, if untreated, usually fatal infection characterized by progressive immunodeficiency, a long clinical latency period and opportunistic infections. The hallmark of HIV disease is infection of, and viral replication within, T-lymphocytes expressing the CD4 antigen, a critical component of normal cell-mediated immunity. Qualitative defects in CD4 responsiveness and progressive depletion in CD4+ cell counts increase the risk for opportunistic infections such as Pneumocystis carinii jiroveci pneumonia (PCP), and neoplasms such as non-Hodgkin's lymphoma and Kaposi's sarcoma. HIV infection can also disrupt blood monocyte, tissue macrophage, neutrophil, and B-lymphocyte (humoral immunity) function, predisposing to infection with encapsulated bacteria and Gram-negative bacilli. Direct attack of CD4+ cells in the central and peripheral nervous systems can cause HIV meningitis, peripheral neuropathy and dementia.

- Nearly 1 million people in the United States and 40 million people worldwide are infected with HIV. Without treatment, the average time from acquisition of HIV to an AIDS-defining opportunistic infection is about 10 years; survival then averages 1-2 years. However, there is tremendous individual variability in these time intervals, with some patients progressing from acute HIV infection to death within 1-2 years, and others not manifesting HIV-related immunosuppression for >20 years after HIV acquisition. Antiretroviral therapy and prophylaxis against opportunistic infections has markedly improved the overall prognosis of HIV disease.

2. HIV Disease Stages

Viral Transmission

- HIV infection is acquired primarily by sexual intercourse (anal, vaginal, infrequently oral), exposure to contaminated blood (primarily needle transmission) or maternal-fetus (perinatal) transmission. Sexual practices with the highest risk of transmission include unprotected receptive anal intercourse (especially with mucosal tearing), unprotected receptive vaginal intercourse (especially during menses) and unprotected rectal/vaginal intercourse in the presence of genital ulcers (eg, primary syphilis, genital herpes, chancroid). Lower risk sexual practices include unprotected insertive anal/vaginal intercourse and oral-genital contact. The mode of transmission does not affect the natural history of HIV disease.

Acute (Primary) HIV Infection

- In most patients, a symptomatic flu-like syndrome occurs 1-4 weeks after HIV transmission. Termed acute (or primary) HIV, this is accompanied by extremely high HIV RNA levels (often >1 million copies/mL) and usually also a moderate decline in the CD4+ cell count. Acute HIV infection is confirmed by demonstrating a high viral load in the absence of HIV antibody. Most experts recommend treatment with antiretroviral therapy during this period, although the duration of such therapy is not clear.

Seroconversion

- Development of a positive HIV antibody test usually occurs within 4 weeks of acute infection, and in nearly 100% by 6 months.

Asymptomatic HIV Infection

- Asymptomatic HIV infection lasts a variable amount of time (average 8-10 years), and is accompanied by a gradual decline in CD4+ cell counts and a relatively stable HIV RNA level (sometimes referred to as the viral "set point").

- Findings include thrush or vaginal candidiasis (persistent, frequent or poorly responsive to treatment), cervical dysplasia/carcinoma *in situ*, herpes zoster (recurrent episodes or involving multiple dermatomes), oral hairy leukoplakia, peripheral neuropathy, diarrhea or constitutional symptoms (eg, low-grade fevers, weight loss). Previously referred to as AIDS-related complex, or ARC.

AIDS

• AIDS is defined by a CD4+ cell count <200/mm³, a CD4+ cell percentage of total lymphocytes <14% or the presence of one of several AIDS-related opportunistic infections. Some of the more common opportunistic infections include *Pneumocystis carinii* pneumonia, cryptococcal meningitis, recurrent bacterial pneumonia, *Candida* esophagitis, CNS toxoplasmosis, tuberculosis, non-Hodgkin's lymphoma, CMV disease and disseminated *Mycobacterium avium-intracellulare* (MAI) infection.

Advanced HIV Disease

• Patients with CD4+ cell counts <50 cells/mm3 are considered to have advanced HIV disease. Most AIDS-related deaths occur at this point. Common late-stage opportunistic infections are caused by CMV disease (retinitis, colitis), disseminated *Mycobacterium avium-intracellulare* (MAI), HIV-associated wasting and HIV dementia.

3. Acute (Primary) HIV Infection

General Concepts

• Acute clinical illness associated with *primary acquisition of HIV*, occurring *1-4 weeks after viral transmission* (range: 6 days to 6 weeks). Symptoms develop in 50%-90%, but are *often mistaken for the flu* or other nonspecific viral syndrome and not diagnosed.

ID Board Pearls

• *More severe symptoms* may *correlate with more rapid HIV disease progression.*

• As a general rule, *patients will recover spontaneously without treatment*, reflecting development of an effective immune response and *depletion of susceptible CD4+ cells.*

Differential Diagnosis

• *Differential diagnosis* includes EBV, CMV, influenza, viral hepatitis, enteroviral infection, secondary syphilis, toxoplasmosis, HSV with erythema multiforme, drug reaction, Behçet's disease and acute SLE. (Figure 1)

Signs and Symptoms

General Concepts

• Signs and symptoms usually *reflect hematogenous dissemination of virus to lymphoreticular and neurologic sites*:

   * Fever (96%)

   * Lymphadenopathy (74%)

   * Pharyngitis (70%): Typically non-exudative (unlike EBV, which is usually exudative)

   * Rash (70%): Maculopapular viral exanthem of the face and trunk is most common, but can involve the extremities, palms and soles; mucocutaneous ulceration involving mouth, esophagus or genitals

   *Arthralgia/myalgia (54%)

   *Diarrhea (32%)

*Neurologic symptoms (12%): *Headache is most common;* neuropathy, Bell's palsy and meningoencephalitis are rare.

Laboratory Findings

General Concepts

CBC
- *Lymphopenia* followed by lymphocytosis (common).

- *Atypical lymphocytosis is usually absent/mild* (unlike EBV, where atypical lymphocytosis may be 20%-30% or higher).

- Elevated transaminases in some (but not all patients).

- *Isolated "cytopenias" common* (leukopenia, thrombocytopenia).

- Depressed CD4+ cell count. Can rarely be low enough to induce opportunistic infections.

- HIV antibody. *Usually negative,* although persons with prolonged symptoms of acute HIV may have positive antibody tests if diagnosed late during the course of illness.

- HIV RNA (or "viral load"): *invariably high-titer positive.*

Figure 1

Diagnosing suspected HIV infection

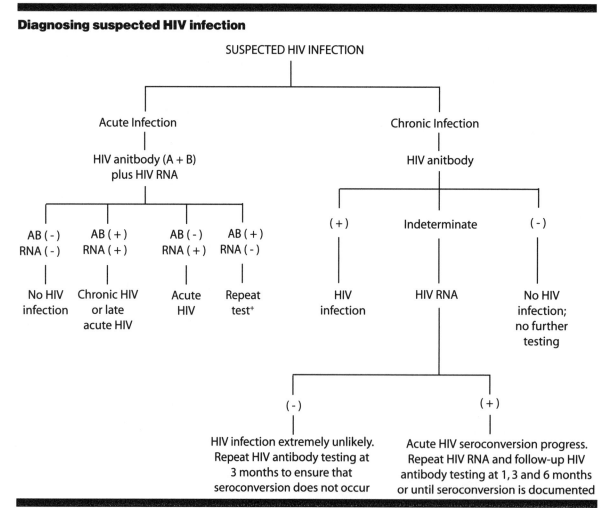

From Sax PE. HIV Essentials. *Royal Oak, MI: Physicians' Press; 2007*

4. HIV Antibody Testing

ID Board Pearls

- Heterophile usually negative, although rarely positives have occurred; therefore, a positive heterophile does not exclude the diagnosis of acute HIV

Confirming the Diagnosis of Acute HIV Infection

General Concepts

- Obtain HIV antibody test after informed consent to exclude prior disease.

- Order *viral load test* (HIV RNA PCR), preferably RT-PCR (lower limit of 400 copies/mL). HIV RNA confirms acute HIV infection prior to seroconversion. Most individuals will have very high viral loads (>100,000 copies/mL).

- For any positive test result, repeat both HIV RNA and do follow-up antibody testing at 1, 3 and 6 months until HIV antibody turns positive. p24 antigen can also be used to establish the diagnosis, but is less sensitive than HIV RNA PCR.

- Order other tests/serologies as indicated. May include throat cultures for bacterial/viral respiratory pathogens, heterophile tests, EBV VCA IgM/IgG, CMV IgM/IgG, HHV-6 IgM/IgG and hepatitis serologies as appropriate to establish a diagnosis for the patient's symptoms.

ID Board Pearls

- Be suspicious of a *false-positive test if the viral load is low* (<20,000 copies/mL).

General Concepts

- *Most patients produce antibody to HIV within 6-8 weeks of exposure; half* will have a *positive antibody test in 3-4 weeks,* and nearly 100% will have detectable antibody by *6 months*.

ELISA
- Usual screening test. *All positives are confirmed with Western blot* or other more specific tests.

Western Blot
- CDC criteria for interpretation:

    * *Positive*: At least 2 of the following bands: p24, gp41, gp160/120

    * *Negative*: No bands

    * *Indeterminate*: Any HIV band, but does not meet criteria for positivity

Test Performance

- *The 2-step HIV antibody testing is highly accurate.*

    * ELISA negative: (ELISA sensitivity 99.7%, specificity 98.5%). No further testing is required, unless acute or recently acquired HIV suspected; in such cases, obtain an HIV RNA test as noted above

    * ELISA positive confirmed with Western blot: The probability that ELISA and Western blot are both false-positives is extremely low (<1 per 140,000 in one series of blood donors)

    * Unexpected ELISA/Western blot result: Repeat test to exclude clerical/computer error

Indeterminate Western Blot

- Causes include seroconversion in progress; advanced HIV disease with loss of antibody response; cross-reacting antibody from pregnancy, blood transfusions, organ transplantation; autoantibodies from collagen vascular disease; infection with HIV-2; influenza vaccination; or recipient of HIV vaccine.

• Approximately 4%-20% of reactive ELISAs are then read as "indeterminate" on the confirmatory Western blot. This is *usually due to a single p24 band or weak other bands*.

• *In low-risk patients, an indeterminate result almost never represents true HIV infection;* options include repeating the test in 2-3 and 6 months (if still indeterminate, reassure) or ordering a viral load test (if negative, reassure; if viral load is high, seroconversion is in progress) or both.

5. Initial Assessment of HIV-infected Patients

General Concepts

Clinical Evaluation

• History and physical examination should *focus on diagnoses associated with HIV infection. Most of these conditions also occur commonly in patients without HIV.*

• However, the *severity, frequency and duration* of these conditions are usually increased in HIV disease.

Dermatologic (HSV)

• Severe *herpes simplex* (oral/anogenital); *herpes zoster* (VZV) (especially recurrent, cranial nerve, or disseminated); *molluscum contagiosum; staphylococcal abscesses; tinea* nail infections; *Kaposi's sarcoma* (from HHV-8 infection); petechiae (from ITP); *seborrheic dermatitis; new or worsening psoriasis; eosinophilic pustular folliculitis;* severe cutaneous drug eruptions (especially sulfonamides).

Oropharyngeal

• Oral candidiasis; oral hairy leukoplakia (from EBV); Kaposi's sarcoma (frequently on palate/gums); gingivitis/periodontitis; warts; apthous ulcers (especially esophageal/perianal).

Constitutional Symptoms

• Fatigue, fevers, *chronic diarrhea*, weight loss.

Lymphatic

• Persistent, *generalized lymphadenopathy*.

Others
• Active TB (especially *extrapulmonary*).

• Non-Hodgkin's lymphoma (*especially CNS*).

• Myopathy.

ID Board Pearls

- *Unexplained leukopenia and/or anemia, thrombocytopenia* (including ITP) should suggest HIV.

- Otherwise unexplained miscellaneous neurologic conditions (Bell's palsy, other cranial/peripheral neuropathies, Guillain-Barré syndrome, mononeuritis multiplex, aseptic meningitis, cognitive impairment) should suggest HIV.

Baseline Laboratory Testing

CD4+ Cell Count (Lymphocyte Subset Analysis):

General Concepts

- The absolute CD4+ cell count is calculated by multiplying the lymphocyte count (obtained on a routine differential) by the percentage of lymphocytes that are CD4+ (measured by flow cytometry).

- Cell counts remain stable over 5-10 years in 5% of patients, while others may show rapid declines (>300 cells/year).

- *Since variability exists within individual patients and between laboratories, it is useful to repeat any value before making management decisions.*

ID Board Pearls

- Acute HIV infection is characterized by *a marked decline in CD4+ cell count, followed by a gradual rise associated with clinical recovery.*

- Chronic HIV infection shows *progressive decline* (~50-80 cells/year) in CD4+ cell count without treatment, *followed by more rapid decline 1-2 years prior to opportunistic infection* (AIDS-defining diagnosis).

Uses of CD4+ Cell Count

General Concepts

- Gives context of *degree of immunosuppression for interpretation of symptoms* and signs.

- Used to guide therapy: most guidelines support CD4+ <350/mm³ as a threshold for consideration of initiating antiretroviral therapy.

- Prognosis in these patients is markedly influenced by performance status, presence/history of opportunistic infections or neoplasms, and HIV RNA.

- In the current treatment era, CD4+ cell counts <50 do not carry nearly as grim a prognosis as they did prior to combination antiretroviral therapy; many therapy-naïve patients can have dramatic clinical, immunologic and virologic responses to treatment.

ID Board Pearls

- All guidelines state that therapy should be started with CD4+ count <200, regardless of HIV RNA.

- For prophylaxis against PCP, toxoplasmosis and MAC/CMV infection, CD4+ cell counts of 200/mm³, <100/mm³ and <50/mm³ are used as threshold levels, respectively.

- Provides estimate of risk of death: CD4+ cell counts <50/mm³ are associated with a markedly increased risk of death (median survival, 1 year), although some patients with low counts survive >3 years even without antiretroviral therapy.

Assays and Interpretation

- Tests, sensitivities and dynamic range: 3 assays are FDA-approved, each with advantages and disadvantages. Any assay can be used to diagnose acute HIV infection and guide/monitor therapy, but the same test should be used to follow patients longitudinally.

  * RT-PCR Amplicor®: Sensitivity, 400 copies/mL; dynamic range, 400-750,000 copies/mL

  * RT-PCR Ultrasensitive 1.5®: Sensitivity, 50 copies/mL; dynamic range, 50-50,000 copies/mL

  * bDNA Versant 3.0®: Sensitivity, 75 copies/mL; dynamic range, 75-500,000 copies/mL

- Correlation between *viral load* and CD4+ count: Viral load assays correlate inversely with CD4+ cell counts, but do so imperfectly (eg, some patients with high CD4+ counts have relatively high viral loads and vice versa). For any given CD4+ count, higher viral loads correlate with more rapid CD4+ decline.

- Significant change in *viral load* assay is defined by *at least a 2-fold (0.3 log$_{10}$) change in viral RNA* (accounts for normal variation in clinically stable patients), *or a 3-fold (0.5 log$_{10}$) change in response to new antiretroviral therapy* (accounts for intra-laboratory and patient variability).

- For example, if a viral load result is 50,000 copies/mL, then the range of possible actual values is 25,000-100,000 copies/mL, and the value needed to demonstrate antiretroviral activity is 17,000 copies/mL or less.

Indications for Viral Load Testing

General Concepts

- *Usually performed in conjunction with CD4+ cell counts.* Indicated for the diagnosis of acute HIV infection and for initial evaluation of newly diagnosed HIV.

- Also recommended 2-8 weeks after initiation of antiretroviral therapy, and every 3-4 months in all HIV patients (Figure 2).

ID Board Pearls

- *In response to antiretroviral therapy, changes in viral load generally precede changes in CD4+ cell count.*

Figure 2

Indications for initiating antiretroviral therapy

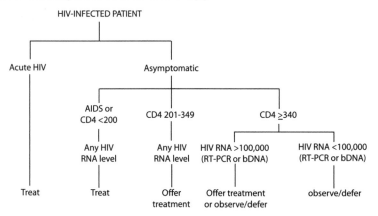

Combination antiretroviral therapy has led to dramatic reductions in HIV-related morbidity and mortality for patients with severe immunosuppression (CD4 <200/mm^3) or a prior AIDS-defining illness. Treatment of asymptomatic patients is far more controversial, many of whom live years before developing any HIV-related symptom. As a result, not all asymptomatic patients with HIV require antiretroviral therapy. Potential benefits of starting antiretroviral therapy with relatively high CD4+ cell counts include reduction in HIV RNA, prevention of immunodeficiency, delayed time to onset of AIDS, and decreased risk of drug toxicity, viral transmission, and selecting resistant virus. Potential risks of early antiretroviral therapy include reduced quality of life (from side effects/inconvenience), earlier development of drug resistance (with consequent transmission of resistant virus), limitation in future antiretroviral choices, unknown long-term toxicity of antiretroviral drugs, and unknown duration of effectiveness.

The primary goals of therapy are prolonged suppression of viral replication to undetectable levels (HIV RNA <50-75 copies/mL), restoration/preservation of immune function, and improved clinical outcome. Once initiated, antiretroviral therapy is usually continued indefinitely.

From Sax PE. HIV Essentials. Royal Oak, MI: Physicians' Press; 2007

6. Antiretroviral Therapy

General Concepts

- *Advances in antiretroviral therapy have led to dramatic reductions in HIV-related morbidity and mortality* for patients with severe immunosuppression (CD4+ count <200) or a prior AIDS-defining illness. All such patients should therefore be treated.

- *Treatment of asymptomatic patients, however, is far more controversial*, as many of them live years before developing any HIV-related symptom.

- Potential benefits of early antiretroviral therapy include easier control of viral replication, reduction in viral load, prevention of immunodeficiency, delayed time to onset of AIDS, and decreased risk of drug toxicity, viral transmission and selecting resistant virus.

- Potential risks of early antiretroviral therapy include reduced quality of life (from side effects/inconvenience), earlier development of drug resistance (with consequent transmission of resistant virus and limitation in future antiretroviral choices), unknown long-term toxicity of antiretroviral drugs and unknown duration of effectiveness.

- Once initiated, antiretroviral therapy is usually continued indefinitely, although research is ongoing to define the role of intermittent treatment.

Choice of initial antiretroviral therapy treatment with at least 3 active agents is now the standard of care (Table 1 and Table 2).

- *Advantages*. Most clinical data and longest follow-up for viral suppression.

- *Disadvantages*. Complexity, high pill burden, long-term toxicity and drug interactions may compromise future protease inhibitor (PI) regimens.

ID Board Pearls

- The primary goals of therapy are to *prolong survival and improve quality of life*. Studies show that this *is most reliably accomplished with suppression of viral replication to undetectable levels*

(viral load <50-75 copies/mL), which allows for the most robust increase in CD4+ cell counts.

Antiretroviral Treatment Failure

General Concepts

- Decisions about when and how to change antiretroviral therapy are highly controversial. There are several overlapping definitions of drug failure, including virologic failure, immunologic failure and clinical failure; these are discussed further below.

- Virologic failure generally precedes immunologic failure, and immunologic failure generally precedes clinical failure.

- Changes due to drug toxicity are more straightforward.

- If the patient has an HIV RNA level <50-75 *copies/mL* (virologic suppression), often a single drug substitution from the same drug class is appropriate.

Criteria for Virologic Failure

- Less than a 0.5-0.75 $\log_{10}$ reduction in plasma HIV RNA by 4 weeks after starting therapy, or <1 $\log_{10}$ reduction by 8 weeks.

- *Failure to suppress plasma HIV RNA to undetectable levels within 4-6 months of starting therapy.* The degree of initial decrease in plasma HIV RNA and overall trend in decreasing viremia should be considered before changing therapy. For example, a patient with a viral load >750,000 copies/mL before therapy who stabilizes after 6 months of therapy at a level that is detectable but <10,000 copies/mL may not warrant an immediate change in therapy, so long as the trend is still downward.

ID Board Pearls

- *Repeated detection of virus in plasma after initial suppression to undetectable levels, suggesting the development of resistance.* The degree of plasma HIV RNA increase should be considered. For example, it may be reasonable to consider close,

Table 1

Antiretroviral Components Recommended for Treatment of HIV-1 Infection in Treatment-Naïve Patients: DHHS Guidelines[a]

SELECT NRTI PAIR PLUS EITHER NNRTI OR PI

	NRTI Pair	NNRTI	PI
Preferred	• Tenofovir/ emtricitabine[b,d]	• Efavirenz[c]	• Atazanavir + ritonavir • Fosamprenavir + ritonavir (2x/d) • Lopinavir/ritonavir[d] (2x/d) • Lopinavir/ritonavir[d] (1x/d) • Duranavir + ritonavir
Alternative	• Zidovudine/lamivudine[b,d] • Didanosine + (emtricitabine or lamivudine) • Abacavir/lamivudine (if negative for HLAB*5701)	• Nevirapine[e]	• Atanavir[f] • Fosamprenavir (2x/d) • Fosamprenavir + ritonavir (1x/d) • Saquinavir + ritonavir

Adapted from: Sax PE, Cohen CJ, Kuritzkes DR. *HIV Essentials.* Sudbury, MA: Jones & Bartlett; 2009.
Adapted from: Panel on Antiretroviral Guidelines for Adults and Adolescents. *Guidelines for the use of antiretroviral agents in HIV-1 infected adults and adolescent.* Department of Health and Human Services. *November 3, 2008; 1-139.* Available at http://www.aidsinfor.nih.gov/ContentFiles/AdultandAdolescentGL.pdf. *Accessed on March 23, 2009.*

[a] A combination antiretroviral regimen in treatment-naïve patients generally containing 1 NNRTI + 2 NNRTI's, or a single or ritonavir-boosted PI + 2 NRTIs. Selection of a regimen for an antiretroviral-naïve patient should be individualized based on virologic efficacy, toxicities, pill burden, dosing frequency, drug-drug interaction potential and comorbid conditions.
[b] Emtricitabine may be used in place of lamivudine and vice versa.
[c] Efavirenz is not recommended for use in the first trimester of pregnancy or in sexually active women with child-bearing potential who are not using effective contraception.
[d] Co-formulated.
[e] Nevirapine should be initiated in women with CD4+ count >250 cells/mm³ or in men with CD4+ count >400 cells/mm³ because of increased risk of symptomatic hepatic events.
[f] Atazanavir must be boosted with ritonavir if used in combination with tenofovir.

Table 2

Initial Antiretroviral Components Regimens: International AIDS Society-USA Treatment Guidelines

SELECT NRTI PAIR PLUS EITHER NNRTI OR PI

	NRTI Pair[a]	NNRTI	PI
Preferred	• Tenofovir/emtricitabine[b,c] • Zidovudine/lamivudine[b,c] • Abacavir/lamivudine[b,c] • Didanosine + lamivudine[b,c]	• Efavirenz[d] • Nevaripine[e]	• Atazanavir • Darunavir + ritonavir • Lopinavir/ritonavir[c] • Atazanavir + ritonavir • Saquinavir + ritonavir • Fosamprenavir + ritonavir

Adapted from: Sax PE, Cohen CJ, Kuritzkes DR. *HIV Essentials.* Sudbury, MA: Jones & Bartlett; 2009.
Adapted from: Panel on Antiretroviral Guidelines for Adults and Adolescents. *Guidelines for the use of antiretroviral agents in HIV-1 infected adults and adolescent.* Department of Health and Human Services. November 3, 2008; 1-139. Available at http://www.aidsinfor.nih.gov/ContentFiles/AdultandAdolescentGL.pdf. Accessed on March 23, 2009.

[a] *Triple-NRTI regimens are no longer recommended as initial therapy because of insufficient antiretroviral potency compared with a regimen containing efavirenz. However, for patients requiring treatment with regimens that preclude use of NNRTI's or PI's, a combination consisting of zidovudine, abacavir and lamivudine may be considered.*
[b] *Emtricitabine may be used in place of lamivudine and vice versa.*
[c] *Co-formulated.*
[d] *Efavirenz is not recommended for use in the first trimester of pregnancy or in sexually active women with child-bearing potential who are not using effective contraception.*
[e] *Nevirapine should be initiated in women with CD4+count >250 cells/mm³ or in men with CD4+ count >400 cells/mm³ because of increased risk of symptomatic hepatic events.*

short-term observation in a patient whose plasma HIV RNA increases from undetectable to low level detectability (50-5000 copies/mL) at 4 months. Most patients who fall into this category, however, will likely show progressive increases in plasma viremia and require a change in therapy.

- *Any reproducible significant increase* (more than 3-fold) *from the nadir of plasma HIV RNA not caused by intercurrent infection, vaccination or test methodology.*

Risk Factors for Virologic Failure

- Risk factors include low drug levels (due to poor adherence, enhanced metabolism from drug interactions or diminished absorption); high baseline viral load or low baseline CD4+ cell counts (patients with advanced disease are at greater risk of failing therapy); slow viral load response, genetic factors (heterozygotes for mutant CCR5 may be more likely to respond); baseline viral resistance (due to prior antiretroviral therapy [common] or primary acquisition of a highly drug resistant strain [uncommon]); and inadequate potency of the regimen (for example, mono- or dual-nucleoside therapy).

- The optimal management of virologic failure in patients who are otherwise doing well (with good CD4+ restoration and clinical status) is not well established. One approach is to change therapy as soon as virologic failure is evident, since continued treatment with nonsuppressive regimens selects for additional resistance mutations. Another approach is to change therapy only for immunologic or clinical failure, given the discordance between virologic failure and clinical failure ("CD4+/viral load disconnect"); increased pill burden/side effects associated with subsequent regimens; the perception that changing treatment too soon may exhaust future options; and lack of guarantee that changing regimens improves prognosis. Our general approach is to change early with HIV RNA rebound in patients who have multiple other treatment options—where many alternative therapies exist—and to defer changing when extensive antiretroviral resistance is present. A review of the patient's adherence to the antivirals is a key component of any evaluation of treatment failure. Resistance testing (discussed below) is also a central component of choosing new regimens.

Immunologic Failure

- Immunologic failure is defined by a progressive decline in CD4+ cell count. When HIV RNA has also rebounded or is increasing, a change in therapy is recommended based on results of resistance testing and previous antiretroviral regimen. For patients who have continued virologic suppression but declining CD4+ cell counts, the optimal management strategy is uncertain; epidemiologic studies suggest that these patients generally have a good prognosis and treatment changes are not mandatory.

Clinical Failure

- Clinical failure is defined as HIV disease progression (eg, constitutional symptoms, opportunistic infections, recurrent bacterial pneumonia). Change in therapy is recommended based on results of resistance testing and previous antiretroviral regimen.

- Antiretroviral treatment failure can be defined in various ways. These include virologic failure (inability to achieve virologic suppression or occurrence of virologic rebound), immunologic failure (progressive CD4+ decline) and clinical failure (HIV disease progression). Causes of treatment failure include inadequate adherence, preexisting drug resistance, regimen complexity, side effects and suboptimal pharmacokinetics. All of these factors can lead to persistent viral replication and evolution of drug resistance.

- Therapeutic goals for patients who have experienced treatment failure vary depending on the treatment history; subsequent regimens generally need to be individualized, with the help of resistance testing. Such testing can identify drugs that are likely to be active in patients with prior treatment failures, although other factors, such as regimen tolerability, drug-drug interactions and achievable plasma concentrations are also important. Developing an individualized, optimized antiretroviral regimen ensures that each patient receives drugs with the greatest chance of achieving success. This strategy has been adopted in several recent clinical trials in order to demonstrate greater efficacy of the test drug over the best regimen derived from approved agents, sometimes called an optimized background regimen.

- Poor medication adherence is the most common cause of treatment failure. With poor adherence, sub-inhibitory drug levels occur, allowing ongoing viral replication and often the emergence of resistant virus. Such resistant variants are likely preexisting mutants that have escaped drug control or host immune failure. The level of adherence required to prevent treatment failure varies depending on the regimen used. In the early protease inhibitor era, there was a sharp increase in failure rates when adherence fell below 95%. A more recent analysis suggests that lower levels of adherence are required when using NNRTI-based regimens, likely due to the longer plasma half-life of nevirapine and efavirenz compared with PIs. One potential limitation of this analysis for the current treatment era is that it involved unboosted PIs, which have less favorable pharmacokinetics than PIs given with low-dose ritonavir.

- For patients with virologic failure due to noncompliance, the first step is to establish how much of the combination regimen is being taken. Often a patient will have stopped an entire regimen simultaneously, due either to poor tolerability or psychosocial issues. In this context, virologic failure usually occurs without the development of antiretroviral drug resistance, as viremia occurs in the absence of selective pressure of the antivirals. Starting a new regimen (one with the goal of fewer side effects) or restarting the same regimen with a renewed emphasis on the importance of adherence may result in treatment of virologic suppression.

Types of Treatment Failure
- *Virologic failure* is most strictly defined as the inability to achieve or maintain virologic suppression. In a treatment-naïve patient, the HIV RNA level should be <400 copies/mL after 24 weeks or <50 copies/mL by 48 weeks after starting therapy. Virologic rebound is seen when there is repeated detection of HIV RNA after virologic suppression in either treatment-naïve or treatment-experienced patients.

- *Immunologic failure* can occur in the presence or absence of virologic failure, and is defined as a failure to increase the CD4+ cell count by 25-50 cells/mm^3 above baseline during the first year of therapy, or as a decrease in CD4+ cell count to below baseline count while on therapy.

- *Clinical failure* is the occurrence or recurrence of HIV-related events after at least 3 months on potent antiretroviral therapy, excluding events related to an immune reconstitution inflammatory syndrome (IRIS).

- *Usual sequence of treatment failure.* Virologic failure usually occurs first, followed by immunologic failure and finally by clinical progression. These events may be separated by months or years and may not occur in this order in all patients.

- *Goals after virologic failure.* When patients have detectable HIV RNA on treatment, clinicians should attempt to identify the cause of their lack of response and set a new treatment goal. Patients with limited or intermediate prior treatment experience, such as those failing their first antiretroviral regimen, should be treated with the intention of achieving a HIV RNA level below the limit of quantification using ultrasensitive HIV RNA assays (<50 copies/mL with RT-PCR or <75 copies/mL using bDNA) in order to prevent the selection of additional resistance mutations. Provided that medication adherence issues and regimen tolerability have been addressed, the regimen should be changed sooner rather than later.

- On the other hand, achieving an undetectable HIV RNA level in patients with an extensive prior treatment history may not be possible. The main goals in these patients should be partial suppression of HIV RNA below the pretreatment baseline level, which in turn leads to the preservation of immune function and the prevention of clinical progression. A likely explanation for this phenomenon is that continued antiretroviral therapy in the face of resistance selects for less fit virus, ultimately leading to less immunologic damage. It is well documented that such patients on treatment have a slower CD4 cell decline than those not on therapy that have wild-type virus. Consequently, even with extensive drug resistance and virologic rebound, antiviral therapy should be continued, since stopping therapy is associated with higher rates of disease progression. (From *Sax PE, Cohen CJ, Kuritzkes DR*. HIV Essentials. *Sudbury, MA: Jones & Bartlett; 2009*.)

Resistance Testing and Selection of New Antiretroviral Therapy

General Concepts

- In cases of virologic failure, resistance testing has become standard practice to help guide appropriate choices in therapy. The two types of tests available are resistance genotype and resistance phenotype .

- *Genotypic assays* characterize nucleotide sequences of the reverse transcriptase/protease portions of the virus and identify resistance mutations associated with various drugs.

- *Phenotypic assays* attempt to grow the virus (or more accurately, a genetic construct of the patient's virus) in the presence of drugs, providing a more intuitively applicable measurement of resistance (similar to that done with bacteria).

- **Compared to phenotypic assays**, genotypic assays are faster (1-2 weeks vs. 2-3 weeks for results), less expensive ($400 vs. $1000), and have less inter-laboratory variability; however, mutations do not always correlate with resistance and results are sometimes difficult to interpret.

ID Board Pearls

- *Genotype testing is used for most patients*. Reserve the use of *phenotype* testing for instances in which interpretation of the genotype is *highly complex or confusing*.

Morphologic and Metabolic Abnormalities Associated with HIV and Its Treatment

General Concepts

Lipodystrophy Syndrome
- The prevalence of this syndrome varies widely

(5%-75%), depending on the definition used; most clinical cohort studies suggest that 30%-60% of patients on HIV treatment will have some subjective alteration in body habitus.

- The most common manifestation is *subcutaneous fat atrophy, which occurs most prominently in the face, limbs and buttocks*; the appearance engendered by marked fat atrophy can give the appearance of wasting even when a patient has a good CD4+ cell count and a suppressed HIV RNA level.

- Fat accumulation, manifesting as an *increase in visceral abdominal fat, a dorsocervical fat pad or breast enlargement is less common*, but can also be quite disfiguring. Patients may have predominantly fat atrophy, accumulation or a mixed picture.

- The optimal treatment awaits definition. Experimental options include cosmetic surgery (collagen or polylactate injections, liposuction), insulin sensitizing agents, growth hormone, metformin and aggressive treatment of hyperlipidemia.

ID Board Pearls

- *Risk factors* identified in some studies for this syndrome *include treatment with NRTI/protease inhibitor combinations, older age, longer duration of HIV infection and AIDS, and lower CD4+ nadir*. All of the PIs and NRTIs have been implicated. The current paradigm is that treatment factors interface with host factors; that NRTIs induce fat wasting through mitochondrial toxicity, protease inhibitors lead to fat accumulation, and the 2 together accelerate fat cell apoptosis.

Metabolic Abnormalities

General Concepts

- *The predominant metabolic abnormalities associated with treatment are hyperlipidemia, insulin resistance and elevated lactate*. The hyperlipidemia and insulin resistance are most strongly linked to PI-based therapy. Since hypertriglyceridemia is often marked, initial use of a fibrate (gemfibrozil 600 mg BID or fenofibrate 67 mg

QD) is recommended, followed if necessary by a statin. Pravastatin (at a starting dose of 20 mg QD) is the preferred statin for patients on PIs, since it is not metabolized through the CYP3A4 cytochrome p450 pathway; atorvastatin can be used cautiously as well.

Lactic Acidosis/Hepatomegaly with Fatty Degeneration (Hepatic Steatosis)

ID Board Pearls

- Simvastatin and lovastatin are contraindicated with PIs.

General Concepts

- Clinical presentation *includes nonspecific GI complaints (abdominal distension/pain, nausea, vomiting), weakness, weight loss and sometimes dyspnea.*

- In addition to elevated serum lactate levels, patients may have an anion gap metabolic acidosis, and elevated liver transaminases (with concomitant hepatic steatosis), CPK, LDH, lipase and amylase.

- Treatment includes withdrawal of NRTIs and supportive care as needed, including hemodialysis and mechanical ventilation.

ID Board Pearls

- *This is a rare but potentially fatal complication* most often associated with prolonged use of NRTIs, in particular d4T.

7. Overview of Opportunistic Infections in HIV Disease

General Concepts

- Patients with HIV disease are at risk for infectious complications not seen in immunocompetent patients. Such opportunistic infections occur in proportion to the severity of immune system dysfunction (reflected by CD4+ cell count depletion and duration at such levels). While community acquired infections (eg, pneucoccal pneumonia) can occur at any CD4+ cell count, the "classic" HIV-related opportunistic infections (PCP, toxoplasmosis, cryptococcus, disseminated *M avium intracellulare* complex, CMV) do not occur until CD4+ cell counts are dramatically reduced. Specifically, it is rare to encounter PCP in HIV patients with CD4+ count >200/mm³ for a prolonged period of time.

Prevention of Opportunistic Infections

- The guidelines for prevention of opportunistic infections (OIs) have been extensively revised over the past few years to reflect the major effect potent antiretroviral therapy has on risk for OIs.

- As a general rule, *response to immunizations is improved with higher CD4+ cell counts.* As a result, for patients with low CD4+ counts, it may be optimal to initiate antiviral therapy first and defer immunization until the CD4+ count has increased to >200 cells/mm³.

Pharmacologic Prophylaxis of Opportunistic Infections in HIV

General Guidelines

- If possible, give vaccines early in the course of HIV infection, while the immune system may still respond.

- Alternatively, to increase the likelihood of response in patients with *advanced HIV disease*, vaccines should be administered *after* retroviral *therapy has increased CD4+ cell count* >200. Vaccines should be given when patients are clinically stable, not acutely ill (eg, give during a routine office visit, rather than during hospitalization for an OI).

- *Live vaccines* (eg, oral polio, oral typhoid, yellow fever) are *generally* contraindicated, but measles vaccine is well-tolerated in children, and MMR (measles, mumps, rubella) vaccine is recommended for adults as described below.

P (carinii) jiroveci Pneumonia (PCP)

- *Indications:* CD4+ <200/mm^3, oral thrush, constitutional symptoms, or previous history of PCP.

- *Preferred prophylaxis.* TMP-SMX 1 DS tablet PO QD or 1 SS tablet PO QD. 1 DS tablet PO 3 times a week is also effective, but daily dosing may result in fewer missed doses.

Alternate prophylaxis

- *Dapsone* 100 mg PO QD (preferred as second-line by most; more effective than aerosolized pentamidine when CD4+ cell count <100; may also partially protect against toxoplasmosis), or

- *Atovaquone* 1500 mg PO QD (comparably effective to dapsone and aerosolized pentamidine; more GI toxicity vs. dapsone, but less rash), or

- *Aerosolized pentamidine* 300 mg via Respirgard II nebulizer® once monthly (exclude active pulmonary TB first to avoid nosocomial transmission).

- *Without prophylaxis*, 80% of AIDS patients develop PCP, and 60%-70% relapse within 1 year after the first episode. Prophylaxis with TMP-SMX also reduces the risk for bacterial infections and cerebral toxoplasmosis. Among patients with prior non-life threatening reactions to TMP-SMX, 55% can be successfully rechallenged with 1 SS tablet daily, and 80% can be rechallenged with gradual dose escalation using TMP-SMX elixir (8 mg TMP + 40 mg SMX/mL) given as 1 mL for 3 days, then 2 mL for 3 days, then 5 mL for 3 days, then 1 SS tablet PO QD. Macrolide regimens for MAI (azithromycin, clarithromycin) add to efficacy of PCP prophylaxis. Primary and secondary prophylaxis may be discontinued if CD4+ cell counts increase to >200 cells/mm^3 for 3 months or

longer in response to antiretroviral therapy (ie, immune reconstitution).

- Prophylaxis should *be resumed if the CD4+ cell count decreases to <200/mm^3*.

Toxoplasmosis

General Concepts

- *Indications:* CD4+ count <100/mm^3 with positive toxoplasmosis serology (IgG).

- *Preferred prophylaxis:* TMP-SMX 1 DS tablet PO QD.

- *Alternate prophylaxis:*

  * Dapsone 50 mg PO QD + pyrimethamine 50 mg PO weekly + folinic acid 25 mg PO weekly, or

  * Dapsone 100 mg + pyrimethamine 50 mg twice weekly (no folinic acid), or

  * Atovaquone 1500 mg PO QD

- *Primary prophylaxis* can be discontinued if CD4+ cell counts increase to >200/mm^3 for at least 3 months in response to antiretroviral therapy.

- *Secondary prophylaxis* (chronic maintenance therapy) may be discontinued in patients who responded to initial therapy, remain asymptomatic and whose CD4+ counts increase to >200/mm^3 for 6 months or longer in response to antiretroviral therapy. Secondary prophylaxis should be restarted if the CD4+ count decreases to <200/mm^3.

- Some experts would obtain an MRI of the brain as part of the evaluation prior to discontinuation of secondary prophylaxis.

ID Board Pearls

- The incidence of toxoplasmosis in *seronegative patients is too low to warrant chemoprophylaxis*.

Tuberculosis (*M tuberculosis*)

General Concepts

- *Indications.* **Any CD4+ cell count with PPD induration ≥5 mm, history of positive** PPD without prior treatment or close contact with active case of TB. Must exclude active disease (chest x-ray mandatory).

- *Preferred prophylaxis.* INH 300 mg PO QD for 9 months + pyridoxine 50 mg PO QD x 9 months.

- *Alternate prophylaxis.* Rifampin 600 mg PO QD for 2 months + pyrazinamide 20 mg/kg PO QD for 2 months.

- Consider prophylaxis for skin test-negative patients when the probability of prior TB exposure is >10% (eg, patients from developing countries, IV drug abusers in some cities, prisoners). However, a trial testing this strategy in the United States did not find a benefit for empiric prophylaxis. INH prophylaxis delayed progression to AIDS and prolonged life in Haitian cohort with positive PPD treated for 6 months.

- Rifampin plus pyrazinamide for 2 months was effective in a multinational clinical trial; watch for possible increased risk of hepatotoxicity. Rifabutin may be substituted for rifampin in rifampin-containing regimens.

ID Board Pearls

- Rifampin *should not* be given to patients receiving *amprenavir, indinavir, lopinavir + ritonavir, nelfinavir, saquinavir or delavirdine*.

Atypical Mycobacteria
M avium-intracellulare (MAI)

General Concepts

- *Indications:* CD4+ count <50/mm³.

- *Preferred prophylaxis:*

  * Azithromycin 1200 mg PO once a week

(fewest number of pills; fewest drug interactions; may add to efficacy of PCP prophylaxis), or

  * Clarithromycin 500 mg PO BID (more effective than rifabutin; associated with survival advantage; resistance detected in some breakthrough cases)

- Alternate prophylaxis. Rifabutin (less effective).

  * Macrolide options (azithromycin, clarithromycin) preferable to rifabutin. Azithromycin is preferred for patients on protease inhibitors due to simplicity and fewer drug interactions. Primary prophylaxis may be discontinued if CD4+ cell counts increase to >100/mm³ for 3 months or longer in response to anti-retroviral therapy. Secondary prophylaxis may be discontinued for CD4+ cell counts that increase to >100/mm³ for 6 months or longer in response to antiretroviral therapy if patients have completed 12 months of MAI therapy and have no evidence of disease

ID Board Pearls

- *Resume MAI prophylaxis for CD4+ count <100/mm³.*

Pneumococcus (*S pneumoniae*)

General Concepts

- *Indications.* Generally recommended for all patients with CD4+ >200/mm³.

- *Preferred prophylaxis.* Pneumococcal polysaccharide (23 valent) vaccine (same dose as for normal hosts). Revaccinate at 5 years.

ID Board Pearls

- Incidence of invasive pneumococcal disease is >100-fold higher in HIV patients. *Reimmunize if initial vaccine is given when CD4+ count <200/mm³, but is now >200/mm³ due to antiretroviral therapy.*

Influenza

General Concepts

- *Indications.* Generally recommended for all patients.

- *Preferred prophylaxis.* Influenza vaccine.

- Optimally between October and January.

ID Board Pearls

- *Give annually inactivated whole virus and split virus vaccine* (same dose as for normal hosts).

Hepatitis B

General Concepts

- *Indications.* All susceptible (anti-HbcAb negative and anti-HBsAg negative) patients.

- *Preferred prophylaxis.* Hepatitis B recombinant DNA vaccine (same dose as for normal hosts).

ID Board Pearls

- *Response rate is lower than in HIV-negative controls. Repeat series if no response is achieved, especially if CD4+ count was low during initial series and is now increased.*

Hepatitis A

General Concepts

- *Indications.* All susceptible patients who are also infected with hepatitis C; rubella vaccine (same dose as for normal hosts) infected with hepatitis C; HAV-susceptible seronegative gay men or travelers to endemic areas; any chronic liver disease.

- *Preferred prophylaxis.* Hepatitis A vaccine (same dose as for normal hosts).

ID Board Pearls

- *Response rate is lower than in HIV-negative controls.*

H influenzae

General Concepts

- *Indications.* Not generally recommended for adults.

- *Preferred prophylaxis. H influenzae* type B polysaccharide vaccine (same dose as for normal hosts).

ID Board Pearls

- Incidence of *H influenzae* disease is increased in HIV patients, *but two-thirds are caused by non-type B strains. Unclear whether vaccine offers protection.*

Measles, Mumps, Rubella

- *Indications.* Patients born after 1957 and never vaccinated; patients vaccinated between 1963 and 1967.

- *Preferred prophylaxis.* MMR (measles, mumps, rubella) vaccine (same dose as for normal hosts).

Travel Vaccines (same dose as for normal hosts)

- *Indications.* Travel to endemic areas.

- All considered *safe except oral polio, yellow fever and live oral typhoid.*

Treatment of Opportunistic Infections

- Antiretroviral therapy (ART) and specific antimicrobial prophylactic regimens have led to a dramatic decline in HIV-related opportunistic infections.

- Opportunistic infections occur predominantly in patients not receiving ART (due to undiagnosed HIV infection or non-acceptance of therapy) or in the period after starting ART (due to lack of eliciting a previously absent inflammatory host response). Surprisingly, despite high rates of virologic failure, the rate of opportunistic infections in patients actually taking their prescribed regimen remains quite low.

  * This is presumably due to continued immunologic response seen despite virologic failure, a phenomenon that may be linked to impaired "fitness" (virulence) of resistant HIV strains.

8. Postexposure Prophylaxis

General Concepts

- The CDC estimates that more than 600,000 significant exposures to blood-borne pathogens occur yearly. Of 56 confirmed cases of HIV acquisition in healthcare workers, more than 90% involved percutaneous exposure, with the remaining cases due to mucous membrane/skin exposure. Estimates of *HIV seroconversion rates after percutaneous and mucous membrane exposure to HIV-infected blood are 0.3% and 0.09%*, respectively; lower rates of transmission occur after non-intact skin exposure.

- By comparison, the risks of seroconversion after percutaneous exposure to hepatitis B and hepatitis C viruses are 30% and 3%, respectively.

- Factors for increased risk of HIV transmission after percutaneous exposure includes deep injury (OR 16.1), visible blood on device (OR 5.2), source patient is terminally ill (OR 6.4) or needle in source patient's artery/vein (OR 5.1); AZT prophylaxis reduces the risk of transmission (OR 0.2).

Recommendations

- *Initiate postexposure prophylaxis (PEP) as soon as possible after exposure (preferably within hours) and continue PEP for 4 weeks* if tolerated.

- Seek expert consultation *if viral resistance is suspected*.

- Offer pregnancy testing to all women of childbearing age not known to be pregnant.

- Advise exposed persons to seek medical evaluation for any acute illness during follow-up.

- *Perform HIV-antibody testing and HIV viral load testing for any illness compatible with an acute retroviral syndrome* (eg, pharyngitis, fever, rash, myalgia, fatigue, malaise, lymphadenopathy).

- Precautions include sexual abstinence or use of condoms; refraining from donating blood, plasma, organs, tissue or semen; and discontinuation of breast-feeding after high-risk exposures.

- Evaluate exposed persons taking PEP within *72 hours after exposure, and monitor for drug toxicity for at least 2 weeks*. Approximately 50% will experience nausea, malaise, headache or anorexia, and about one-third will discontinue PEP due to drug toxicity.

- Lab monitoring should include (at a minimum) a CBC, serum creatinine, liver function tests, serum glucose (if receiving a PI to detect hyperglycemia) and monitoring for crystalluria and hematuria (if indinavir is prescribed).

ID Board Pearls

- *All guidelines suggest PEP should be administered as soon as possible after exposure, but there is no absolute window after which PEP should be withheld following serious exposure.* Because clear-cut efficacy data for patient selection and PEP regimens are lacking, most experts rely on CDC guidelines, which emphasize the type of exposure and potential infectivity of the source patient. There are no formal guidelines for nonoccupational PEP, but it is reasonable to consider PEP for serious exposures (eg, rape victims, shared needle use). Occupationally-acquired HIV infections and PEP failures should be reported to the CDC.

- *Perform HIV-antibody testing for at least 6 months postexposure (at baseline, 6 weeks, 3 months and 6 months).*

- Advise exposed persons to *use precautions to prevent secondary transmission during follow-up, especially during the first 6-12 weeks*, when most HIV-infected patients will seroconvert.

9. Further Reading

Books

Bartlett JG. *A Pocket Guide to Adult HIV/AIDS Treatment*. Baltimore, MD: U.S. Department of Health and Human Services; 2007.

Bartlett JG, ed. *The Johns Hopkins Hospital Guide to Medical Care of Patients with HIV Infection*. 10th ed. Philadelphia, PA: Lippincott Williams & Wilkins; 2002.

Dolin R, Masur H, Saag MS, eds. *AIDS Therapy*. 2nd ed. New York, NY: Churchill Livingstone; 2003.

Sax PE, Cohen CJ, Kuritzkes DR. *HIV Essentials*. Sudbury, MA; Jones & Bartlett; 2009.

Wormser GP. *AIDS and Other Manifestations of HIV Infection*. 4th ed. London, England: Elsevier Academic Press; 2004.

Journal Articles

Aberg JA. Management of dyslipidemia and other cardiovascular risk factors in HIV-infected patients: case-based review. *Top HIV Med*. 2006;14:134-139.

Bernstein WB, Little RF, Wilson WH, et al. Acquired immunodeficiency syndrome-related malignancies in the era of highly active antiretroviral therapy. *Int J Hematol*. 2006;84:3-11.

Breen RA, Swaden L, Ballinger J, Lippman MC. Tuberculosis and HIV co-infection: a practical therapeutic approach. *Drugs*. 2006;66:2299-2308.

Cespedes MS, Aberg JA. Neuropsychiatric complications of antiretroviral therapy. *Drug Saf*. 2006;29:865-874.

Cingolani A, Fratino L, Scoppettuolo G, Antinori A. Changing pattern of primary cerebral lymphoma in the highly active antiretroviral therapy era. *J Neurovirol*. 2005;11:38-44.

Crum-Cianflone NF. Immune reconstitution inflammatory syndromes: what's new? *AIDS Read*. 2006;16:199-206,213,216-217.

del Rio C. Current concepts in antiretroviral therapy failure. *Top HIV Med*. 2006;14:102-106.

Egger M, May M, Chene G, et al. Prognosis of HIV1-infected patients starting highly active antiretroviral therapy: a collaborative analysis of prospective studies. *Lancet*. 2002;360:119-129.

French N, Kaleebu P, Pisani E, Whitworth JA. Human immunodeficiency virus (HIV) in developing countries. *Ann Trop Med Parasitol*. 2006;100:433-454.

Geretti AM. Clinical implications of HIV drug resistance to nucleoside and nucleotide reverse transcriptase inhibitors. *AIDS Rev*. 2006;8:210-220.

Ghafouri M, Amini S, Khalili K, Sawaya BE. HIV-1 associated dementia: symptoms and causes. *Retrovirology*. 2006;3:28.

Grubb JR, Moorman AC, Baker RK, Masur H. The changing spectrum of pulmonary disease in patients with HIV infection on antiretroviral therapy. *AIDS*. 2006;20:1095-1107.

Henry K. The case for more cautious, patient focused antiretroviral therapy. *Ann Intern Med*. 2000;132:306-311.

Hirsch MS, Brun-Vezinet F, D'Aquila RT, et al. Antiretroviral drug resistance testing in adult HIV-1 infection: recommendations of an International AIDS Society-USA Panel. *JAMA*. 2000;283:2417-2426.

Hogan MT. Cutaneous infections associated with HIV/AIDS. *Dermatol Clin*. 2006;24:473-495.

Honda KS. HIV and skin cancer. *Dermatol Clin*. 2006;24:521-530.

Kaplan JE, Masur H, Holmes KK. Guidelines for preventing opportunistic infections among HIV-infected persons—2002. Recommendations of the U.S. Public Health Service and the Infectious Diseases Society of America. *MMWR Recomm Rep*. 2002;51(RR-8):1-52.

Kourtis AP, Lee FK, Abrams EJ, Jamieson DJ, Bulterys M. Mother-to-child transmission of HIV-1: timing and implications for prevention. *Lancet Infect Dis*. 2006;6:726-732.

Lai AR, Tashima KT, Taylor LE. Antiretroviral medication considerations for individuals coinfected with HIV and Hepatitis C virus. *AIDS Patient Care STDS*. 2006;20:6778-6792.

Lawn SD, Wilkinson RJ. Immune reconstitution disease associated with parasitic infections following antiretroviral treatment. *Parasite Immunol*. 2006;28:625-633.

Lehloenya R, Meintjes G. Dermatologic manifestations of the immune reconstitution inflammatory syndrome. *Dermatol Clin*. 2006;24:549-570.

Lima MA, Koralnik IJ. New features of progressive multifocal leukoencephalopathy in the era of highly active antiretroviral therapy and natalizumab. *J Neurovirol*. 2005;11:52-57.

Lin D, Tucker MJ, Rieder MJ. Increased adverse drug reactions to antimicrobials and anticonvulsants in patients with HIV infection. *Ann Pharmacother*. 2006;40:1594-1601.

Macneal RJ, Dinulos JG. Acute retroviral syndrome. *Dermatol Clin*. 2006;24:421-429.

Maggi P, Maserati R, Antonelli G. Atherosclerosis in HIV patients: a new face for an old disease? *AIDS Rev*. 2006;8:204-209.

Manzardo C, Del Mar Ortega M, Sued O, Garcia F, Moreno A. Central nervous system opportunistic infections in developed countries in the highly active antiretroviral therapy era. *J Neurovirol*. 2005;11:72-82.

Medina F. Perez-Saleme L, Moreno J. Rheumatic manifestations of human immunodeficiency virus infection. *Infect Dis Clin North Am*. 2006;20: 891-912.

Niu MT, Stein DS, Schnittman SM, et al. Primary human immunodeficiency virus type 1 infection: review of pathogenesis and early treatment intervention in humans and animal retrovirus infections. *J Infect Dis*. 1993;168:1490-1501.

Panel on Antiretroviral Guidelines for Adults and Adolescents. Guidelines for the use of antiretroviral agents in HIV-1-infected adults and adolescents. Department of Health and Human Services. November 3, 2008;1-139. Available at http://www.adisinfo.nih.gov/ContentFiles/Adultan dAdolescent GL.pdf. Accessed on March 23, 2009.

Perno CV, Svicher V, Ceccherini-Silberstein F. Novel drug resistance mutations in HIV: recognition and clinical relevance. *AIDS Rev*. 2006;8: 179-190.

Petropoulou H, Tratigo A, Katsambas AD. Human immunodeficiency virus infection and pregnancy. *Clin Dermatol*. 2006;24:536-542.

Phillips AN, Gazzard BG, Clumeck N, et al. When should antiretroviral therapy for HIV be started? *BMJ*. 2007;334:76-78.

Rosen MJ, Narasimhan M. Critical care of immunocompromised patients: human immunodeficiency virus. *Crit Care Med*. 2006;34:S245-S250.

Sax PE. Opportunistic infections in HIV disease: down but not out. *Infect Dis Clin North Am*. 2001; 15:433-455.

Scosyrev E. An overview of the human immunodeficiency virus featuring laboratory testing for drug resistance. *Clin Lab Sci*. 2006;19:231-245.

Sidiq H, Ankoma-Sey V. HIV-related liver disease: infections versus drugs. *Gastroenterol Clin North Am*. 2006;35:487-505.

Smith D. The long-term consequences of antiretroviral therapy. *J HIV Ther*. 2006;11:24-25.

Steininger C, Puchhammer-Scotkl E, Popow Kraupp T. Cytomegalvirus disease in the era of highly active antiretroviral therapy (HAART). *J Clin Virol*. 2006;37:1-9.

Subramanian S, Mathai D. Clinical manifestations and management of cryptococcal infection. *J Postgrad Med*. 2005;51:S21-S26.

Sudano I, Spieker LE, Noll G, Corti R, Weber R, Luscher TF. Cardiovascular disease in HIV infection. *Am Heart J*. 2006;151:1147-1155.

The Antiretroviral Therapy (ART) Cohort Collection. Prognostic importance of initial response in HIV-1 infected patients starting potent antiretroviral therapy: analysis of prospective studies. *Lancet*. 2003;362:679-686.

Updated U.S. Public Health Service Guidelines for the Management of Occupational Exposures to HBV, HCV, and HIV and Recommendations for Postexposure Prophylaxis. MMWR Recomm Rep. 2001;50(RR-11):1-52.

USPHS Task Force Recommendations for use of antiretroviral drugs in pregnant HIV-1-infected women for maternal health and interventions to reduce perinatal HIV-1 transmission in the United States. *MMWR*. 2002;51(RR18):1-38.

Valenti WM. Hepatitis C update. *AIDS Read*. 2007;17:19-22.

Valle R, Haragsim L. Nephrotoxicity as a complication of antiretroviral therapy. *Adv Chronic Kidney Dis*. 2006;13:314-319.

Waters L, Nelson M. New therapeutic options for hepatitis C. *Curr Opin Infect Dis*. 2006:19:615-622.

Wojna V, Nath A. Challenges to the diagnosis and management of HIV dementia. *AIDS Read*. 2006;16:615-616.

Yoon CJ. Progressive multifocal leukoencephalopathy in the era of highly active antiretroviral therapy. *AIDS Read*. 2006;16:304-306, 309

Chapter 7: Immunodeficiencies for the ID Boards

Burke A. Cunha, MD

Contents

1. Overview

General Concepts

- Primary congenital immunodeficiencies are rare.

- *Immunologically-mediated* recurrent infections have *characteristic histories and infection patterns* due to specific microorganisms that suggest the nature of the immune defect.

- Historical Clues are repeated infections by encapsulated organisms or unusually severe or persistent infections with low-virulence "hallmark" organisms.

  * Invasive aspergillosis

  * Toxoplasma meningoencephalitis

  * *Pneumocystis (carinii) jiroveci* pneumonia (PCP)

ID Board Pearls

- *Pattern of organ involvement or the type of microorganism* should suggest a defect in humoral immunity (HI) or cell-mediated immunity (CMI).

2. Determining the Immune Defect

Defects in Humoral Immunity (HI)

Children with HI Defects

- *Recurrent* sinopulmonary infections

- *Recurrent* diarrhea

- *Recurrent* meningitis

- *Recurrent* cellulitis

- *Recurrent* bacteremias

Adults with HI Defects

- Family history of severe infections

- *Autoimmune diseases*

- Family history of recurrent infections

- *B-cell malignancies*

Children/Adults with HI Defects

- Unusually *severe* infections with *common* organisms, such as:

  * *Giardia*

  * Enteroviruses

  * *Mycoplasma pneumoniae*

  * *Granulocyte defects*

- Recurrent infections with *encapsulated* organisms, such as:

  * *Neisseria meningitidis*

  * *Streptococcus pneumoniae*

  * *Haemophilus influenzae*

- Recurrent infections with:

  * *S aureus*

3. Clinical Approach

* *B cepacia*

* *Serratia*

* *Nocardia*

* *Aspergillus*

Defects in Cell-Mediated Immunity (CMI)

General Concepts

Children with CMI Defects
• Unusual infections

• *Invasive* fungal infections

Older Children/Adults with CMI Defects
• History of *anergy*

• *Multiple malignancies*

General Concepts

Adults with CMI Defects
• Prone to *recurrent infections* due to *intracellular* organisms.

ID Board Pearls

• Severe varicella

• Severe reactions to live vaccines

• Common CMI pathogens:

* HSV

* Listeria

* PCP

* Aspergillus

Determine the Nature of Recurrences

• Rule out *coincidental recurrences* (repeated urinary tract infections or viral upper respiratory infections).

• *Recurrent infections* include >1 pneumonia/year or ≥3 total episodes of pneumonias.

• With recurrent infections, *differentiate reinfection from relapse*

ID Board Pearls

• Eliminate *non-infectious mimics of recurrent infections*

* Sarcoidosis

* Vasculitis

* SLE

* Drug reactions

4. Nonimmune Recurrent Infections

Periodic Reinfections

• Recurrent group A streptococcal pharyngitis

• Recurrent group A streptococcal cellulitis

• Cystitis (reinfection)

Congenital and Structural Abnormalities

• Recurrent meningitis

  *Myelomeningocele

  *Dural sinus leak

• Genitourinary structural abnormalities

• Recurrent pneumonias *(right middle lobe syndrome)*

Acquired Abnormalities

• *Device-associated infections* (removal required for cure)

• Prosthetic valve endocarditis

• CNS shunt infections

• Inadequate or inappropriate antibiotic therapy

• Chronic prostatitis

• Arteriovenous shunt infections

• Undrained abscesses

• Infected stents/stones

• Semi-permanent central IV line infections (Hickman-Broviac catheters)

5. Immune-Based Recurrent Infections

Immunologically-Based Recurrent Infections

Characteristic *pattern of organ involvement*

• Recurrent sinopulmonary infections

• Recurrent skin abscesses *(pyodermas)*

• *Unusual response to antigens or vaccines*

  * GVH response to blood transfusions

  * Anergy

  * *Failure to develop antibodies to protein and polysaccharide vaccines*

• *Severe infections with encapsulated organisms*

  * *Streptococcus pneumoniae*

  * *Haemophilus influenzae*

  * *Neisseria meningitidis*

• *Severe infections with intracellular organisms*

  * *Pneumocystis carinii* pneumonia (PCP)

  * Invasive aspergillosis

  * *Toxoplasma*

  * *Mycobacterium avium-intracellulare* (MAI)

ID Board Pearls

• *Unusually* severe/recurrent infections *with common organisms*

  * Mycoplasma

  * Giardia

  * *Persistent or chronic infection*

  * Severe or recurrent *enteroviral* meningoencephalitis

  * *Progressive* EBV virus infection

6. Screening Tests for Suspected Immunodeficiency Syndromes

Screening Tests for Suspected HI (Antibody/Phagocyte/Complement) Defects

Tests for HI Defects
• Quantitative serum immunoglobulins identify the most common *antibody defects*.

• *Serum IgA levels* are the *most important* determination.

• HI may also be assessed by measuring IgG antibody titers to protein or polysaccharide vaccines.

• Antibody defects have low or *no titers after immunizations* for:

  * Diphtheria

  * *Haemophilus*

  * Tetanus

  * *Pneumococcus*

Tests for Complement Defects
• CH_{50}

• Serum C_2, C_3, C_4, C_{5-9}

Tests for Phagocytic Defects
• Obtain a white blood cell count/differential to provide a quantitative *number* of circulating phagocytic cells.

• Nitroblue tetrazolium (NBT) reduction test is used to test phagocyte *function*.

Screening Tests for Suspected CMI (T-Lymphocyte/Macrophage) Defects

• *Total lymphocyte count*

• *Anergy testing (PPD, Candida)*

• *T-lymphocyte subsets*

• *HIV serology*

Screening Tests for Neutrophil Defects

• *NBT*

• *$CD1^{1b}/CD^{18}$ by fluorescence*

7. Summaries of Immunodeficiency Syndromes

Legend:

X = X-linked
AR = autosomal recessive
AD = autosomal dominant
? = unknown

Hi Defect

Bruton's Agammaglobulinemia (*X-Linked*): Congenital Agammaglobulinemia (HI Defect)

Defect: B+K kinase

Defect: Xq22

Inheritance: *X-linked*

• *No tonsils or nodes*

• *Asplenic* (Howell-Jolly bodies)

• Presents in childhood

• *Hypogammaglobulinemia*

• Recurrent otitis and sinopulmonary infections

• Associated with *dermatomyositis*

• Recurrent bacteremias

• *Rheumatoid arthritis*

• Recurrent septic arthritis (eg, ureaplasma)

• ↓ *IgA, IgG, IgM*

• Recurrent/chronic enteroviral meningitis

• Infections after first year of life; (15% die of infection before adulthood)

Hyper IgM Syndrome (HI Defect)

Defect: T-cell cannot express CD^{40}L

Inheritance: *X-linked, AR*

• Presents in infancy

• Bruton-like

• *Resembles X-linked agammaglobulinemia*

• PCP

• Cryptococcus

• CMV

• Cryptosporidia

Selective IgA Deficiency (HI Defect)

Defect: 6p21

Inheritance: *AR*

• Presents in childhood

• *Recurrent Giardia diarrhea*

• Recurrent otitis and sinopulmonary infections

• Associated with *rheumatoid arthritis*, *SLE*

• Bronchiectasis

• ↓ *IgA* (normal IgG, IgM)

• Anaphylactic reactions to blood transfusions or gamma globulin

Common Variable Immune Deficiency (CVID) (HI Defect)

Defect: ?

Inheritance: ?

• Atrophic gastritis or *pernicious anemia*

• Death from lymphoreticular malignancies

• Presents in childhood. Onset at any age.

• *Lymphocytosis*

• *Splenomegaly (25%)*

- $\downarrow/N\,IgA,\ \downarrow IgG,\ \downarrow/N\,IgM$

- *Alopecia areata*

- *Cryptosporidia*

- Recurrent pneumonias and bronchiectasis

- Hemolytic anemia

- Verruca vulgaris

- *Generalized adenopathy*

- *Resembles X-linked agammaglobulinemia, but with normal tonsils*

Duncan's Syndrome: *X-Linked* Lymphoproliferative Syndrome (HI Defect)

Defect: ?

Inheritance: *X-linked*

- Overwhelming infection and death

- B-cell lymphomas

- Presents in childhood

- $\downarrow$ *EBNA titers*

- *Males* complicated with *EBV* infection

- *Hypogammaglobulinemia*

- Acquired hypogammaglobulinemia

- *Aplastic anemia*

Selective IgM Deficiency (HI Defect)

Defect: ?

Inheritance: ?

- *Atopic*

- Presents in adults

- *Recurrent pneumococcal pneumonia and meningitis*

- *Splenomegaly*

Hypogammaglobulinemia with Thymoma (HI Defect)

Defect: ?

Inheritance: ?

- RBC aplasia

- Anemia

- Presents in infancy

- Eosinopenia

- Severe diarrhea

Hyperimmunoglobulinemia E Syndrome (Job's Syndrome) (HI Defect)

Defect: ?

Inheritance: *AD*

- *"Cold" S aureus abscesses* (skin, abdomen, pelvis)

- *Chronic mucocutaneous candidiasis*

- Presents in infancy

- Mild eosinophilia

- *Deep set eyes with hypertelorism*

- $\uparrow\uparrow\uparrow IgE$

- *Coarse facies*

- *Recurrent S pneumoniae/H influenzae pneumonias*

- *Severe eczema*

- Hyperextensible joints

- Hyperkeratosis

- Pathogenic bone fractures (bones fragile)

- *Double rows of teeth* (primary and secondary)

Cyclic Neutropenia (HI Defect)

Defect: ?

Inheritance: *AR*

- *Fever and chills during neutropenia*

- Presents in childhood

- *Cycles in multiples of 7 days; (usually 21-day cycles)*

CMI Defects

DiGeorge Syndrome (thymic apasia) (CMI Defect)

Defect: 22qII locus

Inheritance: *AD*

- Persistent *oral candidiasis*

- *Fatal reactions to live vaccines*

- Presents in infancy

- Antibody responses impaired

- *Interrupted aortic arch*

- May die in infancy of congenital heart disease

- *Thymic and parathyroid aplasia*

- Mild cases may live to adulthood

- *Congenital heart disease* (PDA, TA, ASD/VSD)

- *Avoid live vaccines*

- Anti-mongolian eye slant

- Fatal graft vs. host reactions to blood products

- *Low set/notched ears*

- Use radiated blood products

- Neonatal *hypocalcemic seizures*

- $\uparrow IgE$

Nezelof's Syndrome (CMI Defect)

Defect: ?

Inheritance: ?

- Presents in childhood

- *Lymphopenia*

- Verruca vulgaris

- *Same as DiGeorge syndrome, but no facial abnormalities; small thymus*

Chronic Mucocutaneous Candidiasis (CMI Defect)

Defect: ?

Inheritance: ?

- Do not develop disseminated/invasive candidiasis

- Not anergic

- Presents in childhood

- Death occurs during early adulthood of non-candidal infection

- *Associated with endocrinopathies* (hypothyroidism and hypoparathyroidism, DM, PA)

Chédiak-Higashi Syndrome (CMI Defect)

Defect: Defect in phagolysome formation (CHS1/LYST)

Inheritance: *AR*

- *Neutropenia*

- Chemotactic defect

- Presents in childhood

- *Bleeding* secondary to platelet defects

- *Partial oculocutaneous albinism*

- Lymphoma-like syndrome in young adults

- *Nystagmus*

- *Characteristic giant lysosomal granules in WBCs*

- Spinocerebellar degeneration

- *Peripheral neuropathy*

- Gingivitis

- Autonomic dysfunction

- Aphthous ulcers

- Hepatosplenomegaly

- Pyogenic (skin, respiratory tract) infections

CMI/HI Defects

Severe Combined Immunodeficiency Disease (SCID) (CMI/HI Defects)

Defect: IL-2 receptor B-Chain Absent

Inheritance: *X-linked* recessive

- Lymphoreticular malignances

- Anergy

- Neonatal viral infections often fatal (HSV, CMV, RSV)

- *Eosinophilia*

- Presents in childhood

- *Hypogammaglobulinemia*

- *VZV, PCP*

- *Lymphopenia*

- Recurrent oral candidiasis

- Avoid live virus vaccines (may be fatal)

- Recurrent diarrhea

- $\downarrow$ *IgM* ($\downarrow$ IgG, $\downarrow$ IgA)

- Recurrent otitis and sinopulmonary infections

SCID with ADA Deficiency (CMI/HI Defects)

Defect: ?

Inheritance: *AR*

- Anergy

- *Absent ADA*

- Presents in childhood

- *Eosinophilia*

- Recurrent oral candidiasis

- *Hypogammaglobulinemia*

- Recurrent diarrhea

- *Lymphopenia*

- *No thymus*

- *Rib and scapular deformities*

Ataxia-Telangiectasia (CMI/HI Defect)

Defect: ?

Inheritance: *AR*

- *Progressive bronchiectasis*

- $\downarrow IgA/IgE$ ($\downarrow$ IgG)

- Presents in childhood

- Lymphoreticular malignancies

- Recurrent oral candidiasis

- Lymphopenia

- Recurrent diarrhea

- $\uparrow$ AFP

- Recurrent pneumonias

- $\downarrow CD_3/CD_4$

Wiskott-Aldrich Syndrome (CMI/HI Defect)

Defect: XpII

Inheritance: *X- linked recessive*

- Lymphoreticular malignancies

- $\downarrow IgM$ ($\uparrow$ IgA, $\uparrow$ IgE)

- Presents in infancy

- *Thrombocytopenia and bleeding problems*

- *Severe eczema*

- *Small platelets*

- Recurrent otitis or sinopulmonary infections

- Bacteremias

- Anergy (late); death in childhood from infections or malignancies

Granulocyte Defects

Chronic Granulomatous Disease (CGD) Granulocyte Defect)

Defect: NAPDH Oxidase

XL defect: p91 phox

AR defect: p22 phox, p67 phox, p47 phox

Inheritance: *X-linked*

- *Draining lymph nodes with sinus tracts*

- *Recurrent abscesses of lungs, skin, liver*

- *Hepatosplenomegaly*

- Gingivitis

- Aphthous ulcers

- Diffuse granuloma formation

- Osteomyelitis

- Associated with *discoid lupus*

- Pyogenic infections

- *Serratia*

- *Reduced superoxide generation*

- Presents in childhood

- Infections with *catalase positive organisms*

  * *S aureus*

  * *B cepacia*

  * *Nocardia*

  * *Aspergillus*

Myeloperoxidase Deficiency (Granulocyte Defects)

Defect: Myeloperoxidase

Inheritance: 3 *AR*

- *Most common 1° phagocyte disorder*

- Clinical infection rare

- Candida infection (especially in DM)

8. Therapy of Congenital Immunodeficiency

HI Defects

Immunoglobulin therapy is useful in patients with:

• Agammaglobulinemia

• Antibody deficiencies with near-normal immunoglobulin concentrations

• Wiskott-Aldrich syndrome

• Severe combined immunodeficiency

• X-linked immunodeficiency with increased IgM

• Intravenous immunoglobulin contains primarily IgG. A dose of 400 mg/kg per month should be given to approximate physiologic IgG levels.

CMI Defects

• CMI defects may be treated by *bone marrow transplantation*.

• *Prolonged immunosuppression* may result in subsequent malignancies.

• HIV patients may have relapsing or recurrent infections.

   * *Pathogens predicted by the CD4 count.*

   * *Prompt treatment of opportunistic infection in AIDS patients minimizes further helper T-lymphocyte loss.*

   * *Antigenic-induced stimulation of the immune system should be avoided if possible.*

ID Board Pearls

• It is not possible to replace defects in secretory IgA with immunoglobulin therapy.

   * *Serum immunoglobulin contains very little IgA.*

* Immunoglobulin therapy *is contraindicated in IgA deficiency because of the high frequency of anti-IgA antibodies.*

9. Further Reading

Cohen J, Powderly WG. *Infectious Diseases*. 2nd ed. New York, NY: Mosby; 2004.

Grieco MH. *Infections in the Abnormal Host*. New York, NY: Yorke Medical Books; 1980.

Gorbach SL, Bartlett JG, Blacklow NR. *Infectious Diseases*. 3rd ed. New York, NY: Lippincott Williams & Wilkins; 2004.

Mandell GL. Principles and Practice of Infectious Diseases. 6th ed. Philadelphia, PA: Churchill Livingstone, 2005.

Virella G, Goust JM, Fudenberg HH, eds. *Introduction to Medical Immunology*. 2nd ed. New York, NY: Marcel Dekker; 1990.

Chapter 8:
Zoonoses for the ID Boards

Dennis J. Cleri, MD, FACP, FAAM, FIDSA
Anthony J. Ricketti, MD, FCCP
John R. Vernaleo, MD, FACP

Contents

1. Overview

The spotted fever rickettsioses have a worldwide distribution. Some patients develop an eschar at the site of the tick bite, but rarely in Rocky Mountain Spotted Fever (*Rickettsia rickettsii*). In addition, except for *C burnetii*, these organisms cause vasculitis. The treatment for most diseases is doxycycline. Chloramphenicol is equally as effective, although not generally the drug of choice.

Although *C burnetii* was placed with the order Rickettsiales, it has been reclassified to the gamma subdivision of the Proteobacteria, along with *Legionella* and *Francisella*, based upon the sequencing of the 16s rDNA encoding gene. Its small cell variant allows it to survive in the environment. Its large cell variant resides in macrophages, which are unable to kill the bacteria.

Ticks transmit these diseases, as well as protozoa, other bacteria, and viruses. Toxic local reactions are common. Anaphylaxis has been reported after *Rhipicephalus sanguineus* bite.

Rickettsial diseases are of particular importance to the infectious disease practitioner in the differential diagnosis of fever in the international traveler. These are summarized in Table 1.

Table 1

Epidemiology and Distinguishing Rashes of Selected Rickettsial and Related Arthropod-Borne Diseases

Disease	Pathogen	Vector	Geographic Distribution	Incubation Period	Rash / Complications
Epidemic Typhus (louse-borne typhus) and recurrent disease	*Rickettsia prowazekii*	Body lice or recurrent disease, years after the initial infection	Central Africa, South America	10–14 days	**No Eschar;** Erythematous, macules, petechiae on trunk beginning in axilla Multiorgan failure, acute renal failure; shock, ischemia or gangrene of distal fingers and toes
Murine typhus	*Rickettsia typhi* (*R felis* causes a typhus-like illness)	Rat fleas	Tropical and subtropical — worldwide	1–2 weeks	**No Eschar;** Poorly visible exanthem on trunk; Most cases mild-untreated fatality rate 4%; aseptic meningitis, deafness, deep vein thrombosis; renal and hepatic insufficiency; CNS complications
Rocky Mountain Spotted Fever ("The most severe of all of all tick-borne rickettsioses.")	*Rickettsia rickettsii*	*Dermacentor* and *Amblyomma* ticks	North and South America	2–14 days (average: 7 days)	**Eschar rare;** Few patients have rash initially; usually begins on wrist and ankles and may be diffuse or petechial Deafness, seizures, confusion, focal neurologic deficits; untreated — 23% mortality; with treatment —3-7% mortality
Mediterranean spotted fever (boutonneuse fever)	*Rickettsia conorii*	*Rhipicephalus* (dog tick) and *Haemaphysalis* ticks	Mediterranean and Caspian areas, Middle East, Indian subcontinent, Africa	6 days	**Inoculation eschar** ('*tache noire*') at tick bite (72% of cases), generalized maculopapular rash 1–7 days following the onset of fever CNS, retinal, peripheral gangrene, respiratory distress, multiorgan failure, 2–4% mortality

(continued)

Epidemiology and Distinguishing Rashes of Selected Rickettsial and Related Arthropod-Borne Diseases

Disease	Pathogen	Vector	Geographic Distribution	Incubation Period	Rash / Complications
Rickettsialpox (Kew Garden's fever)	*Rickettsia akari*	Mouse mites	North and South America, Asia	7 days	**Eschar** starts as papule with tender lymphadenopathy; papular rash becomes vesicular; 20–40 lesions
					Self-limited disease
Scrub typhus	*Orientia tsutsugamushi*	Larval trombiculid (chigger) mites	Southeast Asia, western Oceania, eastern Australia, China, western Russia	6–21 days (usually 10–12 days)	**50% have eschar;** rash is macular, pale, transient and easily missed
					80% with fever and generalized lymphadenopathy; pneumonitis, meningoencephalitis, DIC, hemorrhage, renal failure in untreated cases
African tick bite fever (Tick bite fever – 1911)	*Rickettsia africae*	*Amblyomma* ticks	Sub-Saharan Africa, Caribbean, *R africae* isolated from ticks on Reunion Island (Indian Ocean)	5–7 to 10 days	**1 or more eschars** with lymphadenitis; 30% with vesicular cutaneous rash and mouth blisters
					Self-limited, mild disease with no fatalities
Similar disease to African tick bite fever	*Rickettsia parkeri* or closely related species		South America and rare case in North America		
Spotted fever	*Rickettsia massiliae*	*Rhipicephalus sanguineus*	Africa, Europe, America		Fever, night sweats, **1 or more eschars**, acute visual loss (chorioretinitis), maculopapular rash on the palms and soles. May be resistant to rifampin.

2. *Rickettsia rickettsii* (Rocky Mountain Spotted Fever)

Synonyms

• Rocky Mountain Spotted Fever

• Tick typhus

• Tobia fever (Columbia)

• São Paulo fever or febre maculosa (Brazil)

• Fiebre manchada (Mexico)

Causative Organisms

• *Rickettsia rickettsii*

Epidemiology

• Ticks are both the vector and reservoir: ticks pass the pathogen both trans-stadially and transovarially

• Transmission through vertebrate hosts (horizontal transmission) also occurs

• *Dermacentor variabilis* (American dog tick) in eastern, Midwestern and far west U.S.

  * Also transmits the toxin of tick paralysis

• *Dermacentor andersoni* (Rocky Mountain wood tick) in the western U.S.

  * Also caries Colorado tick fever

  * Also transmits the toxin of tick paralysis

• *Rhipicephalus sanguineus* (brown dog tick) in Mexico

  * Also transmits Mediterranean spotted fever (MSF) due to *Rickettsia conorii*, the most important tick-borne disease in North Africa

• *Amblyomma americanum* (lone star tick) eastern and western U.S.

  * Tick also carries *Ehrlichia chaffeensis*, and possibly *Babesia cervi* and southern tick-associated rash illness (STARI)

  * Transmits the toxin of tick paralysis (Also transmitted by *Ixodes scapularis*, and *I pacificus*)

• *Amblyomma cajennense* in Central and South America

Key Clinical Features

• The tick-bite is painless

• Infection occurs after the tick feeds for 6–10 hours

• Ticks may feed up to 2 weeks

• Incubation period: 2–14 days

• Initial symptoms prior to the rash: fever, myalgia, headache

• Gastrointestinal symptoms (nausea, vomiting, diarrhea, abdominal pain and tenderness) may present before the rash appears

• Rash:

  * Few patients develop the rash on the first day of symptoms

  * About half of patients develop the rash within the first 3 days of illness

  * Almost 90% of patients develop a rash within 3–5 days

  * 10–15% of patients do not develop a rash – more in older patients and African American patients

  * Rash usually begins on the wrists and ankles. Involvement of the palms and soles is considered typical but may occur in less than half of patients

  * Progression of the rash is usually centripetal

  * The rash may begin on the trunk, be diffuse and/or petechial

* 4% of patients develop skin necrosis or gangrene, especially of digits

* Eschar ('*tache noire*') is rare but has been reported

* Conjunctivitis (30%)

* Lymphadenopathy (27%)

• Neurologic findings

　* Severe headaches

　* Meningismus, focal neurologic deficits, deafness, ataxia, is less frequent

　* Seizures and coma in less than 10% of patients

　* Confusion

　* Transient deafness

• Retinal involvement: retinal vein engorgement, arterial occlusion, flame hemorrhage and papilledema without increased intracranial pressure

• Systemic symptoms and multiorgan involvement

　* 25% or less of patients

　　• Hepatomegaly

　　• Splenomegaly

　　• Jaundice

　　• Pneumonia (one third of patients will have a cough)

　　• Myocarditis and/or arrhythmia

　　• Edema

　　• Shock

　　• Renal failure in severe disease

Key Differential Diagnostic Features

• Differential Diagnosis

　* Typhoid fever

　* Murine and epidemic louse borne typhus

　* Measles

　* Rubella

　　• Rubella is suggested by postauricular lymph nodes and lack of toxicity

　* Upper or lower respiratory tract infection

　* Gastroenteritis

　* Acute abdomen

　* Enteroviral infections

　* Meningococcemia

　* Disseminated gonorrhea

　* Secondary syphilis

　* Leptospirosis

　* Vasculitis

　* Idiopathic thrombocytopenic purpura (ITP)

　* Thrombotic thrombocytopenic purpura (TTP)

　* Infectious mononucleosis

　* Drug eruptions

　* Ehrlichioses

　* Spotted fever group rickettsial infection

- Differentiating from other rickettsial diseases

  * *R parkeri*

    - Milder disease

    - Eschar present

    - Transmitted by bite from Gulf Coast tick (*Amblyomma maculatum*)

    - 50% of cases confused with RMSF

Key Laboratory/Radiology Features

Specific Laboratory Findings

- Weil-Felix text (*Proteus* OX-19 and OX-2 agglutination) is unreliable

- Indirect immunofluorescence (IFA) the best, most widely available test

  * Sensitivity poor in first 10–12 days of illness

  * 94% sensitivity with seroconversion from 14–21 days

- Direct immunofluorescence of skin biopsies (3–4 mm punch biopsy with the petechial lesion in the center) has a 70% sensitivity and 100% specificity, but not readily available

- Dot-enzyme immunoassay

- Polymerase chain reaction (PCR) for DNA only useful in late infections and post-mortem

- Direct culture may be achieved by guinea pig, embryonated egg, or cell culture inoculation, but is hazardous and not routinely available

Nonspecific Laboratory Findings

- Cerebrospinal fluid

  * Lymphocytic pleocytosis

  * Elevated protein

  * Increased pressure

- Hyponatremia present in 50% of cases

- Transaminases and CPK are often elevated

- Thrombocytopenia is common but WBC and Hgb remain normal

- Chest x-rays show no infiltrates

- EKG changes (ST and nonspecific ST-T wave changes)

  * Ventricular arrhythmia suggests myocarditis

- In advanced disease

  * Elevated creatinine and BUN

  * Hypotension resulting in acute tubular necrosis

Therapy

Empiric

- Decision to treat is always based on clinical suspicion – doxycycline should always be included in the initial therapeutic regimen

- Therapy is always started before laboratory confirmation

- Therapy often includes treatment for meningococcemia and *Staphylococcus aureus* sepsis

Definitive/Specific

- Doxycycline 100 mg twice daily for at least 7 days and 2 days after the patient becomes afebrile

- Chloramphenicol may be preferred during pregnancy, especially during the first and second trimesters in order to avoid effects on fetal bone and dental development

- Retrospective data suggests that chloramphenicol may be less effective than doxycycline

- Doxycycline is recommended in children of all ages, as 1 course of therapy is unlikely to stain teeth

- Duration of therapy: 3 days after defervescence – therapy usually is between 5–7 days

Prognostic Factors

- 23% mortality unless treated early

- 3%–7% mortality with treatment

- Higher mortality in children under 4 and adults over 40 years of age

- A significant number of survivors suffer with headaches

- Some survivors have persistent EEG abnormalities

Further Reading

Books and Book Chapters

Cunha BA, ed. *Tickborne Infectious Diseases – Diagnosis and Management*. New York, NY: Marcel Dekker; 2000.

Sexton DJ, Walker DH. Spotted fever group rickettsioses. In: Guerrant RL, Walker DH, Weller PF, eds. *Tropical Infectious Diseases – Principles, Pathogens, & Practice*. 2nd ed. v.1. Philadelphia, PA: Elsevier Churchill Livingstone; 2006:539-547.

Walker DH, Raoult D. *Rickettsia rickettsii* and other spotted fever group Rickettsiae (Rocky Mountain spotted fever and other spotted fevers). In: Mandell GL, Bennett JE, Dolin R, eds. *Mandell, Douglas, and Bennett's Principles and Practice of Infectious Diseases*. 6th ed. v.2. Philadelphia, PA: Elsevier Churchill Livingstone; 2005:2287-2295.

Woodward TE, Cunha BA. Rocky Mountain spotted fever. In: *Tickborne Infectious Diseases – Diagnosis and Management*. New York, NY: Marcel Dekker; 2000:121-137.

Journal Articles

Chen LF, Sexton DJ. What's new in Rocky Mountain spotted fever? *Infect Dis Clin N Am*. 2008;22:415-432.

Clark RP, Hu LT. Prevention of Lyme disease and other tick-borne infections. *Infect Dis Clin N Am*. 2008;22:381-396.

Goddard J, Varela-Stokes AS. Role of the lone star tick, *Amblyomma americanum* (L.), in human and animal diseases. *Vet Parasitol*. 2008; Oct 28 [Epub ahead of print]

Jensenius M, Fournier P-E, Raoult D. Rickettsioses and the international traveler. *Clin Infect Dis*. 2004;39:1493-1499.

Klasco R. Colorado tick fever. *Med Clin North Am*. 2002;86:435-440.

Paddock CD, Finley RW, Wright CS, et al. *Rickettsia* parkeri rickettsiosis and its clinical distinction from Rocky Mountain spotted fever. *Clin Infect Dis*. 2008; 47:1889-1196.

Parola P, Labruna MB, Raoult D. Tick-borne r ickettsioses in America: unanswered questions and emerging diseases. *Curr Infect Dis Rep*. 2009;11:40-50.

3. *Rickettsia akari* (Rickettsialpox, Kew Gardens fever)

Synonyms

• Rickettsialpox

• Kew Gardens fever

Causative Organisms

• *Rickettsia akari*

Epidemiology

• Differs from other rickettsial diseases as it is transmitted by mouse-mite bite (*Liponyssoides sanguineus*)

• Mites become infected by feeding on mice (*Mus musculus*)

• New York City dogs have a high seroprevalence – ticks or fleas may also transmit the disease

• High seroprevalence in intravenous drug abusers in Baltimore

• Initially described in New York City (Kew Gardens housing complex – Kew Gardens fever)

• Reported (or suggested by serologic studies) in eastern Europe, Korea, Turkey, France, Italy, Costa Rica, New Guinea, and South Africa

Key Clinical Features

• Incubation period: 7 days

• Typical cases (92%)

  * Fever

  * Eschar

    • Starts as a papule

    • Vesicle appears in the center of the papule

    • Vesicle dries, turns brown to black

  * Tender lymphadenopathy draining the eschar

  * Rash

    • Appears on 3rd or 4th day

    • Papular rash that becomes vesicular

    • Vesicles dry and then leave a black crust

    • Total usually 20–40 skin lesions

    • Palms and soles spared

Key Differential Diagnostic Features

• Skin eschars may confuse the disease with cutaneous anthrax

• Smallpox

• Varicella and zoster

• Herpes simplex

• Other rickettsial diseases (Queensland tick typhus, African tick-bite fever)

Key Laboratory/Radiology Features

• Transient leucopenia

• Transient thrombocytopenia

• Diagnosis by serology

  * IgG and IgM detected 7–15 days after the onset of symptoms

  * Cross reactions with *Rickettsia rickettsii*

• Immunochemistry for identification of organisms in skin biopsies

• Polymerase chain reaction

• Culture (in cell culture systems) from eschar biopsy where organisms are most abundant

Therapy

Empiric

- Therapy should include specific therapeutic recommendations; primarily doxycycline

Definitive/Specific

- Doxycycline 200 mg/day for 7 days

- Chloramphenicol is considered an alternate therapy

- Azithromycin

Prognostic Factors

- Benign, self-limited disease – almost all patients recover without sequelae

Further Reading

Books and Book Chapters

Raoult D. *Rickettsia akari* (Rickettsialpox). In: Mandell GL, Bennett JE, Dolin R, eds. *Mandell, Douglas, and Bennett's Principles and Practice of Infectious Diseases*. 6th ed. v.2. Philadelphia, PA: Elsevier Churchill Livingstone; 2005:2295- 2296.

Journal Articles

Madison G, Kim Schluger L, Braverman S, et al. Hepatitis in association with rickettsialpox. *Vector Borne Zoonotic Dis*. 2008;8:111-115.

Paddock CD, Koss T, Eremeeva ME, et al. Isolation of Rickettsia akari from eschars of patients with rickettsialpox. *Am J Trop Med Hyg*. 2006;75:732-738.

4. *Coxiella burnetii* (Q fever)

Synonyms

- Q fever

- *Rickettsia burnetii*

- *Rickettsia diaporica*

Causative Organisms

- *Coxiella burnetii*

  * Gram-negative cell wall – intracellular pathogen

  * Spore stage exists – able to withstand harsh environments

  * Large and small variants

Epidemiology

- Most common animal reservoirs: cattle, sheep, goats

- Organisms shed in urine, feces, milk and birth products, especially placenta of infected sheep

- Dogs and cats reported as a source of infection

- Also found in arthropods, fish, birds, rodents, marsupials, horses, dogs, cats, swine, camels and other domestic livestock

- Worldwide distribution

- Humans infected by aerosols

  * Contaminated straw

  * Living along a roadside where sheep traveled

  * Occupational disease of those in direct contact with animals

  * Handling contaminated laundry

  * Laboratory exposure

  * Ingestion of contaminated raw milk

* Skinning infected rabbits

• Isolated from human breast milk and placentas — at least 1 case of human vertical transmission

• Ticks and other arthropods may transmit infection

    * Transmitted percutaneously after crushing a tick between the fingers

• Transmitted by blood transfusion

• Very few reports of human-to-human transmission

• HIV+ patients have a 13 times higher incidence of infection and are more symptomatic than the general population

• Sexual transmission in humans – a case of Q fever orchitis after intercourse with partner who developed Q fever 15 days later

Key Clinical Features

• Incubation period: 20 days (range: 14–39 days)

• Most primary infections are asymptomatic

    * Symptomatic infections are more frequent in adults than children

• 3 most common clinical presentations of primary infection are:

    * (1) Self-limited flu-like illness

    * (2) Hepatitis (more frequent in younger patients)

    * (3) Pneumonia (more frequent in older patients)

    * Clinical presentations appear to be geographic in nature (ie, pneumonia more common than hepatitis in eastern Canada; in southern Spain, hepatitis is common while pneumonia is rare)

• Produces an acute and sometimes chronic disease

• Usually a self-limited febrile illness (2–14 days average)

    * Most common form of disease

    * Endemic areas: 11%–12% of population are antibody positive

    * Age and dose important

    * Many patients asymptomatic

• Complications

    * Pneumonia

        • May present as an atypical pneumonia

        • Rapidly progressive pneumonia mimics Legionnaire's disease

        • Pneumonia as an incidental finding in the febrile patient

        • 5% of patients have splenomegaly

        • Fever and severe headache suggest meningitis but CSF is unremarkable — organism has been isolated from this CSF

        • Rarely fatal

    * Chronic Q fever

        • Duration of symptoms prior to diagnosis (1–14 months: average 5.6 months)

        • Fever absent in 18% of cases

    * Endocarditis

        • Usually affects abnormal or prosthetic valves (90% of cases)

        • May infect clots in left ventricular aneurysms

- Patients have defect in cell-mediated immune response to pathogen

- Clinical manifestations

  * Clubbing of fingers

  * Hypergammaglobulinemia

  * Splenomegaly and hepatomegaly in 50% of patients

  * Purpuric rash secondary to leukocyto-clastic vasculitis in 20% of patients

  * Arterial emboli in 1/3 of patients

  * Relapses may occur years after therapy

  - Infection of a vascular prosthesis

  - Infection of aneurysms

* Myocarditis (rare)

* Pericarditis

* Osteomyelitis

* Chronic lung disease and interstitial pulmonary fibrosis

* Prolonged fever

* Purpuric eruptions

* Hepatitis

  - One of the most common manifestations

  - More common in sheep and goat breeding areas

  - Clinical presentations:

    * Infectious hepatitis

* FUO with granulomas in the liver – typical doughnut granuloma with dense fibrin ring surrounded by a central lipid vacuole

* Osteomyelitis

* Neurologic manifestations

  - Symptoms

    * Severe headache most common symptom

    * Residual disease

      - Weakness

      - Myelitis

      - Peripheral neuritis

      - Recurrent meningismus

      - Blurred vision

      - Residual paresthesias

      - Sensory loss

      - Behavioral disturbance

      - Cerebellar signs

      - Cranial nerve palsies

      - Extrapyramidal disease

      - Miller-Fisher variant of Guillain-Barre syndrome (areflexia and ophthalmoparesis)

      - Demyelinating polyradiculoneuritis

  - Encephalitis or aseptic meningitis 0.2%–1.3% of cases

  - Confusional states

  - Dementia

- Extrapyramidal disease

- Optic neuritis

- Chronic fatigue syndrome

    * Hematologic complications

        - Bone marrow necrosis

        - Histiocytic hemophagocytosis

        - Hemolytic anemia

        - Disease-simulating lymphoma

        - Transient hypoplastic anemia

        - Reactive thrombocytosis

        - Thrombocytopenia (rare)

        - Splenic rupture

    * Erythema nodosum

    * Glomerulonephritis

Key Differential Diagnostic Features

- May mimic Legionnaire's disease

- Pneumonic tularemia

- Hepatitis must be differentiated from Hodgkin's disease and infectious mononucleosis as the doughnut ring granuloma are seen in both

- Important cause of FUO

- Culture-negative endocarditis especially in patients with prosthetic valves

Key Laboratory/Radiology Features

- Although the organism may be cultured, culture is usually not attempted because of the high risk of infectivity in the laboratory and lack of sensitivity of the techniques

- Pneumonia

    * Diagnosis confirmed by serology

        - Microagglutination

        - Complement fixation – most commonly used test

        - Microimmunofluorescence

        - Indirect immunofluorescence

            * IgM antibodies may persist for almost 2 years

        - ELISA

        - Cross reactions with *Bartonella* and *Legionella micdadei* antibodies

    * PCR may be used for diagnosis

    * WBC usually normal in 2/3 of the patients; 1/3 have elevated WBCs

    * Hepatic transaminases elevated in all patients

    * Bilirubin usually normal, jaundice rare

    * Inappropriate ADH syndrome rare

    * Chest x-rays variable

        - Nonsegmental and segmental pleural-based opacities

        - Multiple rounded opacities very typical of Q fever pneumonia

        - Pleural effusion 35% of cases – usually small but may be large

        - Atelectasis

        - Increase in reticular markings

        - Hilar adenopathy

- Chronic Q fever

  * Endocarditis

    - Vegetations characteristic

      * Subacute and chronic inflammatory infiltrates

      * Many large foamy cells

      * Organisms readily seen on electron microscopy

    - Diagnosis confirmed by serology

  * Hypergammaglobulinemia

  * Elevated ESR

  * Anemia

  * Microscopic hematuria

- Meningoencephalitis

  * 50% of patients will have CSF pleocytosis (18-1392 cells/mm^3) with mononuclear cell predominance in almost all cases

  * CSF protein increased; CSF glucose normal

Therapy

Empiric

- Doxycycline

- Therapy is always started before laboratory confirmation

- Atypical presentations of Q fever, scrub typhus, murine typhus, human monocytic ehrlichiosis, and bartonellosis may present with fevers of more than one week's duration. Even without confirmation of the diagnosis, treatment with doxycycline should be initiated in patients with the appropriate epidemiologic risks

Definitive/Specific

- Doxycycline is the treatment of choice for pneumonia

  * Some strains resistant to doxycycline in vitro

  * Chloramphenicol has been used as an alternate

  * Co-trimoxazole (trimethoprim-sulfamethoxazole) and ketolide telithromycin also effective

  * Quinolones and rifampin most effective agents in a fibroblast-infected susceptibility testing system

    - Consider use in meningitis

  * May fail to respond to macrolides

  * Rifampin has been added to therapy in difficult cases with success

  * Delayed defervescence is seen in spite of therapy with doxycycline in patients presenting with jaundice, relative bradycardia and absence of headache. This is also seen in scrub and murine typhus

- Endocarditis usually requires more than 1 drug: doxycycline plus another agent

  * Valve replacement should be dictated by hemodynamics only

  * Duration of treatment unknown – possibly indefinitely

  * Doxycycline with rifampin or ciprofloxacin for 2 years

  * Doxycycline with pefloxacin or ofloxacin

  * Theoretical use of doxycycline with chloroquine or amantadine

  * Doxycycline and hydroxychloroquine used with success – duration of therapy: 1.5–3 years

- Serology should be performed during therapy

* Treatment success seen with

  - Falling ESR

  - Correction of anemia

  - Correction of hypergammaglobulinemia

  - Antibody titers reduced

    * IgM disappears first followed by IgA

    * IgG remains positive for years

- Hepatitis may be treated with doxycycline or an alternative agent

  * 2 weeks therapy with doxycycline or alternative drug is usually sufficient

  * Occasionally, longer periods of therapy required

Further Factors

- Coexisting conditions may worsen the prognosis of pneumonia

Further Reading

Books and Book Chapters

Marrie TJ. Q fever. In: Marrie TJ, ed. *Community Acquired Pneumonia*. New York, NY: Kluwer Academic/Plenum Publishers; 2001:571-587.

Marrie TJ, Raoult D. *Coxiella burnetii* (Q fever). In: Mandell GL, Bennett JE, Dolin R, eds. *Mandell, Douglas, and Bennett's Principles and Practice of Infectious Diseases*. 6th ed. v.2. Philadelphia, PA: Elsevier Churchill Livingstone; 2005:2296-2303.

Marrie TJ, Raoult D. Update on Q fever, including Q fever endocarditis. In: *Current Clinical Topics in Infectious Diseases*. 22. Malden, MA: Blackwell Publishing; 2002:97-124.

Journal Articles

Bernit E, Pouget J, Janbon F, et al. Neurological involvement in acute Q fever: a report of 29 cases and review of the literature. *Arch Intern Med*. 2002;162:693-700.

Botelho-Nevers E, Raoult D. Fever of unknown origin due to rickettsioses. *Infect Dis Clin N Am*. 2007;21:997-1011.

Fournier PE, Etienne J, Harle JR, et al. Myocarditis, a rare but severe manifestation of Q fever: report of 8 cases and review of the literature. *Clin Infect Dis*. 2001 May 15;32:1440-1447.

Healy B, Llewelyn M, Westmoreland D, et al. The value of follow-up after acute Q fever infection. *J Infect*. 2006;52:e109-e112.

Karakousis PC, Trucksis M, Dumler JS. Chronic Q fever in the United States. *J Clin Microbiol*. 2006;44:2283-2287.

Levy PY, Carrieri P, Raoult D. *Coxiella burnetii* pericarditis: report of 15 cases and review. *Clin Infect Dis*. 1999;29:393-397.

Marrie TJ. *Coxiella burnetii* (Q fever) pneumonia. *Clin Infect Dis*. 1995:21 (suppl 3):S253-S264.

Musso D, Raoult D. *Coxiella burnetii* blood cultures from acute and chronic Q-fever patients. *J Clin Microbiol*. 1995;33:3129-3132.

Tissot-Dupont H, Raoult D. Q fever. *Infect Dis Clin N Am*. 2007;22:505-514.

5. *Rickettsia prowazekii* (Epidemic typhus, Louse-borne typhus)

Synonyms

- Epidemic typhus

- Louse-borne typhus

- Exanthematic typhus

- Historical typhus

- Classic typhus, sylvatic typhus

- Red louse disease

- Jail fever

- The infection of military camps (Zavorziz, 1676)

- Recrudescent epidemic typhus (Brill-Zinsser disease)

Causative Organisms

- *Rickettsia prowazekii*

Epidemiology

- Transmitted by the human body louse (*Pediculus humanus corporis*)

  * In general, lice are host-specific

  * Lice feces contains ammonium compounds which attract other lice

  * Feed on blood 5 times daily with a lifespan of 4–12 weeks

    • Acutely subject to dehydration, and may only rehydrate through a blood meal

  * Lice will leave the febrile host and seek a noninfected afebrile person

    • Killed in clothing if washed in hot water (above 50° C)

*Infection does not occur directly from the bite but from contamination of bite sites, mucous membranes or conjunctivae with infected louse feces or infected crushed louse bodies

* Infections through aerosols of louse fecal dust reported

* Lice become infected with the pathogen, rupture louse gut epithelial cells, releasing blood, causing the sick louse to turn red, which die within 1 week

- Human transmission by close physical contact between hosts

- Sexual transmission of lice

- Classically a disease of the winter months with the wearing of heavy clothing and poor personal hygiene

- Outbreaks during periods of war, famine and social upheaval

- Permanent foci of lice infestation now found in regions of cold weather, poverty and homeless communities

- Occurs in areas of extreme poverty world-wide including tropical areas

- Reactivation of disease (Brill-Zinsser disease) with waning immunity or stress sometimes years later UNRELATED to louse infestation

- Patients with chronic asymptomatic bacteremia, life-long carriage of *R prowazekii* and recurrent (Brill-Zinsser) disease may make it impossible to eradicate epidemic typhus

- Potential bioterrorist agent

  * Stable in dried louse feces – remains viable for up to 100 days

  * May be spread by aerosol — naturally occurring feces is dry and powdery with less than 2% water content

- Extrahuman reservoirs

  * Antibodies for *R prowazekii* found in both domestic and wild animals in Africa and France, livestock in Mexico, donkeys in South America and Egypt

  * Does the above represent cross-reaction with other organisms?

  * *R prowazekii* strains isolated from *Hyalomma* spp. ticks

  * *R prowazekii* isolated from flying squirrels (*Glaucomys volans*) in the U.S.

Key Clinical Features

- Both primary and recrudescent disease may be asymptomatic and go undetected or present with clinical disease

- Incubation period: 10–14 days

- Prodrome: 1–3 days of malaise before the abrupt onset of severe headache and fever (39–40° C)

- Some patients assume a crouching position because of myalgias

- Severe myalgia (100%), arthralgia, malaise, anorexia, chills

- CNS symptoms: photophobia, drowsiness, confusion, delirium, coma, seizures in 80% of cases

  * Meningeal irritation

  * Cerebral thrombosis from vasculitis a rare complication

  * Hearing loss

- Rashes considered typical, but some reports state it is present in only 20%–40% of cases (especially in African cases with dark-skinned patients)

- Cough 38%–70% of patients

- Nausea and vomiting 43%–57% of patients

- Diarrhea 13% of patients

- Multiple organ dysfunction

- Splenomegaly reported in 1 series

- Vascular compromise

  * Shock in 7% of patients

  * Ischemia and gangrene of distal fingers, toes and other sites

- Rash characteristics

  * Nonconfluent erythematous and blanching

  * Nonblanching macules, petechiae and sometimes purpura (1/3 of cases)

  * Distribution: trunk starting in axilla that spreads centrifugally to the extremities

  * Occasionally found on soft palate and conjunctiva (15%)

  * Eschars absent

- Brill-Zinsser Disease

  * Appears as sporadic cases years after primary disease

  * Unrelated to louse infestation

  * Similar but milder symptoms – rarely fatal

Key Differential Diagnostic Features

- Should be part of the differential diagnosis in any severe outbreak of unexplained fever in unhygienic conditions, war, social catastrophe, jails, cold environments, poverty, or internment camps

Key Laboratory/Radiology Features

- IgM antibodies excludes the diagnosis of Brill-Zinsser disease and indicates acute infection

- Patients with Brill-Zinsser disease have IgG antibodies

- Chest x-rays often have infiltrates from primary pneumonia or secondary bacterial pneumonia

- Thrombocytopenia (40%)

- Transaminases abnormal (63%)

- Hyperbilirubinemia (20%)

- Increased BUN (31%)

- Diagnostic tests

    * Weil-Felix test was the standard but it is no longer used – of historical interest

        - Patients with Brill-Zinsser disease have no agglutinating antibodies by this test

        - Cross-reactivity with other rickettsial diseases

    *More sensitive tests

        - Plate microagglutination

        - Indirect immunofluorescence

        - Western blot with cross-adsorption tests will differentiate *R prowazekii* from *R typhi*

        - Cell culture will isolate the organism (L929 fibroblast cell monolayers) and microscopic identification by Gimenez or immunofluorescence stain

        - Quantitative real-time PCR

Therapy

Empiric

- Doxycycline

- Treatment must be initiated on suspicion, prior to confirmation of diagnosis

- <u>Failure to show response within 24–48 hours of specific therapy is presumptive evidence that epidemic typhus is not the diagnosis</u>

Definitive/Specific

- Doxycycline for both primary disease and Brill-Zinsser disease

- Chloramphenicol is alternate therapy

- Fluoroquinolones should not be used

- Beta lactams, aminoglycosides, and sulfonamides are ineffective

- Although there is a long history of vaccine development, at present, there is no commercially available vaccine

- Preventive therapy aimed at eradication of the vector

    * Insecticide (10% DDT or 1% malathion, or 1% permethrin)

Prognostic Factors

- Mortality without treatment up to 60%

- Mortality in antibiotic era: 4%

- Highest mortality

    *Patients over the age of 60 years

    *Poor nutritional status

6. *Rickettsia typhi* (Murine typhus)

Further Reading

Books and Book Chapters

Raoult D, Walker DH. *Rickettsia prowazekii* (epidemic typhus, louse-borne typhus). In: *Mandell GL, Bennett JE, Dolin R, eds. Mandell, Douglas, and Bennett's Principles and Practice of Infectious Diseases*. 6th ed. v.2. Philadelphia, PA: Elsevier Churchill Livingstone; 2005:2303-2306.

Journal Articles

Azad AF. Pathogenic rickettsiae as bioterrorism agents. *Clin Infect Dis*. 2007;45 (Suppl 1):S52-S55.

Bechah Y, Capo C, Mege JL, et al. Epidemic typhus. *Lancet Infect Dis*. 2008;8:417-426.

Brouqui P, Raoult D. Arthropod-borne diseases in homeless. *Ann N Y Acad Sci*. 2006;1078:223-235.

Raoult D, Roux V. The body louse as a vector of reemerging human diseases. *Clin Infect Dis*. 1999;29:888-911.

Synonyms

• Murine typhus

• Endemic typhus

• Flea-borne typhus

Causative Organisms

• *Rickettsia typhi*

• *Rickettsia felis*

* Detected in cat fleas and opossums in Texas and southern California

* Causes typhus-like illness in patients from Texas, Mexico, France and Brazil

Epidemiology

• Worldwide zoonosis

• Associated with rat and cat fleas

* *Rattus rattus* and *Rattus norvegicus*

* Opossums (*Didelphis marsupialis*) and cats most important reservoirs in Texas and California

* *Xenopsylla cheopis* rat flea

* *Ctenocephalides felis* cat flea

* Both horizontal and transovarial transmission in fleas

* Transmitted to humans by inoculation of infected flea feces into a pruritic flea bite

* Few infected patients actually report a flea bite or flea exposure

• Especially important in subtropical and coastal areas

• Important in south Texas and southern California

- Outbreaks in areas housing displaced persons

- Cases occur all year

  * Peak in Texas in spring and summer

  * Peak in California in summer and fall

Key Clinical Features

- Incubation period: 1–2 weeks

- Abrupt onset of symptoms

  * Fever (96–100%)

  * Chills (44%–87%)

  * Severe headache (45%–88%)

  * Myalgia (33%)

  * Nausea (33%)

  * Rash (18% at presentation, but eventually 50%–80% of patients develop rash)

    - Onset of rash usually 1 week into febrile illness

    - Petechiae (<10%)

    - Macular or maculo-papular (78%)

    - Distribution

      * Trunk (88%)

      * Extremities (>45%)

      * Palms and soles reported but infrequent

- As disease progresses:

  * Nausea (48%), vomiting (40%) and anorexia (35%)

  * Abdominal pain (11%–60%)

  * Cough (35%)

- Hepatomegaly (24%–29%) and splenomegaly (5%–24%)

- Neurologic symptoms (45%)

  * Confusion (2%–13%)

  * Stupor

  * Seizures

  * Ataxia

  * Other focal findings

- Childhood disease usually mild

- Complications infrequent

  * Respiratory failure

  * Renal insufficiency

  * Hepatic insufficiency

  * 10% require ICU admission

  * 4% of adult hospitalized patients die

  * Culture-negative endocarditis reported

  * Splenic rupture

  * CNS complications occur 10 days to 3 weeks into disease

    - Papilledema

    - Hemiparesis

    - Facial nerve palsy

Key Differential Diagnostic Features

- Must be considered in the differential diagnosis of diseases occurring in returning travels

- May mimic

  * Vector-borne infections

    - Rocky Mountain Spotted Fever

    - Ehrlichiosis

    - Anaplasmosis

    - West Nile Virus fever

    - Babesiosis

    - Dengue

  * Non-vector-associated infections

    - Typhoid fever

    - Meningococcal sepsis

    - Leptospirosis

    - Viral and bacterial meningitis

    - Measles

    - Toxic shock syndrome

    - Secondary syphilis

    - Kawasaki syndrome

Key Laboratory/Radiology Features

- Early mild leukopenia (18%–50%) in first 7 days of illness

- Anemia (18%–75%)

- Elevated ESR (59%–89%)

- Thrombocytopenia in first 7 days of illness (19%–48%)

- Later increased WBCs in 33% of patients

- Prothrombin time prolonged but DIC is rare

- Most frequent abnormality: elevated AST (38%–92%)

- Other liver enzymes (alkaline phosphatase, ALT, LDH

- Hypoproteinemia (45%)

- Hypoalbuminemia (46%–89%)

- Hyponatremia (mild – 60%)

- Hypocalcemia (79%)

- CSF usually normal or mild pleocytosis (10–640 cells/mm^3) with mononuclear predominance and mild increase in protein in the presence of symptoms suggests viral meningitis or leptospirosis

- CSF will be strongly positive for *R typhi* IgM

- Weil-Felix agglutination testing no longer used

- Immunohistologic demonstration of the organism in tissue

- Serologic testing: 50% positive in 1 week and nearly all patients positive in 15 days

  * Serologic test rarely diagnostic at the onset of symptoms

  * Indirect fluorescent antibody – "gold standard"

  * Solid-phase immunoassay

- Culture should not be attempted because the organism represents a significant biohazard

- PCR diagnosis using peripheral blood, buffy coat, plasma (fresh or frozen), tissue specimens, and arthropods

Therapy

Empiric

- Therapy is always started before laboratory confirmation

- Patients usually respond to appropriate therapy within 3 days

- Doxycycline must always be included in empiric therapy when this is part of the differential diagnosis and is the recommended treatment for suspected cases

- Atypical presentations of Q fever, scrub typhus, murine typhus, human monocytic ehrlichiosis and bartonellosis may present with fevers of more than 1 week's duration. Even without confirmation of the diagnosis, treatment with doxycycline should be initiated in patients with the appropriate epidemiologic risks

Definitive/Specific

- Doxycycline (also suggested therapy for late trimester pregnancy)

    * Delayed defervescence is seen in spite of therapy in patients presenting with jaundice, relative bradycardia and absence of headache. This is also seen in Q fever and scrub typhus

- Chloramphenicol (IV) is an alternate therapy (and suggested therapy for early trimester pregnancy)

- Continue antibiotics for 2–3 days after defervescence

- Fluoroquinolones have been used in clinical trials and may be an alternative therapy

- Steroids have been used in severe CNS disease

Prognostic Factors

- Case-fatality rate

    * Mortality 1% with use of appropriate antibiotics

    * Mortality 4% without antibiotics

- Severity worse when appropriate therapy delayed

- More severe disease associated with trimethoprim-sulfamethoxazole treatment

- Disease more severe in:

    * Elderly

    * Men

    * African origin

    * High WBC

    * Hepatic dysfunction

    * Renal dysfunction

    * G6PD deficiency

- More severe liver disease and jaundice associated with:

    * Hemolytic disorders (G6PD deficiency)

    * Hemoglobinopathies

    * Thalassemia

Further Reading

Books and Book Chapters

Dumler JS, Walker DH. *Rickettsia typhi* (Murine typhus). In: Mandell GL, Bennett JE, Dolin R, eds. *Mandell, Douglas, and Bennett's Principles and Practice of Infectious Diseases*. 6th ed. v.2. Philadelphia, PA: Elsevier Churchill Livingstone; 2005:2306-2309.

Journal Articles

Zimmerman MD, Murdoch Dr, Rozmajzi PJ. Murine typhus and febrile illness, Nepal. *Emerg Infect Dis*. 2008;14:1656-1659.

Civen R, Ngo V. Murine typhus: an unrecognized suburban vector borne disease. *Clin Infect Dis*. 2008;46:913-918.

7. *Orientia tsutsugamushi* (Scrub typhus, previously *Rickettsia tsutsugamushi*)

Synonyms

- In Japanese, "tsutsuga" means something small and dangerous, and "mushi" means creature

- Scrub typhus

- Summer-type scrub typhus (transmitted by *Leptotrombidium deliense* mite)

- Autumn-winter scrub typhus (caused by less virulent *O tsutsugamushi* transmitted by *L scutellare* mite)

- Insect disease bush typhus (as it was called during the Battle of Buna-Gona, New Guinea Campaign – November 16, 1942-January 22, 1943)

- *Rickettsia tsutsugamushi*

Causative Organisms

- *Orientia tsutsugamushi*

Epidemiology

- Found in an area bounded by Japan, Eastern Australia and Eastern Russia

  * Includes Indian subcontinent, China and the entire Far East

- Approximately 1 million infections per year documented

- Rodents act as reservoirs

- Transmitted by the larval form of the trombiculid mite (chigger) which acts as both a reservoir and vector

- No person-to-person transmission

Key Clinical Features

- Incubation: 6–21 days (usually 10–12 days)

- Eschar at site of chigger feeding with regional tender lymphadenopathy

  * Eschar begins as papule that enlarges, undergoes central necrosis and develops a black crust with an erythematous halo

- Macular or maculopapular rash on trunk that later extends to arms and legs appears 5–8 days after the onset of fever

- Signs and symptoms:

  * Fever (100%)

  * Eschar (60%)

  * Chills (39%)

  * Cough (24%)

  * Dyspnea (18%)

  * Headache (21%)

  * Diarrhea (18%)

  * Generalized lymphadenopathy (33%) and splenomegaly are common

  * Rash (21%)

- Complications

  * Some patients develop CNS signs: tremors, delirium, nervousness, or nuchal rigidity during the 2nd week into the infection

  * Renal failure (9%), in one case secondary to acute tubular necrosis from direct invasion of the pathogen

  * Guillain-Barré syndrome

  * Transverse myelitis

  * Respiratory failure – interstitial pneumonia

* Acute reversible hearing loss

* Myocarditis (3%) — cardiomegaly reversible
  in surviving patients

* Acute fulminant myocarditis with cardiogenic
  shock with 50% mortality

* Septic shock (3%)

* Gastric vascular bleeding and duodenal ulcer
  bleeding

  • Endoscopy reveals superficial mucosal
    hemorrhage, multiple erosions and ulcers
    without any predilection for site

  • Endoscopic lesions directly related to skin
    lesions and severity of disease

• HIV and Scrub typhus coinfection: may increase
  or decrease HIV viral load

Key Differential Diagnostic Features

• Routine laboratory tests are of no value in
  differentiating scrub typhus from the other
  diseases in the differential diagnosis

• Differential diagnosis includes

  * Rickettsial pox

  * Mediterranean spotted fever

  * Dengue

    • Dengue associated with hemorrhage,
      especially bleeding from the gums which
      is not seen in scrub typhus

    • Low platelet counts and low WBCs were
      more strongly associated with dengue

  * Leptospirosis

  * Murine typhus

* Hemorrhagic fever with renal syndrome
  (HFRS) (from Hantavirus)

  • On presentation, none of the patients with
    scrub typhus demonstrated hemorrhagic
    manifestations

  • Scrub typhus patients > HFRS patients

    * Skin lesions

    * Eschar

    * Regional lymphadenopathy

    * Maculopapular rash

  • HFRS patients >Scrub typhus patients

    * Retro-orbital pain

    * Lumbar back pain

    * Flank tenderness

    * Proteinuria

    * Occult blood in the urine

    * Significantly lower platelet counts

Key Laboratory/Radiology Features

• Leukopenia (19%)

• Leukocytosis (34%)

  * In buffy coats, mononuclear cells stained
    positive for the organism in 3 of 7 patients
    using immunoalkaline phosphatase method
    prior to and 2 days into therapy

• Elevated AST (81%) and ALT (75%)

• Thrombocytopenia (44%) can be severe enough
  to cause bleeding

• Albuminuria (88.9%) in septic shock

- Direct and indirect bilirubin usually elevated in septic shock

- Indirect immunofluorescent antibody assay – "gold standard"

    * Antibody titers are not diagnostic early in the disease

- Nested PCR on buffy coat but may give a false negative

    * Rate of detection: before antibiotics — 90.5%; 3 days of either doxycycline or rifampin — 60.5%; 4 days of antibiotics — 10%

- Immunohistochemical staining cutaneous lesions

- Elevated AST, ALT and alkaline phosphatase are frequently found in scrub typhus but not diagnostic

- Interstitial pneumonia (especially common in autopsy series)

- Cardiac lesions (endocardial or pericardial in 80% of autopsy series

- Chest x-rays abnormal in 59%–72% of patients

    * Bilateral diffuse reticulonodular opacities

    * Unilateral or bilateral hilar adenopathy (25%–27%)

    * Pleural effusions (12%–43%)

    * Septal lines

    * Consolidations uncommon

- Central nervous system

    * Autopsy studies: meningoencephalitis with "typhus nodules" (cluster of microglial cells) and hemorrhage

- Abdominal involvement on CT

    * Splenomegaly

    * Periportal areas of low attenuation

    * Gallbladder wall thickening

    * Lymphadenopathy

    * Splenic infarct

    * Ascites

Therapy

Empiric

- Doxycycline

- Atypical presentations of Q fever, scrub typhus, murine typhus, human monocytic ehrlichiosis, and bartonellosis may present with fevers of more than one week's duration. Even without confirmation of the diagnosis, treatment with doxycycline should be initiated in patients with the appropriate epidemiologic risks

Definitive/Specific

- Doxycycline is the drug of choice

    * Delayed defervescence is seen in spite of therapy in patients presenting with jaundice, relative bradycardia and absence of headache. This is also seen in Q fever and murine typhus

- Chloramphenicol is alternative therapy

- Other drugs: rifampin and azithromycin

- Ciprofloxacin should not be used

Prognostic Factors

• Infection during pregnancy causes spontaneous abortion

• Relapses occur after short treatment courses

• Untreated, mortality 3–60%

Further Reading

Books and Book Chapters

Raoult D. Scrub typhus. In: *Mandell GL, Bennett JE, Dolin R, eds. Mandell, Douglas, and Bennett's Principles and Practice of Infectious Diseases.* 6th ed. v.2. Philadelphia, PA: Elsevier Churchill Livingstone; 2005:2309-2310.

Journal Articles

Blacksell SD, Bryant JN, Paris DH, et al. Scrub typhus serologic testing with the indirect immuno-fluorescence method as a diagnostic gold standard: a lack of consensus leads to a lot of confusion. *Clin Infect Dis.* 2007;44:391-401.

Hsu YH, Chen HI. Pulmonary pathology in patients associated with scrub typhus. *Pathology.* 2008;40:268-271.

Jeong YJ, Kim S, Wook YD, et al. Scrub typhus: clinical, pathologic, and imaging findings. *Radiographics.* 2007;27:161-172.

Kim DM, Byun JN. Effects of antibiotic treatment on the results of nested PCRs for scrub typhus. *J Clin Microbiol.* 2008;46:3465-3466.

Kim DM, Kang DW, Kim JO, et al. Acute renal failure due to acute tubular necrosis caused by direct invasion of *Orientia tsutsugamushi. J Clin Microbiol.* 2008;46:1548-1550.

Lai CH, Huang CK, Weng HC, et al. Clinical characteristics of acute Q fever, scrub typhus, and murine typhus with delayed defervescence despite doxycycline treatment. *Am J Trop Med Hyg.* 2008;79:441-446.

Lee KL, Lee JK, Yim YM, et al. Acute transverse myelitis associated with scrub typhus: case report and a review of the literature. *Diagn Microbiol Infect Dis.* 2008;60:237-239.

Liu YX, Feng D, Zhang Q, et al. Key differentiating features between scrub typhus and hemorrhagic fever with renal syndrome in northern China. *Am J Trop Med Hyg.* 2007;76:801-805.

Mahajan SK, Bakshi D. Acute reversible hearing loss in scrub typhus. *J Assoc Physicians India.* 2007;55:512-514.

Phimda K, Hoontrakul S, Suttinont C, et al. Doxycycline versus azithromycin for treatment of leptospirosis and scrub typhus. *Antimicrob Agents Cheother.* 2007;51:3259-3263.

Sittiwangkul R, Pongprot Y, Silviliarat S, et al. Acute fulminant myocarditis in scrub typhus. *Ann Trop Paediatr.* 2008;28:149-154.

Thap LC, Supparanond W, Treeprasertsuk S, et al. Septic shock secondary to scrub typhus: characteristics and complications. *Southeast Asian J Trop Med Public Health.* 2002;33:780-786.

Tsay RW, Chang FY. Serious complications in scrub typhus. *J Microbiol Immunol Infect.* 1998;31:240-244.

Walsh DS, Myint KS, Kantipong P, et al. *Orientia tsutsugamushi* in peripheral white blood cells of patients with acute scrub typhus. *Am J Trop Med Hyg.* 2001;65:899-901.

Watt G, Jongsakul K, Chouriyagune C, et al. Differentiating dengue virus infection from scrub typhus in Thai adults with fever. *Am J Trop Med Hyg.* 2003;68:536-538.

Watt G, Parola P. Scrub typhus and tropical rickettsioses. *Curr Opin Infect Dis.* 2003;16:429-436.

8. Tick Paralysis

Synonyms

• Tick toxicosis

Causative Organisms

• Ticks that transmit *R rickettsii* and other rickettsial diseases

    * Vector in Australia: *Ixodes holocyclus*

    * Vector in North America: *Dermacentor andersoni* and *D variabilis*

Epidemiology

• 60 species of ticks cause tick paralysis

    * In North America, 6 species of ticks

        • *Dermacentor andersoni*

        • *D variabilis*

        • *A americanum*

        • *A maculatum*

        • *Ixodes scapularis*

        • *I pacificus*

    * In Europe, Crete, South America and Australia additional species of ticks

        • *Rhinencephalus*

        • *Hyalomma*

        • *Boophilus*

        • *Haemaphysalis*

    * Most cases occur from engorged pregnant females that have fed for 5 days, although tick paralysis has been reported associated with feeding male ticks

    * Disease is the result of a toxin (holocyclotoxin) produced in the salivary glands. Toxins differ among tick species, but experimental evidence suggests cross protection using a single experimental vaccine

• The same ticks that transmit *R rickettsii* cause tick paralysis (tick toxicosis), 1 of the 8 most common tick-borne diseases in the United States. It is believed to have been first described in Australia

• More common in females (76% of patients)

• More common in children (82% of patients)

• Most frequent tick locations are: scalp, behind the ear, neck and groin

Key Clinical Features

• Some cases present with a prodrome (12–36) hours before the onset of flaccid paralysis. Typically, in children there is irritability and lethargy followed by bilateral leg weakness. The child appears uncoordinated. The prodrome consists of:

    * Paresthesias

    * Restlessness

    * Irritability

    * Fatigue

    * Myalgias

• Most characteristic findings in North American cases

    * Symmetric and flaccid paralysis

    * Diminished or complete lack of reflexes

    * Normal sensory examination and mental status

    * Sphincter function normal

    * Normal cerebrospinal fluid

    * No autonomic dysfunction

- Unusual clinical syndromes

  * Bell's palsy

  * Extraocular muscle paralysis and/or diplopia

  * Upper or lower limb weakness

  * Ataxia

  * Myoclonus

  * Chorea

- Presents as an acute symmetric ascending flaccid paralysis over 12–24 hours

  * Disease progresses from lower extremities to upper extremities to lower cranial nerves, to upper cranial nerves, and finally the respiratory muscles fail

  * Mental status remains normal until respiratory failure

- Disease evolves over hours or days

- Australian cases

  * Hypertension associated with *I holocyclus* tick paralysis

  * Pupillary changes seen more often with Australian cases

  * Focal weakness seen more often with Australian cases or with tick in the subclavian fossa

- NO fever

- Pain is usually absent but has been rarely reported

- Complications: myocarditis

Key Differential Diagnostic Features

- Guillain-Barré syndrome

  * Leg pain absent in tick paralysis but may be present in 20% of children with Guillain-Barré syndrome

  * Weakness in Guillain-Barré evolve more slowly than in tick paralysis

- Miller-Fisher variant (ophthalmoplegia, ataxia, areflexia without muscle weakness)

- Botulism

- Myasthenia gravis

- Periodic paralysis

- Diphtheria

- Heavy metal poisoning

- Porphyria,

- Solvent inhalation

- Electrolyte abnormalities

- Cerebellar ataxia

  * Acute cerebellar ataxia in young children often caused by

    - Varicella

    - Coxsackie

    - Epstein-Barr virus

    - *Borrelia burgdorferi*

    - Mycoplasma

    - Systemic lupus and other inflammatory disorders

- Spinal cord compression

- Transverse myelitis

- Poliomyelitis and other enteroviruses that mimic polio

- Organophosphate poisoning

- CMV polyradiculomyeitis

- Encephalomyelitis

  * West Nile fever

  * Other viral encephalitis

Key Laboratory/Radiology Features

- No significant diagnostic laboratory findings

- Pathophysiology

  * Australian cases: presynaptic decrease in acetylcholine release

  * North American cases: both decreased nerve conduction and decrease in acetylcholine release

Therapy

Definitive/Specific

- Remove the tick

- An antiserum has been used in Australian cases

  * The hyperimmune antiserum is prepared in dogs

  * Acute allergic reactions and serum sickness is common

Prognostic Factors

- Australian cases: Often progresses for 24–48 hours after tick removal

  * Recovery may take days to weeks

- North American cases: Improves as soon as tick is removed

  * Recovery in 24 hours

- 10%–12% mortality from respiratory failure once bulbar weakness appears

- If the tick is removed before the appearance of bulbar involvement, patients recover within hours or days

Further Reading

Books and Book Chapters

Torres JM, Schlossberg D. Tick paralysis. In: In: Cunha BA, ed. *Tickborne Infectious Diseases – Diagnosis and Management*. New York, NY: Marcel Dekker, 2000:103-110.

Journal Articles

Edlow JA, McGillicuddy DC. Tick paralysis. *Infect Dis Clin North Am*. 2008;22:397-413.

Parola P, Paddock CD, Raoult D. Tick-borne rickettsioses around the world: emerging diseases challenging old concepts. *Clin Microbiol Rev*. 2005:18:719-756.

ID Board Pearls

• *Rickettsia rickettsii*
(Rocky Mountain Spotted Fever)

   * Digital infarction may be a presentation of Rocky Mountain spotted fever. This, in combination with meningeal-neurologic findings and an atypical vasculitic rash, may more strongly suggest meningococcemia and *Staphylococcus aureus* sepsis.

   * Early treatment of Rocky Mountain spotted fever may prevent diagnosis by IFA, and IFA cannot distinguish among the spotted fever rickettsial diseases.

   * Only 70% of patients with Rocky Mountain spotted fever report a tick bite.

   * 3 additional tick-borne diseases (*Rickettsia parkeri*, *Rickettsia africae*, and *Rickettsia massiliae*) have been identified in addition to the suggestion that variation in *R rickettsii* genotypes may be the explanation for wide variations in fatality rates.

   * *Rickettsia massiliae* is the ONLY pathogenic rickettsia prevalent in Africa, Europe, and America.

• *Rickettsia akari* (Rickettsialpox, Kew Gardens fever)

   * Rickettsialpox should be included in the differential diagnosis of acute hepatitis.

• *Coxiella burnetii* (Q fever)

   * Blood cultures (by cell culture) will isolate *C burnetii* from 17% of untreated patients with acute Q fever and from 53% of untreated patients with chronic Q fever, but will remain negative in patients being actively treated for the disease.

   * 60% of those infected with *C burnetii* are asymptomatic.

   * Most patients who develop chronic Q fever manifest the disease (1) months to years after the initial infection; (2) commonly present as culture-negative endocarditis (75%–100% of cases); and most patients have predisposing conditions (ie, valvular heart disease, vascular abnormalities, immunosuppression).

   * Some authors recommend serologic screening every 4 months for 2 years after acute Q fever infection in order for early diagnosis of asymptomatic chronic Q fever and endocarditis, thus affording early treatment and avoiding valve replacement.

   * No test can guarantee cure of Q fever endocarditis.

   * A few as 1 organism by inhalation may cause infection with *C burnetii*.

• *Rickettsia prowazekii* (Epidemic typhus, Louse-borne typhus)

   * The rash of epidemic typhus is usually NOT found on the face, palms or soles.

   * Prothrombin time is usually normal in epidemic typhus.

• *Rickettsia typhi* (Murine typhus)

   * In Hawaii, there is no seasonal distribution in the incidence of murine typhus.

• *Orientia tsutsugamushi* (Scrub typhus)

   * PCR may not be positive during the first 5 days of symptomatic illness with *Orientia tsutsugamushi* infection.

   * PCR from eschar effective in making the diagnosis even after antibiotic therapy

• Tick paralysis

    * In patients with tick paralysis, especially in North America, it is essential to look for more ticks if there is no improvement or a worsening of symptoms after the tick is removed.

    * In patients with tick paralysis and fever, other tick-borne infections should be considered, as fever is not seen in tick paralysis.

    * In tick paralysis, it has been suggested that the closer the tick is to the central nervous system (especially on the back of the neck or head) the shorter the incubation period. The tick's location may produce localized weakness: Bell's palsy caused by a tick behind the ear or in the external auditory canal; weakness of the frontalis and orbicularis oculi cause by ticks on the forehead; and upper (unilateral brachial plexus neuropathy) or lower limb weakness caused by ticks on the upper arm or genitalia respectively.

    * Antibiotic prophylaxis is not indicated after a tick-bite. Patients should be cautioned as to the symptomatology of a possible rickettsial-related or other tick-borne infections.

II. Ehrlichiosis and Related Diseases

1. **Overview**

2. *Ehrlichia chaffeensis* **(Human Monocy-totropic Ehrlichiosis)**

3. *Anaplasma phagocytphilum* **(Human Granulocytic Anaplasmosis, formerly Human Granulocytic Ehrlichiosis ([***Ehrlichia phagocytophila*** group])**

4. *Ehrlichia canis*

5. *Ehrlichia ewingii* **and** *Ehrlichia muris* **(Murine typhus)**

6. *Neorickettsia sennetsu* **(Sennetsu Neorickettsiosis, formerly** *E sennetsu* **([Sennetsu Ehrlichiosis])**

1. Overview

Ehrlichia and *Anaplasma* species are Gram-negative intracellular bacteria of the Anaplasmataceae family. They are characterized by (1) their natural nonhuman hosts (*E chaffeensis*: deer, dogs, other canids; *E ewingii*: dogs and deer; and, *A phagocytphilum*: deer, livestock, and rodents); (2) principal target cell (macrophages – *E chaffeensis* and *A phagocytphilum*; granulocytes – *E ewingii* and *N sennetsu*); (3) the formation of morula (clustered inclusion bodies in host cell vacuoles), and, (4) their transmission by arthropod vectors. *N sennetsu* appears to be limited to human hosts. Most patients report a tick bite within the previous month. Early signs and symptoms of these diseases tend to be nonspecific and mimic mostly benign self-limited viral illnesses, especially mononucleosis. Doxycycline is both the empiric and definitive treatment.

2. *Ehrlichia chaffeensis* (Human Monocytotropic Ehrlichiosis)

Synonyms

• Human monocytotropic ehrlichiosis

Causative Organisms

• *Ehrlichia chaffeensis*

Epidemiology

• Tick-transmitted disease

  * *Amblyomma americanum* (Lone Star tick)

  * *Dermacentor variabilis*

  * *Ixodes pacificus*

  * In ticks, the pathogen is transmitted trans-stadially (between developmental stages) but not transovarially

• Mammalian hosts:

  * Deer (especially the white-tailed deer)

  * Dogs

  * Coyotes

• Peak months: May–July

• Reported in most states

• 75% of cases male

Key Clinical Features

• Incubation period: 7 days

• In one study, 11% of FUO cases displayed seroconversion

• 41%–63% of clinical disease results in hospitalization

• Mild to severe disease in immunocompetent host averaging 23 days in duration

• Symptoms – Most commonly sudden onset of fever, chills, generalized myalgia, and severe headache

* Fever (97%)

* Chills (67%)

* Headache (81%)

* Myalgia (68%)

* Malaise (84%)

* Nausea (48%) usually later in the disease

* Anorexia (66%) usually later in the disease accompanied by weight loss

* Vomiting (37%)

* Diarrhea (25%) with more severe disease

* Abdominal pain (22%)

* Rash (36%) – maculopapular or occasionally petechial (less frequently in transplant patients)

* Cough (26%) with more severe disease

* Shortness of breath (23%) with more severe disease

* Lymphadenopathy (25%) with more severe disease

* Confusion (20%) with more severe disease

• Complications

  * Pneumonia

  * ARDS with 18% requiring mechanical respiratory support

  * Meningoencephalitis

  * Anemia in patients ill more than one week

  * Gastrointestinal bleeding

  * Coagulopathy (DIC)

* Acute renal insufficiency that may require dialysis

* Culture-negative endocarditis

* Toxic-shock-like syndrome

* Immunosuppressed patients have had fulminant disease

* More severe disease in HIV-infected patients

Key Differential Diagnostic Features

• Rocky Mountain Spotted Fever

* Patients with ehrlichiosis are less likely to have a rash and rarely have a petechial rash

* Patients with ehrlichiosis are more likely to have leukopenia and lymphopenia

• Early disease may mimic other common infections

* Viral or bacterial respiratory infections

* Urinary tract infections

* Sepsis

* Bacterial or viral meningitis

* Gastroenteritis

• A positive history of a tick bite

* Rocky Mountain Spotted Fever

* Colorado tick fever

* Babesiosis

* Lyme disease

* Tularemia

• Other diseases in the differential diagnosis

* Meningococcemia

* Toxic shock syndrome

* Leptospirosis

* Hepatitis

* Enteroviral infections

* Influenza

* Murine typhus

* Q fever

* Typhoid fever

* Bacterial sepsis

* Endocarditis

* Kawasaki disease

* Collagen-vascular diseases

* Leukemia

Key Laboratory/Radiology Features

• Routine labs

* Leukopenia (60%) (more leukopenia in transplant patients)

* Thrombocytopenia (68%)

* Elevated liver enzymes (AST – 86%; ALT – 80%) (less frequently in transplant patients)

* Abnormal renal function (BUN – 38%; creatinine – 29%) (more frequent in transplant patients)

* Peripheral smears

  • Morulae observed in <7% of patients, most often in immunocompromised patients with overwhelming infection

  • The morulae are a darker color than that of the nucleus

• CSF findings in severe disease

  * Lymphocytic pleocytosis

  * Elevated protein

  * Cells with morulae

• Chest x-ray

  * 50% of patients have infiltrates

• Culture in cell culture systems a research technique only

• Serologic testing the principle diagnostic method

  * Indirect immunofluorescence assay (IFA)

• Immunohistologic demonstration of the organism is not reliable due to sampling difficulties

• PCR on peripheral blood appears to give the most sensitive and timely results

  * 60%–85% sensitivity

  * PCR often positive while serology is negative in the acute illness

Therapy

Empiric

• Doxycycline

• Delay in treatment will prolong hospitalization and longer length of illness

• Atypical presentations of Q fever, scrub typhus, murine typhus, human monocytic ehrlichiosis, and bartonellosis may present with fevers of more than one week's duration. In patients with the appropriate epidemiologic risks, even without confirmation of the diagnosis, doxycycline treatment should be initiated

Definitive/Specific

• Doxycycline 100 mg twice daily for 7–10 days

• Rifampin demonstrates low *in vitro* MICs; fluoroquinolones demonstrate variable *in vitro* susceptibility

• *In vitro*: doxycycline and rifampin highly active, but fluoroquinolones variable

• *In vitro*: no activity demonstrated for beta-lactams, cotrimoxazole, macrolides or telithromycin

• *In vitro* resistance to chloramphenicol but patients treated with this drug become afebrile faster than patients treated with non-tetracycline antibiotics

Prognostic Factors

• Higher incidence of disease in older individuals

• More severe disease and higher mortality in the elderly

• Delay in diagnosis and treatment increases severity of disease and risk of death

• Mortality: 1%–2% to as high as 5.3% (early reports)

3. *Anaplasma phagocytphilum* (Human Granulocytic Anaplasmosis, formerly Human Granulocytic Ehrlichiosis ([*Ehrlichia phagocytophila* group])

Further Reading

Books and Book Chapters

Bakken JS, Dumler JS Ehrlichiosis. In: Cunha BA, ed. *Tickborne Infectious Diseases – Diagnosis and Management*. New York, NY; 2000:139-168.

Dumler JS, Aguero-Rosenfeld ME. Microbiology and laboratory diagnosis of tickborne diseases. In: Cunha BA, ed. *Tickborne Infectious Diseases – Diagnosis and Management*. New York, NY; 2000:15-54.

Walker DH, Dumler JS. *Ehrlichia chaffeensis* (human monocytotropic ehrlichiosis), *Anaplasma phagocytphilum* (human granulocytotropic anaplasmosis) and other Ehrlichieae. In: Mandell GL, Bennett JE, Dolin R, eds. *Mandell, Douglas, and Bennett's Principles and Practice of Infectious Diseases*. 6th ed. v.2. Philadelphia, PA: Elsevier Churchill Livingstone; 2005:2310-2318.

Journal Articles

Hamburg BJ, Storch GA, Micek ST, et al. The importance of early treatment with doxycycline in human ehrlichiosis. *Medicine* (Baltimore). 2008;87:53-60.

Paddock CD, Childs JE. *Ehrlichia chaffeensis*: a prototypical emerging pathogen. *Clin Microbiol Rev*. 2003;16:37-64.

Paddock CD, Folk SM, Shore GM, et al. Infections with *Ehrlichia chaffeensis* and *Ehrlichia ewingii* in persons coinfected with human immunodeficiency virus. *Clin Infect Dis*. 2001;33:1586-1594.

Prince LK, Shah AA, Martinez LJ, et al. Ehrlichiosis: making the diagnosis in the acute setting. *South Med J*. 2007;100:825-828.

Thomas LD, Hongo I, Block KC, et al. Human ehrlichiosis in transplant recipients. *Am J Transplant*. 2007;7:1641-1647.

Synonyms

- Human granulocytic ehrlichiosis

- *Ehrlichia phagocytophila* group

- *Ehrlichia equi* (this genus and species has been used interchangeably with *E phagocytophila*)

Causative Organisms

- *Anaplasma phagocytphilum*

    * Order *Rickettsiales*, family *Anaplasmataceae*

    * Life cycle alternates between arthropod (tick) reservoir and mammalian hosts

    * Lives in granulocyte endosomes: vacuoles allow bacteria to form colonies (morulae) that may be seen with Romanowsky-stained (Wright stain or Giemsa stain) peripheral blood smears

Epidemiology

- *Ixodes persulcatus*-complex (ticks) act as the vector for *A phagocytphilum*, *Borrelia burgdorferi*, and *Babesia microti*

- *I scapularis* are vectors in the northeastern and upper Midwest U.S.

- *I pacificus* are vectors along the northern Pacific coast

- Ticks (as are the host, the white-footed mouse) are not infrequently co-infected with *B burgdorferi*

- 5% of humans with *A phagocytphilum* either had a history of erythema migrans or serologic evidence of *B burgdorferi* infection

- *A phagocytphilum* cycles between ticks and nonhuman vertebrate and invertebrate hosts

  * Important reservoirs: white-footed mouse (*Peromyscus leucopus*), deer mouse (*P maniculatus*), and white tailed deer (*Odocoileus virginianus*)

- In ticks, *A phagocytphilum* is transferred both by trans-stadial (between feeding stages – larva to nymph to adult tick) and transovarially

- Seroprevalence rates for *A phagocytphilum* in the U.S.: 8.9%–36%

- *A phagocytphilum* infection identified in Europe

- Possible transplacental transmission has been reported

- Acquired by individuals butchering white tailed deer either by direct contact or aerosolization

- *A phagocytphilum* remains viable in refrigerated blood up to 18 days

- Humans are generally a dead-end host as the infection does not persist for long

- Peak incidence in July and November at peak activity of nymphal and adult stages of the *I scapularis* tick in the eastern U.S.

- Perinatal transmission has been documented

- Nosocomial transmission and transmission through cutaneous and mucocutaneous contact with blood or bloody respiratory secretions (during endotracheal intubation of the index case)

- Limited evidence of transmission through blood transfusion

Key Clinical Features

- Nonspecific, nonfatal, mild, self-limited illness to fatal disease

- Age and comorbid conditions determine severity of illness

- Incubation period: 1–2 weeks after tick exposure

- Initial symptoms: fever, rigors, myalgia and headache

- Common symptoms

  * Fever

  * Headache

  * Myalgias and malaise

  * Rigors

- Less frequent symptoms

  * Anorexia

  * Nausea

  * Cough

- Uncommon symptoms

  * Abdominal pain

  * Change in mental status

  * Rash

- Complications

  * Opportunistic infections (sometimes fatal), especially in immune compromised patients

    - Herpes simplex esophagitis

    - *Candida albicans* pneumonia and esophagitis

    - Invasive pulmonary aspergillosis

Key Differential Diagnostic Features

• Infectious Agents

    * Viral syndromes, especially enteroviral infections

    * Epstein-Barr virus infection

    * Human herpes virus 6 infection

    * Parvovirus B-19 infection

    * Viral hepatitis

    * West Nile Virus infection

    * Disseminated gonococcal infection

    * Bacterial endocarditis

    * Meningococcemia

    * *Mycoplasma pneumoniae* infection

    * Post-group A streptococcal infection

    * Secondary syphilis

    * Septic shock

    * Typhoid

• Non-infectious

    * Allergic drug reactions

    * Immune complex disease

    * Kawasaki disease

    * Thrombotic thrombocytopenic purpura

    * Toxic hemophagocytic and macrophage activation syndromes

• Other vector-borne zoonoses to be considered in these patients exposed to insects and ticks

    * Babesiosis

    * Bartonellosis

    * Colorado tick fever

    * Human monocytic ehrlichiosis

    * Leptospirosis

    * Lyme disease

    * Murine typhus

    * Q fever

    * Rat-bite fevers

    * Rocky Mountain Spotted Fever

    * Tularemia

    * Dengue

    * Malaria

    * Tick-borne encephalitis

• Hematologic abnormalities may suggest leukemia and lymphoma as morulae may be confused with Auer rods

Key Laboratory/Radiology Features

• Thrombocytopenia, leucopenia with normal bone marrow biopsies

• Leukopenia with left shift

• Leukopenia and thrombocytopenia correct themselves in the second week of the illness

- Elevation of transaminases

- Confirmation of diagnosis

    * Wright or Giemsa-stained peripheral blood
      smear during the early phase of infection
      (morulae seen in 20%–80% of patients in the
      first week of infection)

    * Polymerase chain reaction amplification of
      A phagocytphilum-specific DNA in acute
      phase peripheral blood — 67%–90%
      sensitivity

    * Isolation of organism in promyelocytic
      leukemia cell cultures inoculated with acute
      phase blood

    * Indirect fluorescent antibody (IFA) for IgM
      and IgG with 4-fold rise in titer common and
      sensitive test

        • Antibodies persist for months in seroreac-
          tive patients

Therapy

Empiric and Definitive/Specific

- All patients with suspected or proven disease
  should be treated with doxycycline 100 mg twice
  daily, either IV or PO for 4–5 days

- Rifampin has been recommended as alternate
  therapy in children (20 mg/kg up to 600 mg in
  2 divided doses) and adults (300 mg twice daily)
  for 5–7 days

- No vaccines are available

- *In vitro*: doxycycline and rifampin highly active,
  but fluoroquinolones active

- *In vitro*: no activity demonstrated for beta-lactams,
  cotrimoxazole, macrolides or telithromycin

- *In vitro resistance to chloramphenicol*

Prognostic Factors

- Age

- Comorbid conditions especially immune
  compromise

- Complicating opportunistic infections

- Septic or toxic shock-like syndrome

- Complicating conditions

    * Respiratory insufficiency

    * Rhabdomyolysis

    * Pancarditis

    * Renal failure

    * Hemorrhage

    * Neurologic complications

        • Brachial plexopathy

        • Demyelinating polyneuropathy

- Case fatality rate 0.2%–1%

- Immunity to reinfection probably exists,
  although at least 1 patient has had a documented
  reinfection

Further Reading

Journal Articles

Bakken JS, Dumler S. Human granulocytic anaplasmosis. *Infect Dis Clin N Am*. 2008;22:433-448.

Centers for Disease Control and Prevention (CDC). *Anaplasma phagocytphilum* transmitted through blood transfusion – Minnesota, 2007. *MMWR*. 2008;57:1145-1148.

Dhand A, Nadelman RB, Aguero-Rosenfeld M, et al. Human granulocytic anaplasmosis during pregnancy: case series and literature review. *Clin Infect Dis*. 2007;45:589-593.

Dumler JS, Madigan JE, Pusteria N, et al. Ehrlichiosis in humans: epidemiology, clinical presentation, diagnosis, and treatment. *Clin Infect Dis*. 2007;45 (Suppl 1):S45-S51.

Hotopp JCD, Lin M, Madupu R, et al. Comprative genomics of emerging human ehrlichiosis agents. *PLoS Genet*. 2006;2:e21.

Krause PJ, Wormser GP. Nosocomial transmission of human granulocytic anaplasmosis. *JAMA*. 2008;300:2308-2309.

Muffly T, McCormick TC, Cook C, et al. Human granulocytic ehrlichiosis complicating early pregnancy. *Infect Dis Obstet Gynecol*. 2008;2008:359172.

4. *Ehrlichia canis*

Synonyms

• Canine tropical pancytopenia

• Canine monocytic ehrlichiosis

• Canine ehrlichiosis

• Venezuelan human *Ehrlichia* (a strain of *E canis*)

Causative Organisms

• *Ehrlichia canis*

Epidemiology

• Vectors: *Ixodes persulcatus* (Russia), *I turdis*, *Haemaphysalis flava*, *H longicornis* ticks

• *Rhipicephalus sanguineus* (brown dog tick) in temperate regions especially in the U.S. and South America

• Infection documented in the U.S., Israel, Brazil, Vietnam, and serologic and molecular evidence of infection in Central and South America, the Caribbean, parts of Africa, southern Europe and southeast Asia

• Host: dogs and humans, pumas (Brazil) and small mammals (*Apodemus agrarius, Crosidura lasiura*)

• Chronically infected dogs appear to be the most important reservoir

Key Clinical Features

• May be asymptomatic in healthy individuals with morulae being visible on the peripheral smear

• May present as milder but similar clinical signs and symptoms as human monocytic ehrlichiosis

Key Differential Diagnostic Features

• Same as for human monocytic ehrlichiosis

• In dogs, the severity of the disease depends upon the host's immune status, age and breed

Key Laboratory/Radiology Features

• Mild thrombocytopenia

• Mild leukopenia

• Anemia

• Relative lymphocytosis caused by low numbers of neutrophils

• Diagnosis by PCR and Western blot

• *E canis* cross reacts serologically with *E chaffeensis* and *E ewingii*

Therapy

Empiric and Definitive/Specific

• Doxycycline

• *In vitro*: doxycycline and rifampin highly active, but fluoroquinolones variable

• *In vitro*: no activity demonstrated for beta-lactams, cotrimoxazole, macrolides or telithromycin

Prognostic Factors

• Many infections asymptomatic or mild

Further Reading

Journal Articles

Branger S, Rolain JM, Raoult D. Evaluation of antibiotic susceptibilities of *Ehrlichia canis*, *Ehrlichia chaffeensis*, and *Anaplasma phagocytphilum* by real-time PCR. *Antimicrob Agents Chemother*. 2004;48:4822-4828.

Filoni C, Catao-Dias JL, Bay G, et al. First evidence of feline herpesvirus, calicivirus, parvovirus, and Ehrlichia exposure in Brazilian free-ranging felids. *J Wildl Dis*. 2006;42:470-477.

Kim CM, Yi YH, Yu DH, et al. Tick-borne rickettsial pathogens in ticks and small mammals in Korea. *Appl Environ Microbiol*. 2006;72:5766-5776.

Perez M, Bodor M, Zhang C, et al. Human infection with *Ehrlichia canis* accompanied by clinical signs in Venezuela. *Ann N Y Acad Sci*. 2006;1078:110-117.

Perez M, Rikhisa Y, Wen B. *Ehrlichia canis*-like agent isolated from a man in Venezuela: antigenic and genetic characterization. *J Clin Microbiol*. 1996;34:2133-2139.

Unver A, Perez M, Orellana N, et al. Molecular and antigenic comparison of *Ehrlichia canis* isolates from dogs, ticks, and a human in Venezuela. *J Clin Microbiol*. 2001;39:2788-2793.

Vinasco J, Li O, Alvarado A, et al. Molecular evidence of a new strain of *Ehrlichia canis* from South America. *J Clin Microbiol*. 2007;45:2716-2719.

Zhang X, Luo T, Keysary A, et al. Genetic and antigenic diversities of major immunoreactive proteins in globally distributed *Ehrlichia canis* strains. *Clin Vaccine Immunol*. 2008;15:1080-1088.

5. *Ehrlichia ewingii* and *Ehrlichia muris*

Synonyms

• None

• Shizuoka isolates (probably a different species of *Ehrlichia* more closely related to *E chaffeensis* than *E muris*)

Causative Organisms

• *Ehrlichia ewingii* and *Ehrlichia muris*

Epidemiology

• Reported mostly in immunocompromised patients

• *E ewingii* found in *Amblyomma americanum* (Lone Star tick) in the eastern U.S.

• *E muris* found in *Ixodes* species ticks (*Ixodes persulcatus* in Russia) and *Haemaphysalis flava* ticks and *Apodemus argenteus*, *A speciosus* and *Eothenomys kageus* mice in Japan

• Dogs (in Japan) also found to be seropositive for *E muris*

Key Clinical Features

• *E ewingii* causes a similar but milder disease than human monocytic ehrlichiosis

  * A subset of HIV infected patients have been described in detail

    • Milder disease than seen in HIV patients with *E chaffeensis* infection

    • Fever (100%)

    • Malaise (50%)

    • Myalgia (50%)

    • Headache (25%)

    • Nausea and vomiting (25%)

    • Leukopenia (75%)

    • Thrombocytopenia (75%)

    • Anemia (75%)

    • Pancytopenia (25%)

    • Elevated AST and ALT (<50%)

    • Hyponatremia (75%)

    • Rashes

      * Diffusely erythematous

      * Morbilliform

      * Scattered petechiae

      * Macules

  * Non-HIV infected patients

    • Immunosuppressed (75%)

    • Headache (100%)

    • Myalgia (25%)

    • Stiff neck (25%)

    • Morulae on peripheral smear (25% — immunosuppressed patient)

    • Leukopenia (25%)

    • Abnormal liver enzymes (25%)

    • Abnormal CSF — 1 of 3 patients had pleocytosis

• *E muris* antibodies found in 1% of populations surveyed in Japan, but it did not appear to be associated with human disease

• In Russia, there was an association between an acute febrile illness and positive *E muris* antibody titers

Key Differential Diagnostic Features

• Same as for human monocytic ehrlichiosis

Key Laboratory/Radiology Features

• Indirect immunofluorescence cross reacts with *E chaffeensis* sera

• PCR – requires species specific primers

• Western blot – *E ewingii* and *E canis* cross react

• In HIV-infected patients, morulae were seen in 50% of patients with *E ewingii* infection: 5% of mature and immature neutrophils and in rare eosinophils

Therapy

Empiric and Definitive/Specific

• Doxycycline: Same as for human monocytic ehrlichiosis

Prognostic Factors

• *E ewingii*: produces milder disease – prognosis good

Further Reading

Books and Book Chapters

Walker H, Dumler JS. *Ehrlichia chaffeensis* (human monocytotropic ehrlichiosis), *Anaplasma phagocytphilum* (human granulocytotropic anaplasmosis) and other Ehrlichieae. In: Mandell GL, Bennett JE, Dolin R, eds. *Mandell, Douglas, and Bennett's Principles and Practice of Infectious Diseases*. 6th ed. v.2. Philadelphia, PA: Elsevier Churchill Livingstone; 2005:2310-2318.

Journal Articles

Buller RS, Arens M, Hmiel SP, et al. *Ehrlichia ewingii*, a newly recognized agent of human ehrlichiosis. *N Engl J Med*. 1999;34:148-155.

Inayoshi M, Naitou H, Kawamori F, et al. Characterization of *Ehrlichia* species from *Ixodes ovatus* ticks at the foot of Mt. Fuji, Japan. *Microbiol Immunol*. 2004;48:737-745.

Paddock CD, Folk SM, Shore GM, et al. Infections with *Ehrlichia chaffeensis* and *Ehrlichia ewingii* in persons coinfected with human immunodeficiency virus. *Clin Infect Dis*. 2001;33:1586-1594.

6. *Neorickettsia sennetsu* (Sennetsu Neorickettsiosis, formerly *Ehrlichia sennetsu* ([Sennetsu Ehrlichiosis])

Synonyms

- Sennetsu Neorickettsiosis – generally confined to western Japan and Malaysia

- Sennetsu ehrlichiosis

- Sennetsu rickettsiosis

- *Ehrlichia sennetsu*

- "Hyuga" fever

Causative Organisms

- *Neorickettsia sennetsu*

Epidemiology

- *N sennetsu* like *E chaffeensis* infects monocyte-macrophages

- *N sennetsu* infects trematodes, the cercariae of which may infect snails and aquatic insects

- Other fish, mammals and birds may be reservoirs

- Arthropods including a fish parasite metacercaria of fluke (*Stellantchasmus falcatus*) is the suspected vector as disease is associated with eating raw fish

Key Clinical Features

- Incubation period: ~2 weeks after exposure

- Sudden onset of fever and chills

- Fatigue/lethargy

- Backache and joint pains

- Headache

- Myalgia

- Sore throat

- Anorexia

- Sleeplessness

- Drenching sweats

- Constipation

- Generalized lymphadenopathy especially postauricular and posterior cervical lymphadenopathy

  * Lymphadenopathy noted 5–7 days after the onset of symptoms

  * Lymphadenopathy is tender

- Rash is rare

Key Differential Diagnostic Features

- Infectious mononucleosis

- Scrub typhus

Key Laboratory/Radiology Features

- Increases in serum transaminases

- Leukopenia

- Both a relative and absolute lymphocytosis with the appearance of atypical cells

- RBC and platelet counts remain normal in most cases

- C-reactive protein becomes positive

- Alpha-2 globulin fraction increases

- Diagnosis by PCR, and culture in selected laboratories

- Indirect fluorescent antibody test, direct fluorescent antibody

- Mice are highly susceptible to *N sennetsu* and are used to isolate the organism in specialized laboratories

Therapy

Empiric and Definitive/Specific

• Doxycycline: Same as for human monocytic ehrlichiosis

• Susceptible to ciprofloxacin

• Resistant to macrolides, penicillin, aminoglycosides and chloramphenicol

Prognostic Factors

• Never fatal in the normal host

Further Reading

Books and Book Chapters

Dummler JS, Walker DH. Ehrlichioses and anaplasmosis. In: Guerrant RL, Walker DH, Weller PF, eds. *Tropical Infectious Diseases – Principles, Pathogens, & Practice*. 2nd ed. v.1. Philadelphia, PA: Elsevier Churchill Livingstone; 2006:564-573.

Stricklan GT, Olson JG. Ehrlichiosis. In: Strickland GT, ed. *Hunter's Tropical Medicine and Emerging Infectious Diseases*. 8th ed. Philadelphia, PA; WB Saunders Company, 2000:445-448.

Journal Articles

Fukuda T, Yamamoto S. Neorickettsia-like organism isolated from metacercaria of a fluke, *Stellantchasmus falcatus*. *Jpn J Med Sci Biol*. 1981;34:103-107.

Hoilien CA, Ristic M, Huxsoli DL, et al. Rickettsia sennetsu in human blood monocyte cultures: similarities to the growth cycle of *Ehrlichia canis*. *Infect Immun*. 1982;35:314-9.

Rikihuisa Y. The tribe Ehrlichieae and ehrlichial diseases. *Clin Microbiol Rev*. 1991;4:286-308.

Tachibana N, Kobayashi V. Effect of cyclophosphamide on the growth of *Rickettsia sennetsu* in experimentally infected mice. *Infect Immun*. 1975;12:625-629.

ID Board Pearls

• *Ehrlichia chaffeensis* (Human Monocytotropic Ehrlichiosis)

  * Ownership of dogs increases the risk of acquiring disease.

  * An atypical lymphocytosis may be observed during the recovery phase (2nd week) of illness.

  * Bone marrow examination during the acute illness may reveal hyperplasia (75%), hypoplasia (13%), and small noncaseating granulomas or histiocyte aggregates in many patients.

  * Chloramphenicol does not have *in vitro* activity against *Ehrlichia chaffeensis*. Both therapeutic successes and failures have been reported.

  * No post therapy relapse has been reported with doxycycline.

  * PCR sensitivity reduced by doxycycline treatment of both *E chaffeensis* and *A phagocytphilum* infection.

• *Anaplasma pharogycophilum* (Human Granulocytic Anaplasmosis, formerly Human Granulocytic Ehrlichiosis ([*Ehrlichia phagocytophila* group])

  * Persistently elevated antibody levels for *A phagocytphilum* should be interpreted as evidence of past infection and not reinfection or unresolved infection.

  * There is no evidence that untreated *A phagocytphilum* progresses to chronic infection, even in the presence of positive antibody titers.

  * Routine examination of peripheral blood smears for the diagnosis of human monocytic ehrlichiosis has identified less than 10% of

patients with *E chaffeensis*. This is in contrast to *A phagocytphilum*, where morulae are identified in 0.5%–40% of patients. A 2-hour examination of blood smears by an experienced technician will often identify infected cells. Examination of bone marrow or employing immunofluorescence or immunocytochemical staining of peripheral smears offers no advantage. Buffy coat examination may increase detection.

* Serologic surveys suggest that from 15%–36% of populations in endemic areas may have been infected.

• *Ehrlichia canis*

* Morulae have persisted for 1 year in the peripheral blood of an asymptomatic subject infected with the Venezuelan human ehrlichia believed to be an *E canis* variant.

• *Ehrlichia ewingii* and *Ehrlichia muris*

* The most common serologic method used, the indirect immunofluorescence assay may erroneously identify *E ewingii* infection as *E chaffeensis*.

* Significant numbers of wild mice in Japan are seropositive to *E muris*, BUT rats appear resistant to the infection and have been seronegative.

• *Neorickettsia sennetsu* (Sennetsu Neorickettsiosis, formerly *Ehrlichia sennetsu* ([Sennetsu Ehrlichiosis])

* During the initial stages of infection with *N sennetsu*, there is a neutrophilia.

* Although the Romanowsky, Giemsa or Diff-Quick – stained peripheral-blood buffy coat is of value in identifying morulae in the cytoplasm of leukocytes, it is of limited value in diagnosing *N sennetsu*.

* There have been no fatalities reported with this disease

III. Corynebacteria and Related Species

1. **Overview**

2. ***Rhodococcus equi (Corynebacterium equi)***

1. Overview

Rhodococcus equi is a Gram-positive, pleomorphic, coccobacillus soil saprophyte that is principally a veterinary pathogen. The organism's most important but not exclusive veterinary disease is bronchopneumonia in foals. The first case of human infection was reported 42 years ago, and it has become an important pathogen in immune compromised and compromised HIV patients.

2. Rhodococcus equi (Corynebacterium equi)

Synonyms

- *Corynebacterium equi*

Causative Organisms

- *Rhodococcus equi*

  * Pleomorphic, Gram-positive coccobacilli – obligate aerobe

    • Intracellular pathogen that infects macrophages

  * Veterinary medicine

    • First isolated from pneumonia in foals in 1923

    • Submaxillary lymphadenitis in swine

    • Ulcerative lymphangitis in cows

    • Found in animal feces (including wild birds) and rarely in human feces

    • Isolated from other animals, including cats and dogs

  * Appears as a diphtheroid and may be mistaken for a contaminant

  * May be acid-fast, causing confusion with *Mycobacterium* species, especially when isolated in a patient with a cavitary pneumonia

  * Intracellular organism that is difficult to eradicate

  * Grouped with aerobic Actinomycetes (which includes *Mycobacterium*, *Norcardia*, *Gordonii*, *Tsukamurella* ([formerly *Rhodococcus aurianticus*]), and *Corynebacterium*)

  * Other related organisms isolated from humans, particularly immunocompromised patients include: *R rhodochrous*, *R fascians* (*R luteus*) and *R erythropolis*

Epidemiology

- Isolated from air, soil and water

  * Highest concentration in air, in warm, dry, and windy weather

  * Isolated with increased frequency from herbivore habitats, especially horse and horse farms

- Worldwide distribution except Antarctica

- Infects principally immunosuppressed patients

  * Most cases (2/3) AIDS patients with CD4+ count <300

    • Patients may have concurrent *Pneumocystis jiroveci*, *Mycobacterium avium-intracellulare*, and/or oral and/or esophageal candidiasis

- In immunocompetent patients, especially children, infection is usually extrapulmonary – often associated with:

  * Trauma

  * Contamination

  * Contact with horses

  * Contact with soil

Key Clinical Features

- Reported rarely in children under the age of 18 years

  * 1/3 are immunocompromised

  * In the pre-HAART era, most patients were HIV/AIDS

- Disease rare in immunocompetent adult hosts

  * Pneumonia (80% of all cases)

- 20% of pulmonary infections accompanied by extrapulmonary sites of infection

  * Nonpulmonary cases secondary to trauma or ingestion

    - 25% if extrapulmonary disease is without evidence of pulmonary disease

    - Endophthalmitis secondary to trauma

    - Lymphadenitis

    - Mandibular, long bone and vertebral osteomyelitis

    - Orbital implant infection

    - Otitis media with mastoiditis

    - Ingestion, dissemination to regional lymph nodes

      * Pelvic masses

      * Peritonitis

      * Mesenteric adenitis

      * Infected colonic polyps

  * Nonpulmonary disease only manifesting as fever and bacteremia – patients with malignancies, neutropenia or had received chemotherapy

    - Central venous catheters often present

- Most common disease is interstitial pneumonia that, if left untreated, progresses to consolidation and then cavitary disease over 2–4 weeks

  * Pleural effusion and empyema a common complication

  * Less common complications

    - Mediastinitis

- Cardiac tamponade

- Endobronchial masses

- Pneumothorax

- Mediastinitis

- HIV/AIDS patients have bacteremia especially in the pre-HAART era

- Less common complications secondary to bacteremia especially in the compromised patient results in dissemination of infection to the:

  * Brain

  * Bone marrow

  * Thyroid (including thyroid abscess in an HIV-infected patient)

  * Skin

  * Retroperitoneum

  * Kidney

  * Lymph nodes

    - Caseating granulomas have been described in some nodes

- Bacteremia without pulmonary infection has been described in AIDS patients

- Nonpulmonary presentations

  * Peritonitis secondary to peritoneal dialysis

  * Mycetoma of the foot with dissemination to lymph nodes, lungs, and brain

  * Bacteremia with soft tissue mass in pelvis with enlarged axillary nodes

  * Bloody diarrhea with bacteremia

  * Tumor-like lesions in soft tissues (pelvis, thigh, bronchi)

* Purulent pericarditis

* Skin infections secondary to trauma

• Non-HIV compromised patients

    * Pneumonia

    * Paravertebral abscesses

    * Peritonitis secondary to peritoneal dialysis

    * Skin infections secondary to trauma

      • Skin lesions may ulcerate

    * Eye infections secondary to trauma

      • One infection progressed to meningitis

Key Differential Diagnostic Features

• Must be differentiated from other causes of cavitary pneumonia in AIDS patients

    * Invasive pulmonary aspergillosis

    * Mycobacterial diseases especially *Mycobacterium tuberculosis*

    * Bacterial pneumonia especially from *Pseudomonas aeruginosa*

• Necrotizing pneumonia may be confused with pulmonary tuberculosis or nocardiosis in any patient

• Must be differentiated from soft-tissue tumors

• Lung abscess, especially in immunocompromised (transplant) patients, especially where routine laboratory culture demonstrates diphtheroids

• May be confused with *Para-streptomyces abscessus* as both share similar pathologic characteristics including intrahistiocytic localization

Key Laboratory/Radiology Features

• Chest x-rays

    * Infiltrates

    * Consolidation

    * Nodules – single or multiple

    * Cavitation –single or multiple

      • More frequent in upper lobes

      • Usually occurs 2–4 weeks into the disease

      • Thick walled

      • Contain air-fluid levels

    * Pleural effusions or empyema

    * Mediastinal enlargement

    * CTs of chest may be of more assistance in the diagnosis

• Diagnosis by culture

    * Obtain cultures directly from infected areas

    * *R equi* is slow growing and may be overgrown in mixed cultures

    * May appear as "diphtheroids"

    * Takes 48 hours until colonies take on typical large mucoid morphology and pink color does not appear for 4–7 days

    * Blood cultures

      • Positive in 50% of HIV patients

      • Positive in 25% of solid organ transplant patients

- Positive in 30% of immunocompetent patients

* Other sites to culture

- Joint fluid — in cases of *R equi* septic arthritis

- Pleural effusion

- Peritoneal fluid

- Dialysate

- Abscess aspirates

- CSF

- Brain

- Pharyngeal exudates

- Stool

- Urine

- Skin

- Wounds

- Bone biopsy

- Lymph nodes

- Intravenous catheters

- Autopsy specimens

Therapy

Empiric

- 2 drug regimens with a macrolide, rifampin and/or a fluoroquinolone may be started while awaiting susceptibility testing

- Monotherapy ineffective

- Oral therapy may be used for localized non-CNS disease in an immunocompetent host

Definitive/Specific

- In human isolates, beta-lactam resistance linked to virulence factors

    * 50% resistant to beta-lactams and clindamycin

    * Beta-lactam susceptible isolates may acquire resistance

    * Beta-lactams not recommended for treatment

- Ciprofloxacin and norfloxacin not recommended: 16% and 18% resistance respectively

- Penicillins NOT recommended even if susceptible

- Monotherapy is NOT recommended

- Synergy demonstrated with

    * Macrolides and rifampin

    * Macrolides and tetracycline

    * Rifampin and tetracyclines

    * Imipenem and aminoglycosides

- Recommended therapy

    * Combinations of 2 or 3 agents is the treatment of choice

        - In an immunocompromised host, these agents should include 2 or 3 of the following:

            * Vancomycin

            * Imipenem or meropenem

            * Rifampin

            * Fluoroquinolone

            * Aminoglycoside

            * Macrolide

- Treat IV for 2–3 weeks or until clinical improvement, followed by

- Oral agents should be continued until cultures are negative

- 2–6 months therapy advised for

  * Immunocompromised hosts

  * Bone and joint infections

  * CNS infections

  * Pulmonary infections

- HIV and immunocompromised patients should receive long-term antimicrobial therapy with a macrolide plus rifampin or a quinolone, or doxycycline plus rifampin

* Imipenem (most effective in animal studies)

* Antipseudomonal aminoglycoside (ie gentamicin)

* Erythromycin

* Vancomycin (most effective in animal studies)

* Rifampin (most effective in animal studies)

  - Some rifampin resistant isolates have been reported

  - OR until the patients improve clinically and cultures are negative

  - HIV patients may require life-long therapy

Prognostic Factors

- Relapses are common

Further Reading

Books and Book Chapters

Cornish N, Washington JA. *Rhodococcus equi* infections: clinical features and laboratory diagnosis. In: Remington JS, Swartz MN, eds. *Current Clinic Topics in Infectious Diseases 19*. Malden, MA: Blackwell Science, Inc; 1999:198-215.

Meyer DK, Reboil AC. Other Coryneform bacteria and *Rhodococcus*. In: Mandell GL, Bennett JE, Dolin R, eds. *Mandell, Douglas, and Bennett's Principles and Practice of Infectious Diseases*. 6th ed. v.2. Philadelphia, PA: Elsevier Churchill Livingstone; 2005:2465-2478.

Touchie C. *Rhodococcus equi* and *Bordetella bronchiseptica*. In: Marrie TJ, ed. *Community Acquired Pneumonia*. New York, NY: Kluwer Academic/Plenum Publishers;2001:877-884.

Journal Articles

Cronin SM, Abidi MH, Shearer CJ, et al. *Rhodococcus equi* lung infection in an allogeneic hematopoietic stem cell transplant recipient. *Transpl Infect Dis*. 2008;10:48-51.

Munoz P, Palomo J, Guinea J, et al. Relapsing in *Rhodococcus equi* infection in a heart transplant recipient successfully treated with long-term linezolid. *Diag Microbiol Infect Dis*. 2008; 60:197-199.

Nichols WG, Prentice J, Houze Y, et al. Fatal pulmonary infection associated with a novel organism, "*Para-streptomyces abscessus*". *J Clin Microbiol*. 2005;43:5376-5379.

Perez MG, Vassilev T, Kemmerly SA. *Rhodococcus equi* infection in transplant recipients: a case of mistaken identity and review of the literature. *Transpl Infect Dis*. 2002;4:52-56.

ID Board Pearls

- In the severely immunocompromised patient (especially HIV patients), infection with tuberculosis in less likely to result in cavitation rather than dissemination. If cavitation is present in these patients, *Rhodococcus equi* infection should be suspected.

- Air-fluid levels are seen in *R equi* cavities, but are not usually seen in cavities from *Mycobacterium tuberculosis*.

- Hemoptysis is reported in 15% of *R equi* pulmonary infections.

- Relapsing *R equi* (co-infected with *Cryptococcus neoformans*) in a heart transplant patient was successfully treated for the *R equi* infection with 6 months of linezolid and fluconazole. Other newer successful combinations have been IV ertapenem and oral rifampin after failure of vancomycin treatment.

1. **Overview**

2. ***Bacillus anthracis* (Anthrax)**

1. Overview

Bacillus anthracis is a spore-forming, Gram-positive bacillus that causes acute disease in herbivores and man. Spores are found worldwide except in Antarctica. The spore may survive for many years, presenting an environmental as well as a bioterrorism threat. Robert Koch was first to identify the organism in 1875, and Louis Pasteur produced the first animal vaccine (for sheep) in 1881. The most famous strains are the Ames strain (released as a bioterrorist weapon in 2001) and the Vollum (or Vellum) strain, used as a test weapon by the British on Gruinard Island in 1942.

2. *Bacillus anthracis* (Anthrax)

Synonyms

• The Sixth Plague of the book of Exodus

• Black bane

• Malignant pustule

• Woolsorters disease

• Siberian ulcer

• Bacteridie (Davaine – 1864)

Causative Organisms

• *Bacillus anthracis*

Epidemiology

• Acquired from contact with anthrax-infected animals or contaminated animal products

• Herbivores naturally infected after ingesting spores from contaminated soil

• Carrion birds and mammalian predators (jackals, hyenas and lions) are resistant to infection

• Three routes of human infection: (1) inhalation; (2) cutaneous; (3) gastrointestinal

Inhalation anthrax

• Naturally occurring disease is rare – goat hair mill or wool or tannery workers, laboratory accidents – last naturally occurring case in the U.S. in 1976

  * A single case should be considered a possible bioterrorist attack

• Lethal dose (LD_{50}): 2500-55,000 spores; LD_{10}: 100 spores (in monkey experiments) with 1–3 spores sufficient to cause infection, but fatal infectious dose in humans based upon the fatal inhalation cases in New York City and Connecticut is probably very low

Cutaneous anthrax

• Most common form of naturally occurring disease — ~2000 cases/year worldwide

• Usually associated with exposure to anthrax-infected animals

• Organisms in contact with skin, especially but not necessarily at a cut or abrasion

Gastrointestinal anthrax (2 forms of disease – oral-pharyngeal and abdominal)

• Uncommon, but outbreaks reported in Africa and Asia with rare cases in the U.S. with ingestion of an infected animal, especially if the meat is raw or undercooked

Key Clinical Features

Inhalation anthrax

• Incubation: 2–43 days (Sverdlovsk)

• Incubation in monkeys experimentally infected: 58 and 98 days

• Initial symptoms nonspecific: fever, shortness of breath, cough, headache, vomiting, chills, weakness, and abdominal and chest pain — all lasting a few hours to a few days, with all laboratory studies remaining nondiagnostic

• In some patients this is followed by a brief period of recovery, while other patients progress directly to fulminant infection

• In the fulminant stage of disease, there is a sudden onset of fever, dyspnea, sweating and shock

  * In some cases, lymphadenopathy and expansion of the mediastinum results in stridor – the chest x-ray at this stage shows widening of the mediastinum

  * Cyanosis, hypotension, hypothermia, and rapid progression to death in 24–36 hours• Hemorrhagic meningitis in 50% of patients

Table 2

Initial Signs and Symptoms: Inhalation Anthrax

Signs and Symptoms	% Patients	Signs and Symptoms	% Patients
Fever and chills	100	Sweats	70
Fatigue, malaise, lethargy	100	Cough - minimal	90
Nausea and vomiting	90	Dyspnea	80
Chest discomfort or pleuritic chest pain	70	Myalgias	60
Headache	50	Confusion	40
Abdominal pain	30	Sore throat	20
Rhinorrhea	10	Hypotension <110 mm Hg	10
Fever >37.8°C	70	Tachycardia >100/min	80

* Meningismus

* Delirium and obtundation

Cutaneous anthrax

• Incubation: as late as 12 days (Sverdlovsk); mean incubation in 2001 U.S. attacks: 5 days (range 1–10 days); classic disease described an incubation period of 1–6 days; others have reported incubation periods from 12–19 days

• Usually affects hands, arms, neck and face

• Begins as a pruritic macule or papule that enlarges and progresses to a large ulcer by day 2

• This is followed by the appearance of a ring of 1–3 mm to 1–2 cm vesicles that discharge clear or serosanguineous fluid – satellite vesicles may develop

• Develops into a <u>painless</u> black eschar with extensive local gelatinous nonpitting edema

• Eschar dries and falls off in 1–2 weeks

• Accompanied by lymphangitis and painful lymphadenitis with systemic symptoms

• Complications

    * An infant in 2001 had rapid progression to systemic disease, microangiopathic hemolytic anemia with renal involvement and hyponatremia

Gastrointestinal anthrax

• Symptoms develop 1–6 or 2–5 days after eating contaminated meat (mean incubation period was 42 hours (range 2 hours – 144 hours)

• Oral-Pharyngeal disease

    * Fever >39° C

    * Ulcers in the posterior oropharynx, severe sore throat

• Tonsillar ulcers: 72% (unilateral in 85% of these cases)

• Evolution of oral lesions: (1) edema and congestion; (2) central necrosis and ulceration producing a white patch by the end of the first week; (3) patch becomes a pseudomembrane

• In some patients, the lesions did not progress through all stages

• Airway compromise from lymphadenopathy and neck swelling developed in some cases

* Esophageal ulceration with dysphagia

* Regional lymphadenopathy with edema and sepsis

* Marked neck swelling

• Abdominal disease

    * One report put incubation period between 15 and 72 hours

    * 91% gastrointestinal complaints; 9% oropharyngeal complaints

    * In one report, children died within 48 hours of onset of symptoms

    * Initial symptoms: fever > 39° C, anorexia, nausea, vomiting, malaise progressing to bloody diarrhea

    * Progresses to severe abdominal pain (with rebound tenderness), hematemesis, melanotic stools and/or bloody stools and diarrhea; watery diarrhea less frequently

    * Abdominal pain decreases as ascites develops – ascites is typically voluminous

    * Intestinal lesions usually in terminal ileum or cecum

* Progresses to an acute abdomen and/or sepsis

* Massive ascites in some cases

Meningitis

• May complicate any of the 3 forms of the disease or rarely present without any other organ involvement

Key Differential Diagnostic Features

Inhalation anthrax

• Influenza — if widened mediastinum present, suspect anthrax

• Early disease resembles viral upper respiratory infections

• Tularemia — will also produce widened mediastinum

Cutaneous anthrax

• Ulceroglandular tularemia

• Scrub typhus

• Rickettsial spotted fevers

• Rat-bite fevers

• Plague

• Ecthyma – usually without edema or systemic disease

• Ecthyma gangrenosum – usually in neutropenic patients

• Arachnid bites (brown recluse spider) - this is almost always painful with necrosis

• Vasculitis

• Staphylococcal furuncle – this is usually painful

• Orf – no gelatinous edema and a scab forms but without an eschar

• Syphilitic chancre

• Burn wound

• Milker's nodule

Gastrointestinal anthrax

• Oral-Pharyngeal disease

* Diphtheria

* Peritonsillar abscess

• Abdominal disease

* May be confused with nonulcerative hemorrhagic lesions associated with septicemic anthrax

* Gastroenteritis

* Acute surgical abdomen

Key Laboratory/Radiology Features

Inhalation anthrax – Presenting findings

• Average WBC:	9800/mm^3
• >70% neutrophils:	70%
• Bands >5%:	80%
• Elevated AST and ALT:	90%
• Hypoxia:	60%
• Metabolic acidosis:	20%
• Elevated creatinine:	10%

• Hemorrhagic pleural effusions

- Radiology – Chest x-ray

    * Any abnormality: 100%

    * Mediastinal widening: 70%

    * Infiltrates or consolidation: 70%

    * Pleural effusion: 80%

- Chest CT

    * Any abnormality: 100%

    * Mediastinal lymphadenopathy,
      widening of the mediastinum: 70%

    * Pleural effusions: 80%

    * Infiltrates or consolidation: 60%

Cutaneous anthrax

- Gram-stain positive for organisms on fluid
  discharged from vesicles

- If Gram-stain negative, perform a punch biopsy
  for immunohistochemical staining and PCR

- Blood cultures should be obtained

Meningitis

- Hemorrhagic CSF with polymorphonuclear pleocytosis

- CSF Gram-stain often positive

Gastrointestinal anthrax

- Oral-Pharyngeal disease

    * + Gram-stain on oropharyngeal swab

    * + culture of oropharyngeal lesion

    * Blood cultures often negative

    * PCR and immunostaining may be of value

- Abdominal disease

    * Abdominal x-rays nonspecific or may suggest
      obstruction

    * Mediastinal widening in chest x-rays in some
      patients

    * Surgical findings: mesenteric adenopathy,
      serosanguineous to hemorrhagic ascites, bowel
      ulceration, edema and necrosis

    * Stool cultures have grown *B anthracis*

    * Culture of blood and ascitic fluid

    * PCR and immunostaining

Diagnosis

- Gram-stain: broad, encapsulated, Gram-positive
  bacilli

- Blood culture or culture of potentially infected
  specimens

- Standard blood cultures may become positive in
  6–24 hours

- In inhalational anthrax, sputum cultures and
  Gram-stains often nondiagnostic

- Severe cases – Gram-positive bacilli will be seen
  on the blood smear

- Hemorrhagic mediastinitis; hemorrhagic thoracic
  lymphadenitis; hemorrhagic meningitis

- Direct fluorescent antibody staining of infected
  tissue

- PCR

- Immuno-histochemical staining

- Gamma-phage

- Nasal swabs in human inhalational anthrax of
  unknown value

- Serologic testing only useful for retrospective study

- All confirmatory test performed by the <u>Laboratory Response Network for Bioterrorism</u>

Therapy

Empiric

- Empiric therapy is the same as definitive therapy where anthrax is suspected

- A licensed vaccine is available and given to US military active-duty and reserve personnel

- Post exposure prophylaxis for 60 days with antibiotics recommended for those potentially exposed to airborne anthrax

    * Ciprofloxacin

    * Doxycycline

    * Amoxicillin

Definitive/Specific

- Antibiotics indicated in cutaneous disease, as even though it does not change the resolution of the cutaneous lesions, it prevents systemic complications

- Doxycycline is the preferred tetracycline

- For inhalational anthrax: FDA approved penicillin, doxycycline and ciprofloxacin

    * 2 or 3 drug regimens were recommended in 2001 inhalational anthrax cases

    * Initial recommendations were ciprofloxacin OR doxycycline PLU.S. 1–2 other drugs (vancomycin, penicillin, ampicillin, chloramphenicol, imipenem, clindamycin, clarithromycin)

    * Some advocated the use of clindamycin in the combination for its ability to decrease bacterial toxin production

    * Penicillin or ampicillin should not be used alone because of the possibility of an inducible beta-lactamase

- *In vitro* activity demonstrated for clindamycin, rifampin, imipenem, aminoglycosides, chloramphenicol, vancomycin, cefazolin, tetracycline, linezolid, and macrolide antibiotics

- Doxycycline and fluoroquinolones not recommended for CNS disease

- Human polyclonal anthrax immunoglobulin exists in the U.S. Strategic National Stockpile

Prognostic Factors

Inhalation anthrax

- Untreated mortality rate: 97%–100%

- Mortality rate: 40%–89%

- Mortality rate with intensive care: 45%

Meningitis

- Mortality rate: near 100%

Cutaneous anthrax

- Without antibiotics – mortality 10%-20%

- Mortality with treatment: ≤1%

Gastrointestinal anthrax

- Children have a more fulminant course with higher mortality

- Untreated mortality: 25%–75%

• Treated: mortality in one study: 13%

    * Patients who died had incubation periods of <24 hours

    * Other reports indicate that most deaths occurred with incubation periods of <48 hours with death in <48 hours

• Oral pharyngeal and abdominal disease – mortality very high due to difficulty in recognizing early disease

Further Reading

Books and Book Chapters

Walker DH. Anthrax. In: Guerrant RL, Walker DH, Weller PF, eds. *Tropical Infectious Diseases – Principles, Pathogens, & Practice*. 2nd ed. v.1. Philadelphiam, PA: Elsevier Churchill Livingstone; 2006:448-453.

Journal Articles

Beatty ME, Ashford DA, Griffin PM, et al. Gastrointestinal anthrax: review of the literature. *Arch Intern Med*. 2003;163:2527-2531.

Cleri DJ, Vernaleo JR, Rabbat MS, et al. Anthrax Disease Caused by *Bacillus anthracis*. *Infectious Diseases Practice*. 1995;19:77–79.

Grabenstein JD. Vaccines: countering anthrax: vaccines and immunoglobulins. *Clin Infect Dis*. 2008;46:129-136.

Inglesby TV, O'Toole T, Henderson DA, et al. Anthrax as a biological, 2002, updated recommendations for management. *JAMA*. 2002;287:2236-2252.

Spencer RC. *Bacillus anthracis*. *J Clin Pathol*. 2003;56:182-187.

Swartz MN. Recognition and management of anthrax – an update. *N Engl J Med*. 2001;345:1621-1626.

ID Board Pearls

• 25% of the fatal cases of inhalational anthrax in Sverdlovsk had evidence of focal, hemorrhagic and necrotizing lesions similar to tuberculous Ghon's complexes.

• Rarely, the primary lesion of inhalational anthrax appears in the nasal mucosa or sinuses.

• In patients with cutaneous anthrax of the face, edema may become massive with the development of multiple bullae accompanied by systemic toxicity. These lesions should NOT be incised or debrided as this will increase the risk of bacteremia.

• Anthrax eschars dry and fall off leaving little or no scaring.

• ALL patients with oropharyngeal anthrax developed neck swelling; <u>in 75% of the patients, the neck swelling was unilateral.</u>

• No pus was found in patients who underwent incision and drainage for tonsillar abscess.

V. Zoonotic Gram-Negative Bacilli

1. Overview

Campylobacter jejuni and *Campylobacter coli* are the most common causes of bacterial diarrhea worldwide. These organisms are part of the normal gastrointestinal flora of wild and domestic animals including poultry and pets. *Campylobacter* species are a major cause of traveler's diarrhea with symptoms that may be more severe than salmonellosis or shigellosis.

Brucellosis is a major zoonotic infection worldwide. It is caused by Gram-negative coccobacilli of the genus *Brucella*, and affects cattle, sheep, goats, other livestock, and sea mammals. Since the discovery of *Brucella melitensis* by Sir David Bruce in 1887, several species have been identified, including *B abortus* (which infects cattle), *B melitensis* (which infects sheep and goats), *B suis*, *B neotomae*, *B ovis,* and *B canis*. In some countries where *B abortus* has been eradicated, *B melitensis* (in southern Europe) and *B suis* (in South America) have emerged as causes of infection in cattle. Although brucellosis has been controlled in most industrialized nations, it remains a major problem in the Mediterranean region, western Asia, Africa and Latin America, causing livestock abortions, decreased milk production, sterility and veterinary care costs. *B melitensis* is the principal cause of human brucellosis. *B abortus*, *B suis* and *B canis* cause most of the remainder of human disease.

Yersinia pestis and *Yersinia pseudotuberculosis* became separate species ~20,000 years ago. Unlike *Y pestis*, *Y pseudotuberculosis* appears to be toxic to fleas, including causing the fleas to have diarrhea. *Y pseudotuberculosis* is a member of the *Enterobacteriaceae* family, a zoonotic pathogen that has the ability to survive in the environment with minimal nutritional requirements and at extremes of temperature, especially as a fecal contaminant. In animal models, the organism localizes in extracellular sites in association with platelets, inducing thrombosis. They also exhibit the property of survival in phagocytes, suppressing the inflammatory response in spite of causing tissue necrosis.

2. *Campylobacter jejuni*

Synonyms

- Once known as *Vibrio fetus*; that species is now *Campylobacter fetus*

- *Vibrio jejuni* (now *Campylobacter jejuni*)

- Winter dysentery or black scours in cattle (*C jejuni*)

Causative Organisms

- *Campylobacter jejuni*

- *Campylobacter coli*

- *Campylobacter upsaliensis* (believed to be under-identified because it is slower growing and may not grow as well on certain selective media) causes sporadic gastrointestinal disease in humans

- *Campylobacter fetus* (more likely to cause bacteremia, especially in a debilitated host)

Epidemiology

Campylobacter jejuni

- In the U.S., the most important risk factor is handling chicken (50%-70% of infections in the U.S., Europe and Australia attributed to eating chicken)

- International travel is a risk factor

- High prevalence in wild and domestic animals including rodents and birds; especially animals with diarrhea; and/or, under 6 months old

  * Prevalence of *Campylobacter* species in household pets especially cats and birds: 42.9% in the cats and 41.5% in the dogs. *Campylobacter upsaliensis* was the species most commonly isolated and *Campylobacter jejuni* was the second most commonly isolated

- Consumption of unpasteurized milk and cheese is the most frequent cause of outbreaks – milk becomes contaminated from colonized cow feces and teats

- Consumption of sausages or red meat

- Cultured from surface water – infections associated with consumption of untreated water – 1 outbreak in Japan traced to tap water

- *Campylobacter*-associated diarrhea is common in developing countries and the second-leading cause of pediatric diarrhea

- Peak human infections in summer months which is coincident with seasonality of infections in chickens and livestock

- Higher incidence of infection in developing countries

- 2–7 times more frequent in industrialized countries than *Salmonella*, *Shigella* or *Escherichia coli* O157:H7 infections

- Grossly underreported with only 1 in 38 cases diagnosed

- Person-to-person spread unlikely and outbreaks in day-care centers or mental institutions very rare

- Homosexual men have a 40-times greater incidence of infection as compared the general population

Campylobacter fetus

- Colonizes cattle and sheep

- Age a major risk factor

- Many patients debilitated, but 21% have no immunosuppression

Key Clinical Features

Campylobacter jejuni

Clinical presentations

- During outbreaks, 50% of patients with + stool cultures are asymptomatic

- Most disease self-limited – usually resolves without treatment in 1 week

* Acute onset

* Diarrhea – loose or watery or bloody (8–10 movements/day)

* Fever (>90% of patients) – may be low grade and lasts for 1 week

* Diarrhea may be minimal with abdominal cramps and pain being the predominant symptom

• Severe invasive disease in some cases

• Some patients develop a relapsing diarrhea which lasts several weeks

Complications

• Cellulitis (rare)

• Dissemination

  * Bacteremia <1% of patients

  * Gastrointestinal

    • Cholecystitis

    • Pancreatitis

    • Peritonitis

    • Gastrointestinal hemorrhage

  * Extraintestinal (rare)

    • Meningitis

    • Endocarditis

    • Septic arthritis

    • Osteomyelitis

    • Sepsis, especially neonatal sepsis (bacteremia in <1% of patients most likely in immunocompromised patients)

• Immune

  * Guillain-Barré

    • Guillain-Barré syndrome affects 1–2 persons/100,000 population in the general population

    • *C jejuni* responsible for 30% of Guillain-Barré syndrome cases

    • Neurologic symptoms occur 1–3 weeks after the onset of diarrhea

  * HLA-B27 histocompatibility group antigen positive patients are predisposed to develop reactive arthritis several weeks after infection

    • 1 study reported 7% incidence of reactive arthritis and 1% incidence of reactive tendonitis, enthesopathy or bursitis

  * Uveitis

  * Hemolytic anemia

  * Hemolytic uremic syndrome

  * Carditis

  * Encephalitis

Campylobacter fetus

Clinical presentations

• More often causes bacteremia and sepsis

• Outbreaks rare

• Mostly infects debilitated patients

• Causes intermittent diarrhea or diffuse abdominal pain

• Gastrointestinal disease resembles that of *C jejuni*

Complications

• Cellulitis most frequent extraintestinal presentation in septicemic patients

• Endovascular medical device-related infections: 20% infection rate in bacteremic patients

• Prosthetic joint infections

• Prosthetic heart valves

Campylobacter upsaliensis

• Acute gastroenteritis/acute and intermittent chronic diarrhea with lower rates of fever, acute diarrhea and rectal bleeding

Key Differential Diagnostic Features

• Indistinguishable from other pathogens, such as *Salmonella*, *Shigella* and *Yersinia* species

• May be mistaken for a surgical abdomen

• Early inflammatory bowel disease

• Signs and symptoms of *Campylobacter* bacteremia lack any specificity

Key Laboratory/Radiology Features

• Fecal leukocytes and RBCs in stools of 75% of patients

• WBC may be elevated

• Other laboratory tests usually normal

• Diffuse colonic inflammation seen on endoscopy

• Diagnosis made by culturing the organism from stool or blood

  * *C jejuni* – diagnosis by <u>stool cultures</u>; blood cultures rarely positive

  * *C fetus* - diagnosis by <u>blood culture</u>; stool cultures rarely positive

• PCR and ELISA (species-specific assays to detect antigen in stool)

• Darkfield or phase contrast microscopy on fresh stool may detect the typical <u>darting motility</u> of *Campylobacter* species, especially in acute illness

• PCR

Therapy

• A recent study from Taiwan reported 93.4% resistance to tetracycline and 90.2% resistance to ciprofloxacin, but only 3.3% resistant to erythromycin

• French study of bacteremic isolates: 32% resistant to fluoroquinolones and 8% resistant to erythromycin

• Antibiotic therapy indicated

  * High fever

  * Bloody stools

  * Illness for >1 week

  * Pregnancy

  * HIV infection or other immunocompromised condition

Empiric

• Amoxicillin-clavulanic acid or imipenem: blood isolates usually susceptible

• Empiric treatment with fluoroquinolones for *C fetus* bacteremia associated with increased risk of a fatal outcome

• Gentamicin should be included in a multidrug regimen to treat severe disease and/or endovascular infection

Definitive/Specific

- Macrolides (erythromycin, azithromycin or clarithromycin) or fluoroquinolones for prolonged or severe symptoms

- Also susceptible to aminoglycosides, chloramphenicol, clindamycin, nitrofurans, imipenem

- Dual resistance to macrolides and fluoroquinolones reported

- Normally resistant to and should not be treated with tetracyclines, amoxicillin, ampicillin, metronidazole, cephalosporins, and always resistant to vancomycin, rifampin and trimethoprim

- Alternate therapy: doxycycline, clindamycin

Prognostic Factors

- In bacteremic patients, failure to administer appropriate antibiotic strongly associated with fatal outcome: 88% mortality within 30 days

- Treatment with 3rd generation cephalosporin associated with increased mortality

- 30-day mortality rate for *Campylobacter* bacteremia: 15%

Campylobacter jejuni

- Overall case-fatality rate: 0.05/1000 infections

- Diarrhea is usually self-limited

- Guillain-Barré syndrome occurs between <1 case/1000 infections to 30 times for every 100,000 cases of *Campylobacter* infections with a case-fatality ratio near 10%

Campylobacter fetus

- Leading cause of *Campylobacter* bacteremia

- Almost all patients survive with antibiotic therapy

- Independent risk factors for death: malignancy, isolated fever

Further Reading

Books and Book Chapters

Blaser MJ, Allos BM. Campylobacter jejuni and related species. In: Mandell GL, Bennett JE, Dolin R, eds. *Mandell, Douglas, and Bennett's Principles and Practice of Infectious Diseases*. 6th ed. v.2. Philadelphia, PA: Elsevier Churchill Livingstone; 2005:2548-2557.

Journal Articles

Allos BM. *Campylobacter jejuni* infections: update on emerging issues and trends. *Clin Infect Dis*. 2000;32:1201-1206.

Centers for Disease Control and Prevention (CDC), *Campylobacter jejuni* infection associated with unpasteurized milk and cheese—Kansas, 2007. *MMWR*. 2009;57:1377-1379.

Hannu T, Mattila L, Rautelin *H. Campylobacter*-triggered reactive arthritis: a population-based study. *Rheumatology* (Oxford). 2002;41:312-318.

Pacanowski J, Lalande V, Lacomb K, et al. *Campylobacter bacteremia*: clinical features and factors associated with fatal outcome. *Clin Infect Dis*. 2008;47:790-796.

Wierzba TF, Abdel-messih IA, Gharib B, et al. *Campylobacter* infection as a trigger for Guillain-Barre syndrome in Egypt. *PLoS One*. 2008;3:e3674.

3. Brucella species

Synonyms

- Gastric remittent fever

- Mediterranean fever, Neapolitan fever, Country fever of Constantinople

- New fever of Crete

- Malta fever

    * Named derived from Melita (honey), the Roman name for the Isle of Malta

    * Melitococcie (French)

- Gibraltar fever, Rock fever of Gibraltar

- Cyprus fever

- Undulant fever

- Typhomalarial fever

- Intermittent typhoid

- *Micrococcus melitensis*

- *Brucella rangiferitarandi* (*Brucella suis* biotype 4 isolated from reindeer and Eskimos)

- *Moraxella melitensis*, *Alkaligenes melitensis* (*Brucella melitensis*)

- *Moraxella duplex* was believed at one time to be *Brucella suis* biotype 5

Causative Organisms

- *Brucella melitensis* – the most common cause of human brucellosis

- *Brucella abortus* – (cattle) – causes human disease

- *Brucella ovi*s – (sheep)

- *Brucella canis* – (dogs – first isolated in kennel-bred dogs) – causes human diseases

- *Brucella suis* – (swine) – causes human disease

- *Brucella pinnipediae* (seals) and *Brucella ceteceae* (mink whales, dolphins and porpoises): both species were referred to as *Brucella maris*

- *Brucella neotomae* – (desert wood rat)

Epidemiology

- Worldwide distribution but remains endemic in the Mediterranean basin, Arabian gulf, the Indian subcontinent, parts of Mexico and Central and South America – 500,000 cases/year

- Significant disease among rural and nomadic peoples

- Significant human disease where *B melitensis* is endemic in sheep and goats

- Consumption of raw milk or unpasteurized dairy products

    * Camel milk believed to be the most important source of transmission in the Middle East and Mongolia

    * Consumption of undercooked animal meats (especially liver) has been implicated in infection

    * Asymptomatic family members of an index case should be investigated for infection

- Occupational disease of shepherds, abattoir workers, veterinarians, dairy industry personnel, microbiologists – direct contact with an infected cow documented in one case

- Transmitted through human breast milk resulting in meningitis

- Human-to-human transmission reported

- Environmental –airborne transmission

- Blood transfusion

Table 3

Clinical Presentation: *B melitensis*

Signs and Symptoms	% Patients	Signs and Symptoms	% Patients
Fever	77.8	Seizures	0.2
Joint pain	21	Splenomegaly	17.2
Low back pain	14	Hepatomegaly	10.2
Night sweats	3.6	Hepatosplenomegaly	15.1
Cough, shortness of breath or hemoptysis	3.3	Lymphadenopathy	10–20%
Testicular pain, scrotal swelling, burning on urination	2	Jerky limb movements	0.1
GI symptoms: anorexia, diarrhea, constipation, abdominal pain, nausea, vomiting, anorexia, jaundice	Up to 70 in some studies	Burning sensation in the feet	0.1
Headache	2.2	Swollen hand	0.2
Fatigue	1.3	Weight loss	0.8
Skin papules or mouth ulcers	1.4–5		

- Laboratory accidents

  * Ingestion

  * Inhalation

  * Mucosal or skin contact

Key Clinical Features

- Infective dose low — as few as 10 organisms

- Incubation period: 7 days – 3 months, but may be as long as 10 months

- Asymptomatic bacteremia

- Fever may be the only sign of disease

- *B melitensis* more often associated with acute infections while other *Brucella* species tend to present with subacute or more prolonged disease

- Undulating fever typical: temperature remains normal during the early part of the day, then rises during the evening

Complications

• Genitourinary complications

    * Epididymo-orchitis

    * Hydrocele

    * Urinary tract infection

    * Interstitial nephritis, pyelonephritis, IgA nephropathy

    * Glomerulonephritis resulting in end-stage renal disease

• Skeletal system (10%–80% of patients)

    * Sacroiliitis and spondylitis most frequent

    * Joint effusions, especially in hips, knees and ankles

    * Post infectious spondylarthritis, bursitis, tenosynovitis

    * Prosthetic joint infections

• Gastrointestinal system (up to 80% of patients have GI complaints)

    * Chronic liver disease

    * Multifocal liver and lung nodules with necrosis – fatal disease reported

    * Splenic abscess

    * Acute cholecystitis

    * Colitis and acute ileitis

    * Spontaneous bacterial peritonitis

• Pulmonary

    * Pneumonia and bronchitis

    * Lung nodules

    * Lung abscess

    * Miliary disease

    * Hilar adenopathy

    * Pleural effusions and empyema

• Implantable pacemaker and cardioverter-defibrillator infections

• Eye lesions

    * Immune uveitis (chronic iridocyclitis, nummular keratitis, multifocal choroiditis, optic neuritis)

    * Endophthalmitis

    * Dacryoadenitis

• Cardiovascular

    * Endocarditis

    * Deep vein thrombosis

• Abscesses

• Hematologic complications (infrequent)

    * Thrombocytopenia with cutaneous purpura

    * Bleeding from mucosa

    * Hypersplenism

    * Hemophagocytosis

• Neurologic

    * Transient ischemic attacks

    * Meningitis and meningoencephalitis

    * Myelitis-radiculoneuritis

    * Brain and epidural abscesses

    * Meningovascular syndromes

    * Cranial nerve palsies

Table 4

Principal Differentials Considered

Principal Differential Considered	% Patients	Principal Differential Considered	% Patients
Enteric fever	34	Malaria	16
Arthritis	9.5	Brucellosis	14.6
FUO	8.3	Epididymo-orchitis, bilateral hydrocele, urinary tract infection or pyelonephritis	2.2
Tuberculosis	1	Chronic liver disease, splenic abscess or acute cholecystitis	1.4
Endocarditis	1.5	Bronchitis, pneumonia	1.2
Skin rashes, Stevens-Johnson syndrome or cellulitis	1.5	Meningitis	1.1
HIV infection	.5	Enteric fever and brucellosis	5.5
Pulmonary tuberculosis and brucellosis	.1	Rheumatic arthritis and brucellosis	.1
Chorea	.1	Peripheral neuritis	.1

* Aggressive mood and seizures from chronic neurobrucellosis of 2.5 years duration

* Ventriculo-peritoneal shunt infection

• Rashes (5% of patients)

  * Papules

  * Ulcers

  * Abscess

  * Erythema nodosum

* Petechiae

* Purpura

* Vasculitis

Key Differential Diagnostic Features

• Clinical presentations of brucellosis are nonspecific and inclusion in the differential diagnosis is dependent upon epidemiology

• Diagnosis is dependent upon laboratory confirmation

Key Laboratory/Radiology Features

- Anemia, leukopenia, thrombocytopenia, abnormal coagulation profiles – usually mild

- Blood cultures – isolation of the organism is the gold standard

    * May not become positive for days or weeks

    * Rate of isolation from routine blood cultures may be as low as 15%

    * Sensitivity: 91% for acute brucellosis and 74% for chronic disease using lysis centrifugation techniques

- Bone marrow cultures – granulomas found in 75% of bone marrows

- Joint effusions grow *Brucella* less than 50% of time – pleocytosis in joint fluid with mostly lymphocytes

- Speciation by standard microbiologic methods

- ELISA may be of value – a single report indicates a 100% sensitivity and 99.2% specificity

- PCR may detect organisms in patients with negative cultures – primers available for *B abortus* and *B melitensis*

- Serologic tests of value

    * Rose Bengal Plate Agglutination Test – used as rapid screening: 99% sensitivity

    * Standard tube agglutination

    * Immunocapture agglutination

    * Latex agglutination

    * Complement fixation, ELISA

    * Fluorescence polarization assay

Therapy

Empiric and Definitive/Specific

- Treatment of uncomplicated non-pregnant adults (See Skalsky et al for details)

    * First line therapy

        - WHO/FAO 1986: doxycycline + rifampicin - both for 6 weeks

        - Ioannina 2007: doxycycline 6 weeks + streptomycin 2–3 weeks

        - 2008 meta analysis: doxycycline 6 weeks + rifampicin 6 weeks + gentamicin 2 weeks OR doxycycline 6 weeks + gentamicin 2 weeks

    * Alternative therapy

        - WHO/FAO 1986: tetracycline 6 weeks + streptomycin 2–3 weeks

        - Ioannina 2007: doxycycline 6 weeks + rifampicin 6 weeks

        - 2008 meta analysis: doxycycline 6 weeks + streptomycin 2 weeks

    * Second-line therapy

        - WHO/FAO 1986: no recommendation

        - Ioannina 2007: doxycycline 6 weeks + gentamicin 1 week

        - 2008 meta analysis: doxycycline + rifampicin 6 weeks or tetracycline 6 weeks + gentamicin or streptomycin 2 weeks

    * Optional (poor evidence)

        - WHO/FAO 1986: co-trimoxazole

        - Ioannina 2007: cotrimoxazole + doxycycline + other antibiotic 6 weeks OR ofloxacin or ciprofloxacin + doxycycline/rifampicin 6 weeks

- 2008 meta analysis: co-trimoxazole + doxy-cycline/rifampicin 6 weeks

* Not recommended

- WHO/FAO 1986: No recommendation

- Ioannina 2007: Azithromycin or meropenem

- 2008 meta analysis: monotherapy or < 30 days of treatment or quinolone with or without rifampicin or doxycycline

- High rates of relapse with cotrimoxazole alone

- Neurobrucellosis: doxycycline plus rifampin plus ceftriaxone with steroids in selected cases – no controlled studies as to the efficacy of steroids

- Other therapeutic recommendations

  * Doxycycline and streptomycin for 45 days (first choice)

  * Doxycycline and rifampin (second choice)

  * Rifampin and cotrimoxazole or gentamicin (children under the age of 8 years)

  * Rifampin (pregnant women)

  * Prosthetic joint infections treated successfully with prolonged therapy with streptomycin, rifampicin, and doxycycline and 2 stage surgical exchange of prosthesis

Prognostic Factors

- Antibiotic therapy shortens duration of illness, and reduces relapses and risk of complications

- Usually a self-limited disease

- Majority of deaths caused by cardiac complications

- Fatal systemic disease with multifocal liver and lung nodules

Further Reading

Books and Book Chapters

Young EJ. *Brucella* species. In: Mandell GL, Bennett JE, Dolin R, eds. *Mandell, Douglas, and Bennett's Principles and Practice of Infectious Diseases*. 6th ed. v.2. Philadelphia, PA: Elsevier Churchill Livingstone; 2005:2669-2674.

Journal Articles

Celebi G, Kulah C, Kilic S, et al. Asymptomatic Brucella bacteraemia and isolation of *Brucella melitensis* biovar 3 from human breast milk. *Scand J Infect Dis*. 2007;39:205-208.

Corbel MJ. Brucellosis: an overview. *Emerg Infect Dis*. 1997;3:213-221.

Dhand A. Ross JJ. Implantable cardioverter-defibrillator infection due to *Brucella melitensis*: case report and review of brucellosis of cardiac devices. *Clin Infect Dis*. 2007;44:e37-e39.

Mantur BG, Amarnath SK, Shinde RS. Review of clinical and laboratory features of human brucellosis. *Indian J Med Microbiol*. 2007;25:188-202.

Pappas G, Akritidis N, Bosikovski M, et al. Brucellosis. *N Engl J Med*. 2005;352.2325-2336.

Pappas G, Akritidis N, Christou L. Treatment of neurobrucellosis: what is known and what remains to be answered. *Expert Rev Anti Infect Ther*. 2007;5:983-990.

Park KW, Kim D-M, Park CY, et al. Fatal systemic infection with multifocal liver and lung nodules caused by *Brucella abortus*. *Am J Trop Med Hyg*. 2007;77:1120-1123.

Skalsky K, Yahav D, Bishara J, et al. Treatment of human brucellosis: systematic review and meta-analysis of randomized controlled trials. *BMJ*. 2008;336:701-704.

Solera J. Treatment of human brucellosis. *J Med Liban*. 2000;48:255-263.

4. *Francisella tularensis* (Tularemia)

Synonyms

• Rabbit fever (U.S.)

• Deer-fly fever (U.S.)

• Market-men's disease (U.S.)

• Wild hare disease (yato-byo) (Japan)

• O'Hara's disease (Japan)

• Water-rat trappers' disease (Russia)

• Plague-like disease in rodents

• Pahvant Valley fever

• *Bacterium tularense*

• *Pasteurella tularensis*

• *Citellus beecheyi* (Richardson – 1911)

Causative Organisms

• *Francisella tularensis*

    * Fastidious, Gram-negative, pleomorphic coccobacillus

    * 4 major subspecies

        • *F tularensis* subsp. *tularensis* (type A) – the most virulent subtype

          * Isolated in North America – a single case in Europe

          *2 subpopulations — AI and AII

            • Type AI found in central U.S. associated with the eastern cottontail rabbit and the American dog tick (*Dermacentor variabilis*) and the Lone Star tick (*Amblyomma americanum*)

            • Type AII found in western U.S. associated with the wood tick (*Dermacentor andersoni*) and the deer fly (*Chrysops discalis*) and the mountain cottontail rabbit.

        • *F tularensis* subsp. *holarctica* (type B)

          * Milder disease

          * Found in all areas of the Northern Hemisphere

        • *F tularensis* subsp. *mediasiatica*

          * Milder disease

          * Isolated from animals from central Asia

        • *F tularensis* subsp. *novicda* – rarely isolated. A single isolate was reported from the Southern Hemisphere

        • *F philomiragia*

Epidemiology

• Potential bioterrorist weapon

• Isolated from over 200 vertebrate, invertebrate, insect and arthropod species

    * Most common ticks in U.S.: (*Dermacentor variabilis, Amblyomma americanum, Dermacentor andersoni*)

    * Mosquito-borne transmission most common mode in Scandinavia

    * Most cases in U.S. are rabbit and deer associated

• Outbreaks of disease can be years apart

• <u>Human-to-human transmission does not occur</u>

• Geographic patchy distribution over the entire Northern Hemisphere

* In the U.S., most cases from Arkansas, South Dakota, Missouri and Oklahoma; no cases from Hawaii

• 2 ecologic cycles: terrestrial and aquatic

   * Terrestrial: *F tularensis* subsp. *tularensis* - associated with rabbits and ticks in a dry environment

   * Aquatic: *F tularensis* subsp. *holarctica* – associated with hares, small rodents, mosquitoes, ticks near streams, ponds, lakes and rivers

      • May persist for long periods in water associated with protozoa

      • Natural reservoir in water voles (Russia) and muskrats (Canada)

      • Waterborne transmission reported in Russia, especially in flooded areas

• Birds are susceptible to *F tularensis* and may be a reservoir

• Arthropods are vectors but do not appear to be reservoirs

   * Bacteria circulates in a tick-animal cycle

   * Mosquitoes may be a vector in Russia and Sweden

   * Tabanid flies have acted as a vector

• 2 major sources of transmission in the U.S.: tick bite transmission and contact with rabbits

   * Tick-borne tularemia

      • Peaks in the summer

      • Predominantly west of the Mississippi

   * Rabbit-associated tularemia

      • Peaks in the winter during rabbit hunting season

Key Clinical Features

• Incubation period: 3–6 days (range: few hours to 2–3 weeks)

• General features:

   * Abrupt onset of fever and chills

   * Muscle pain

   * Headache

   * Dry cough common in all forms

   * Rashes common in all forms

      • Papular skin rash

      • Erythema nodosum

• Ulceroglandular or glandular tularemia (~75% of patients)

   * From direct contact with infected animals or vector-borne infection

   * Papule at point of entry progresses to a slow healing ulcer with a crust

   * At the same time, axillary or inguinal nodes enlarge depending on the site of the ulcer – untreated, nodes can enlarge to the size of hen's eggs with suppuration being common

   * Untreated, these fistulae heal after weeks or months

   * Pneumonia occurs in 30% of these patients

   * Glandular tularemia the same as ulceroglandular disease except there is no visible primary lesion

• Oropharyngeal tularemia

   * From ingestion of contaminated food or water

   * Ulcerative tonsillitis or pharyngitis, most often right-sided with prominent lymphadenopathy of adjacent nodes

* In some areas, more often in children

* A cluster of cases of ulcerative tonsillitis or pharyngitis should suggest food or water-borne disease

• Oculoglandular tularemia

* A special form of ulceroglandular disease with the primary lesion in the conjunctiva

* Conjunctivitis combined with preauricular adenopathy

* Transmitted from contact of contaminated hands with the eye

• Typhoidal tularemia (~25% of patients)

* No focal symptoms

* May be contracted through inhalation as well as all other modes of transmission

* Prolonged high fevers with relative bradycardia

* Gastrointestinal and pulmonary symptoms common

* Disease may be self-limited, especially with *F tularensis* subsp. *holarctica*

* Patients may suffer septicemic complications

* Pneumonia occurs in 80% of these patients

• Respiratory tularemia

* Primary lung disease occurs after inhalation of aerosols (laboratory workers, aerosolization from gardeners after running over an infected rabbit while mowing a lawn or parkway center median with a ride-on power mower, or as the result of a bioterrorist attack)

* Severe respiratory insufficiency and necrotizing pneumonia

* Sudden onset of fever, chills, temperature to 104° F with relative bradycardia, nonproductive cough, pleuritic chest pain, profuse diaphoresis

• Cough may produce mucopurulent sputum or hemoptysis

* Signs and symptoms may be nonspecific, mild and last for days or weeks when accompanying ulceroglandular disease

* Chest x-ray: infiltrates, hilar adenopathy, pleural effusion

• Apical or miliary disease resembling tuberculosis

• Single or multilobar infiltrates or consolidation

• Hilar adenopathy with or without infiltrates

• Mediastinal adenopathy

• Abscesses with cavitation

• Residual calcific and fibrotic lesions

• ARDS

• Ovoid densities are rare

* *F tularensis* subsp. *holarctica* has caused discrete infiltrates

Key Differential Diagnostic Features

• Diagnosis is often made on epidemiology and clinical presentation

• Differential Diagnosis for Ulceroglandular Tularemia

* Anthrax

• Ulcer often in the neck, hands or arms

• Painless ulcer with gelatinous raised edge

- Satellite vesicles

- Regional lymphadenopathy may or may not be present; when present, minimum enlargement that is painless

- Initially no fever or systemic symptoms

  * Sporotrichosis

    - Ulcer on the fingers, hands, arms

    - Initial painless papule

    - Nodular lymphangitis with skip areas

    - Regional adenopathy may or may not be present

    - Initially no fever or systemic symptoms

  * *Mycobacterium marinum*

    - Ulcers on the fingers and hands

    - Verrucous nodules

    - Nodular lymphangitis

    - Initially no fever or systemic symptoms

  * Differences of ulceroglandular tularemia from Anthrax, Sporotrichosis and *Mycobacterium marinum*

    - In tularemia, the regional nodes are painfully enlarged out of proportion to the ulcer size

    - In tularemia, there is initially fever and systemic symptoms

    - In tularemia, submaxillary and anterior cervical nodes involved

- Differential Diagnosis for Oculoglandular Tularemia

  * Lymphogranuloma venereum

- Inguinal or generalized adenopathy

- No periorbital edema

- No conjunctivitis

- The cornea is clear

  * Adult inclusion conjunctivitis (*Chlamydia trachomatis* serotypes D–K)

    - Lymphadenopathy may or may not be present

    - No periorbital edema

    - Hemorrhagic and mucopurulent conjunctivitis with a predisposition for the lower lid

  * Herpes zoster

    - Ptosis and/or ophthalmoplegia is seen that is not seen in the other infections

    - The cornea may or may not be clouded

    - Dendritic ulcers may be present

  * Epidemic keratoconjunctivitis (Adenovirus types 8 and 19)

    - Hemorrhagic conjunctivitis

    - Cloudy corneal infiltrates

  * Listeria

    - The cornea may or may not be clear

    - Corneal ulcer may be present

  * Differences of oculoglandular tularemia and the above differential diagnosis

    - In tularemia, there is submaxillary, and anterior cervical lymphadenopathy which is seen in Listeria infections but may or may not be present in the other diseases

    - In tularemia, there is periorbital edema which is usually absent in the other infections

- In tularemia, there is a unilateral follicular, purulent ulcer

- The cornea is clear

- Differential Diagnosis for Oropharyngeal Tularemia

  * Oropharyngeal tularemia

    - Majority of patients have tularemic pneumonia

    - Painful pharyngeal ulcers

    - Anterior adenopathy, submandibular nodes may be normal

  * Group A streptococcal pharyngitis

    - Painful exudative pharyngitis

    - Anterior cervical adenopathy

    - Increase or normal WBC

    - Peripheral eosinophilia

    - Normal serum transaminases

  * Infectious mononucleosis

    - Painful tonsillar enlargement

    - Posterior cervical adenopathy

    - Normal or decreased WBC

    - Elevated serum transaminases

  * Diphtheria

    - Adherent bluish white membrane

    - Painless pharyngitis

    - Anterior and submandibular adenopathy

    - Normal or elevated WBC

    - Normal transaminases

- Differential Diagnosis for Typhoidal Tularemia

  * Tularemic Pneumonia

    - Pleuritic chest pain

    - Severe headache

    - Unilateral or bilateral hilar adenopathy

  * Q fever

    - Severe headache

    - Relative bradycardia

    - Serum transaminases elevated

    - Lower lobe infiltrates

  * Psittacosis

    - Severe headache

    - Relative bradycardia

    - Serum transaminases elevated

    - Lower lobe infiltrates with consolidation

  * Mycoplasma

    - Unilateral lower lobe infiltrates

    - Pleural effusions may or may not be present

    - Bilateral hilar adenopathy may or may not be present

  * Legionella

    - Relative bradycardia

    - Pleuritic chest pain may or may not be present

    - Pleural effusion may or may not be present

    - Asymmetrical, rapidly progressive multilobar infiltrates

• Serum transaminases elevated

• Differential Diagnosis for Typhoidal Tularemia

* Typhoid fever

• Relative bradycardia

• Salmonella in bone marrow smears

* Brucellosis

• Brucella/granulomas in bone marrow

* Typhoidal infectious mononucleosis

* Malaria

* Miliary tuberculosis

• AFB in bone marrow granulomas

* Typhoidal tularemia

• Necrotizing granuloma in bone marrow

Key Laboratory/Radiology Features

• Diagnosis confirmed by

* Serology: agglutination test

• Antibody levels (including IgM) may remain elevated for years

* ELISA tests available but have no advantage over agglutination tests

* Polymerase chain reaction

• High sensitivity and specificity for primary ulceroglandular tularemia lesions

• More sensitive than culture

* Culture:

• HIGH RISK OF LABORATORY-ACQUIRED INFECTION requires a biosafety level 3 laboratory for isolation

• Most easily cultured from ulcers

• May be cultured from blood, node aspirates, gastric aspirates, respiratory secretions

• Inoculation into guinea pigs and subsequent cultures

* Skin tests no longer used

* Lymphocyte stimulation tests not at the practical stage of development

* Meningitis: CSF: mononuclear pleocytosis, elevated protein, low glucose

* Immunofluorescence used to identify organism in tissue samples and used to confirm the identity of isolates

* Transportation of isolates to a reference laboratory for identification is STRICTLY controlled by US federal regulations

Therapy

Empiric

• Empiric therapy can include any of the recommendations for specific therapy

• Fluoroquinolones or doxycycline have the broadest spectrum against the organisms in the wide differential diagnosis

• Should be included in the differential diagnosis of FUO and treatment for diseases in the differential should include antibiotics for tularemia

Definitive/Specific

• Gentamicin or tobramycin 5 mg/kg IV in divided doses every 8 hours for 7–14 days

* Relapse rates higher than with streptomycin

• Streptomycin considered drug of first choice by some authors

* 7.5–10 mg/kg IM every 12 hours for 7–14 days

* Other regimens have been recommended

* Jarisch-Herxheimer-like reaction has been rarely reported

• Chloramphenicol for complicating meningitis

* Relapse rates significantly higher than streptomycin

• Milder disease has been treated with doxycycline 200 mg daily for 14 days but treatment failures have been reported

• Quinolones may be an effective alternative especially in mild to moderate disease (ciprofloxacin 400 mg IV BID for 7-14 days or levofloxacin 500 mg IV QD for 7-14 days)

• Some authors recommend duration of therapy to be at least 14 days

• Postexposure prophylaxis in a bioterrorist mass exposure

* Doxycycline 100 mg twice daily

* Ciprofloxacin 500 mg twice daily

• Antibiotic prophylaxis

* After potential exposures of unknown risk is not indicated

* After laboratory exposure: Streptomycin IM or 14 days of oral doxycycline or ciprofloxacin

Prognostic Factors

• In pre-antibiotic era, mortality was 3.6%–33% (other estimates 5%–15% to peaks of 30%-60%)

• With treatment, mortality 2.2%–3.8%

• Complications:

* Can progress rapidly, especially in immuno-compromised patient from septic shock and death

* Meningitis

* Endocarditis

* Prosthetic joint infection

* Rhabdomyolysis especially in the typhoidal form of disease

* Hepatitis and jaundice

* Encephalitis

* Osteomyelitis

* Splenic rupture

* Pericarditis

* Disseminated intravascular coagulation

* Renal failure

* Peritonitis

* Thrombophlebitis

• Tularemia should be part of the differential diagnosis in all patients with FUO

• After treatment, patients may remain debilitated for months. This is associated with late lymph node suppuration and fatigue

• Poor outcomes associated with

* Advanced age of patient

* Coexisting medical conditions

* Symptomatic a month or more before treatment initiated including delay in diagnosis and inappropriate antibiotics

* Advanced pleuropulmonary disease

* Typhoidal tularemia

* Renal failure

- Recovery confers life-long immunity although rare re-infections have been reported

- Vaccines

    * Killed vaccines are ineffective

    * Live vaccine is available and may be considered for individuals at high risk

Further Reading

Books and Book Chapters

Cunha BA. Tularemia. In: Cunha BA, ed. *Tickborne Infectious Diseases – Diagnosis and Management.* New York, NY: Marcel Dekker; 2000:251-268.

Cunha BA, Johnson DH. Tularemia. In: Marrie TJ, ed. *Community Acquired Pneumonia.* New York, NY: Kluwer Academic/Plenum Publishers; 2001:841-848.

Penn RL. *Francisella tularensis* (Tularemia). In: Mandell GL, Bennett JE, Dolin R, eds. *Mandell, Douglas, and Bennett's Principles and Practice of Infectious Diseases.* 6th ed. v.2. Philadelphia, PA: Elsevier Churchill Livingstone; 2005:2674-2685.

Journal Articles

Eliasson H, Broman T, Forsman M, et al. Tularemia: current epidemiology and disease management. *Infect Dis Clin N Am.* 2006;20:289-311.

Nigrovic LE, Wingerter SL. Tularemia. *Infect Dis Clin N Am.* 2008;22:489-504.

5. *Yersinia pestis* (Plague)

Synonyms

- The great dying

- The great pestilence

- *Pasteurella pestis*

- Pasteurellosis

- Black death (bubonic plague)

    * Black death of Europe – the second pandemic (1300s-1600s)

- Pestis siderans (septicemic plague)

- Plague of Athens (430–426 BC)

- Antonine plague (166–270 AD)

- Justinian plague (542–590 AD) – the first plague pandemic

- Modern pandemic (3rd pandemic) (1855 or 1894-1900s)

Causative Organisms

- *Yersinia pestis*

Epidemiology

- Principally a zoonosis of rodent (over 200 species)

- Carnivores also have become infected

- Except for sparrows, birds do not develop disease

- Transmitted from animal to animal by infected flea bites

    * Flea pathophysiology

        - Fleas attach to infected rodents and acquire the infection

        - *Y pestis* produces coagulase causing blood clots in the flea paraventricularis, preventing the fleas from being satiated

- As rodents die, flea abandons the rodent for the nearest warm body

- The flea attaches and regurgitates bacilli into the new victim

* 1500 species of fleas and *Hyalomma detritium* tick

* *Xenopsylla cheopis* flea efficiently transmits disease

* *X cheopis* and *Nosopsyllus fasciatus* responsible for plague epidemics in the 16th an 17th century England along with the human flea, *Pulex irritans*

- Important reservoirs: domestic rats (*Rattus rattus*) and the common sewer rat (*R norvegicus*)

- Risk factors for plague epidemics

    * Urbanization

    * War

    * Societal upheavals

    * Natural disasters

- Risk factors in U.S.

    * Failure to store garbage in covered rodent-proof containers

    * A garden within 90 meters of the home

    * Unused out-buildings

    * Nearby wrecked cars

    * Lumber or wood piles

    * Discarded tires

    * Trash piles

    * Failure to control fleas on pets

    * Rat population exceeds 4 per square meter

* Handling infected animals

* Sick domestic cats from endemic areas

- Between 1977 and 1988, cats-associated plague resulted in 23 cases and 5 deaths

    * Persons who participate in outside activity in endemic areas

    * Medical personnel caring for infected patients

    * Laboratory workers

    * Veterinarians and their assistants

    * Travelers to plague-endemic areas

    * Pet owners from endemic areas

- Agent of bioterrorism used throughout history

    * Effective aerosol dose: 100–500 organisms

    * Will survive for an hour and may travel up to several kilometers

Key Clinical Features

- Aerosolized (bioterrorism) incident – Primary inhalation plague pneumonia

    * In a bioterrorist attack:

        - Cases will present simultaneously or sequentially at different locations, in both endemic an nonendemic areas

        - Death would rapidly follow onset of symptoms

        - Patients complain of fever, cough productive of bloody, watery or purulent sputum, chest pain, and shortness of breath

        - Cyanosis, organ failure and death in one to 5 days

    * In primary inhalation disease

- Incubation period depends on inoculum: a few hours for large inoculums but more typically 24–60 hours

- Incubation period for hematogenous plague pneumonia is the same

* <50% of patients have lymphadenopathy

- Sudden onset of fever, chills and painless cough

- Sputum is thin, watery, blood-tinged with plague bacilli easily seen on Gram-stain of sputum (Gram-negative rod)

* Bipolar staining only seen with Wright, Giemsa or Wayson stain

- Death within 24 hours

• Subclinical plague

* During periods of outbreaks of plague in endemic areas, hemagglutination titers rise from 4.7% baseline (nonepidemic years) to 46.8 % during epidemic years

• Plague Pharyngitis

* Inhalation or ingestion results in acute tonsillitis with inflamed anterior cervical nodes

* Lymph node aspirates and throat cultures are positive for *Y pestis*

* Asymptomatic individuals in endemic areas have been found to have positive throat cultures

* Pharyngeal colonization is not prolonged

• Pestis minor

* Mild febrile illness

* Localized lymphadenopathy

- Spontaneously draining nodes signal recovery

• Must differentiate from lymphogranuloma venereum

* Recover without treatment

• Cutaneous Manifestations

* 25% of Vietnamese patients had skin lesions at or near the bubo or flea bite

- Vesicles

- Eschars

- Papules

- Less frequently cellulitis, abscesses, ulcerations

- Ecthyma gangrenosum rare

- In early or late bubonic plague – sicker patients develop moist gangrenous skin resembling a carbuncle

- Septicemic patients develop purpura which sloughs near death (the "Black Death")

• Bubonic plague

* Most common presentation of disease acquired from an infected flea bite resulting in local painless lymphadenopathy

* At the site of the bite, the lesion may be macular, papular vesicular, pustular or develop an eschar

* Incubation period: 10 hours to 10–14 days (average: 3–6 days)

* Simultaneously with the painless lymphadenopathy, there is a sudden onset of fever (38.5°–40° C)

* Nodes rapidly enlarge from 1–10 cm and become tender

- Enlarging abdominal nodes may produce symptoms mimicking an acute abdomen

- Nodes may continue to enlarge during recovery

- Lymphadenitis and confluent necrosis of nodes results in serosanguineous effusion and bleeding

- Complications of lymphadenitis

    * Limb edema

    * Staphylococcal, pneumococcal, *Pseudomonas* spp. and other bacterial superinfections

* In nonmeningitis patients: insomnia, delirium, stupor, weakness, staggering gait, vertigo, slurred speech and memory loss occurs

- Septicemic plague (Pestis siderans)

    * Primary septicemic plague (without lymphadenopathy)

        - Occurs more frequently over the age of 60 years

    * 25% of bubonic plague patients have bacteremias with 10 or more organisms/mm^3

    * Tendency to become hypotensive

    * Patients rapidly become moribund

    * Lower temperatures as compared with patients with bubonic plague

    * High-grade bacteremia with organisms visible in peripheral blood smears

    * Disease progresses so rapidly that nodes do not have the opportunity to enlarge

- Pneumonic plague (Demic plague) – see Aerosolized (bioterrorism) incident - Primary inhalation plague pneumonia

- Plague meningitis

    * Most commonly occurs between 9th and 17th day of bubonic disease that is inadequately treated

    * May develop without adenopathy

    * Patients with axillary buboes are at increased risk – 1/3 of patients with axillary buboes develop plague meningitis

    * Hunters, veterinarians and veterinarian assistants are at particular risk because they handle infected animals

        - Plague bacilli growing in animal tissue acquire an antiphagocytic capsule and are believed to be more virulent

    * Symptom: fever, headache, Kernig's sign, seizures, vestibulocerebellar symptoms, and coma

- Pediatric plague – (southwest) U.S.

    * Ages between 8–10 years with male predominance

    * 15.8% mortality

    * Most cases bubonic plague

    * 16% develop pneumonia

    * 11% develop meningitis

    * 18% develop sepsis

Key Differential Diagnostic Features

- Differential diagnosis

    * Tularemia – the most important zoonosis that may be confused with plague

        - Similar incubation periods (tularemia 2–10 days)

- Both have the skin, lungs, oral and gastrointestinal mucosa as portals of entry

  * Tularemia skin entry point - an ulcer or pustule which is much less common in plague

- Adenopathy common in both diseases

- Tularemia usually does not result in an elevated WBC

- *Francisella tularensis* is rarely cultured

- *F tularensis* may become an indolent or self-limited disease

  * 5%–33% mortality untreated; 0%–8% mortality treated

- Both diseases are commonly complicated by pneumonia or meningitis

- Tularemia more frequently causes pericarditis

- Plague more frequently complicated by shock

* Reye's syndrome – Clinical similarities with plague found early in the disease

  - Hypoglycemia, once thought to be the hallmark of Reye's syndrome actually occurs infrequently

  - Reye's syndrome and plague patients both exhibit elevated liver enzymes and prothrombin times

* Differential diagnosis of lymphadenopathy of plague

  - Acute lymphadenitis

    * *Staphylococcus aureus* infections of node or region draining involved node

    * Streptococcal infections of one or region draining involved node

* *Pasteurella* species (ie, *Pasteurella multocida*)

* Primary or secondary syphilis (regional or generalized lymphadenopathy with moderately enlarged nodes that are rubbery, discrete and not tender)

- Acute cervical lymphadenitis

  * Group A streptococcal pharyngitis – plague pharyngitis resembles acute bacterial tonsillitis

  * Botulism

  * Diphtheria

  * Viral upper respiratory infections

  * *Neisseria gonorrhea* pharyngitis

  * Primary syphilis

- Inguinal lymphadenitis

  * Lymphogranuloma venereum

  * Chancroid

  * Granuloma inguinale

* Gastrointestinal disease or acute abdomen

  - Acute surgical abdomen

  - *Capnocytophaga canimorsus* sepsis

* Other febrile illnesses: early stages of plague may be confused with

  - Typhus

  - Relapsing fever

  - Dengue

  - Malaria

- Plague pneumonia differential diagnosis

  * Primary (inhalation) pneumonia – 2% of cases in U.S.

  * Secondary pneumonia from bubonic or septicemic disease 12% of cases

- Plague meningitis differential diagnosis

  * May present without lymphadenopathy but with all the typical findings of bacterial meningitis (fever, headache, meningismus, Kernig's sign, seizures, vestibulocerebellar symptoms, coma)

  * Spinal fluid may be yellow, pleocytotic, abnormal chemistries and positive Gram's stain

Key Laboratory/Radiology Features

- Organisms may be cultured from all sources on MacConkey agar and cystine heart agar with 8% sheep blood and brain-heart infusion broth: ideal growth temperature is 28° C–30° C and not 37° C. Blood cultures must be held at least 10 days

- WBC range from 10,000–20,000 cells/mm³ with occasional patients having leukemoid reactions (WBC> 100,000 cells/mm³)

- Disseminated intravascular coagulopathy with fibrin split products

- Some patients develop enlarged livers with elevated liver enzymes, elevated bilirubin and prothrombin times

  *Patients with liver abnormalities and hypoglycemia may be mistaken for Reye's syndrome

- In plague meningitis, Gram stain of CSF often reveals Gram-negative rods

  *CSF is yellow with pleocytosis and typical chemistries of bacterial meningitis

- Serologic diagnosis for retrospective diagnosis only

  *Passive hemagglutination tests

  *Complement fixation

  *ELISA

- PCR

  *89% sensitivity in culture positive patients

  *80.7 % sensitivity in ELISA for F-1 antigen positive patients

  *100% specificity in culture, antigen, and antibody negative patients

- Monoclonal antibody against F-1 antigen has as high as a 100% sensitivity and specificity

- X-ray findings

  *Patchy bronchopneumonia

  *Segmental or lobar pneumonia

  *Cavities may be present

  *Affected lungs may display consolidation within hours or days

  *Multilobed progressive unilateral or bilateral disease

  *Lobes may swell from edema or hemorrhage with bowing fissures mimicking *Klebsiella* pneumonia

  *Pleural effusions and air bronchograms may be present

Therapy

Empiric

- When plague is in the differential diagnosis, treatment should include doxycycline or gentamicin

Definitive/Specific

- Treatment of choice for all forms of disease except meningitis: streptomycin (1 gram IM twice daily or 10–20 mg/kg/day in 2 divided doses in children up to the adult dose) for 7–10 days

- Gentamicin 2 mg/kg loading dose followed by 1.7 mg/kg every 8 hours intravenously (adjusted for renal function after the loading dose) is considered either first or second choice for therapy for all disease other than plague meningitis

- Uncomplicated cases in adults

    * Doxycycline 200 mg IV loading followed by 100 mg IV or by mouth twice daily or

    * Ciprofloxacin 500 mg by mouth or 400 mg IV twice daily

- Antimicrobial susceptibility testing is essential

    * 13% of strains from Madagascar were resistant

- For plague meningitis – chloramphenicol (50–100 mg/kg IV in 4 divided doses after a 25 mg/kg loading dose in children) is the drug of choice and continued for at least 7 days up to the maximum adult dose (1 gram IV every 6 hours)

- Chemoprophylaxis is indicated for individuals exposed to aerosolized bacilli (bioterrorism, laboratory accident, household and face-to-face contacts of primary or secondary plague pneumonia patients) with oral doxycycline 100 mg twice daily or oral ciprofloxacin 500 mg twice daily either for at least 7 days

Prognostic Factors

- 27% mortality with hypotension

- 33% mortality with septicemic plague even with treatment

- 40%–70% mortality in untreated patients

- Prompt appropriate treatment: 5%–18% mortality

Further Reading

Books and Book Chapters

Butler T. *Plague and other* Yersinia *infections*. London, England: 1983.

Butler T, Dennis DT. *Yersinia* species including plague. In: Mandell GL, Bennett JE, Dolin R, eds. *Mandell, Douglas, and Bennett's Principles and Practice of Infectious Diseases*. 6th ed. v.2. Philadelphia, PA: Elsevier Churchill Livingstone; 2005:2691-2701.

Cleri DJ, Marton R, Rabbat M, Vernaleo J: Pneumonia caused by *Yersinia pestis* Plague pneumonia. In: Marrie TJ, ed. *Community Acquired Pneumonia*. New York, NY: Kluwer Academic/Plenum Publishers;2001:777-799.

Journal Articles

Butler T. A clinical study of bubonic plague: observations of the 1970 Vietnam epidemic with emphasis on coagulation studies, skin histology and electrocardiograms. *Am J Med*. 1972;53:268-276.

Cleri DJ, Ricketti A, Panesar M, et al. Plague (*Yersinia pestis*) – Parts I and II. *Infect Pract Clin*. 2004:259-265 and 271-275.

Cunha CB, Cunha BA. Impact of plague on human history. *Infect Dis Clin N Am*. 2006;20:253-272.

Koirala J. Plague: disease, management, and recognition of act of terrorism. *Infect Dis Clin N Am*. 2006;20:273-287.

6. *Yersinia pseudotuberculosis*

Synonyms

• Malassez's bacillus

• Vignal's bacillus

• *Bacillus pseudotuberculosis rodentium*

Causative Organisms

• *Yersinia pseudotuberculosis*

Epidemiology

• Worldwide distribution but particularly in temperate climates of the northern hemisphere especially in countries with cold climates

• Enteropathogen of cattle, deer, sheep, goats, pigs, birds, rodents, lagomorphs

   * Pet and stray cats and dogs become infected in cold months and excrete up to 10^4 bacteria per gram of feces

   * Cause of mastitis in cows

• Transmitted by direct contact with infected animals including a pet-dog bite

• Worldwide – infection linked to milk (including pasteurized milk), water and pork

• Transmitted in the entire chain of pork production

• Linked to salads, vegetable production (carrots, iceberg lettuce, vegetable juice)

• Found in soil and water (including well water) where implicated lettuce was grown with hares and deer as the suspected animal reservoir – transmitted after drinking from a mountain stream probably contaminated by infected rats

• Incidence: .6-5/100,000 population (Finland)

• Periodic outbreaks in daycare centers and schools

Key Clinical Features

Clinical Presentation

• Incubation period: 3–7 days

• Fever (93%) and abdominal pain (83%) caused by mesenteric lymphadenitis

• Diarrhea (21%) and vomiting (23%)

• Joint and back pain (50%)

Complications

• Small-bowel gangrene

• Multiple abscesses in immunosuppressed patients

• Erythema nodosum (in one outbreak, >80%)

• Reactive arthritis

   * 30% incidence of joint pain and 4 of the 33 (12%) fulfilled criteria for reactive arthritis (in a serotype O:3 outbreak in Finland)

   * Other outbreaks (serotypes O:1a and O:3): incidence 68%–100%

   * Much less common in children than adults

   * Polyarticular disease most common: predominance of small joints of hands and feet

   * Joints affected: hands, wrist, feet, knees, ankles, shoulder, Achilles tendon pain, heel pain, sacroiliitis, chest pain

   * Back and neck symptoms

   * HLA-B27 positive in patients tested

   * Duration of symptoms: 1-6 months

• Sepsis in patients with: HIV (serotype O:1), malignancy, cirrhosis, diabetes, aplastic anemia, thalassemia, and iron overload (patients with alcoholism, asplenia, hemochromatosis and heavy tobacco use)

* Sepsis presenting as high fever, fatigue, loss of appetite, has been reported in a healthy woman accompanied by elevated liver enzymes and a rash followed by desquamation

- Multiple hepatic abscesses

- Chronic prostatitis/recurrent urinary tract infections

- Nephritis

- Iritis

- Infected abdominal aortic aneurysm with adjacent lymphadenopathy

Key Differential Diagnostic Features

- Indistinguishable from acute appendicitis

Key Laboratory/Radiology Features

- Culture of blood, stool and other lesions

- Serologic studies: some serologic studies tended to cross-react with other pathogens; immunoblotting appeared reliable

- PCR may be used for typing of isolates

Therapy

Empiric and Definitive/Specific

- Sepsis has been successfully treated with ceftriaxone and imipenem

- Usually susceptible to tetracyclines and streptomycin but resistant to ampicillin

Prognostic Factors

- Sepsis: 75% mortality in spite of antibiotic therapy

Further Reading

Books and Book Chapters

Butler T, Dennis DT. *Yersinia* species, including plague. In: Mandell GL, Bennett JE, Dolin R, eds. *Mandell, Douglas, and Bennett's Principles and Practice of Infectious Diseases*. 6th ed. v.2. Philadelphia, PA: Elsevier Churchill Livingstone; 2005:26912701.

Journal Articles

Brubaker RR. Factors promoting acute and chronic disease caused by yersinia. *Clin Microbiol Rev*. 1991;4:309-324.

Fukushima H, Gomyoda M, Ishikura S, et al. Cat-contaminated environmental substances lead to *Yersinia pseudotuberculosis* infection in children. *J Clin Microbiol*. 1989;27:2706-2709.

Hadou T, Elfarra M, Alauzet C, et al. Abdominal aortic aneurysm infected with *Yersinia pseudotuberculosis*. *J Clin Microbiol*. 2006;44:3457-3458.

Hannu T, Mattila L, Nuorti JP, et al. Reactive arthritis after an outbreak of *Yersinia pseudotuberculosis* serotype O:3 infection. *Ann Rheum Dis*. 2003;62:866-869.

Jalava K, Hakkinen M, Valkonen M, et al. An outbreak of gastrointestinal illness and erythema nodosum from grated carrots contaminated with *Yersinia pseudotuberculosis*. *J Infect Dis*. 2006;194:1206-1209.

Laukkanen R, Martinez PO, Siekkinen KM, et al. Transmission of *Yersinia pseudotuberculosis* in pork production chain from farm to slaughterhouse. *Appl Environ Micrbiol*. 2008;74:5444-5450.

Paglia MG, D'Arezzo S, Festa A, et al. *Yersinia pseudotuberculosis* septicemia and HIV. *Emerg Infect Dis*. 2005;11:1128-1130.

Seddik H, Ahtil R, En-Nouali H, et al. Small-bowel gangrene revealing *Yersinia pseudotuberculosis* infection. *Gastroenterol Clin Biol*. 2008 Nov 6 [Epub ahead of print].

Stolzel F, Pursche S, Bruckner S, et al. *Yersinia pseudotuberculosis* causing abscesses in a 31-year-old patient in the post-immunosuppression period after allogeneic HSCT. *Bone Marrow Transplant.* 2008 Nov 3 [Epub ahead of print].

Tauxe RV. Salad and pseudoappendicitis: *Yersinia pseudotuberculosis* as a foodborne pathogen. J Infect Dis. 2004;189:761-763.

ID Board Pearls

- *Campylobacter jejuni and Campylobacter fetus*

  * Seasonal outbreaks of *C jejuni* infections observed in industrialized countries are not seen in developing nations.

  * Beta-lactamase enzyme is commonly seen in *C jejuni*, but not in *C fetus*. *C jejuni* is inhibited by clavulanic acid, but NOT by tazobactam or sulbactam. Amoxicillin-clavulanic acid is effective against most, if not all strains of *C jejuni*.

- *Brucella species*

  * Although cardiovascular complications only involve 2% of cases, it accounts for most of the deaths from brucellosis.

  * Not only may patients develop asymptomatic bacteremias, but brucella may be asymptomatically excreted in human breast milk.

- *Francisella tularensis*

  * For tularemia, seroconversion (agglutination test) does not occur until into the 3rd week or later into the disease.

  * False positive serology for tularemia occurs with brucellosis.

  * Third generation cephalosporins exhibit in vitro susceptibility for tularemia but often fail clinically.

  * Relapse may occur with any antibiotic treatment of tularemia except streptomycin.

  * *Francisella tularensis* is easily killed by heating but not by cold or freezing.

  * Automated laboratory identification systems are unreliable for the identification of *F tularensis* and should not be used for that reason, and they may generate aerosols.

VI. Rat-Bite Fevers

• *Yersinia pestis* (Plague)

* "Blains": untreated patients may develop a generalized papular rash of the hands, feet and pectoral areas. If the patient survives, these evolve into vesicles and pustules resembling smallpox.

• *Yersinia pseudotuberculosis*

* *Y pseudotuberculosis* can cause skin infections with lymphangitis similar to sporotrichosis.

1. **Overview**

2. **Streptobacillus moniliformis (Haverhill Fever)**

3. **Spirillum minus**

1. Overview

Besides *Streptobacillus moniliformis* and *Spirillum minus*, the ubiquitous *Rattus rattus* and *R norvegicus*, and rodents in general, are responsible for over 85 diseases or groups of diseases that infect man. These include Arenaviridae, Bunyaviridae, orthopoxviruses, Lyssavirus, hepatitis E virus, multiple bacteria including rickettsia and anaplasma, protozoa, dermatophytic fungi, microsporidia, helminths, ectoparasites and ticks. Plague is the best known of these diseases, but we often forget that *S moniliformis* is both associated with rat bites and ingestion, and *Sp minus* should be considered in the differential diagnosis of travelers, especially from the Far East.

2. *Streptobacillus moniliformis* (Haverhill fever)

Synonyms

• Rat-bite fever

• Haverhill fever
  (erythema arthriticum epidemicum)

• *Actinomyces muris*

• *Actinobacillus multiformis*
  (AKA *Actino-moniliformis*)

• *Haverhillia multiformis*

• *Haverhillia moniliformis*

• *Streptothrix muris ratti*

• *Actinobacillus putorii* (isolated from a boy after a weasel bite (Dick and Tunnicliff – 1918)

Causative Organisms

• *Streptobacillus moniliformis*

  * Gram-negative pleomorphic short coccobacillary rods with bulbous swellings

  * May stain Gram-positive and is often missed as debris

Epidemiology

• Part of the normal flora of the oropharynx, trachea and nasal secretions of wild and laboratory rats, mice, gerbils and other rodents

• Half of healthy laboratory rats and some mice have *S moniliformis* colonizing their conjunctivae, and pharynx

• Weasels, squirrels, dogs, cats (including house pets) and pigs have been identified as sources of infection (greyhounds, in particular)

• The bacterium is excreted in rat urine

• Healthy animal carriers do not appear to pass the disease amongst themselves

• Distribution is worldwide

• The risk of developing rat-bite fever after receiving a bite from an infected animal is believed to be 10%

• Human infections result either from rat bites (*rat-bite fever*) or ingestion of contaminated milk, water or food (*Haverhill fever*)

Key Clinical Features

• Rat-bite fever

  * Incubation period: 1–4 days to 10 days (extreme range: 1–22 days) but rarely more than 10 days

  * Abrupt onset of fever, chills, severe headache, vomiting, and severe migratory arthritis

  * The rash begins 2–4 days after the onset of fever

    • Petechial or measles-like nonpruritic rash over the extremities including the palms and soles, and blisters

    • The rash may be macular, morbilliform, vesicular, pustular, or hemorrhagic pustular

    • Rare patients have rashes limited to macules on the fingers

    • The rash may dramatically desquamate

  * The rat bite is usually healed and regional lymphadenopathy is rare or absent.

• Haverhill fever

  * Haverhill fever patients have more severe vomiting and complain of pharyngitis.

• Rash

  * Rash appears over the palms, soles and extremities 2 to 4 days after the onset of fever.

  * It is nonpruritic, maculopapular, morbilliform, petechial, vesicular, hemorrhagic vesicular, or pustular

* Hemorrhagic pustules and cutaneous abscesses have been reported

* The lesions evolve to become purpuric and then confluent and sometimes desquamate

* Patients may present with only acrally distributed purpuric macules on the fingers

* Other skin lesions and arthritis follow 2 days later.

• Arthritis complicates a large number of cases: 50%–88% have polyarthritis, and a minority develop septic arthritis concurrently or a few days after the rash

* Knee joints are most commonly affected followed by ankles, elbows, wrists, shoulders and hips

* Most cases resolve in 2 weeks, but chronic arthritis may persist for years with periods of exacerbation and remission

* A patient with a subcutaneous hand abscess presented with remitting seronegative symmetrical synovitis and pitting edema

* 50% of patients will develop an asymmetric migrating polyarthritis affecting the knees, shoulders, elbows, wrists and hands, while the bitten area seems to heal

* Joint effusions are more common in adults than children and are exceedingly painful

* Synovial fluid has a high white cell count

• Untreated patients may become afebrile in 3–5 days with full recovery in 2 weeks

• Untreated patients may remain ill for months

• Complications

* Endocarditis is an infrequent complication that occurs on previously damaged valves. Endocarditis on a normal valve has been reported in an HIV+ patient

* Myocarditis

* Pericarditis

* Massive pericardial effusion

* Pneumonia

* Hepatitis

* Nephritis

* Amnionitis

* Anemia

* Subglottic mass with bilateral parotid swelling

* Brain abscess (with *Actinobacterium meyerii*)

* Meningitis

* Abscesses in the liver, spleen, kidney and female genital tract

* Diarrhea and weight loss is accentuated in infants and children

* Occasionally, there are relapses occurring at irregular intervals over weeks or months in untreated patients and rarely in treated patients

* Infrequently, though, untreated patients may remain ill for months

* Arthritis can persist for up to 2 years

Key Differential Diagnostic Features

• Benign viral infections

• Meningococcemia

• Enteric fever

• Drug reactions

• Rocky Mountain Spotted Fever

• Secondary syphilis

- Uniarticular or polyarticular arthritis suggests

    * Rheumatoid arthritis

    * Disseminated gonorrhea

    * Lyme disease

    * Brucellosis

    * Septic arthritis

    * Rheumatic fever

    * Vasculitic disease

Key Laboratory/Radiology Features

- White blood cell counts reach 30,000/mm^3

- Diagnosis by the isolation from blood, joint fluid or abscesses

- Organisms may be seen in blood smears, pus, or joint fluid with Giemsa, Gram or Wayson stains

- Bacteria may be cultured from blister fluid

- ELISA for antibody detection

- PCR

- Radiographic abnormalities are seen in the growth plates of secondary growth centers of developing children

Therapy

Empiric

- Depends upon what is considered in the differential diagnosis but should include one of the primary (penicillin) or secondary drugs (doxycycline)

- The most important considerations are meningo-coccemia, Rocky Mountain Spotted Fever, and septic complications

Definitive/Specific

- Drug of choice: Intravenous therapy: penicillin G; oral therapy: amoxicillin-clavulanate

- Secondary drug in penicillin allergy: doxycycline

- Prophylaxis after rat bites recommended: amoxi-cillin-clavulanate or doxycycline

- Organisms are susceptible to penicillin, cephalosporins, aminoglycosides, tetracyclines, erythromycin and clindamycin

- L forms are resistant to penicillin and susceptible to tetracycline

- Other successful regimens have included imipenem and ofloxacin, rifampin and clin-damycin, and clarithromycin

Prognostic Factors

- Mortality: 7%–10% to 10%–15% in untreated patients

- Patients with pericarditis or endocarditis have a 53% mortality

- In children, the disease may be so rapidly fatal that bite-marks will be fresh

Further Reading

Books and Book Chapters

Washburn RG. *Streptobacillus moniliformis* (Rat-bite fever). In: Mandell GL, Bennett JE, Dolin R, eds. *Mandell, Douglas, and Bennett's Principles and Practice of Infectious Diseases*. 6th ed. v.2. Philadelphia, PA: Elsevier Churchill Livingstone; 2005:2708-2710.

Journal Articles

Dendle C, Wooley IJ, Korman TM. Rate-bite fever septic arthritis: illustrative case and literature review. *Eur J Clin Microbiol Infect Dis*. 2006;25:791-797.

Elliott SP. Rate bite fever and *Streptobacillus moniliformis*. *Clin Microbiol Rev*. 2007;20:13-22.

Stehle P, Dubuis O, So A, et al. Rat bite fever without fever. *Ann Rheum Dis*. 2003;62:894-896.

Shenk SH, Ricketti AJ, Muddasir SM, et al. Rat-bite fevers: *Streptobacillus moniliformis* and *Spirillum minus*. *Infectious Disease Practice for Clinicians*. 2006;30:509-514.

Stehle P, Dubuis O, So A, et al. Rat bite fever without fever. *Ann Rheum Dis*. 2003;62:894-996.

3. *Spirillum minus*

Synonyms

Rat-bite fever from *Spirillum minus* is also known as

- Sodoku

- Sokosho

***Spirillum minus* has been known as**

- *Spirillum minor*

- *Spirocheta morsus muris*

- *Sporozoa muris*

Causative Organisms

- *Spirillum minus*

  * Motile spiral-shaped bacteria with bipolar flagella that stain with silver stains

  * With darkfield microscopy, they demonstrate the classic "darting motility

  * Most often, the organism is considered Gram-negative

Epidemiology

- Principally causes disease in Asia and Japan, rarely in the U.S.

- Naturally found in rats (25%), mice, guinea pigs, wild and domestic cats, ferrets, bandicoots and other carnivores that feed on infected rodents

- Disease is acquired by rat or rodent bite

Key Clinical Features

- Incubation period: 5–30 days (usually 5–10 days)

- Initial bite wound heals, but in 1-4 weeks becomes swollen, purple, and painful with concomitant lymphangitis and lymphadenitis

* The bite wound progresses to a "chancre-like" ulceration with induration and eschar formation

* Contact with a rodent may result in an ulcer in an atypical area

• Symptoms of sepsis accompany the wound inflammation (fever, chills, headache, malaise)

    * Hyperreflexia

    * Myalgia

    * Arthralgia

    * Hyperesthesia

    * Edema

• Rash – initial symptoms accompanied by a red-brown to purple macular rash (rarely urticarial) over the extremities, trunk, face and scalp

    * The rash fades over prolonged afebrile periods

• Fever – rises to 103° F–104° F over 3 days, remains elevated for 3 days then returns to normal

• Fever returns 3–9 to 5–10 days later and recurs

• Complications

    * Endocarditis

    * Myocarditis

    * Pleurisy

    * Hepatitis

    * Splenomegaly

    * Meningitis and meningoencephalitis

      • Headaches

      • Psychological instability

      • Irritability

      • Scanning reveals diffuse ischemia

      • Fatal cases preceded by delirium

    * Epididymitis

    * Conjunctivitis

    * Anemia

• Complications of treatment: patients are at risk for Jarisch-Herxheimer reactions

Key Differential Diagnostic Features

• *Borrelia* spp.

• Malaria

• Lymphoma

• Other relapsing diseases

Key Laboratory/Radiology Features

• White blood cell counts: 10,000-20,000/mm³

    * Eosinophilia with leukocytosis during relapses

• The organisms cannot be cultured but will reproduce in 1–3 weeks after mouse or guinea pig intraperitoneal injection

• Serology is generally not available

• Kahn reactions and *Proteus* OXK agglutination are sometimes positive

• Diagnosis is made by direct visualization of the organism in blood, exudates of lymph nodes by staining with Giemsa, or Wright stains, or the use of darkfield microscopy

    * The organisms are visualized in peripheral blood only during febrile episodes

Therapy

Empiric

- Depends upon what is considered in the differential diagnosis but should include one of the primary (penicillin) or secondary drugs (doxycycline)

Definitive/Specific

- Drug of choice: intravenous therapy: penicillin G for 10–14 days; oral therapy: amoxicillin-clavulanate

- Secondary drug in penicillin allergy: doxycycline

- Prophylaxis after rat bites recommended: amoxicillin-clavulanate or doxycycline

Prognostic Factors

- Untreated, the disease spontaneously remits in 1–2 months

- Few cases remain symptomatic for years

- 6%–10% mortality in untreated cases

Further Reading

Books and Book Chapters

Washburn RG. *Spirillum minus* (Rat-bite fever). In: Mandell GL, Bennett JE, Dolin R, eds. *Mandell, Douglas, and Bennett's Principles and Practice of Infectious Diseases*. 6th ed. v.2. Philadelphia, PA: Elsevier Churchill Livingstone; 2005:2810.

Journal Articles

Shenk SH, Ricketti AJ, Muddasir SM, et al. Rat-bite fevers: *Streptobacillus moniliformis* and *Spirillum minus*. *Infect Pract Clin*. 2006;30:509-514.

ID Board Pearls

- *Streptobacillus moniliformis*

  * Young *Streptobacillus moniliformis* cultures may appear Gram-positive.

  * On primary cultures, *Streptobacillus moniliformis* may appear as obligate anaerobes.

  * Rat-bite fever strains of *Streptobacillus moniliformis* are antigenically distinct from Haverhill fever strains.

  * For *Streptobacillus moniliformis*, single serum agglutinin titers of 1:80 are considered diagnostic. However, these titers may persist for up to 2 years and be as high as 1:1280.

  * Growth of *Streptobacillus moniliformis* is inhibited by sodium polyanethol sulphonate, a common adjunct to most commercially available blood culture systems.

  * 25% of patients with S*treptobacillus moniliformis* have a false positive serologic test for syphilis.

- *Spirillum minus*

- 50% of patients with Spirillum minus have a false positive serologic test for syphilis.

- Spirillum minus cannot be grown on artificial media.

VII. Zoonotic Spirochetal Infections

1. Overview

2. *Leptospira* Species (including Weil's disease)

3. *Borrelia* Species (*B recurrentis, B hermsii*) (Relapsing fever)

1. Overview

The principle spirochetal diseases that infect man include *Treponema pallidum* subsp. *pallidum* (syphilis), *T pallidum* subsp. *pertenue* (yaws), *T pallidum* subsp. *endemicum* (endemic syphilis – bejel), *T carateum* (pinta), *Leptospira* species, *Borrelia* species (relapsing fever), *B burgdorferi* (Lyme disease) and *Spirillum minus* (rat-bite fever – sodoku). They share the facts that they spread hematogenously; Jarisch-Herxheimer reactions are known to occur with the treatment (syphilis, relapsing fever, Lyme disease, leptospirosis, and *Spirillum* rat-bite fever); they are recurrent and/or have a chronic phase (syphilis, non-syphilitic treponemes, leptospirosis, borreliosis, Lyme disease, and *Spirillum minus*); and are treatable by antibiotics. Of these, we will discuss leptospirosis and borreliosis, both of which develop such a high-grade bacteremia that the organisms are visible on the peripheral blood smear.

2. Leptospira Species (including Weil's disease)

Synonyms

• Weil's disease

• Akiyami (Japan)

• Autumn fever

• French disease (named by German physicians in WWI)

• *Spirochaeta interrogans*

• *Spirochaeta icterohaemorrhagiae* (Inada et al — 1916)

• *Spirochaeta icterogenes* (Uhlenhuth and Fromme — 1915, 1916)

• *Leptospira biflexa* (Prior to 1989, Leptospira were divided into 2 species: *L interrogans* and *L biflexa*)

Causative Organisms

(Most common) Pathogenic *Leptospira* species

• More than 250 pathogenic serovars exist

• May remain viable for months in water at room temperature, but survival decreased to hours in domestic sewage

• *Leptospira interrogans*

  * Pathogenic Serovars

    • Icterohaemorrhagiae – most pathogenic (found in rats and isolated from water in the tropics and U.S.)

    • Copenhageni

    • Canicola

    • Pomona (found in cattle)

    • Australis

    • Autumnalis

- Pyrogenes

- Bratislava

- Lai

- *Leptospira noguchii*

  * Pathogenic serovars

  - Panama

    - Pomona

- *Leptospira santarosai* serovar Bataviae

- *Leptospira borgpetersenii*

  * Pathogenic serovars

    - Ballum (especially found in mice and rats)

    - Hardjo (especially found in cattle — where it sometimes causes mastitis, abortion, and premature calves)

    - Javanica

- *Leptospira kirschneri*

  * Pathogenic serovars

    - Bim

    - Bulgarica

    - Grippotyphosa

    - Cynopteri

- *Leptospira weilii*

  * Pathogenic serovars

    - Celledoni

    - Sarmin

- *Leptospira* genomospecies I serovar Sichuan

- *Leptospira faeni* serovar Hurtsbridge

- *Leptospira meyerii* serovar Sofia

Epidemiology

- Worldwide distribution

- 3 epidemiologic patterns

  * Temperate climates where human infection is the result of direct contact with infected animals

  * Tropical climates where many animals are carriers and human infection results from contact with the environment where there is widespread contamination

  * Rodent-borne infection in urban environment

- Outbreaks in South America associated with El Nino-related excessive rainfall and flooding

- Outbreaks associated with other floods

- Associated with rice harvesting in China

- Peak seasons: rainy season in tropical areas; late summer and fall in temperate regions

- Highest incidence in U.S.: Hawaii

- Highest incidence in tropics because of increased survival of pathogen in warm and humid conditions

- Source of infection: direct or indirect contact (contaminated soil or water) with urine or tissue from infected animals

  * Humans or animals may be maintenance hosts – species where the infection is transferred from animal-to-animal by direct contact, usually at an early age

  * Chronic renal tubular infection in infected animals

* Rodents (especially rats) and small mammals most important carriers

* Dogs (with increased incidence of infection in North America), cats, livestock

* Dogs are a significant reservoir in tropical countries

* Wild or feral animals

* Animals become infected in infancy and excrete pathogen either continually or intermittently for life

• Recreational (especially associated with water sports; walking barefoot on damp ground or gardening with bare hands) or vacation exposure becoming more important – detailed itineraries necessary to ascertain risks of acquiring infection

• Occupation exposure (farm workers, veterinarians, animal handlers, butchers, meat inspectors, exterminators, hunters, sewer workers, miners, septic tank cleaners, gamekeepers, fish farmers, canal workers, rice field worker, and taro, banana, sugar cane, and livestock farmers – especially dairy farmers)

• Children handling puppies and kittens

• Portal of entry

* Cuts or abrasions in the skin

* Conjunctiva

* Intact skin after prolonged immersion in water

* Water-borne transmission with contaminated water supplies

* Inhalation of contaminated water or aerosols

* Less frequently from animal bites

* Human-to-human transmission and human sexual transmission

* Isolated from human breast milk and transmitted from mother to infant by breast milk

* Excretion of pathogen in human urine months after recovery recorded

Key Clinical Features

• Although serovar icterohaemorrhagiae causes most of the severe disease in humans, this is not invariable and any serovar may be responsible for any of the clinical syndromes

• Weil's disease: most severe form of infection

• Mean incubation period: 10 days

Anicteric leptospirosis

• Most cases are subclinical or only mildly symptomatic and patients do not seek medical attention

• Cases that come to medical attention usually present with sudden onset of fever

* Fever may be biphasic and recur after remission of 3–4 days

• Other symptoms

* Chills

* Abdominal pain

* Conjunctival suffusion

* Headache may be severe and resemble dengue fever with retro-orbital pain and photophobia

* Intense myalgia of the lower back, thighs, calves

• Infrequently, patients present with a transient rash lasting <24 hours – pretibial maculopapular

• Less frequent findings: lymphadenopathy, splenomegaly and hepatomegaly

• Symptoms last about 1 week until antibodies appear

• Aseptic meningitis ≤25% of all cases of leptospirosis – more frequent in younger patients

- Respiratory symptoms in >50%–67% of patients

- Myocarditis strongly associated with severity of pulmonary symptoms

Icteric leptospirosis

- 5%–10% of all patients with leptospirosis

- Severe rapidly progressive disease

- Patients present late in the course of disease

- Complications

    * Acute renal failure (16%–40%)

    * Necrotizing pancreatitis noted at autopsy in some patients

        - Pulmonary complications not related to severity of jaundice

        - Symptoms include cough, dyspnea, hemoptysis

        - ARDS

        - Intraalveolar hemorrhage in the majority of patients even without symptoms

        - Pulmonary hemorrhage may cause death

        - As low as 17% of jaundiced patients had pulmonary symptoms in Brazil

- Myocarditis (10%–40%)

- Infection in pregnancy has caused abortion and fetal death in some but not all patients

- Cerebrovascular accident

- Rhabdomyolysis

- Thrombotic thrombocytopenic purpura

- Acute acalculous cholecystitis

- Erythema nodosum

- Aortic stenosis

- Kawasaki disease-like syndrome

- Reactive arthritis

- Epididymitis

- Nerve palsies

- Male hypogonadism

- Guillain-Barré syndrome

- Cerebral arteritis mimicking Moyamoya disease

Ophthalmologic disease

- Conjunctival suffusion in the majority of patients

- Pathognomonic sign of Weil's disease: conjunctival suffusion and scleral icterus

- Anterior uveitis (unilateral or bilateral) in minority of cases after recovery sometimes presenting weeks or months after recovery

- Clinical findings may include panuveitis, anterior chamber cells, vitreous opacities, vasculitis, and some patients may have these physical findings without visual abnormalities

Chronic or Latent Disease

- May produce chronic symptoms similar to Lyme disease

- Single case of late-onset meningitis after icteric disease

- Uveitis may be late onset and the result of an immune response to reinfection

- Persistent headaches for long periods after acute disease in a few patients

Key Differential Diagnostic Features

- Yellow fever

- Dengue fever

- Kawasaki disease

- Moyamoya disease (progressive stenosis and occlusion of the terminal portion of the bilateral carotid arteries as well as arterial collateral vessels – genetic predisposition (80% concordance in identical twins and 10% incidence in affected relatives, and an ethnic predisposition for the Asian population). The disease is associated with the development of dilated, fragile collateral vessels at the base of the brain, which are termed Moyamoya vessels

Key Laboratory/Radiology Features

Routine laboratory testing

- Urinalysis: proteinuria, pyuria with or without hematuria and hyaline or granular casts

- Darkfield microscopy will allow visualization of the organisms directly in the blood or urine

- Direct detection by immunofluorescence staining, immunoperoxidase staining, silver staining

- Serology by ELISA for leptospiral antigen in urine under development

- PCR

- Microscopic agglutination test (serology) – best test for epidemiologic surveys

Anicteric leptospirosis

- 64%–67% have chest x-ray changes

Icteric leptospirosis

- No hepatocellular necrosis in survivors – liver function studies return to normal in survivors

- Serum bilirubin levels may remain high for weeks

- Only moderate rises in AST and ALT and minor elevation of Alk Phos

- Serum amylase rises in patients with acute renal failure but symptoms of pancreatitis are uncommon

- Thrombocytopenia ≥50% of patients, but is usually transient and not from DIC

- Pulmonary involvement may be very variable – Brazil: only 33% with x-ray changes

- Fatal disease is often preceded by renal failure, liver failure, pneumonia, and hemorrhage

Radiographic findings

- Diffuse small opacities – may be widely disseminated or may coalesce in areas of consolidation resulting in increased severity of symptoms

- Pleural effusions

- Patchy infiltrates representing pulmonary hemorrhage

EKG changes with myocarditis

- T wave abnormalities

- Repolarization abnormalities

- Arrhythmia

Therapy

Empiric and Definitive/Specific

- Prophylaxis: PO doxycycline

- Mild disease: PO doxycycline, ampicillin, or amoxicillin

- Severe disease: IV penicillin G, ceftriaxone, or ampicillin

Prognostic Factors

- Anicteric leptospirosis — mortality extremely rare

- Icteric leptospirosis — mortality 5%–15%

* Respiratory insufficiency associated with death (Brazil)

* Myocarditis may be fatal (54% mortality with myocarditis)

* Repolarization abnormalities and arrhythmias a poor prognostic sign

Ophthalmologic disease

• Visual abnormalities may persist for years after acute disease

Chronic or Latent Disease

• Usually good prognosis

Further Reading

Books and Book Chapters

Levett PN. Leptospirosis. In: Mandell GL, Bennett JE, Dolin R, eds. *Mandell, Douglas, and Bennett's Principles and Practice of Infectious Diseases.* 6th ed. v.2. Philadelphia, PA: Elsevier Churchill Livingstone; 2005:2789-2795.

Journal Articles

Hashikata H, Liu W, Mineharu Y, et al. Current knowledge on the genetic factors involved in moy-amoya disease. *Brain Nerve.* 2008;60:1261-1269.

Kuroda S, Houkin K. Moyamoya disease: current concepts and future perspectives. *Lancet Neurol.* 2008;7:1056-1066.

Levett PN. Leptospirosis. *Clin Microbiol Rev.* 2001;14:296-326.

3. *Borrelia* Species (*B recurrentis, B hermsii*) (Relapsing fever)

Synonyms and Causative Organisms

Borrelia hermsii

• Tick-borne relapsing fever (TBRF)

• At least 15 species of *Borrelia* cause disease, each associated with its own tick vector that inhabit caves, decaying wood, rodent burrows and animal shelters

• Endemic relapsing fever

Borrelia recurrentis

• Louse-borne relapsing fever (LBRF)

• *Borrelia duttonii* – strains from east and central Africa

• *Borrelia persica (B usbekistanica* and *B sogdianum)* — strains from Asia

• *Borrelia hispanica* — strains from Spain

• *Borrelia crocidurae (B microti* and *B merionesi)* — strains from Senegal

• *B hermsi, B turicatae, B parkeri* – strains from western US

Epidemiology

• *Borrelia hermsii*

* Worldwide distribution – isolated areas in the southwest Pacific have reported no cases although in some of these areas, infected ticks are present

• The last major outbreak was after WWII

• Recently, the disease has been limited to the Andean foothills and Ethiopia, southern Sudan, and Rwanda

* *Ornithodoros* species soft ticks

* Each species of tick has its own host and habitat

* They will travel less than 50 yards independently

* Ticks are night feeders, with painless bite, with blood meal lasting only 5-20 minutes

* Adult ticks can survive without taking a blood meal for up to 15 years in specific environments and still maintain the borrelial infection

* Infection in humans is achieved via tick saliva or feces, both of which are released during a blood meal

* Some species of ticks pass the infection transovarially

* Animal reservoirs: rodents (chipmunks, squirrels, rats, mice) rabbits, owls, and lizards

* Campers

• *Borrelia recurrentis*

* *Pediculus humanus* — human body louse — vector

* Humans are the only host

* Person-to-person transmission by the human body louse

* Disease is transmitted by crushing the louse, releasing the *Borrelia* which are capable of penetrating intact skin or mucous membranes

* Because the bacteria penetrates the midgut, multiplies in the hemolymph of the arthropod, and does not penetrate the louse tissue, it cannot infect man by bite or saliva, or pass the organism transovarially

* Although it was once thought that infection could not be passed through louse feces, new evidence indicates that *B recurrentis* is passed in louse feces

* Occurs in epidemics associated with war, famine, overcrowding, natural disasters

Key Clinical Features

• During febrile periods, bacteremia reaches 100,00 organisms/mm^3 of blood and during afebrile periods, these organisms are sequestered in organs

• Bacteremia and fever recur when *Borrelia* undergo immune antigenic modification and reinvade the bloodstream

Clinical disease

• Prodrome is rare in both diseases

• Both diseases have an acute onset of fever and rigors, severe headache, myalgias, arthralgias, and lethargy

• In both diseases, initial physical findings include conjunctival suffusion, petechiae, diffuse abdominal tenderness and in some cases organomegaly

• Less frequent findings: nuchal rigidity, rales and rhonchi, lymphadenopathy and jaundice

• Hemorrhage more common with LBRF (petechiae, epistaxis, hemoptysis, hematuria, hematemesis

• Rash in both diseases may be truncal in distribution, and petechial, macular or papular

• Tick-borne relapsing fever

  * Incubation: 7 days (4–18 days)

  * Duration of first febrile attack: 3 days

  * Afebrile intervals: 7 days

  * Duration of relapses: 2–3 days

  * Number of relapses: 3 (range: 0–13)

  * Maximum temperature 105° F

  * Splenomegaly: 41%; Hepatomegaly 17%

  * Jaundice:7%

* Rash: 28%

* Respiratory symptoms: 16%

* CNS complications: 9%

• Louse-borne relapsing fever

  * Incubation: 8 days (4–18 days)

  * Duration of first febrile attack: 5.5 days

  * Afebrile intervals: 9 days

  * Duration of relapses: 2 days

  * Number of relapses: 1–2 (range: 1–5)

  * Maximum temperature 101° F–102° F

  * Splenomegaly: 77%; Hepatomegaly 66%

  * Jaundice:6%

  * Rash: 8%

  * Respiratory symptoms: 34% — cough

  * CNS complications: 30%

• Complications

  * Iritis and iridocyclitis

  * Pneumonia and bronchitis

  * Otitis media

  * Acute respiratory distress syndrome

  * Hepatitis

  * Hepatic necrosis

  * Miliary splenic abscesses

  * Neurologic complications: coma, cranial nerve palsies, hemiplegia, meningitis, seizures

  * Central nervous system hemorrhages, perivascular infiltrates and degenerative lesions

* Myocarditis associated with arrhythmias

* Gastrointestinal and renal hemorrhagic lesions

* The primary febrile episode may end in a crisis with fatal hypotension and shock

* Pregnancy: increased maternal and fetal mortality

Key Differential Diagnostic Features

• In epidemics, can be confused with coexisting typhus

• Malaria

• Typhoid fever

• Hepatitis

• Leptospirosis

• Rat-bite fever

• Colorado tick fever

• Dengue

• Neurologic disease may be confused with neurologic complications of Lyme disease, especially in the face of cross-reacting serology

Key Laboratory/Radiology Features

• WBCs to 25,000 cells/mm^3

• ESR elevated up to 110 mm/hour

• CSF pressure is elevated when neurologic symptoms are present with 15–2200 cells/mm^3, elevated protein (160 mg/dL), with a normal CSF glucose level

• CSF smear or animal inoculation may reveal spirochetes in 12% of patients

• Visualization of the organisms on the peripheral blood smear (Wright or Giemsa stained thick and thin smears or dark field wet mounts reveal organisms 70% of the time)

• Organisms rarely seen during afebrile periods

• Increased yield by staining smears with acridine orange smears by fluorescence microscopy or buffy coat smears

• Serology (agglutination, complement fixation, immobilizing antibodies)

• Proteus OXK agglutination positive; OX-19 and OX-2 are usually but not invariably negative

Therapy

Empiric and Definitive/Specific

• Doxycycline is the treatment of choice except in pregnant patients

• Doxycycline prophylaxis recommended after exposure

• Erythromycin or macrolide preferred treatment for pregnant women and children under the age of 8 years

• Penicillin and chloramphenicol also effective therapy

• TBRF treated for longer periods of time because of higher rates of failure than LBRF

• Meningitis or encephalitis: IV penicillin G, cefotaxime, or ceftriaxone for 2 or more weeks

• Jarisch-Herxheimer reaction affects ~80% of patients treated for LBRF *Borrelia recurrentis* infection and carries ~5% mortality – may be prevented by administration of (sheep) anti-tumor necrosis factor-alpha Fab

Prognostic Factors

Tick-borne relapsing fever

• Mortality: 2%–5%

Louse-borne relapsing fever

• Mortality: 4%–40%

• Mortality may reach 70%–80% in untreated cases

Further Reading

Books and Book Chapters

Rhee KY, Johnson, Jr WD. *Borrelia* species (relapsing fever). In: Mandell GL, Bennett JE, Dolin R, eds. *Mandell, Douglas, and Bennett's Principles and Practice of Infectious Diseases*. 6th ed. v.2. Philadelphia, PA: Elsevier Churchill Livingstone; 2005:27952798.

Journal Articles

Badger MS. Tick talk: unusually severe case of tick-borne relapsing fever with acute respiratory distress syndrome-case report and review of the literature. *Wilderness Environ Med*. 2008;19:280-286.

Centers for Disease Control and Prevention (CDC). Acute respiratory distress syndrome in persons with tickborne relapsing fever—three states, 2004-2005. *MMWR*. 2007;56;1073-1076.

Cooper PJ, Fekade D, Remick DG, et al. Recombinant human interleukin—10 fails to alter proinflammatory cytokine production or physiologic changes associated with the Jarisch-Herxheimer reaction. *J Infect Dis*. 2000;181:203-209.

Dworkin MS, Schwan TG, Anderson DE Jr, et al. Tick-borne relapsing fever. *Infect Dis Clin North Am*. 2008;22:449-468.

Fekade D, Knox K, Hussein K, et al. Prevention of Jarisch-Herxheimer reactions by treatment with antibodies against tumor necrosis factor alpha. *N Engl J Med*. 1996;355:347-348.

Houhamdi L, Raoult D. Excretion of living *Borrelia recurrentis* in feces of infected human body lice. *J Infect Dis*. 2005;19:1898-1906.

Roux V, Raoult D. Body lice as tools for diagnosis and surveillance of reemerging diseases. *J Clin Microbiol*. 1999. 37:596-599.

4. Infectious Disease Clinical Pearls

- Primary cultures for *Leptospira* species may take up to 13 weeks to grow, but subcultures will grow in 2 weeks or less.

- Patients treated with penicillin should be closely monitored for Jarisch-Herxheimer reactions.

- Syphilis serology is positive 5%–10% of the time in patients infected with *Borrelia* species. Lyme serology may also be falsely positive.

- Jarisch-Herxheimer reaction, if it is to occur, will begin within 2 hours of beginning treatment for *Borrelia* relapsing fever, which can be fatal. Prevention with prior administration of steroids or interleukin-10 is ineffective.

- Surveillance of body lice (utilizing PCR) may be used as a tool to detect reemerging infections (*Rickettsia prowazekii*, *Bartonella quintana*, and *Borrelia recurrentis*).

VIII. Bartonella Species

1. **Overview**

2. ***Bartonella bacilliformis* (Oroya fever and Verruga Peruana)**

3. ***B quintana* and *B henselae* (Bacillary Angiomatosis and Peliosis)**

4. ***B henselae, B clarridgeiae, Afipia felis* (agents of Cat Scratch Disease)**

5. ***Neisseria animaloris* spp. nov. and *Neisseria zoodegmatis* spp. nov., (Eugonic fermenters [EF organisms – infections following dog bites])**

6. **Infectious Disease Clinical Pearls**

1. Overview

Bartonella are alphaproteobacteria closely related to *Brucella* and *Agrobacterium*. Although trench fever was the first clinical manifestation of *Bartonella* infection to be recognized, a similar disease was described during the Middle Ages. Infection may only be induced in primates. Insects and arthropods transmit the organism. Domestic cats are reservoirs of *Bartonella* and transmit the disease through scratches or bites, lice, or indirectly by their fleas.

2. *Bartonella bacilliformis* (Oroya fever and Verruga Peruana)

Synonyms

• Oroya fever

• Verruga peruana

• Carrion's disease

Causative Organisms

• *Bartonella bacilliformis*

Epidemiology

• Transmitted by sandfly bite (*Lutzomyia verru-carum* – formerly *Phlebotomus* species)

• Disease limited to Andes Mountains above 1–3 km altitude

• Recent cases in the high rain forests (probably transmitted by *L columbiana*)

• No nonhuman vertebrate hosts for *B. bacilliformis*

• Humans (who remain persistently bacteremic for months after recovery) are the reservoir for *B bacilliformis*

• Survivors of acute infection may have persistent bacteremia and act as a reservoir of disease

Key Clinical Features

Oroya fever

• 3–12 week incubation period after inoculation (1-30 week range; mean 2 months)

• Mild disease – slowly developing mild febrile illness that may go unnoticed lasting less than a week

   * First manifestation will be rash

• Severe disease

   * Sudden onset of high fever, chills, diaphoresis, anorexia, prostration, headache

   * Altered mental status associated with development of severe anemia from bacterial invasion of RBCs

   * Severe myalgia, abdominal pain, emesis, jaundice, lymphadenopathy

   * Hepatosplenomegaly

• Duration of illness: 1–6 weeks

• 2–20 weeks after recovery (or without preceding illness) arthralgia, fever and a series of verrucae appear as painless erythematous papules, sessile or subdermal nodules or large angioma like lesions (verruga peruana)

• Complications

   * Seizures

   * Delirium, meningoencephalitis

   * Obtundation

   * Respiratory distress

   * Pericardial effusion

   * Myocarditis

   * Acute respiratory distress

   * Anasarca

   * Acute renal failure

   * Microthrombosis and severe anemia resulting in cardiac dysfunction (including angina), and hepatic and gastrointestinal dysfunction

   * End-organ ischemia and failure

   * Survivors have a increased susceptibility and infections with toxoplasmosis, salmonella, staphylococci, *Mycobacterium tuberculosis*, amoebae, *Histoplasma*, *Pneumocystis*, herpesvirus and hepatitis B

   * 15% of survivors have persistent bacteremia

* Infection during pregnancy – causes transplacental infection and may cause abortion, maternal death and/or fetal death

Verruga peruana

• If not treated with antibiotics, eruptive disease may occur weeks to months after the acute infection

• Crops of skin lesions develop that evolve from miliary to nodular to mulaire (bullous, blood-filled, with a tendency to bleed and ulcerate)

• Mucosal lesions occur

• Healing occurs with recurrences over a period of weeks to 3–4 months resulting in fibrosis of lesions

• Nodules develop and recede at different sites simultaneously

Key Differential Diagnostic Features

Oroya fever

• Epidemiology (endemic areas in the Andean valleys of Peru, Ecuador and Columbia)

• Differential diagnosis of an acute febrile illness with a pulse deficit

• Typhoid fever

• Malaria

• Brucellosis

• Hepatitis

• Tuberculosis

• Leptospirosis

• Sepsis

• Sylvatic yellow fever

• Typhus

• Paracoccidioidomycosis

• Histoplasmosis

• Hematologic malignancies

• Hemolytic or aplastic anemia

Verruga peruana

• Typical skin lesions

• Same differential as bacillary angiomatosis

    * Pyogenic granuloma

    * Hemangioma

    * Subcutaneous tumors

    * Kaposi's sarcoma

    * Bacillary angiomatosis

Key Laboratory/Radiology Features

Oroya fever

• T-cell ratios reversed

• Giemsa-stained peripheral smears with organisms visible as red-violet rods or rounded forms in RBCs

• IgM and IgG immunoblot assay but have a low specificity

• PCR

• Culture on cell-free media (freshly prepared rabbit-heart infusion agar plates, blood or chocolate agar) with prolonged incubation under special conditions of high humidity

• Blood cultures on agar positive after 6 weeks in 71%–83% of cases

Verruga peruana

• Histology of active lesion demonstrates neovascular proliferation with occasional bacteria

Therapy

Oroya fever and Verruga peruana

Empiric

• Atypical presentations of Q fever, scrub typhus, murine typhus, human monocytic ehrlichiosis, and bartonellosis may present with fevers of more than one-week's duration. Even without confirmation of the diagnosis, patients with the appropriate epidemiologic risks, treatment with doxycycline should be initiated

Definitive/Specific

• For acute disease, IV or oral doxycycline, ciprofloxacin, ampicillin or trimethoprim-sulfamethoxazole

• For verruga peruana or any eruptive disease, rifampin has been the drug of choice in Peru

Prognostic Factors

Oroya fever

• Fatal without treatment 40%–88%

• <10% with treatment

• 30% of hospitalized patients die of opportunistic infections – salmonellosis was the most frequent fatal complication

Verruga peruana

• Not fatal but can be disfiguring

Further Reading

Books and Book Chapters

Walker DH, Maguina C, Minnick M. Bartonelloses. In: Guerrant RL, Walker DH, Weller PF, eds. *Tropical Infectious Diseases – Principles, Pathogens, & Practice*. 2nd ed. v.1. Philadelphia, PA: Elsevier Churchill Livingstone; 2006:454-462.

3. *Bartonella quintana* and *Bartonella henselae* (Bacillary Angiomatosis and Peliosis)

Synonyms

• Trench fever

• 5-day fever or quantin fever

• Wolhynia fever

• Meuse fever

• His-Werner disease

• Shin-bone fever

• Shank fever

• *Bartonia* species

• *Rochalimaea quintana* now renamed *Bartonella quintana*

• *Rickettsia quintana*

• *Rickettsia weigli*

• *Rickettsia wolhynica*

• *Rickettsia pediculi*

• *Rickettsia rocha-limae*

• *Burnetia (Rocha-limae) wolhynica*

• *Wolhynia quintanae*

• BA-TF (organism named by Relman et al, 1990)

• Bacillary angiomatosis

• *Rochalimaea henselae* (first isolated by Koehler et al) now renamed *Bartonella henselae*

• *Rochalimaea elizabethae* now renamed *Bartonella elizabethae*

Causative Organisms

• *Bartonella henselae*

• *Bartonella quintana*

- *Bartonella elizabethae* and *Bartonella clarridgeiae* have rarely caused human disease

Epidemiology

- Worldwide distribution for both *B quintana* and *B henselae*

- Trench fever, etc associated with poor sanitation and hygiene leading to body louse infestation – *B quintana*

  * Spread by the human body louse *Pediculus humanus corporis* feces through breaks in the skin usually induced by the arthropod's injection of proteins which induces pruritus and scratching

  * Persistent human bacteremia helps spread the bacterium to uninfected lice

  * *B quintana* has been isolated from an infected patient with lymphadenopathy who owned a cat. *B quintana* has been isolated from cat fleas and cat dental pulp, and monkey fleas

  * No nonhuman vertebrate hosts for *B quintana*

  * Humans are the reservoir for *B quintana*

- *B henselae*: infects domestic cats including healthy animals, especially in warmer and humid climates and some free range and captive felids in California

- *Ctenocephalides felis*, the cat flea is the common vector for cat-to-cat transmission and may transmit human infection of *B henselae*

- *Ixodes* and *Dermacentor* species ticks are also infected with *Bartonella* species

Key Clinical Features

Trench fever (*B quintana*)

- Incubation period: 15–25 days for natural infection

- Incubation period for experimental infection in human volunteers following the inoculation of a large volume of crushed lice: 6–9 days

- Prodrome: 2 days

- Symptoms – asymptomatic infection to life-threatening sepsis

  * Acute onset of periodic fever of irregular duration, cycles of profuse diaphoresis and chills

  * Pain spreads to the back and limbs with leg pain the most severe

  * Dizziness and headache, which is severe, most often frontal and behind the eyes; occipital headaches accompanied by nuchal rigidity suggesting meningitis

  * Weakness, dyspnea, abdominal pain, diarrhea, constipation, anorexia, nausea

  * Frequent micturition

  * Restlessness, insomnia

  * Fever regresses and recurs every 4–8 (5 days most commonly) days with less severe attacks although occasional cases become weaker and leg pain persists

  * Prolong disability – usually no deaths

- Signs

  * Tongue is furred

  * Conjunctival congestion

  * Decrease in pulse in relation to temperature

Bacillary angiomatosis (epithelioid angiomatosis or bacillary epithelioid angiomatosis)

- First described in HIV patients and now seen in both immunocompetent and immunocompromised patients

- *B quintana* and *B henselae* etiologic agents

- Most often affects the skin

  * May be solitary or multiple

  * Bleed profusely when punctured

  * May be superficial, dermal or subcutaneous

  * Deep lesions may be mobile or fixed

  * Superficial lesions may be red, purple or have no color

  * Oral, anal, conjunctival and gastrointestinal mucosal surfaces may be involved

- Also affects, liver, spleen, bone marrow, and lymph nodes

- Bone lesions and subcutaneous masses most often *B quintana*

- Hepatic and lymph node lesions most often *B henselae*

- Enlarged lymph nodes most often correspond to regional lymphatic drainage from skin lesions

- May be accompanied by disseminated visceral disease

- Occasionally the liver, spleen and lymph nodes may be affected without the patient having skin lesions

Bacillary peliosis

- Originally described involving the liver and spleen of HIV patients, but has been described in other immunocompromised patients, also involving the lymph nodes

- Organs contain blood-filled cystic structures from microscopic to a few millimeters

- Partially endothelialized 'peliotic 'spaces filled with cellular debris and bacilli that stain with Warthin-Starry separated from parenchyma by fibromyxoid tissue

- *B henselae* is the only etiologic agent to date

Chronic bacteremia

- Associated with *B quintana* infection

- Bacteremia may persist for up to 8 years after trench fever. Others have recorded persistent bacteremia for 78 weeks and intermittent bacteremia from 4–58 weeks

Lymphadenopathy

- Afebrile

- Chronic cervical and mediastinal adenopathy

- 1 case associated with coinfection with *Mycobacterium tuberculosis*

- Histology: granulomatous reaction

- *B quintana etiologic* agent

Complications

- Myocarditis – *B henselae*

- Dissemination and encephalitis – *B henselae*

- Inflammatory reactions involving the liver, spleen, lymph nodes, lung and bone marrow without angiomatosis or peliosis – *B henselae*

- Endocarditis – blood culture negative – *B henselae* and *B quintana*

  * 90% have fever and 90% have vegetations on echocardiogram

  * >90% require valve replacement

  * *B quintana* develops in patients without previous valvular injury

  * *B henselae* endocarditis develops in patients with previous valvular disease and is associated with cat scratches or bites, or cat flea exposure

Key Differential Diagnostic Features

Trench fever

• In the homeless population, it may be difficult to recognize symptoms of *B quintana* infection against their multiple health problems

    * Respiratory diseases

    * IV drug abuse

    * Blood borne pathogens

    * Podiatric problems

    * Dermatologic disease

    * Louse-transmitted diseases

• Meningitis

Bacillary angiomatosis

• Pyogenic granuloma

• Hemangioma

• Subcutaneous tumors

• Kaposi's sarcoma

• Distinction from *B bacilliformis*-induced verruga peruana is difficult in patients from endemic areas in the Andean valleys of Peru and Ecuador

Bacillary peliosis

Chronic bacteremia

• Patients are typically asymptomatic

Lymphadenopathy

• One patient had asymptomatic lymphadenopathy

• Another patient on hemodialysis had Sjögren syndrome, mediastinal lymphadenopathy and pancytopenia – *B quintana* was isolated from the bone marrow

• A third patient was HIV-positive and had supraclavicular inflammatory lymphadenitis

Key Laboratory/Radiology Features

Trench fever

• Leukocytosis accompanies fever

• Anemia, especially in the chronically ill

Bacillary angiomatosis and Bacillary peliosis

• Leukopenia

• HIV patients with CD4+ less than 100/mm^3

Chronic bacteremia

• None

Lymphadenopathy

• Normal WBC count but lymphopenia present

• Indirect immunofluorescence the most common serologic test to diagnose *Bartonella* infection

    * *Coxiella burnetii* and *Chlamydia pneumoniae* antibodies cross react with this test

    * Other antibody tests will cross react with *Chlamydia psittaci* and *Chlamydia trachomatis* antigens

• Western blot and cross-adsorption can be used to speciate the organisms and eliminate problems with cross reacting antibodies

• Biopsy specimens will stain for both *B henselae* and *B quintana* with Warthin-Starry staining in patients with both bacillary angiomatosis and peliosis

• Immunohistochemistry: used to detect *B quintina* in tissue and in RBCs by immunofluorescence

- May be cultured on various cell-free media, requires direct plating onto solid media, and usually requires more than 7 days incubation and specialized conditions

    * Primary isolates are usually obtained in 12–14 days, although prolonged incubation for up to 45 days may be necessary

- Homogenized liver, spleen, lymph nodes and skin may be successfully cultured

- Routine antimicrobial testing techniques are inadequate and special techniques must be employed

- PCR often used for identification

- Immunofluorescence and enzyme immunoassay for both *B quintana* and *B henselae*

    * Enzyme immunoassay and radioimmunoprecipitation more sensitive than hemagglutination and immunofluorescence for *B quintana*

- IgM ELISA capture for *B henselae*

Therapy

Empiric

- Doxycycline is recommended for suspected asymptomatic bacteremia

- Clarithromycin or azithromycin

Definitive/Specific

- Clarithromycin or azithromycin or ciprofloxacin for bacillary angiomatosis or peliosis

- Most antibiotics demonstrate in vitro susceptibility

- Some isolates are resistant to penicillin, ampicillin, tetracycline or vancomycin

- Aminoglycosides are most consistently bactericidal in vitro and should be included in therapy for bacteremia and endocarditis

- Chronic bacteremia is successfully treated with doxycycline for 30 days combined with gentamicin for 14 days

- Erythromycin is the recommended treatment for bacillary angiomatosis

- Doxycycline is also recommended for bacillary angiomatosis and an alternative to patients who cannot take macrolides

- Ceftriaxone and fluoroquinolones have been successful in treating bacillary angiomatosis BUT ciprofloxacin therapy has failed

Prognostic Factors

Trench Fever

- Prolonged disability – 4–6 weeks

- Minority of patients develop chronic disease

    * Exhaustion

    * Headaches

    * Recurrent limb pains

    * Irritability

    * Depression

    * Abnormal response to stimuli

    * Tendency to sweat

    * Coldness of extremities

    * Fever

    * Anemia

    * Weight loss

    * Dyspnea on exertion

    * Palpitations

    * Precordial chest pain

* Giddiness

* Arrhythmia

* Acute febrile episodes months later

• Usually no deaths

Bacillary angiomatosis

• Life-threatening in untreated patient

Chronic bacteremia

• Prolonged bacteremia with *B. quintana* both persistent and intermittent has been documented over long periods of time

Lymphadenopathy

• May be associated with or without underlying disease

• Prognosis depends on underlying disease

Complications

• Endocarditis: 11.9% mortality (higher mortality in patients who did not receive at least 14 days or more of aminoglycoside therapy)

Further Reading

Books and Book Chapters

Slater LN, Welch DF. *Bartonella*, including cat-scratch disease. In: Mandell GL, Bennett JE, Dolin R, eds. *Mandell, Douglas, and Bennett's Principles and Practice of Infectious Diseases*. 6th ed. v.2. Philadelphia, PA: Elsevier Churchill Livingstone; 2005:2733-2748.

Journal Articles

Foucault C, Barrau K, Brouqui P, et al. *Bartonella quintana* bacteremia among homeless people. *Clin Infect Dis*. 2002;35:684-689.

Foucault C, Brouqui P, Raoult D. *Bartonella quintana* characteristics and clinical management. *Emerg Infect Dis*. 2006;12:217-223.

Fouch B, Coventry S. A case of fatal disseminated *Bartonella henselae* infection (cat-scratch disease) with encephalitis. *Arch Pathol Lab Med*. 2007;131:1591-1594.

Hoey JG, Valois-Cruz F, Goldenberg H, et al. Development of an IgM capture-based ELISA for detection of acute infections with *Bartonella henselae*. *Clin Vaccine Immunol*. 2008; Dec 3 [Epub ahead of print].

La Scola B, Raoult D. Culture of *Bartonella quintana* and Bartonella henselae from human samples: a 5-year experience (1993-1998). *J Clin Microbiol*. 1999;37:1899-1905.

Maurin M, Raoult D. *Bartonella (Rochalimaea)* quintana infections. *Clin Microbiol Rev*. 1996;9:273-292.

Ohl ME, Spach DH. *Bartonella quintana* and urban trench fever. *Clin Infect Dis*. 2000;31:131-135.

Pipili C, Katsogridakis K, Cholongitas E. Myocarditis due to *Bartonella henselae*. *South Med J*. 2008;101;1186.

4. Bartonella henselae, Bartonella clarridgeiae, Afipia felis (agents of Cat Scratch Disease)

Synonyms

• Oculoglandular syndrome (described by Parinaud in 1899)

Causative Organisms

• *Bartonella henselae*

  * *B. henselae* is the recognized etiologic agent for CSD

• *Bartonella clarridgeiae*, *Afipia felis* and *Bartonella koehlerae*

  * These organisms have been implicated as the cause of CSD in rare cases

Epidemiology

• Worldwide distribution

• In humans, highest prevalence of antibody positivity and bacteremia in warm and humid climates

• Seasonal distribution in the U.S. with most cases between July and January

• Cats are the major reservoir – 50% of domestic cats carry B. henselae antibodies

• Outdoor cats and cats infested with fleas most likely to be infected

• Spread of disease between cats via *Ctenocephalides felis* – the cat flea

• Human infection via cat scratches, bites or from saliva and occasionally from flea bite

  * Clustering of cases in families coincides with the acquisition of a new cat or kitten

  * Evidence of asymptomatic infection in family members of patients (18% overall; 19% in those who liked cats; 1.5% in those who disliked cats)

• Direct conjunctival inoculation with Parinaud oculoglandular syndrome

• Liver and kidney transplantation

Key Clinical Features

• Incubation period: 3–10 days

• Most common manifestations

  * Fever and localized lymphadenopathy only – Most common (95% of patients – this may be an overestimate)

    • Begins with an erythematous papule at site of inoculation that progresses to a vesicle and papular crusted stages

    • Skin lesion persists 1–3 weeks

    • Regional lymphadenopathy develops in 1–3 weeks after inoculation

      * 85% of patients have a single node involved

      * Axillary and epitrochlear (46%)

      * Head and neck (26%)

      * Groin (17.5%)

      * 10% of nodes suppurate requiring drainage

    • Systemic symptoms usually mild (fever, generalized aches, malaise, anorexia, nausea, abdominal pain

      * 1/3 of patients are afebrile and <10% have temperatures >39° C

      * Prolonged fever or fever of unknown origin without lymphadenopathy

  * Hepatosplenic disease

    • Prolonged fever

    • Microabscesses in the liver and/or spleen

- >60% present with abdominal pain (episodic, dull pain over the periumbilical area and or more severe pain in upper quadrants)

- Weight loss

- Chills

- Headache

- Myalgia

- Hepatomegaly or hepatosplenomegaly in >50% of patients

- Symptoms regress in 6 months

• Less common manifestations

* Parinaud oculoglandular syndrome (~5% of patients)

- Symptoms

* Foreign body sensation

* Unilateral eye redness

* Serous discharge

* Increased tear production

- Fever

- Follicular conjunctivitis with necrotic granuloma with ulceration of the conjunctival epithelium

- Regional lymphadenopathy (preauricular, submandibular or cervical nodes)

- Granuloma disappears after several weeks without scarring

* Neuroretinitis, posterior segment ocular disease

- Abrupt onset of typically unilateral painless visual loss

- Optic disc swelling and macular stellate exudate

- 2/3 of patients with neuroretinitis are infected with *B henselae*

* Other ocular complications

- Panuveitis with diffuse choroidal thickening

- Retinal vasoproliferative lesions

- Macular hole

- Vitreal detachment

- Vitritis

- Branch retinal artery and venous occlusions

- Retinal white spots

- Papillitis

- In HIV patients – subretinal mass associated with abnormal vascular network – best seen with fluorescein angiography

* Neurologic disease (~2% of patients)

- Symptoms begin 2–3 weeks after the onset of lymphadenopathy

* Typical symptoms are headache and change in mentation

- Complications

* Encephalitis (most common – 90% of neurologic cases)

- Seizures (46%-80%) common in these patients

- May present as status epilepticus

- Combative behavior (40%)

- Weakness

- Alterations in muscle tone

- Nuchal rigidity

- Extensor plantar responses

- Hypo- or hyperreflexia

  * Aseptic meningitis

  * Radiculopathy

  * Facial nerve palsy

  * Guillain-Barré syndrome

  * Cerebral arteritis

  * Transverse myelitis

  * Epilepsia partialis continua

* Dermatologic disease other than the inoculation papule (~5%)

  - Maculopapular and urticarial eruptions

  - Granuloma annulare

  - Erythema nodosum

  - Erythema marginatum

  - Leukocytoclastic vasculitis

- Other complications

  * Glomerulonephritis usually accompanied by fever and lymphadenopathy

  * Pneumonia, pleural effusion or pleural thickening appearing 1-5 weeks after the lymphadenopathy with recovery in 2 months

  * Osteomyelitis/lytic bone lesions

  * Arthritis/arthralgia (~3% of cases in a study from Israel)

- Begins within 1 week of appearance of lymphadenopathy and persisted longer than the lymphadenopathy (13 weeks vs 9 weeks, median)

- Rheumatoid factor-negative

- Associated more frequently with female gender, >20 years of age and erythema nodosum

- Most frequently affected joints: knees, wrists, ankles and elbows

* Endocarditis

  - ~3% of all cases of endocarditis

  - More common in adult males

  - Insidious presentation

    * Fever

    * Shortness of breath

    * Bibasilar rales

    * Cardiac failure

    * Murmur

    * Aortic valve most commonly involved

    * Vegetations are detected in all patients

* Pseudomalignancy

* Bacillary angiomatosis

* Hematologic complications

  - Thrombocytopenic purpura

  - Hemolytic anemia

  - Development of lupus anticoagulant

  - Prolongation of PTT

- Rare complications

  * Spontaneous splenic rupture

  * Myocarditis

  * Seizures post therapy, deja vu phenomenon preceding seizure and requiring ongoing anti-seizure therapy

  * Persistent lymphadenopathy with pain not responding to antibiotics

  * Panuveitis with retinal detachment, neuroretinitis

  * Mastitis with soreness and erythema of the breast

  * Breast abscesses or granulomas

Key Differential Diagnostic Features

- Abdominal location may mimic malignancy on PET/CT scanning

  * Lymphoma one of the most frequently reported differential diagnosis especially in patients with weight loss, night sweats, and prolonged fever

  * Post-transplant lymphoproliferative disease in children who have undergone renal transplantation and presented with fever, lymphadenopathy and/or organomegaly

  * Solitary breast mass with axillary lymphadenopathy mimicking a breast tumor

  * Kikuchi's disease (a self-limiting histiocytic necrotizing lymphadenitis)

  * Histiocytosis X (in a patient with a solitary soft tissue mass overlying a lytic skull lesion

  * Pancreatic malignancy

  * Biliary malignancy

  * Pharyngeal cancer

- Glomerulonephritis may present as IgA nephritis, acute postinfectious glomerulonephritis or necrotizing glomerulonephritis

Key Laboratory/Radiology Features

- Diagnostic criteria for *B henselae* infection: 3 of the 4 criteria necessary (from Margileth)

  * (1) Cat or flea contact regardless of presence of inoculation site

  * (2) Negative serology for other causes of adenopathy, sterile pus aspirated from a node, a positive PCR assay and/or liver/spleen lesions on CT scan

  * (3) Positive enzyme immunoassay or indirect fluorescence assay with a titer ratio of $\geq$1:64

  * (4) Biopsy showing granulomatous inflammation consistent with CSD or positive Warthin-Starry silver stain

- WBC normal to mildly elevated

- Platelets: normal, elevated, or decreased

- ESR: normal or elevated

- Liver enzymes: usually normal

- CSF: usually normal

- Isolation in culture: 2–6 weeks incubation for primary isolation

  * Poor yield from lymph node cultures

- Skin testing no longer used

- Serology by indirect immunofluorescence and enzyme immunoassay

- Ultrasound of nodes reveal that they are multiple, hypoechoic, highly vascular, with increased echogenicity in surrounding soft tissue

- CT and ultrasound may reveal hepatic and splenic lesions and abdominal lymphadenopathy

- Biopsy of nodes reveals granulomas with multiple microabscesses

- IgM capture-based ELISA for the diagnosis of acute disease

- PCR

- Hepatosplenic disease

  * ESR elevated

  * WBC and platelet counts normal

  * Liver enzymes usually normal

  * Abdominal sonography reveals microabscesses in liver and spleen in 68% of patients – lesions are hypoechoic

  * CT of abdomen: hepatic lesions may be hypoattenuated, isoattenuated or marginally enhanced

  * Liver biopsy reveals granuloma

  * Lesions regress in 6 months – residual calcifications have been rarely reported

- Neuroretinitis, posterior segment ocular disease

  * MRI: unilateral enhancement of the optic nerve-globe junction is a highly specific finding for *B henselae* neuroretinitis

- Neurologic disease

  * Encephalitis

    - CSF may be normal or reveal pleocytosis, and/or elevated protein

    - EEG in acute disease: generalized slowing in 80% of patients with all patients' EEGs returning to normal on follow-up

    - 19% of CTs and MRIs are abnormal – lesions seen in the cerebral white matter, basal ganglia, thalamus and gray matter

- Renal disease

  * Gross or microscopic hematuria

  * Proteinuria

  * Cola-colored urine

  * Normal complement 3 levels

  * Normal renal function

  * Renal biopsies: mesangial hypercellularity, IgA deposition, interstitial infiltrates and/or complement 3 deposition consistent with acute glomerulonephritis

- Orthopedic manifestations

  * Lesions may not be clearly seen on plain x-rays and MRIs or nuclear scans may be required for diagnosis

  * Biopsy reveals necrotizing granulomas with adjacent abscesses

Therapy

Empiric and Definitive/Specific

- In order of decreasing efficacy (efficacy 87%-58%)

  * Rifampin

  * Ciprofloxacin

  * Gentamicin

  * Trimethoprim-sulfamethoxazole

- Azithromycin demonstrated efficacy in another study by reduction in lymph node volume over placebo, but in no other parameter. There was no demonstrated efficacy in disseminated disease

- In the immunocompetent patient with no complications or signs of dissemination, some authors advise no treatment

* Significant lymphadenopathy: antibiotic therapy (azithromycin, rifampin, ciprofloxacin, or trimethoprim-sulfamethoxazole)

* Neuroretinitis and encephalitis: doxycycline plus rifampin; erythromycin with rifampin alternative therapy in children with neuroretinitis

* Hepatosplenic disease in the immunocompetent patient: gentamicin, trimethoprim-sulfamethoxazole, rifampin, or ciprofloxacin. Rifampin may be used alone or in combination with the other drugs

* Endocarditis: aminoglycoside with doxycycline and/or ceftriaxone; surgery may be required

* Immunocompromised patients with disseminated disease: erythromycin, doxycycline, isoniazid, azithromycin, rifampin with therapy continued for at least 3 months

Prognostic Factors

• In the immunocompetent host, untreated CSD is a self-limited disease that resolves in 2–6 months.

  * Mean duration of illness without treatment or treatment with ineffective antibiotics: 14.5 weeks

  * Mean duration of illness with treatment with effective antibiotics: 2.8 weeks

• Prognosis usually excellent in patients with encephalopathy, osteomyelitis, renal disease, and pulmonary disease

Further Reading

Journal Articles

Cherinet Y, Tomilinson R. Cat scratch disease presenting as acute encephalopathy. *Emerg Med J*. 2008;25:703-704.

Florin TA, Zaoutis TE, Zaoutis LB. Beyond cat scratch disease: widening spectrum of *Bartonella henselae* infection. *Pediatrics*. 2008;121:e1413-e1425.

Giladi M, Avidor B, Kletter Y, et al. Cat scratch disease: the rare role of *Afipia felis*. *J Clin Microbiol*. 1998;36:2499-2502.

Magalhaes RF, Pitassi LH, Salvadego M, et al. *Bartonella henselae* survives after the storage period of red blood cells units: is it transmissible by transfusion? *Transfus Med*. 2008;18:287-291.

Margileth AM. Recent advances in diagnosis and treatment of cat scratch disease. *Curr Infect Dis Rep*. 2000;2:643-649.

Palumbo E, Sodini F, Boscarelli G, et al. Immune thrombocytopenic purpura as a complication of *Bartonella henselae*. *Infez Med*. 2008;16:99-102.

Tsuneoka H, Tsukahara M. Analysis of data in 30 patients with cat scratch disease without lymphadenopathy. *J Infect Chemother*. 2006;12:224-226.

5. *Neisseria animaloris* spp. nov. and *Neisseria zoodegmatis* spp. nov., (Eugonic fermenters [EF organisms – infections following dog bites])

Synonyms

- EF-4

- EF-4a and EF-4b

- Eugonic fermenter

Causative Organisms

- *Neisseria animaloris* spp. nov. (EF-4a biotype): +arginine dihydrolase activity

- *Neisseria zoodegmatis* spp. nov. (EF-4b biotype): -arginine dihydrolase activity

Epidemiology

- Commensal bacteria found in the oral cavity of dogs and cats

- Has caused necrotizing pneumonia in domestic cats, a tiger cub, a dog and adult African lion; hepatic abscess and peritonitis in a puppy; and, a retropharyngeal/mandibular abscess in a cat

- Most infections the result of dog and cat bites

- Reports of isolation of the organism(s) from the U.S., Canada and Europe from bite wounds with and without signs of infection, although there is probably a world-wide distribution

Key Clinical Features

- Grown from dog and cat bite wounds without signs of infection

- Abscess and cellulitis from bite wounds

- Cultured from the vagina

Key Differential Diagnostic Features

- Other causes of soft tissue infections and abscesses

Key Laboratory/Radiology Features

- *Neisseria animaloris* spp. nov.: culture – all strains are negative for acid production and acetone production

- *Neisseria zoodegmatis* spp. nov.: most but not all strains produce acid

Therapy

Empiric and Definitive/Specific

- Penicillin and 1st generation cephalosporins should be excluded from empiric therapy for dog and cat bites

In vitro activity

- Susceptible: ampicillin, ceftriaxone, aminoglycosides, chloramphenicol, rifampicin, trimethoprim-sulfamethoxazole, fluoroquinolones

- Intermediate susceptibility reported to erythromycin

- Resistance reported to oxacillin, cephalothin, vancomycin

- May be susceptible or intermediate susceptibility to penicillin

In vivo

- Surgical drainage may be necessary for abscesses

- Infection in animals treated successfully with amoxicillin-clavulanic acid

- Some strains do not appear to produce beta-lactamase

Prognostic Factors

- Good with debridement and treatment

Further Reading

Books and Book Chapters

Steinberg JP, Del Rio C. Other Gram-negative and Gram-variable bacilli. In: Mandell GL, Bennett JE, Dolin R, eds. *Mandell, Douglas, and Bennett's Principles and Practice of Infectious Diseases*. 6th ed. v.2. Philadelphia, PA: Elsevier Churchill Livingstone; 2005:2751-2768.

Journal Articles

Almuzara MN, Figueroa SA, Palombarani SA, et al. Dog bite infections associated with CDC group EF-4a. Report of 2 cases. *Eferm Infecc Microbiol Clin*. 1998;16:123-126.

Baral RM, Catt MJ, Soon L, et al. Successful treatment of a localized CDC Group EF-4a infection in a cat. *J Feline Med Surg*. 2007;9:67-71.

Perry AW, Schlingman DW. Pneumonia associated with eugonic fermenter-4 bacteria in two Chinese leopard cats. *Can Vet J*. 1988;29:921-922.

Talan DA, Citron DM, Abrahamian FM, et al. Bacteriologic analysis of infected dog and cat bites. Emergency Medicine Animal Bite Infection Study Group. *N Engl J Med*. 1999:85-92.

Valentine BA, Porter WP. Multiple hepatic abscesses and peritonitis caused by eugonic fermenter-4 bacilli in a pup. *J Am Vet Med Assoc*. 1983;183:1324-1325.

Vandamme P, Holmes B, Bercovier H, et al. Classification of Centers for Disease Control group eugonic fermenter (EF)-4a and EF-4b as *Neisseria animaloris* sp. nov. and *Neisseria zoodegmatis* sp. nov. respectively. *Int J Syst Evol Microbiol*. 2006;56:1801-1805.

ID Board Pearls

- *B bacilliformis* may be visualized on a Giemsa-stained peripheral smear. *B henselae* and *B quintana* do not produce a sufficiently intense bacteremia to be visualized by light microscopy and peripheral smears.

- During the El Nino weather periods of increased humidity and temperature there is an increased sandfly population with a higher incidence of *B bacilliformis* infections.

- MICs correlate poorly with clinical efficacy of antimicrobial agents for the treatment of *B quintana* infection. Lack of bacteriocidal activity and intraerythrocyte location of the pathogen are believed to be the explanation for this phenomenon.

- Chronic alcoholism is an independent risk factor for *B quintana* endocarditis.

- Before the association with bacillary angiomatosis, peliosis hepatitis was reported in patients with wasting diseases (tuberculosis, advanced malignancies) and the use of anabolic steroids.

- *Bartonella henselae* from asymptomatic carriers may present a risk of transmitting the disease by blood transfusion. Organisms may be isolated from red blood cell units stored at 4° C for 35 days.

- *In vitro* antimicrobial susceptibility does not correlate with clinical efficacy in treating *Bartonella henselae* infections.

IX. Zoonotic Viral Diseases

1. Overview

Poxviridae is made up of 2 subfamilies of double-stranded DNA cytoplasmic viruses – the *Entomopoxvirinae* that infect insects and the *Chordopoxvirinae* that infect vertebrates. The 2 most important members are the smallpox virus (variola) and monkeypox. Variola is strictly a human pathogen and, to the best of our knowledge, no longer exists in nature. The existence of the virus in known and suspected stockpiles makes it a potential bioterrorist weapon. Monkeypox outbreaks associated with infected rodents have occurred in the U.S. Monkeypox is generally a milder disease that mimics smallpox. The other poxviruses are principally zoonotic disease that causes focal skin infection in those individuals handling infected animals. Understanding the wide range of poxvirus diseases and epidemiology will help the clinician differentiate them among themselves, and importantly, from smallpox and the more likely disease, chickenpox.

There are 26 known species of coronavirus infecting 36 animal species. In addition to severe respiratory distress syndrome human coronavirus (SARS-CoV), 4 other human coronaviruses (HCoV-229E, HCoV-OC43, HCoV-NL63, HCoV-HKU1) cause illness. The SARS-like-CoV (SL-CoV) virus from animal hosts has a >99% nucleotide homology with SARS-CoV. From virus sequence data, it appears that the masked (Himalayan) palm civet (*Paguma larvata*) acted as an amplification host. The epidemic strains (including SARS-Urbani) evolved because of civet-human interaction in Chinese animal markets. SL-CoV does not cause disease in humans. HCoV-NL63 and HCoV-HKU1 have a worldwide distribution, and cause respiratory tract infections, especially in the winter months.

Rabies virus is a negative-stranded enveloped Lyssavirus (Lyssavirus type 1). Classical rabies virus is the only naturally occurring Lyssavirus in the Western Hemisphere. There are 7 genotypes and 7 serotypes of Lyssavirus. With the exception of the Lagos bat virus, all have caused human disease.

The viral hemorrhagic fever agents principally fall into 4 families of RNA viruses: the Arenaviridae (Argentine, Bolivian, Brazilian, and Venezuelan hemorrhagic fevers and Lassa fever); the Bunyaviridae (Hantavirus genus, Congo-Crimean hemorrhagic fever from the Nairovirus genus, and Rift Valley fever virus from the Phlebovirus genus); the Filoviridae (Ebola and Marburg viruses) and the Flaviviridae (dengue and yellow fever viruses). Except for Marburg and Ebola viruses, they are widely distributed in nature; many are naturally spread by airborne means; humans are widely susceptible; the differential diagnosis is broad; there is great similarity in clinical presentations making differentiation difficult without sophisticated laboratory support; there are limited prophylactic and therapeutic options; and life-saving supportive therapy often requires an intensive care unit.

2. Rabies

Synonyms

- Rabhas (Sanskrit – refers to the god of death and his dog)

- Hydrophobia (Cornelius Celsus)

Causative Organisms

- Rabies virus

Epidemiology

- Potential rabid animals

    * Foxes, raccoons, skunks, mongooses, bobcats, groundhogs, canids, felines, deer, cattle, horses, monkeys, civets, large and small carnivores

    * Bats are the principal reservoir for rabies throughout the world and have been infected with all the other lyssaviruses except Mokola virus

    * Rabbits and rodents are not epidemiologically important but can be infected

- Worldwide, rabies is most frequently transmitted by the bite of an infected animal: risk 5%–80% after a bite

- Risk after the scratch of an infected animal: 0.1%–1%

- Other modes of transmission

    * Inhalation (from aerosolized infected material in the laboratory or aerosolized virus in caves with many infected bats)

    * Handling and skinning infected carcasses

    * Human-to-human transmission documented

    * Experimentally produced oral transmission

- Cryptogenic rabies (no history of animal bite) is the largest group of human rabies cases in the US (63% from 1958–2001)

* Most cases believed to be of bat origin

* Anecdotal reports of rabies transmission by

  • Lactation

  • Kissing

  • Intercourse

  • Providing health care

  • Transplacental (human)

Key Clinical Features

• Incubation period: The average incubation period (Stage I) is 1–2 months (range: 4 days to 19 years). 75% of symptoms develop 20–90 days after exposure.

• Clinical disease: The prodromal period (Stage II) lasts for 10 days. Patients display anxiety and/or depression. Half the patients have fever and chills and in some patients, gastrointestinal symptoms predominate including nausea, vomiting, diarrhea and abdominal pain. At the bite site or proximally along the nerve radiation, there is itching, pain or paresthesia. Myxedema (mounding of a part of the muscle when hit with the reflex hammer) may be demonstrated. If present, this sign persists throughout the course of disease.

• Symptomatic furious rabies (Stage III) (2–14 days – average survival 5–7 days) manifests itself as furious rabies in 80% of cases. Patients are agitated, hyperactive, waxing and waning alertness, bizarre behavior, hallucinations, aggression, with intermittent lucid periods. There is piloerection, excessive salivation, sweating, priapism, repeated ejaculations and neurogenic pulmonary edema.

  * Hydrophobia begins with difficulty swallowing liquids resulting in pharyngeal and laryngeal spasms and aspiration. As it becomes more severe, the sight of water triggers spasms. Aerophobia (spasms triggered by gently fanning the face) is often present. Seizures occur near death.

• Symptomatic dumb or paralytic rabies patients have a longer average survival (13 days). Patients present with weakness or paralysis in a single limb or may present with quadriplegia. There is pain and fasciculation in the affected muscle groups, and sensory abnormalities in some patients. Some patients have meningeal signs but normal mentation. Cranial nerve abnormalities develop and patients appear expressionless. 20% of patients develop Guillain-Barré syndrome. Some patients survive as long as a month without respiratory support but eventually die with paralysis of respiratory and swallowing muscles.

• Coma (Stage IV) may occur immediately after symptoms appear or up to 2 weeks later.

• Recovery or Death (Stage V): on average, death occurs 18 days after the onset of symptoms. Patients cared for in intensive care units have survived from 25 days to months with respiratory support. Death in these patients is often from myocarditis with arrhythmia or congestive heart failure.

Key Differential Diagnostic Features

• Other causes of viral encephalitis

• Tetanus (when opisthotonos is present)

• Acute inflammatory polyneuropathy

• Transverse myelitis

• Poliomyelitis

• When there is a prolonged incubation period, clinical disease may suggest progressive multifocal leukoencephalopathy

• Spongiform changes in the brain may resemble prion disease

Key Laboratory/Radiology Features

• Nuchal biopsy and saliva – viral antigen and viral RNA can be detected by direct fluorescent antibody test (DFA) and reverse transcription polymerase chain reaction (RT-PCR), respectively

- Chest x-rays demonstrate bronchopneumonia consistent with aspiration and/or respiratory failure

- CT scans of the head reveal nonenhancing symmetrical hypodensities of the basal ganglia

- MRI reveals nonenhancing, ill-defined, mild hyperintensity changes in the brain stem, hippocampus, hypothalamus, deep and subcortical white matter, and deep and cortical gray matter (T-2 weighted) in the conscious patient. The pons may enhance.

- MRI of the brachial plexus in the bitten arm with neuropathic pain will enhance

- CSF is usually normal except in patients with meningismus

    * When abnormal, there is a mononuclear pleocytosis

Therapy

Empiric and Definitive/Specific

- Immediate and proper wound care reduces the risk of rabies by 90%

- All patients should receive rabies vaccine (human diploid vaccine) and rabies immune globulin (RIG) without delay

- Pregnancy is not a contraindication

- There is no time limit after exposure that the vaccine and RIG cannot be given!

- All individuals potentially exposed to the virus (including caregivers) should receive both the vaccine and RIG as soon as possible

- Contacts should be traced to at least 1 week prior to the onset of neurologic symptoms in order to provide them with prophylaxis

- A patient survived rabies without vaccine or RIG after treatment with antiviral agents and induced coma (ketamine, midazolam, ribavirin, and amantadine – the Milwaukee Protocol). She was discharged alert, but with choreoathetosis, dysarthria, and unsteady gait

- Steroids most likely contraindicated as in mouse experiments; they shortened the incubation period and hastened death

Prognostic Factors

- Nearly 100% fatal

- Ketamine-induced coma and ribavirin therapy has failed in other patients

Further Reading

Books and Book Chapters

Cleri DJ, Ricketti AJ, Vernaleo JR. Bioterrorism in critical care. In: *Infectious Diseases in Critical Care*. 3rd ed. Cunha BA, ed. In press.

Journal Articles

CDC. Human rabies—Alberta, Canada, 2007. *MMWR*. 2008;57:197-200.

Cleri DJ, Hamid NS, Panesar M, et al. Rabies (Parts I and II). *Infect Prac Clin*. 2004;28:303-310, 315-318.

Hemachudha T, Sunsaneewitayakul B, Desudchit T, et al. Failure of therapeutic coma and ketamine for therapy of human rabies. *J Neurovirol*. 2006;12:407-409.

Hemachudha T, Wilde H, Willoughby RE Jr, Rupprecht CE. Survival after treatment of rabies. *N Engl J Med*. 2005;353:1068.

Willoughby RE Jr, Tieves KS, Hoffman GM, et al. Survival after treatment of rabies with induction of coma. *N Engl J Med*. 2005;352:2508-2514.

3. Severe Respiratory Distress Syndrome (SARS)

Overview

From November 2002 to July 2003, severe respiratory distress syndrome (SARS) quickly spread from Foshan (Shunde district), Guangdong Province in the People's Republic of China to 33 other countries or regions on five continents. There were 8447 cases, 21% occurring in health care workers (HCWs), and 813 deaths (9.6% overall mortality rate) by the time SARS was contained in July 2003. In the Hong Kong and Hanoi outbreaks, 46% and 63% of cases occurred in HCWs, respectively. The case-fatality rate in 2003 was estimated at 13.2% for patients younger than 60 years, and 50% for patients over 60 years of age. 50% of patients with acute respiratory distress syndrome (ARDS) died. Laboratory-acquired cases resulted in transmission to family contacts. A few patients were "superspreaders" of the virus. In 1 hospital, exposure to a single case resulted in infection in 138 patients and HCWs.

Synonyms

- Severe respiratory distress syndrome (SARS)

Causative Organisms

- Human coronavirus (CoV) group 2b, SARS-CoV is of animal origin

  * SARS-CoV strains from the 2002-2003 outbreak (interestingly referred to as the "late human SARS-CoV" strains based upon presumed evolutionary characteristics) differ from the strains from the 2003-2004 epidemic ("early human SARS-CoV" strains) in

    - Spike protein genetic homogenicity, rate of nonsynonymous mutation, and binding affinity to angiotensin-converting enzyme 2 (ACE-2)

    - Severity of disease

    - Epidemic potential

    - Transmission (animal/human-to-human – early strains (2003-2004 isolates); human-to-human — late strains (2002-2003 isolates)); and,

  - The presence of a 415 nucleotide deletion in some of the late strains

Epidemiology

Human Epidemiology

- There were 2 major SARS outbreaks: (1) the early outbreak originated in Guangdong province in late 2002 (to early 2003) with isolated clusters in Taiwan, Singapore and mainland China from the accidental release of the virus in 2003; and, (2) a second outbreak began in late 2003 to early 2004, again reported from Guangdong province in individuals with animal contacts with different SARS-CoV strains

- Molecular studies separated the human SARS-CoV isolates into early, middle, and late phase outbreak-viruses

  * Human SARS-CoV isolates from 2003-2004 (sporadic cases from the same area of China) were more closely related to animal isolates than human isolates from 2002–2003 (the "pandemic" outbreak). This suggested "an independent species-crossing" event.

- Attack rates range from 10.3%–60%, with a risk of 2.4–31.3 cases/1000 exposure-hours.

- Superspreading events (SSEs) include patients excreting very high titers of virus, aerosol generation, contamination of the environment (fomites), and close contact in healthcare settings. These instances have resulted in as many as 300 infections from a single patient

- Indoor aerosols – airborne spread

- The possibility of rodents and fomites playing a role

- HCWs remained at significant risk even after initiation of infection control precautions. Risk factors include:

  * Performance of high-risk patient care procedures

Key Clinical Features

Table 5

SARS-CoV Infection Signs and Symptoms in Patients at Presentation

Signs and Symptoms	Frequency (results reported from multiple centers)	
	Adult Cases	**Pediatric Cases** (5.5 months to 18 years of age)
Asymptomatic viral colonization	11.5% of "well protected" first line health-care workers who did not seroconvert or later develop disease.	
Fever	99%–100%	98%–100%
Chills and/or rigors	55%–90%	14.5% (Rigor: 8.1%)
Cough (productive nonproductive)	43%–100%	60%–62.9%
Shortness of breath	10%–80%	
Myalgia	20%–60.9%	17.7%
Malaise/lethargy	35%-70%	6.5%
Headache	11%–70%	11.3%
Sputum production	10%–29%	
Sore throat	23.2%–30%	9.7% Independent predictor of severe disease
Coryza	22.5% (not reported in all studies)	22.6%
Nausea and/or vomiting	10–19.6%	41%
Diarrhea	11%-15% Fever and diarrhea, sometimes bloody diarrhea without respiratory symptoms at presentation. Other studies have found 20.3% have watery diarrhea on presentation and 38.4% develop a self-limited diarrhea (most frequently in the first week) sometime during the illness. In the community outbreak in Amoy Gardens, Hong Kong, 73% of 75 patients had watery diarrhea and 97% had positive stools. Hospital-acquired SARS less frequently presents with diarrhea (18.8%).	

* Inconsistent use of personal protective equipment

* Fatigue

* Lack of adequate training

* There is evidence that SARS-CoV was transmitted to HCWs during cardiopulmonary resuscitation

• Other factors that contribute to nosocomial contagion include:

  * ≤1 meter between beds

  * Lack of hand washing facilities

  * Lack of changing facilities for the staff

  * Resuscitation performed on the ward

  * HCWs working while symptomatic

  * Patients requiring oxygen therapy

  * Patients requiring positive airway pressure ventilation

• Recommendations for containing the spread of disease include:

  * Hand washing

  * Appropriate well-fitted facemasks

  * Isolation (airborne precautions)

  * Quarantine of asymptomatic contacts thus significantly decreasing the time from onset of disease to isolation

Complications

• Respiratory complications

  * Patients discharged after SARS-CoV infection frequently have abnormal chest x-rays. These abnormalities include patchy opacification and volume loss.

* CT studies of these patients revealed that 62% developed pulmonary fibrosis.

  • Those who developed CT evidence of pulmonary fibrosis were older (mean age 45 vs. 30.3 years), men (8:7 male:female ratio), were more often admitted to the ICU (26.6% vs. 11.1%), had higher peak LDH levels (438.9 U/l vs. 355.6 U/l), more often required pulsed steroid therapy, had more radiographic opacification, and more abnormal segments on thin-section CT

* CT findings (at ~52 ± 20 days) revealed air trapping (92%), ground glass opacities (90%), reticulation (70%), parenchymal bands (55%), bronchiectasis (18%), consolidation (10%), and honeycombing (8%). A second CT (at ~141 ± 27 days) demonstrated resolution of ground glass and interstitial opacities over time, but air trapping persisted.

* The incidence of spontaneous pneumothorax (in nonventilated patients) is 1.7%. In half of these patients, the pneumothorax was bilateral.

• Cardiovascular complications were seen in the majority of patients

  * Overall, 50.4% of the patients became hypotensive (28.1% in week 1; 21.5% in week 2; and, 14.8% in week 3)

  * Tachycardia that could not be explained because of either fever or hypotension was present in 71.9% of patients (62.8% in week 1; 45.4% in week 2; and, 35.5% in week 3). Tachycardia was weakly associated with steroid therapy during the 2nd and 3rd weeks of illness, and persisted at follow-up in 38.8% of patients

  * Transient bradycardia was seen in 14.9% of patients

  * Reversible cardiomegaly without heart failure occurred in 10.7% of patients

  * Transient atrial fibrillation was seen in one patient

- Acute renal failure (ARF) occurred in 17% of patients admitted with probable SARS

  * The majority of the patients were men (77%), older, and more often had underlying illnesses (diabetes: 38% vs. 6%, $P<0.01$; and, heart failure: 38% vs. 2%, $P<0.001$)

  * There was an increased incidence of respiratory failure (85% vs. 26%, $P<0.001$)

  * Increased incidence of death (77% vs. 8%, $P<0.001$)

  * Complicating the ARF were hypotension (77%) from sepsis, gastrointestinal bleed, ARDS, and rhabdomyolysis (10%-43%)

  * In 1 study, 2 of the 3 patients with rhabdomyolysis died with multiple organ failure

- **Osteonecrosis:** Joint pain is a common complaint after SARS-CoV infection. Osteonecrosis of the hip and knee is a risk for patients receiving steroid therapy. The risk for this complication for low total dose steroid therapy was 0.6%. For higher total dose steroid therapy and for >18 days of therapy, the risk is 9.9%-13%.

- **Bacterial and fungal superinfection,** related to prolonged duration of illness, prolonged ventilator support, and high-dose steroid therapy have been reported. These infections include *Aspergillus* species, *Mucor* species, *Pseudomonas aeruginosa*, *Klebsiella* species, methicillin-resistant *Staphylococcus aureus*, alpha-hemolytic *Streptococcus* species and cytomegalovirus.

- **Endocrine:** Hypocortisolism is found in 39.3% of survivors of SARS-CoV infection. A few patients (3.3%) with hypocortisolism had transient subclinical thyrotoxicosis. Almost 7% were biochemically either centrally or primarily hypothyroid. Most hypothalamic-pituitary-adrenal axis abnormalities returned to normal within 1 year.

- **Hepatitis:** Reactive hepatitis is a common finding in 24% of patients having elevated ALT on admission, and up to 69% developing ALT elevation during the course of their illness. Concomitant hepati-

tis B was not associated with an adverse clinical outcome, but severe hepatitis was. Liver damage appears to be directly caused by SARS-CoV rather than hypoxia.

- **Psychiatric complications** that significantly and negatively affected the quality of life have been seen in other survivors of acute respiratory distress syndrome (ARDS). After intensive care treatment, 17%–43% of patients suffered at least once from clinically significant psychiatric symptoms (point prevalence). Posttraumatic stress disorder (PTSD) was diagnosed in 21%–35% of patients; and, nonspecific anxiety in 23%–48% of patients.

  * HCWs were more likely to suffer from PTSD if there was:

    - a perception of risk to themselves;

    - a significant impact on their work routines;

    - a depressive affect; and,

    - assignment to a high-risk unit unexpectedly

Key Differential Diagnostic Features

- Bacterial community-acquired pneumonias that may result in ARDS and mistaken for SARS-CoV infection

  * *Streptococcus pneumonia*

  * *Haemophilus influenzae*

  * *Moraxella catarrhalis*

  * Community–associated methicillin-resistant *Staphylococcus aureus*

  * Atypical pneumonias (*Legionella* species, etc)

  * The differential diagnosis of viruses that commonly cause ARDS with fever

    - Seasonal influenza (A or B)

    - Parainfluenza virus

Key Laboratory/Radiology Features

Table 6

SARS-CoV Infection: Radiologic and Laboratory Findings in Adult Patients at Presentation

Radiologic and Laboratory Findings	Frequency
Abnormal chest x-ray	78.3%–100% (One report: 35.5% of children have normal chest x-rays at presentation. Another report indicates 97% of children had abnormal chest x-rays.)
Of those with abnormal chest x-rays: Unilateral focal disease: Progressive disease:	56.4% 90%
Detection of infiltrates by CT scan of: 87% positive chest x-ray: 96% positive chest x-rays:	13% detected by chest CT scan 4% detected by chest CT scan
Anemia	Decrease in Hgb by 2 g/dl: 49% Hemolysis: 76%
Lymphopenia	69.6%–90% Wong et al reported 98% developed lymphopenia (absolute counts <1000/mm^3)
CD4 and CD8 lymphocyte counts	Decreases during the early course of disease. Low CD4 and CD8 counts at presentation a poor prognostic sign (associated with admission to the ICU and/or death).
Leukopenia	22%–34.1% Wong et al documented transient leukopenia in 64% of patients during the first week (WBC <4.0x.10^6/dl). 2.5% developed transient neutropenia (absolute count <0.5x.10^6/dl).
Leukocytosis	61% of patients in 2nd and 3rd week of illness (WBC> 11.0x10^6/dl). Elevated absolute neutrophil count an independent predictor of an adverse outcome.
Thrombocytopenia	33–44% (1 study reported thrombocytopenia to be mild and self-limited: platelet counts < 140,000/mm^3). 2.5% with platelet counts < 50,000/mm^3.
Hyponatremia	20.3%–60%
Hypokalemia	25.2%–47%
Hypocalcemia	60%
Increased ALT	23.4%–56%
Increased LDH	47%–87% High peak LDH independent predictor of an adverse outcome
Increased CPK	19%–56%
Prolonged APTT	18%–42.8%
Increased D-dimer	45% (reported from one center)

- Avian influenza

  - Respiratory syncytial virus

  - Adenovirus

  - Varicella

  - Human metapneumovirus

  - Hantavirus

- Other organisms likely to require "mass" critical care, have the potential to spread disease to HCWs, and result in an extensive community epidemic with high morbidity and mortality are:

  * Smallpox

  * Viral hemorrhagic fever

  * Plague

  * Tularemia

  * Anthrax

Therapy

Empiric

- Early positive outcomes using ribavirin and steroids led to widespread use of that combination

- Uncontrolled trials suggest that IFN alfacon-1 (a synthetic interferon) with steroids, protease inhibitors with ribavirin, or convalescent plasma with neutralizing antibody may be useful for treatment

- Other therapies under consideration are reviewed by Cleri et al

Definitive/Specific

- There is no definitive therapy

- Randomized controlled trials are not available to evaluate treatment regimens

Prognostic Factors

- Mortality rates are 6.8% in patients under 60 years, and 43% in older patients

- Increased mortality with:

  * Male sex

  * Comorbid conditions (diabetes, hyperglycemia independent of diabetes, chronic hepatitis, etc). Overall, patients with and without comorbid conditions have 46% and 10% mortality rates, respectively.

  * Advanced age

  * High admission neutrophil count

  * Initial elevated lactic dehydrogenase (LDH)

Further Reading

Journal Articles

Cleri DJ, Ricketti AJ, Vernaleo JR. Severe acute respiratory syndrome (SARS). Submitted for publication to: *Infect Dis Clin N Am*. 2008. B. Cunha, ed.

Gu J, Korteweg C. Pathology and pathogenesis of severe acute respiratory syndrome *Am J Pathol*. 2007;170:1136-1147.

Ho HT, Chang MS, Wei TY, et al. Colonization of severe acute respiratory syndrome–associated coronavirus among health-care workers screened by nasopharyngeal swab. *Chest*. 2006;129:95-101.

Hui DS, Wong KT, Antonio GE, et al. Severe acute respiratory syndrome: correlation between clinical outcome and radiologic features. *Radiology* 2004;233:579-585.

Lam CW, Chan MH, Wong CK. Severe acute respiratory syndrome: clinical and laboratory manifestations. *Clin Biochem Rev*. 2004;25:121-132.

Wong SS, Yuen KY. The management of coronavirus infections with particular reference to SARS. *J Antimicrob Chemother*. 2008;62:437-441.

4. Viral Hemorrhagic Fevers (excluding the Flaviviridae - dengue and yellow fevers)

A. **Filoviridae**

   1. **Marburg hemorrhagic fever**

   2. **Ebola Virus hemorrhagic fever**

B. **Bunyaviridae**

   1. **Rift Valley fever**

   2. **Crimean-Congo hemorrhagic fever**

   3. **Hemorrhagic fever with renal syndrome**

   4. **Hantavirus pulmonary syndrome**

C. **Arenaviridae**

   1. **Lassa fever**

   2. **Argentine hemorrhagic fever**

   3. **Bolivian hemorrhagic fever**

Synonyms

Filoviridae

• Marburg virus — none

• Ebola virus — none

Bunyaviridae

• Rift Valley fever

  * Sandfly fever

  * Phlebotomus fever

  * One of the causes of "abortion storms" among cattle and sheep

• Crimean-Congo hemorrhagic fever virus – none

• Hantavirus – hemorrhagic fever with renal syndrome

  * Korean hemorrhagic fever – Hantaan virus

  * Puumala virus has been implicated in cases of hemorrhagic fever with renal syndrome

  * Related viruses: Dobrava virus, Seoul virus, Puumala virus

• Hantavirus – pulmonary syndrome

Arenaviridae

• Lassa fever

• Argentine hemorrhagic fever

• Bolivian hemorrhagic fever virus

Causative Organisms

• Ebola and Marburg viruses make up the two genera of the Filoviridae, single-stranded negative sense RNA viruses

• The Bunyaviridae are a family of plant and animal spherical enveloped single-stranded negative-sense RNA viruses consisting of 51 species, divided into 5 genera

  * Phlebovirus genus: Rift Valley fever

  * Nairovirus genus: Crimean-Congo hemorrhagic fever virus

  * Hantavirus genus

    • Hantavirus hemorrhagic fever with renal syndrome

    • Hantavirus pulmonary syndrome – hantavirus Sin Nombre

    • 10 other hantaviruses identified as the cause of pulmonary syndrome

- Arenaviridae are single-stranded bisegmented RNA ambisense viruses

  * Lassa fever virus – Lassa fever

  * Junin virus - the cause of Argentine hemorrhagic fever

  * Machupo virus – the cause of Bolivian hemorrhagic fever virus

  * Guanarito virus – the cause of Venezuelan hemorrhagic fever

  * Sabia virus – causes hemorrhagic fever with extensive liver necrosis

  * Whitewater Arroyo virus – causes hemorrhagic fever with liver failure

  * Oliveros virus – hemorrhagic fever

Epidemiology

Filoviridae

- Marburg virus and Ebola virus

  * Person to person transmission probably by droplet

  * Aerosol spread demonstrated in nonhuman primates

  * Handling infected monkeys

  * Source/reservoir in nature remains unknown although asymptomatic fruit bats have been implicated

Bunyaviridae

- Rift Valley fever

  * Mosquito bite

  * Handling infected animal blood or tissue

  * Human-to-human transmission has not been reported

  * Outbreaks associated with heavy rainfall, sustained flooding, and large numbers of mosquitoes.

- Crimean-Congo hemorrhagic fever virus

  * Tick bite (some species of *Hyalomma, Dermacentor, Haemaphysalis* (Middle East) and *Rhipicephalus*)

  * Reported in sub-Saharan Africa, South Africa, Madagascar, the Middle East, European Russia, Pakistan, Afghanistan, central Asian republics, Bulgaria, the former Yugoslavia, northern Greece, XiJiang province of northern China

  * Vertebrates (sheep, goats, cattle, wild herbivores, hares, hedgehogs) including ground-feeding birds are intermediate hosts

- Hantavirus – hemorrhagic fever with renal syndrome

  * Caused by inhalation of infected rodent excreta

  * Distributed in Europe and Asia

  * Rodents develop an asymptomatic infection that persists for months or years

  * The virus sheds in rodent urine, feces and saliva, peaking at 2–10 weeks into the infection and continuing for life

  * Field mouse (*Apodemus agrarius*) reservoir

  * *Rattus rattus* and *R norvegicus* reservoirs

  * *Suncus murinus* — the Indian tree shrew is the only insectivore host

- Hantavirus — pulmonary syndrome

  * Caused by inhalation of infected rodent excreta

  * First reported in the Four Corners region of the U.S. west and now reported in North, Central and South America

* Deer mouse (*Peromyscus maniculatus*) reservoir in U.S.

* *Akodon azarae* most common rodent reservoir (by serosurvey)

* Other rodents associated with other hantaviruses identified that produce the pulmonary syndrome

* Same pathophysiology as hantavirus – hemorrhagic fever with renal syndrome

Arenaviridae

• Lassa virus – Lassa fever

  * Rodent hosts (*Mus musculus* and *Matomys natalensis*)

  * Endemic in west equatorial Africa

  * Multiple cases have been imported into western countries without resulting in secondary cases although one treating physician was found to be IgG antibody positive

  * Antibody prevalence in affected populations: 4%–55%

  * 5%–22% of susceptible individuals seroconvert each year

  * Estimated 3 million first-time and 3 million reinfections per year with 67,000 deaths

  * Most cases occur during the dry season (January–March) but occurs during the rainy season (May–November) in Sierra Leone

  * Acquired by rodent excreta that is either inhaled or contaminates food

  * Person-to-person transmission

• Argentine hemorrhagic fever: Junin virus

  * *Calomys musculinis* rodent natural host

  * Acquired by rodent excreta that is either inhaled or contaminates food

• Bolivian hemorrhagic fever: Machupo virus

  * Endemic in Beni region of northwest Bolivia

  * *Calomys callosus* rodent is the natural host

  * Peak incidence: April–July

  * Acquired by rodent excreta that is either inhaled or contaminates food

  * Person-to-person and nosocomial transmission has occurred

Key Clinical Features

Incubation Periods

• Incubation periods for most pathogens are from 7–14 days, with various ranges

Filoviridae

• Marburg Hemorrhagic Fever: 3–10 days

• Ebola Virus Hemorrhagic Fever: 4–10 days (range 2–21 days)

Bunyaviridae

• Rift Valley Fever: 2–6 days

• Crimean-Congo Hemorrhagic fever

  * After tick bite: 1–3 days (range to 12 days)

  * Contact with contaminated blood: 5–6 days

• Hemorrhagic fever with renal syndrome: 2–3 weeks (range: 2 days–2 months)

• Hantavirus pulmonary syndrome (Sin Nombre virus): 1–2 weeks (range: 1–4 weeks)

Arenaviridae

• Lassa fever: 5–21 days but most cases present within 7–14 days

- Argentine Hemorrhagic fever: 7–14 days

- Bolivian Hemorrhagic fever-Machupo virus: 7–14 days (range 5–19 days)

Other Hemorrhagic Fevers

- Dengue hemorrhagic fever: 2–5 days

- Yellow fever: 3–6 days

- Kyasanur forest hemorrhagic fever: 3–8 days

- Omsk hemorrhagic fever: 3–8 days

- Alkhumra hemorrhagic fever: not determined

- Machupo virus – Bolivian hemorrhagic fever: probably 7–14 days

Contagious Period

- Patients should be considered contagious throughout the illness

Clinical Disease

- Most diseases present with several days of nonspecific illness followed by hypotension, petechiae in the soft palate, axilla and gingiva. Some patients develop neurologic complications

Filoviridae

- Marburg virus

  * Similar to Ebola with a sudden onset of symptoms progressing to multiorgan failure and hemorrhagic fever syndrome

  * Sudden onset of fever, chills, myalgias, headache

  * After 6–8 days, disease progresses to severe hemorrhagic fever

* Some, but not all, of these patients may present with a maculopapular rash by the 5th day of disease

  - Rash is often followed by nausea, vomiting, chest and abdominal pain, sore throat, and diarrhea

* As patients progress, they develop jaundice, pancreatitis, weight loss, delirium, shock, liver failure, massive bleeding and multiorgan failure

* **Key Laboratory and Radiology Findings**

  - Diagnosis by isolation of the virus in a biosafety level 4 laboratory

  - In patients with uveitis, the virus may be isolated from the anterior chamber

  - Antigen detected by PCR and antigen-capture ELISA

  - IgM and IgG antibodies may persist for long periods

  - Direct demonstration of the virus by EM, immunofluorescent staining

- **Ebola virus**

  * Infected patients have a sudden onset of fever, headache, myalgia, abdominal pain, diarrhea, pharyngitis, herpetic lesions of the mouth and pharynx, conjunctival injection and bleeding from the gums

  * The initial faint maculopapular rash that may be missed in dark-skinned individuals evolves into petechiae, ecchymosis and bleeding from venepuncture sites and mucosa

  * Hemiplegia, psychosis, coma and seizures are common

  * Terminal shock

* Key Laboratory and Radiology Findings

- Initial leucopenia and lymphopenia replaced by leukocytosis

- Metabolic acidosis

- Diffuse coagulopathy

- Isolation of the virus in Vero cells in a biosafety level 5 laboratory

- Antigen detected by RT-PCR and antigen-capture ELISA

- IgM and IgG antibodies by ELISA

- No sero-crossreactivity between Ebola and Marburg viruses

- Direct demonstration of the virus by EM, immunofluorescent staining

Bunyaviridae

- Rift Valley fever

  * Livestock commonly abort and have 10–30% mortality

  * Most patients develop a self-limited nonspecific febrile illness

    - Sudden onset of fever, headache, joint and muscle pain, conjunctivitis and photophobia

    - Few patients have a brief initial illness, partial recovery followed by a return of symptoms and a protracted convalescence

  * 5%–10% develop retinal disease 1–3 weeks after their febrile illness

    - Macular exudates, retinal hemorrhages, vasculitis

    - Half of these patients have permanent visual impairment

* 1∞–5% develop CNS complications

  - Encephalitis may develop a week or more into the febrile illness

  - May deteriorate to stupor and coma

  - Survivors have neurologic deficits

* Myocardial necrosis in some fatal cases

* 1% develop typical viral hemorrhagic fever with epistaxis, melena, hematemesis, ecchymosis

* Normal recovery takes 2–3 weeks

* Key Laboratory and Radiology Findings

- In severe cases (1%), DIC, anemia, leucopenia, thrombocytopenia, renal impairment or failure, abnormal liver transaminases, prolonged PT and PTT and the presence of fibrin degradation products

- In patients with encephalitis, there is CSF pleocytosis

- Virus may be isolated by animal inoculation or in cell culture

- Virus may be detected in the patient's blood by RT-PCR

- Antigen-capture ELISA for viral antigen in blood

- Crimean-Congo hemorrhagic fever virus

  * Patients present with sudden onset of fever, chills, headache, dizziness, neck pain, myalgia, eye pain, photophobia, anorexia, sore throat

  * There is lymphadenopathy, tender hepatomegaly (50%)

  * Some patients develop nausea, vomiting, diarrhea, flushing, hemorrhage and gastrointestinal bleeding

* Conjunctival injection and congestion of the pharynx

* Altered mental status including aggressive behavior to coma

* Fever persist from 5–20 days (average 9 days)

* Illness may be biphasic

* Convalescence: 2–4 months

* **Key Laboratory and Radiology Findings**

  • Transient leucopenia

  • Thrombocytopenia prominent and become extremely low early in the illness

  • Anemia

  • Elevated renal function studies and proteinuria during first week of illness

  • Decreased serum protein and albumin

  • Increased AST, ALT, Alk Phos, γ-GT, LDH

  • Virus may be isolated by animal inoculation or in cell culture

  • Virus may be detected in the patient's blood by RT-PCR

  • Antigen-capture ELISA for viral antigen in blood

• Hantavirus – hemorrhagic fever with renal syndrome

  * 5 phases of illness

    • (I) Febrile phase (flu-like illness, back pain, retroperitoneal edema, flushing, conjunctival and pharyngeal injection)

    • (II) Hypotensive phase (may range from mild hypotension to shock and hemorrhage lasting for 1–2 days)

    • (III) Oliguric phase (associated with hypertension, renal failure, pulmonary edema, confusion)

    • (IV) Diuretic phase (may last several months)

    • (V) Convalescence

  * Recovery in most cases believed to be complete

  * Complications

    • Renal rupture in oliguric or early diuretic phase

    • Retroperitoneal hemorrhage (patients with abdominal and back pain)

    • Transient hypopituitarism and intrapituitary hemorrhage (Sheehan's syndrome)

  * **Key Laboratory and Radiology Findings**

    • Patients typically have thrombocytopenia, leukocytosis (often above 30,000 cells/mm^3), hemoconcentration, abnormal clotting profile and proteinuria

    • AST elevated

    • EKG: sinus bradycardia, low voltage and nonspecific ST-T changes

    • Renal shadows absent on abdominal x-rays because of retroperitoneal edema

    • Pulmonary infiltrates not common

    • Renal studies reveal patterns of obstruction or tubular damage

    • Diagnosis made by serology (IgM capture ELISA)

• Hantavirus — pulmonary syndrome

  * Prodromal stage (3–5 days – range: 1–10 days)

* Prodrome is followed by a sudden onset of fever, myalgia, malaise, chills, anorexia, and headache

* Patients go on to develop prostration, nausea, vomiting, abdominal pain and diarrhea

* This progresses to cardiopulmonary compromise with a nonproductive cough, tachypnea, fever, mild hypotension and hypoxia

* Disease progresses at different rates: some patients deteriorate in days, and some over longer periods of time

* Renal failure requiring dialysis has occurred

* Resolution of lung lesions and shock in survivors in 3–6 days

* Complications independent of pulmonary status

  • Low cardiac output – left ventricular contractility may be markedly reduced

  • Elevated systemic vascular resistance

  • Normal or low pulmonary wedge pressure

* **Key Laboratory and Radiology Findings**

  • Independent of pulmonary disease, patients have low cardiac output, elevated systemic vascular resistance, normal to low pulmonary wedge pressures

  • Chest x-rays are initially normal but progress to pulmonary edema and acute respiratory distress syndrome

  • Patients have thrombocytopenia, leukocytosis with left shift, elevated partial thromboplastin times and elevated serum lactic acid and lactate dehydrogenase

  • Hemoconcentration

  • Elevated AST, LDH

• Few go on to develop DIC

• Patients succumb to shock and lactic acidosis

• Diagnosis of Sin Nombre virus infection by ELISA and Western blot assays

• Diagnosis made by serology (IgM capture ELISA)

Arenaviridae

• Lassa fever

  * Onset of disease is gradual with fever, malaise, and myalgia

  * Presents as aseptic meningitis after a prodrome

  * Patients develop conjunctival injection, pharyngitis (with white and yellow exudates) nausea, vomiting and abdominal pain

  * Patients with mild disease improve in 10 days

  * Severely ill patients have facial and laryngeal edema, cyanosis, bleeding and shock

    • Sometimes complicated by pleural or pericardial effusions

  * Complications

    • 20%–30% develop permanent late sensorineural deafness

    • Neurologic complications are a late development: tremors, confusion, seizures, coma

    • Lassa virus crosses the placenta and commonly causes abortion, particularly in the 3rd trimester

    • Orchitis

  * **Key Laboratory and Radiology Findings**

    • Severely ill patients will have mild thrombocytopenia and dysfunctional platelets

- WBCs normal or reduced

- Lymphopenia and thrombocytopenia peak between days 10 and 11 of disease

- Mild elevation of aspartate transaminase is common

- Severe hepatitis is rare

- Diagnosis is made by isolating the virus from blood, throat swabs, or urine in a biosafety level 4 laboratory

- IgM-ELISA antibody testing has replaced indirect fluorescent antibody testing

- Reverse transcriptase PCR positive by day 3 of illness

- Combined ELISA for IgM and viral antigen has a 90% sensitivity within 48 hours of admission

- Serology by immunofluorescent antibody

- Argentine hemorrhagic fever: Junin virus

  * Similar to Lassa fever, encephalopathy more common as is hemorrhagic fever

  * Patients present with a nonspecific illness that becomes severe with hypotension in 3–4 days

  * Petechiae develop on the soft palate, axilla, and gingiva

  * Hemorrhage develops on the 4th day of illness

  * Neurologic findings are more common than with Lassa fever

    - Patients are more irritable, lethargic

    - Muscular hypotonia, hyporeflexia, areflexia

    - Proprioceptive disturbances, inability to ambulate

    - Tremor of the tongue and hands

- Fluctuations in the level of consciousness

- Severely ill patients

  * Bleed from mucous membranes

  * Develop shock

  * Become anuric

  * Seizures and coma

* **Key Laboratory and Radiology Findings**

  - Leukopenia and thrombocytopenia

  - Diagnosis is made by isolating the virus from blood, throat swabs, or urine in a biosafety level 4 laboratory (Vero cells)

  - Cocultivation with peripheral blood mononuclear cells improves sensitivity

  - Viral antigen detection by ELISA or RT-PCR

  - ELISA for serologic diagnosis

- Bolivian hemorrhagic fever: Machupo virus

  * Junin virus vaccine may be cross protective

  * Clinical presentation and disease similar to Lassa fever

* **Key Laboratory and Radiology Findings**

  - Leukopenia and thrombocytopenia

  - Diagnosis is made by isolating the virus from blood, throat swabs, or urine in a biosafety level 4 laboratory (Vero cells)

  - Viral antigen detection by ELISA or RT-PCR

  - ELISA for serologic diagnosis

  - Immunofluorescent antibody testing

Key Differential Diagnostic Features

Filoviridae

• Marburg virus and Ebola virus

  * Other viral hemorrhagic fevers

  * Rickettsioses

  * Malaria

  * Typhoid

  * Leptospirosis

  * Borreliosis

  * Septicemic plague

  * Dysentery

Bunyaviridae

• Rift Valley fever and Crimean-Congo hemorrhagic fever virus

  * Other viral hemorrhagic fevers

  * May be mild disease mistaken for an influenza-like illness

  * Or a more severe disease with a differential diagnosis of the other viral hemorrhagic fevers, particularly the other *Bunyaviridae*

• Hantavirus – hemorrhagic fever with renal syndrome

  * Leptospirosis

  * Murine and louse-borne typhus

  * Pyelonephritis

  * Malaria

  * Other hemorrhagic fevers

  * Post-streptococcal glomerulonephritis

  * Blood dyscrasias

  * Glaucoma

  * Abdominal surgical emergencies

  * Mild cases may be mistaken for influenza

• Hantavirus - pulmonary syndrome (HPS)

  * Acute abdominal emergency

  * Influenza

  * Bacterial pneumonia (may be less likely as HPS has symmetric findings of interstitial infiltrates progressing to alveolar pulmonary edema)

Arenaviridae

• Lassa fever

  * Most febrile illnesses found in west Africa including Marburg and Ebola infections, dengue, Al Kumrah virus infection, Rift Valley fever, Crimean-Congo hemorrhagic fever

  * Malaria

  * Typhoid

  * Bacillary dysentery

  * In patients with neurologic complications, high CSF lymphocyte counts and low CSF glucose will often suggest granulomatous meningitis

• Argentine hemorrhagic fever: Junin virus and Bolivian hemorrhagic fever: Machupo virus

  * Typhoid fever

  * Hepatitis

  * Infectious mononucleosis

  * Leptospirosis

  * Hantavirus pulmonary syndrome

* Dengue

* Dengue hemorrhagic fever

* Rickettsioses

* Malaria in endemic areas

* Intoxications

* Rheumatic diseases

* Blood dyscrasias

Therapy

Empiric

• **Prophylaxis** with ribavirin remains controversial.

• **Treatment** is supportive for all infections. Ribavirin has been used for prophylaxis and treatment of Lassa fever, Sabia virus hemorrhagic fever, Argentine hemorrhagic fever, Bolivian hemorrhagic fever, Rift Valley fever, Congo-Crimean hemorrhagic fever, and Venezuelan hemorrhagic fever. Convalescent serum therapy has been used for Venezuelan hemorrhagic fever. Ribavirin has been used to treat Hantavirus hemorrhagic fever with renal syndrome but does not appear effective in treating Hantavirus pulmonary syndrome. There is no specific therapy for Yellow fever, Ebola or Marburg virus infections. Ribavirin has not shown promise in nonhuman primates with these infections

Definitive/Specific

• There is no definitive treatment

Filoviridae

• Marburg Hemorrhagic Fever and Ebola Virus Hemorrhagic Fever – no antivirals or serum therapy appears to be effective

Bunyaviridae

• Rift Valley fever

* Based upon animal studies, ribavirin and antibody therapy should be attempted

* α-interferon promising in animal studies

• Crimean-Congo hemorrhagic fever

* Ribavirin

* Crimean-Congo virus immune serum may be of benefit

• Hantavirus hemorrhagic fever with renal syndrome

* Ribavirin appears to be effective therapy

• Hantavirus pulmonary syndrome

* Ribavirin is not effective

* A killed vaccine is available but it does not have FDA approval

Arenaviridae

• Lassa fever

* Ribavirin has been recommended for prophylaxis and treatment of Lassa fever, including pregnant women

* Oral ribavirin is believed to be only half as effective as the IV drug

* Post-exposure prophylaxis is recommended by some but not all authorities and evidence of efficacy of ribavirin prophylaxis is limited

• Argentine hemorrhagic fever

* Treatment and prophylaxis same as for Lassa fever

* Ribavirin

* Infusion of convalescent serum during the first 8 days of illness reduces mortality from 15–30% to <1%

* A live-attenuated vaccine is available in Argentina

• Bolivian hemorrhagic fever

* Treatment and prophylaxis same as for Lassa fever

* Ribavirin

Prognostic Factors

Filoviridae

• Marburg virus

* Mortality is 25%–90% (average 25%–30%)

* In fatal cases, there is no antibody response

• Ebola virus

* Mortality rates are 60%–90% for Ebola Zaire and 50% for Ebola Sudan

* Patients usually succumb by day 10

* In fatal cases, there is no antibody response

* Higher mortality in those infected by contaminated needles

Bunyaviridae

• Rift Valley fever

* Mortality 1%

• Crimean-Congo hemorrhagic fever virus

* Survivors develop IgM and IgG responses by day 9 which is absent in most fatal cases

* Mortality rates: 10%–50% with most deaths between 5–14 days

• Hantavirus – hemorrhagic fever with renal syndrome (HFRS)

* Mortality 1%–15%

* No increase in long-term mortality in a study of 1600 Korean War veterans who contracted the infection and only a selective increase in morbidities

• Hypopituitarism with an atrophic pituitary gland and an empty sella has been reported as a late complication

* HFRS from Seoul virus is (1) less severe; (2) more liver involvement; and (3) 1% mortality

• Hantavirus - pulmonary syndrome

* Most deaths occur within 48 hours of admission

* Patients who survive the first 2–3 days of hospitalization, usually recover

* Intensive care improved survival

* Neutralizing antibody response associated with survival

* Mortality: 30%–40%

Arenaviridae

• Lassa Fever

* Lassa fever: 1% mortality (15%–20% mortality for patients requiring hospitalization)

* Mortality correlates with high aspartate transaminase levels

* 100–300,000 infections/year most of which most are mild or asymptomatic (80%)

* Pregnant women have the highest mortality: 16%

* Poor prognostic signs

  • Pharyngitis

  • Tachypnea

  • Bloody diarrhea

  • High fever

• Argentine hemorrhagic fever: Junin virus and Bolivian hemorrhagic fever: Machupo virus

  * Mortality 15%–30% for untreated patients

Further Reading

Books and Book Chapters

Enria D, Mills JN, Flick R, et al. Arenavirus infection. In: Guerrant RL, Walker DH, Weller PF, eds. *Tropical Infectious Diseases – Principles, Pathogens, & Practice*. 2nd ed. v.1. Philadelphia, PA: Elsevier Churchill Livingstone; 2006:734-755.

Peters CJ. Lymphocytic choriomeningitis virus, Lassa virus, and South American hemorrhagic fevers. In: Mandell GL, Bennett JE, Dolin R, eds. *Mandell, Douglas, and Bennett's Principles and Practice of Infectious Diseases*. 6th ed. v.2. Philadelphia, PA: Elsevier Churchill Livingstone; 2005:2090-2098.

Peters CJ, Mills JN, Spiropoulou C, et al. Hantavirus infections. In: Guerrant RL, Walker DH, Weller PF, eds. *Tropical Infectious Diseases – Principles, Pathogens, & Practice*. 2nd ed. v.1. Philadelphia, PA: Elsevier Churchill Livingstone; 2006:762-780.

Peters CJ, Zaki SR. Overview of viral hemorrhagic fevers. Dummler JS, Walker DH. Ehrlichioses and anaplasmosis. In: Guerrant RL, Walker DH, Weller PF, eds. *Tropical Infectious Diseases – Principles, Pathogens, & Practice*. 2nd ed. v.1. Philadelphia, PA: Elsevier Churchill Livingstone; 2006:726-733.

Wahl-Jense V, Feldmann H, Sanchez A, et al. Filovirus infections. In: Guerrant RL, Walker DH, Weller PF, eds. *Tropical Infectious Diseases – Principles, Pathogens, & Practice*. 2nd ed. v.1. Philadelphia, Pa: Elsevier Churchill Livingstone; 2006:784-796.

Watts DM, Flick R, Peters CJ, et al. Bunyaviral fevers: Rift Valley fever and Crimean-Congo hemorrhagic fever. In: Guerrant RL, Walker DH, Weller PF, eds. *Tropical Infectious Diseases – Principles, Pathogens, & Practice*. 2nd ed. v.1. Philadelphia, PA: Elsevier Churchill Livingstone; 2006:756-761.

Journal Articles

Cleri DJ, Ricketti AJ, Porwancher RB, et al. Viral hemorrhagic fevers: current status of endemic disease and strategies for control. *Infect Dis Clin N Am*. 2006;20:359-393.

5. Monkeypox

Synonyms

• None

Causative Organisms

• The orthopoxvirus – monkeypox virus

Epidemiology

• Africa, emerging disease in the U.S. – introduced in 2003 with the importation of African rodents

• Found naturally in the Congo Basin and West Africa

• Contact with animals

  * Monkeys

  * Rodents

    • Gambian rats

    • Elephant shrews

    • Prairie dogs (U.S.) infected after exposure to imported pets from West Africa

    • Rope squirrel

    • Dormouse

• Human-to-human spread documented

  * Secondary attack rate among unvaccinated household contacts: 9.3%

Key Clinical Features

• Incubation period: 7–17 days

  * Exposure to the virus via bites or scratches shortens the incubation period

• Prodrome: 1–4 days for monkeypox; 2–4 days for smallpox; 0–2 days for chickenpox

• Symptomatology for the 3 pox diseases overlap

* Fever is common in all 3 diseases: 90%–100%

* Chills: 70%–90%

* Lymphadenopathy: 60%–90%

* Sweats: 60%–90%

* Headache: 70%

* Muscle pain: 60%–90%

* Sore throat: 58%–70%

* Cough: 55%

* Nausea and vomiting: 20%–50%

* Back pain: 30%–60%

* Runny nose: 20%–40%

* Abdominal pain: 15%

* Wheezing: 10%

* Diarrhea: 10%

* Shortness of breath: 10%

• Rash

  * <25 lesions: 55%

  * 26–100 lesions: 32.5%

  * 101–249 lesions: 5%

  * >250 lesions: 7.5%

• In endemic areas, coinfection with varicella-zoster has been reported

Key Differential Diagnostic Features

• Patients without the typical rash may present as FUO

• Patients with a few lesions may be confused with other pustular diseases

- Patients with many lesions may be confused with smallpox

- Patients with hemorrhagic lesions present a broader differential diagnosis including viral hemorrhagic fevers

- May be confused with chickenpox

- May be confused with buffalopox

Key Laboratory/Radiology Features

- Viral culture – gold standard

- PCR may be used to differentiate from smallpox and other pox viruses

- Immunohistochemical tests of lesions for orthopoxviruses

Therapy

Empiric and Definitive/Specific

- None

- Smallpox vaccine (60%–85%) protective or will ameliorate the severity of monkeypox infection

Prognostic Factors

- 1981–1986: 331 cases in the Democratic Republic of the Congo with 33 deaths

Further Reading

Books and Book Chapters

Damon, I. Orthopoxviruses: vaccinia (smallpox vaccine), variola (smallpox), monkeypox, and cowpox. In: Mandell GL, Bennett JE, Dolin R, eds. *Mandell, Douglas, and Bennett's Principles and Practice of Infectious Diseases*. 6th ed. v.2. Philadelphia, PA: Elsevier Churchill Livingstone; 2005:1742-1753.

Journal Articles

Cleri DJ, Porwancher RB, Ricketti AJ, et al. Smallpox as a bioterrorist weapon: myth or menace? *Infect Dis Clin N Am*. 2006;20:329-357.

Cleri DJ, Ricketti AJ, Vernaleo JR. Fever of unknown origin due to zoonoses. *Infect Dis Clin N Am*. 2007;21:963-996.

Duchini A, Goss JA, Karpen S, et al. Vaccinations for adult solid-organ transplant recipients: current recommendations and protocols. *Clin Microbiol Rev*. 2003;16:357-364.

Johnson N, Fooks A, McColl K. Human rabies case with long incubation, Australia. *Emerg Infect Dis*. 2008;14:1950-1951.

Kolhapure RM, Deolankar RP, Tupe CD, et al. Investigation of buffalopox outbreaks in Maharashtra State during 1992–1996. *Indian J Med Res*. 1997;106:441-446.

6. Other Poxviridae (except Smallpox)

Table 7

SARS-CoV infection Signs and Symptoms in Patients at Presentation

Virus	Synonyms	Hosts	Distri-bution	Trans-mission	Clinical Presentation
Vaccinia virus (Orthopoxvirus) Buffalopox – is the disease in cattle and water buffalo – Pustular lesions on teats and udders of milking buffaloes and calves	Buffalopoxvirus Rabbitpoxvirus	River buffalo – *Bubalis*, cattle humans, no reservoir	World-wide Buffalo-pox endemic Egypt, Indo-nesia, India	Skin abrasion—when human vaccination for smallpox was common, vaccinia virus occasionally infected cattle and water buffaloes	Localized pustular skin lesions that start as macules, become papules, vesicles and pustular. May develop into a black eschar and regional lymphadenitis. Pustular lesions on the hands and face of milkers who are no longer protected by smallpox vaccination. Flu-like symptoms reported with headache, myalgia, and fever sometimes days after the lesion appears
Cowpox virus (Orthopox virus)		Rodents, cats, cattle, zoo and circus animals, especially elephants, humans, cattle, bank voles, field voles, wood mice in Great Britain	Europe, western Asia	Skin abrasions	Incubation: 4–5 days. Lesions progress through macular, popular the pustular stages in 4–5 days then form a hard crust. Localized pustular skin lesions usually restricted to the hands and face; more painful lesions and larger lesions than vaccinia. Localized lymphadenopathy occurs, a brief viremia accompanied by fever and malaise. Lymphangitis, lymphadenitis and fever may persist for days. 6–8 weeks or longer to recover. Permanent scarring occurs
Monkeypox virus (Orthopoxvirus)		Rodents, primates, humans	Western and central Africa, U.S.	Respiratory, oral	Resembles smallpox but milder disease. Smallpox vaccination appears to provide significant (85%) but not complete protection.
Orf virus (Parapoxvirus) Synonyms: contagious pustular dermati-tis, contagious ecthyma, scabby mouth	Contagious pustular dermatitis/ ecthyma virus	Sheep, goats, humans	World-wide	Skin abrasion	Pustular lesions of the skin in humans and skin and oral mucosa in sheep and goats. Lesions are 1–3 cm and progress from bullseye-like (red center, white ring, red halo) to a healing eschar
Bovine papular stomatitis virus (Parapoxvirus)	Stomatitis papular virus Bovine pustular stomatitis	Cattle, humans, occasionally sheep (sheep shearers)	World-wide	Skin abrasion	Pustular lesions on hands in humans and proliferative papules in and around mouths of cattle
Pseudocowpox virus (Parapoxvirus)	Milker's nodules, paravaccinia, pseudocowpox, ring sores	Cattle, humans	World-wide	Skin abrasion	5–7 days incubation. Pustular lesions on hands in humans and teats in milking cows. Forms a hemispheric cherry-red papule that enlarges, becomes firm, elastic and purple reaching 2 cm and may become umbilicated. Lesions are painless but pruritic. Lesions are highly vascular but do not ulcerate. They disappear in 5 weeks. Occasionally localized lymphadenopathy.

continued

Table 7

SARS-CoV infection Signs and Symptoms in Patients at Presentation

Virus	Synonyms	Hosts	Distri-bution	Trans-mission	Clinical Presentation
Tanapoxvirus (Yatapoxvirus) (Clinically, may be confused with monkeypox, tularemia, and anthrax)		Rodents, humans	Eastern and central Africa: Originally described among the population of the Tana River (Kenya) lood plain.	Probably skin abrasion, but exact mode of transmission is unknown. Most lesions on the upper arm, face, neck, and trunk, but rarely on the hands, legs or feet.	Localized pustular skin lesions. Natural incubation period unknown but intradermal inoculation resulted in a lesion in 4 days. Mild fever 2–4 days and sometimes severe headache and backache precedes the lesion. Begins as a small hyperpigmented macule with a central elevation. Nodule and enlarges to 15 mm by the end of the 2nd week. Edema and erythema surrounds the nodule. Tender lymph-adenopathy by the 5th day. The nodule enlarges, ulcerates by the 3rd week and heals with scaring by the 5th or 6th week. Multiple lesions of different ages may be present.
Yabapoxvirus (Yatapoxvirus)	Yaba monkey tumor virus	Monkey, humans	Western Africa	Skin abrasion	Localized pustular skin lesions. Experimental injections into humans produced histiocytomas of the skin, which suppurate. No neoplastic proliferation occurs.
Camelpox (Parapoxvirus)	Contagious ecthyma, amru azuduk disease virus	Camels	Asia, Africa	Probably skin abrasion, but exact mode of transmission is unknown.	Humans may have been infected, but even unvaccinated humans exposed to florid cases have not been infected.
Sealpox (Parapoxvirus)		Seals		Skin abrasion	Localized pustular skin lesions similar to milkers nodules with a mild clinical course

Key Differential Diagnostic Features

• Differential diagnosis

  * Varicella

  * Localized or disseminated herpes zoster

  * Localized or disseminated herpes simplex

  * Impetigo

  * Drug eruptions

  * Erythema multiforme

  * Enteroviral infections

  * Scabies

  * Insect bites

  * Vaccinia

  * Anthrax if an eschar develops

Key Laboratory/Radiology Features

• Electron microscopy will differentiate poxviruses, parapoxviruses and herpes virus group infections

• Viral culture

• Nucleic acid diagnostic techniques

• PCR for orf and parapoxvirus infections

Therapy

• There is no definitive therapy

• Cidofovir shows some promise for the treatment of orthopoxvirus infections

• Ribavirin combined with vaccinia immune globulin for progressive vaccinia

Further Reading

Books and Book Chapters

Damon I. Other poxviruses that infect humans: parapoxviruses, molluscum contagiosum, and tanapox. In: Mandell GL, Bennett JE, Dolin R, eds. *Mandell, Douglas, and Bennett's Principles and Practice of Infectious Diseases*. 6th ed. v.2. Philadelphia, PA: Elsevier Churchill Livingstone; 2005:1753-1756.

Esposito JJ, Fenner F. Poxvirus. In: Knipe DM, Howley PM. *Fields Virology*. 4th ed. v.2. Philadelphia, PA: Lippincott Williams & Wilkins; 2001:2885-2921.

Moss B. Poxviridae: the viruses and their replication. In: Knipe DM, Howley PM. *Fields Virology*. 4th ed. v.2. Philadelphia, PA: Lippincott Williams & Wilkins; 2001:2849-2883.

Tidona CA, Darai G, *The Springer Index of Viruses*. Berlin, Germany: Springer, 2001.

Journal Articles

Cleri DJ, Ricketti AJ, Ramos-Bonner LS, et al Smallpox, monkeypox, & other poxes. *Infect Dis Pract*. 2005;29:395-406.

Cleri DJ, Porwancher RB, Ricketti AJ, et al. Smallpox as a bioterrorist weapon: myth or menace?. *Infect Dis Clin N Am*. 2006;20:329-357.

Strenger V, Muller M, Richter S, et al. A 17-year-old girl with a black eschar. *Clin Infect Dis*. 2009;48:91-92, 133-134.

Trindade GS, Guedes MIC, Drumond BP, et al. Zoonotic vaccinia virus: clinical and immunological characteristics in a naturally infected patient. *Clin Infect Dis*. 2009;48:e37-e40.

7. Herpes B virus

Synonyms

- Simian herpes B virus

- B virus

- *Cercopithecine herpesvirus* 1

- B virus

- "W" isolate named by Sabin in 1934

- *Herpes simiae*

Causative Organisms

- Closely related of human herpesvirus 1 and 2

- Infects 80%–100% of Asian *Macaca* genus monkeys (including and especially rhesus and cynomolgus species native to Asia and northern Africa) and other monkey species causing an asymptomatic or mild disease

  * In macaques, clinically apparent infection resembles human herpes simplex 1 infection with self-limited oropharyngeal or mucocutaneous lesions

- Adult monkey seroprevalence rates – 80%, BUT only 2%–3% of seropositive monkeys shed the virus at any one time

- Induces fatal disease in non macaque primates including man

Epidemiology

- Bites or scratches from infected animals

- Percutaneous (needle stick injury, cage scratch injury, tissue culture-bottle cuts)

- Mucosal inoculation with infected materials from asymptomatic monkeys

- Airborne transmission postulated in at least 2 cases – patients developed fever, pneumonitis, followed by neurologic symptoms

- Human-to-human contact reported once

- Reactivation of herpes B virus infection

- All macaque monkeys should be considered seropositive

- Primate exposure and the decision for post exposure prophylaxis should be made on the following considerations

  * Source of the exposure – macaques are the only primate known to transmit herpes B virus. Other primates should not be considered a risk unless they have the contact with macaques. Immunocompromised, stressed, breeding and sick animals are more likely to shed virus

  * Timeliness and adequacy of first aid for the wound – was the wound cleaned within 5 minutes?

  * Type of wound or exposure – head, torso or neck wounds may result in CNS disease before any other clinical indications and should all be considered high risk

  * Materials that have come in contact with macaques, in addition to direct exposure to the animals

Key Clinical Features

- Asymptomatic cases are considered unlikely – One case with a 10 year latency period was reported, but there is a question as to whether there was a trivial exposure that was not noted

- Incubation period usually 2 days–5 weeks (most cases 3–5 days – other reports, 5–21 days)

- Symptoms begin as a localized vesicular eruption at the site of inoculation

- Symptoms may progress near the site of exposure, be limited to the peripheral nervous system, or be limited to the central nervous system (CNS)

  * Tingling, itching, pain or numbness at site

* Within 3 weeks, paresthesias develop proximally along the inoculated limb accompanied by fever, myalgias, weakness of that extremity, abdominal pain, sinusitis and conjunctivitis

* Lung and liver may become involved

* Some patients develop lymphadenopathy proximal to the inoculation site

* Some patients have NO local symptoms

• May present as a flu-like illness with fever, chills, myalgias without focal findings followed by abrupt onset of CNS symptoms

• The virus spreads along the peripheral nerves to the spinal cord and brain – patients complain of:

* Meningismus, nausea, vomiting, persistent headache, confusion, diplopia, dysphagia, dizziness, dysarthria, cranial nerve palsies and ataxia

* Later in the disease: seizures, hemiplegia, hemiparesis, ascending paralysis, respiratory failure, coma

* Late stage disease appears as brain stem encephalomyelitis to a terminal diffuse encephalomyelitis

• Limited disease with lesions limited to the skin and a self-limited aseptic meningitis reported

• Zosteriform recurrence with encephalitis

• Recurrent vesicular rash

Key Differential Diagnostic Features

• Differs from herpes simplex encephalitis in which focal involvement is more typical

• May appear as simple herpetic or zosteriform lesions in rare cases

• Symptoms may be suggestive of rabies

• The differential diagnosis includes all those illness that cause an ascending myelitis or encephalitis

Key Laboratory/Radiology Features

• Viral culture must only be performed in a Biosafety Level-4 facility

• Cultures must not be sent to the routine diagnostic laboratory but to 1 of the 3 facilities that perform diagnostic testing for Herpes B virus (See suggested reading – *Clin Infect Dis*. 2002;35:1191-1203, page 1194, Table 2)

• PCR although interpretation may be problematic

• Serologic cross-reactivity with human herpes simplex virus 1

• Serologic testing of exposed individuals at the time of exposure and 3-6 weeks later or at the onset of symptoms to send for testing to the B Virus Research and Reference Laboratory at Georgia State University

* A third serum sample should be obtained 3 months later if postexposure prophylaxis is given

* Single samples or serial samples may be tested if the initial sample is not drawn

* Positive titers should be confirmed by Western blot (immunoblot) or competition ELISA as herpes B virus cross-reacts with herpes simplex

Therapy

Empiric and Definitive/Specific

• Immediate and adequate wound or mucosal care the most important factor for reducing the risk of infection

• Postexposure prophylaxis has not been proven to be effective in humans but prevents disease in rabbits

- Acyclovir, valacyclovir, ganciclovir or famciclovir

    * Valacyclovir drug of choice for prophylaxis

    * Acyclovir for treatment without CNS symptoms

    * Ganciclovir drug of choice with CNS symptoms (or all symptomatic patients)

    * Acyclovir drug of choice in pregnant women

- Length of treatment

    * IV therapy continued until symptoms resolve and ≥ 2 sets of cultures are negative after being held 10–14 days

    * "Most experts" believe that therapy should be continued after that period with oral valacyclovir, famciclovir or acyclovir at dosages used for postexposure prophylaxis for 6 months to 1 year followed by suppressive doses for long periods up to life-long therapy

    * There is at least 1 case of reactivation

Prognostic Factors

- 80% mortality without treatment

Further Reading

Books and Book Chapters

Hudnall SD, Stanberry LR. Human herpesvirus infections. In: Guerrant RL, Walker DH, Weller PF, eds. *Tropical Infectious Diseases – Principles, Pathogens, & Practice*. 2nd ed. v.1. Philadelphia, PA: Elsevier Churchill Livingstone; 2006:590-620.

Straus SE. Herpes B virus. In: Mandell GL, Bennett JE, Dolin R, eds. *Mandell, Douglas, and Bennett's Principles and Practice of Infectious Diseases*. 6th ed. v.2. Philadelphia, PA: Elsevier Churchill Livingstone; 2005:1832-1835.

Whitley Richard J. Cercopithecine herpes virus 1 (B virus). In: Fields BN, Knipe DM, Howley PM. *Fields Virology*, 3rd ed. v.2. Philadelphia, PA: Lippincott Williams & Wilkins; 1996:2623-2635.

Journal Articles

Cohen JI, Davenport DS, Stewart JA, et al. Recommendations for prevention of and therapy for exposure to B virus (cercopithecine herpesvirus 1). *Clin Infect Dis*. 2002;35:1191-1203.

Fujima A, Ochiai Y, Saito A, et al. Discrimination of antibody to herpes B virus from antibody to herpes simplex virus types 1 and 2 in human and macaque sera. *J Clin Microbiol*. 2008;46:56-61.

Jainkittivong A, Langlais RP. Herpes B virus infection. *Oral Surg Oral Med Oral Pathol Oral Radiol Endod*. 1998;85:399-403.

Jensen K, Alvarado-Ramy F, Gonzalez-Martinez J, et al. B-virus and free-ranging macaques, Puerto Rico. *Emerg Infect Dis*. 2004;10:494-496.

Jones-Engle L, Engel GA, Heidrich J, et al. Temple monkeys and health implications of commensalism, Kathmandu, Nepal. *Emerg Infect Dis*. 2006;12:900-906.

Nsabimana JM, Moutschen M, Thiry E, et al. Human infection with simian herpes B virus in Africa. *Sante*. 2008;18:3-8.

8. Colorado Tick fever (CTF)

Synonyms

• None

Causative Organisms

• One of the three coltiviruses. It is a member of the nonenveloped, icosahedral multishelled, 60–80 nm, double-stranded (ds) RNA *Reoviridae* family.

  * The other 2 coltiviruses are the Eyach virus (Europe – *Ixodes ricinus* and *I ventalloi* vectors) and the S6-14-03 virus (California ground squirrel and hare hosts — *D variabilis* vector)

Epidemiology

• CTF has been predominantly reported in the Western states and western Canada

• Principally transmitted by the wood tick (*D andersoni* and probably *D variabilis* from the ground squirrel and hare)

  * *Dermacentor* species (principally *D variabilis*) ticks are one of the vectors responsible for transmitting Rocky Mountain spotted fever (*Rickettsia rickettsii*)

  * Also carried by *D occidentalis*, *D albopictus*, *D arumapertus*, *Haemaphysalis leporispalustris*, *Otobius lagophilus*, *I sculptus*, and *I spinipalpis*

  * *I ricinus* and *I ventalloi* appear to be responsible for a similar disease in Europe

• The virus is transmitted between tick stages (trans-stadially) but not transovarially

  * Transmission and amplification occurs between ticks and mammalian hosts (rodents: ground squirrels, chipmunks, marmots and other small mammals, and larger mammals, especially deer)

• Approximately 200–400 cases are reported annually in the U.S.

• In Colorado, 15% of campers were seropositive. This suggests significant subclinical or mild self-limited disease not prompting medical attention or the need for specific diagnosis

• Transmission by transfusion. Along with *Babesia* spp., *R rickettsii*, and *Anaplasma phagocytphilum*, CTF is added to the list of tick-borne transfusion-transmitted diseases

• Transmission from mother to fetus has been suggested by cases of spontaneous abortion and neonatal infection with leucopenia

Key Clinical Features

• Mean incubation period has been estimated at 3–4 days (range: <1–14 days although one reference puts the maximum incubation period at 19 days)

• Typically, there is a sudden onset of fever, chills, severe headache, myalgias, hyperesthesia, weakness and prostration

• Less frequent and less severe are gastrointestinal symptoms (20% of patients)

• The symptom complex has been severe enough in 14% of patients to prompt hospitalization

• Physical Examination: physical findings are nonspecific

  * Injected conjunctivae

  * Erythema of the pharynx

  * Enanthem on the palate

  * Lymphadenopathy and a minimally enlarged spleen are seen in some, but not all patients

  * In 15% of the patients, there is a maculopapular or petechial rash that may be confused with Rocky Mountain Spotted Fever

• Symptoms resolve in 1 week, but 50% of patients have recurrence of fever and symptoms 2 to 3 days later, giving rise to the "saddleback" temperature recordings

- Complications

  * Children experience more complications

  * 5%–10% of all patients develop aseptic meningitis or encephalitis. This occurs almost exclusively in children under the age of 10 years, although it has been reported in adults

  * Hemorrhage, shock and fatalities are rare

  * Other unusual complications:

    - Epididymo-orchitis

    - Pneumonia

    - Hepatitis

    - Pericarditis

    - Myocarditis

    - Gastrointestinal bleeding

    - Disseminated intravascular coagulopathy

Key Differential Diagnostic Features

- Viral meningitis and encephalitis: enteroviruses

- La Crosse virus

- St. Louis encephalitis virus

- Eastern and western equine encephalitis viruses

- Varicella-zoster virus

- Important but less common

  * Rabies virus

  * Powassan virus

  * Lymphocytic choriomeningitis virus

  * Influenza viruses

  * Herpes simplex

  * West Nile virus

- CTF is one of the 4 important causes of tick-borne encephalitis (the others being Rocky Mountain Spotted Fever, Lyme borreliosis, and Powassan encephalitis)

- The coexistence of other tick-borne diseases, particularly Rocky Mountain Spotted Fever must be considered

  * Tick paralysis

  * Hemorrhagic fever with renal syndrome (HTFRS) in CTF endemic areas. The differential diagnosis for HTFRS overlaps with that of CTF.

    - Hemorrhagic scarlet fever

    - Leptospirosis

    - Scrub typhus

    - Murine typhus

    - Hemolytic-uremic syndrome (H.U.S.) (associated with Coxsackieviruses A4, B2, B4, parechovirus 1, and enterohemorrhagic *Escherichia coli* O157:H7)

    - Causes of disseminated intravascular coagulopathy

Key Laboratory/Radiology Features

- Leukopenia

- Thrombocytopenia (less than 150,000/mm^3)

- Initial white blood cell (WBC) counts of 3900/mm^3

  * WBC counts continue to decrease for 5–6 days after the onset of symptoms, often into remission

  * There is a relative neutropenia with a left shift, toxic granulations and lymphocytosis

* Bone marrow reveals an arrested maturation of granulocyte precursors, absent mature forms, many metamyelocytes and myelocytes and decreased megakaryocytes

• Cerebrospinal fluid examinations in patients with meningitis or encephalitis have revealed a monocytosis and elevated protein

• Diagnosis

  * Most cases of CTF are diagnosed by seroconversion (4-fold rise in titers of neutralizing antibodies, complement fixation, immunofluorescent antibodies or enzyme-linked immunoabsorbent testing)

    • Antibodies are usually not detected for the first 2 weeks of the clinical illness

  * Virus isolation is readily achieved in baby mice or Vero or BHK-21 cell cultures up to 6 weeks after refrigeration of the blood clot

  * Rapid diagnosis may be made by direct immunofluorescent examination of peripheral erythrocytes for viral antigen

  * Polymerase chain reaction analysis and viral cultures are more sensitive

Therapy

Empiric

• Empiric antimicrobial therapy should be guided by the differential diagnosis at the time of presentation

• Therapy may include treatment for Rocky Mountain Spotted Fever or other bacterial infections with look-alike rashes and clinical presentations

Definitive/Specific

• There is no specific treatment

Prognostic Factors

• Patients under 20 years of age recover in one week, while 70% of patients over 30 years experience continued fatigue for 3 weeks or more

Further Reading

Books and Book Chapters

Cherry JD. Reoviruses in: Feigin RD, Cherry JD, Demmler GJ, Kaplan SL, eds, *Textbook of Pediatric Infectious Diseases*. vol 2, 5th edition, Philadelphia, PA: WB Saunders; 2003:2102-2106.

Journal Articles

Cleri DJ, Ricketti AJ, Vernaleo JR. Colorado Tick Fever. *Infec Dis Pract*. 2007; 31: 573-577.

Klasco R. Colorado tick fever. *Med Clin North Am*. 86:435-440, 2002.

Romero JR, Simonsen KA. Powassan encephalitis and Colorado tick fever. *Infect Dis Clin N Am*. 2008;22:545-559.

ID Board Pearls

- Poxviruses

  * Camels may acquire a severe generalized rash called camelpox, which is caused by the orthopoxvirus camelpox virus, but it is not generally transmissible to man.

  * Tanapox resembles smallpox, and although the lesions become umbilicated, they never become pustules.

  * Zoonotic vaccinia virus may develop a significant eschar and be mistaken for anthrax.

- Colorado Tick fever (CTF)

  * Peripatetic CTF has been reported in a New York City resident and must be considered in the differential diagnosis of persons returning from an endemic area.

  * Early in the disease, the virus may be detected in both the serum and clotted blood. Pitfalls include freezing the blood sample. CFT virus may be isolated from a refrigerated clotted blood sample after as long as 14 months.

  * Neutralizing antibodies may not be present 10 days into the illness but can be detected by 30 days after the onset of symptoms.

  * Third recurrences of CTF are rare, although some patients experience weeks or months of weakness, and malaise.

  * As thrombocytopenia with hemorrhage is one of the known complications (especially in children), antipyretics that interfere with platelet activity (aspirin) should be avoided.

  * Patients should be advised not to donate blood for 6 months (and probably longer) after recovery.

- Rabies

  * Rabies vaccine is a human diploid cell inactivated vaccine that is not contraindicated for organ-transplant recipients, as the disease has a near 100% mortality. There are specific studies that address the efficacy or safety of this vaccine in these patients.

  * Although 90% of rabies cases develop within 6 months of exposure, long incubation periods over a number of years have been recorded. Animal bite or scratch exposure has been absent in a number of cases. A travel history going back years should be taken and rabies included in the differential diagnosis of encephalitis no matter how remote the possible exposure.

  * The groundhog is the only rodent considered an important vector for rabies.

  * Presenting symptoms may mimic schizophrenia or delirium tremens.

- Herpes B virus

  * Asymptomatic seroconversion after exposure to herpes B virus has not been reported.

  * Herpes B virus is latent in the CNS of macaques and is shed intermittently from the mucosa of infected animals.

  * Macaques are the primates most often found in the monkey temples in south and Southeast Asia where they are important to Hindu and Buddhist culture. Serosurveys of these primates at the world heritage site, Swoyambhu Temple in the Kathmandu valley, found evidence of infection with herpes B virus, rhesus cytomegalovirus, simian virus 40, and simian foamy virus. Herpes B virus as well as these other pathogens become a risk for those visiting these popular areas and in direct contact with their primate inhabitants.

• Viral Hemorrhagic Fever

* Even though antibody-positive rodents have been identified across Australia, neither hantavirus hemorrhagic fever with renal syndrome nor hantavirus pulmonary syndrome has been reported there.

* In hantavirus hemorrhagic fever with renal syndrome, the urine specific gravity is fixed at 1.010 and the kidneys are unable to concentrate urine from 3 weeks to up to 3 months.

* Although recovery from hantavirus hemorrhagic fever with renal syndrome (HFRS) is believed to be complete, antibodies to Seoul virus, one of the viruses that causes HFRS has been linked to hypertensive chronic renal failure.

* Sudden onset of deafness has been associated with Lassa virus seropositivity.

* Patients with Lassa fever may sometimes have a temporary remission before the development of neurologic complications.

* Patients with neurological complications from Lassa fever (tremors, confusion, seizures and coma) often die.

* Persons who have recovered from Lassa fever remain contagious. Viremia persists into the second week of illness, and the virus is found in the urine for 3–9 weeks and in semen for 2–3 months.

* In late Ebola virus infections, viral-infected large abnormal lymphocytes appear with dark cytoplasm (virocytes).

* Only a small number of hemorrhagic fevers result in eye lesions: Rift Valley fever, Kyasanur Forest disease and Omsk hemorrhagic fever (retinal lesions); and, Ebola and Marburg virus infections (uveitis).

Contents

1. **Overview**

2. **New Variant Creutzfeldt-Jakob Disease**

1. Overview

Normal prion proteins (encoded for by the gene on the short arm of human chromosome 20) are a surface protein linked to the cell membrane and have a half-life of 6 hours. Mice lacking normal prion proteins have a complete inability to smell. Abnormal prions are infectious pathogens containing protein but lacking nucleic acid. The abnormal prion protein, besides possessing other properties, accumulates within cells, and is found within cytoplasmic vacuoles and secondary lysosomes. The accumulation of the abnormal prion protein within neurons leads to neuronal death.

All human prion diseases have long incubation periods and are progressive. The typical pathologic process involves neuronal loss, glial proliferation, lack of inflammatory response, and vacuoles (spongiform changes). These diseases include kuru, Creutzfeldt-Jakob disease (CJD) Gerstmann-Straussler-Scheinker syndrome (GSS), and fatal familial insomnia (FFI).

Kuru was the first identified transmissible neurodegenerative disease. It was endemic among the Fore tribes in New Guinea. It is believed to have originated from sporadic cases of CJD-like disease and spread from the practice of ritual cannibalism. The disease is of historic interest.

CJD takes the form of sporadic (85%–90% of cases), familial (5%–15% of cases), iatrogenic (<5% of cases) and new variant disease. CJD is seen worldwide with an incidence and prevalence of 1 case per million population. Disease rates increase between ages 40 to 80 years. The mean age of onset of sporadic CJD is between 57 to 62 years, although the range has been reported between 17 years to patients past 80 years. There are particularly high rates of disease in North Africa, Israel and Slovakia, where there are clusters of familial disease. New variant CJD (nvCJD) appears to be limited to the United Kingdom and France.

Iatrogenic CJD has followed the administration of cadaveric human pituitary hormone, dural graft transplants, and dura mater in radiographic embolization procedures.

GSS syndrome has an incidence between 1–10 cases per million population per year. Almost all cases are familial with autosomal dominant inheritance. Patients present between the ages of 25 and 65 years with progressive cerebellar degeneration.

FFI was first described in Italian families, but cases have been identified worldwide. The disease presents between the ages of 45 and 51 years, progresses rapidly to death in 7–25 months (mean survival: 13 months). Patients present with progressive insomnia with loss of normal circadian rhythm. Patients have dream-like confusion during waking hours, but do not have obvious dementia. There is decreased attention, difficulty concentrating, memory impairment, followed by confusion and hallucinations. Finally, there are motor abnormalities (myoclonus, ataxia, spasticity and hyperreflexia). Dysautonomia (hyperhidrosis, hyperthermia, tachycardia and hypertension) and endocrine abnormalities occur (decreased ACTH secretion, increased cortisol secretion, variations in growth hormone, melatonin and prolactin).

New variant Creutzfeldt-Jakob disease nvCJD first came to attention in 1995. It was recognized by (1) the unusual clustering of a relatively rare disease, (2) a different age distribution from classical CJD, and, (3) the association with an outbreak of bovine spongiform encephalitis.

2. New Variant Creutzfeldt-Jakob Disease

Synonyms

• nvCJD

Causative Organisms

• Infectious pathogens containing protein but lacking nucleic acid

Epidemiology

• First cases reported in the United Kingdom and France in 1995

  * From 1995 to April 2004, 141 cases reported

  * Cases have now been reported from Italy, Ireland and the U.S. (a patient who once lived in the United Kingdom)

  * Epidemiologists estimate that the total number of cases will be between 200 to 3000

  * The greatest number of cases were reported in 2000 (28 cases) and since that year the incidence has been decreasing

• Younger age at onset of symptoms (mean age 26 years: range 12–74 years)

• In the United Kingdom, nvCJD followed an outbreak of bovine spongiform encephalitis

• There is strong evidence that nvCJD arose from a previous infection (bovine-to-human) with bovine spongiform encephalitis

• New government regulations regarding the rendering of beef for consumption were adopted in 1988 through 1990 and are believed to be responsible for the decline in the number of nvCJD cases

Key Clinical Features

- Longer progression of disease (14 months as compared to 4–5 months in patients with spontaneous CJD)

- Early neurobehavioral and psychiatric signs and symptoms

    * Psychiatric symptoms in the absence of dementia or other signs of cortical dysfunction

        • Transient delusions sometimes occur at the onset of the illness including auditory and visual hallucinations

        • As the disease progresses, patients have memory impairment and become more aggressive

        • Psychiatric symptoms persist until dementia is overwhelming

    * Common signs and symptoms

        • Irritability

        • Depression (anxiety, withdrawal, weight loss)

        • Anxiety

        • Psychosis

        • Transient visual and auditory hallucinations and delusions

        • Insomnia and sleep disturbances common later in the disease

- Late neurologic signs (>6 months)

    * Hyperreflexia

    * Myoclonus

    * Cerebellar signs

    * Up-gaze paralysis

    * Incontinence

    * Prominent sensory disturbances

    * Dysesthesias and paresthesias of the face, hands, feet, legs, or hemibody

    * Chorea

    * Dysphagia

    * Hypertonia

    * Clonus

    * Extensor plantar responses

    * Primitive reflexes

- Neuropathology

    * Abnormal prion protein "amyloid" plaques (termed PrP^{Sc}) throughout the cerebrum and cerebellum possessing a dense eosinophilic core and pale periphery. These are also found in a lesser concentration in the basal ganglia and thalamus. Similar plaques are seen in kuru and GSS but not in spontaneous CJD

    * Spongiform changes more prominent in the cerebellum, basal ganglia and thalamus in nvCJD than in spontaneous CJD

    * The prion protein extracted from nvCJD is chemically more similar to that found in bovine spongiform encephalopathy than the prion protein in classical CJD

Key Differential Diagnostic Features

- Alternate diagnosis discovered at autopsy in patients clinically diagnosed as nvCJD included

    * Spontaneous CJD

    * Cerebral vasculitis

    * Alzheimer's disease

    * Limbic encephalitis

* Encephalitis

* Cerebrovascular disease

Key Laboratory/Radiology Features

• CSF is usually normal or unremarkable

• Total CSF protein is normal but the protein profile may be abnormal. One protein is the 14-3-3 protein

* The 14-3-3 protein has not been detected in all cases, but this may be due to inadequate refrigeration of the specimen

• CT scans and MRIs may be normal or only show mild atrophy

* Abnormal thalamic signals have been noted in some patients with both spontaneous CJD and nvCJD

* More recent studies suggest that up to 70% of cases have an increased T_2 signal in the pulvinar of the thalamus

• EEGs were abnormal in 70% of patients but not specific (progressive slowing but no sharp wave complexes as seen in spontaneous CJD)

• Definitive diagnosis is made at post-mortem examination

• Under investigation is the analysis for the pathologic prion protein (PrP^{sc}) in lymphoid tissue (i.e., tonsils, spleen, lymph nodes) making this a valuable diagnostic modality in the future

• A strongly presumptive diagnosis may be made in the appropriate clinical setting accompanied by the demonstration of the PrP^{sc} protein and "florid" plaques in the cerebrum and cerebellum

Therapy

Empiric or Definitive/Specific

• There is no treatment

• Prion therapeutics in experimental models

* Polyanionic compounds (glycosaminoglycans [GAGs])

* Compounds related to GAGs/polysulphate polyanions

* Polycationic compounds

* Tetrapyrrolic compounds

* Polyene antibiotics

* Tetracycline compounds

* Tricyclic and related compounds

* Beta-sheet breaker peptides

* Immunomodulators and immunotherapeutics

Prognostic Factors

• The disease is invariably fatal

Further Reading

Books and Book Chapters

Tyler KL. Prions and prion diseases of the central nervous system. In: Remington JS, Swartz MN, eds. *Current Clinic Topics in Infectious Diseases 19*. Malden, MA: Blackwell Science, Inc; 1999:226-251.

Tyler KL. Prions and prion diseases of the central nervous system (transmissible neurodegenerative diseases). In: *Mandell GL, Bennett JE, Dolin R, eds. Mandell, Douglas, and Bennett's Principles and, Practice of Infectious Diseases*. 6th ed. v.2. Philadelphia, PA: Elsevier Churchill Livingstone; 2005:2219-2235.

Journal Articles

Trevitt CR, Collinge J. A systematic review of prion therapeutics in experimental models. *Brain*. 2006;129 (Pt 9):2241-2265.

ID Board Pearls

- Of all the human prion diseases, only FFI displays dysautonomia, and spongiform degeneration is only rarely seen.

- Patients with nvCJD have bilateral pulvinar hyperintensity on MRI that is bilateral and of greater intensity than any other signal in the thalamus. Patients with spontaneous CJD have less intense signals.

- Patients with nvCJD do not show periodic EEG changes seen in spontaneous CJD.

- Prominent involvement of the cerebellum seen in nvCJD is not usually seen in spontaneous CJD except for the Brownell-Oppenheimer variant and GSS cases.

- nvCJD should be part of the differential diagnosis of any patient with the combination of a progressive neurodegenerative disease with psychiatric symptoms and residence in an area endemic for bovine spongiform encephalitis (the United Kingdom, Ireland).

Chapter 9: Nocardiosis and Actinomycosis for the ID Boards

Nancy Khardori, MD, PhD
Nitin Patel, MD

Contents

1. Overview of Nocardiosis

• Nocardiosis is an uncommon Gram-positive bacterial infection caused by aerobic actinomycetes

• It can be a localized or systemic suppurative disease in humans and animals

• Typically regarded as an opportunistic infection, but approximately one-third of infected patients are immunocompetent

2. Organism

• Most common species:

 * *N asteroides* complex (*N asteroides* sensu stricto, *N farcinica* and *N nova*)

• Other *Nocardia* spp.

 * *N brasiliensis*

 * *N psuedobrasiliensis*

 * *N paucivorans*

 * *N cyriacigeorgica*

 * *N otitidiscaviarum*

 * *N transvelensis*

 * *N veteran*

3. Microbiology

• Filamentous Gram-positive rods, aerobic actinomycetes

• Weakly acid-fast

4. Epidemiology

• Increased incidence in immunocompromised patients, eg, transplants, HIV, chronic steroids, malignancy, etc.

5. Pathogenesis

• Protective immunity is cell-mediated

 * Histopathology – abscess with extensive neutrophil infiltration with necrosis

• Granules/micro colonies composed of dense masses of bacterial filaments extending radially from central core

6. Geographical Distribution

• Worldwide

7. Site of Infection

• Pulmonary – (39%)

• CNS – (9%)

• Systemic – (32%)

• Single site extra pulmonary – (12%)

• Cutaneous – (8%)

8. Clinical Presentation

- Pulmonary

  * Presentation

    - Pneumonia– most common, mostly sub acute, more acute in immunocompromised host

    - Rarely– Laryngitis, tracheitis, bronchitis, sinusitis

    - Spread from lung tissue leading to pericarditis

  * Mediastinitis

  * Superior vena cava syndrome

    - Dissemination is common

  * Symptoms

    - General symptoms: fever, night sweats, weight loss, anorexia

    - Productive cough

    - Hemoptysis

    - Dyspnea

    - Pleuritic chest pain

  * Radiological findings

    - Infiltrates with moderate density

    - Nodules (single/multiple)

    - Thick-walled cavitary lesions

    - Empyema

- *Nocardiosis should be suspected in patients with non-resolving pneumonia.*

  * Asymptomatic particularly in patients with intact immune system

  * Meningitis (uncommon)

  * Brain abscesses (common)

    - Usually supratentorial

    - Multiloculated

    - Single/multiple

  *Symptoms: Headache, meningismus, seizures

- **Cutaneous**

  * Primary cutaneous (subacute cellulitis)

    - Dissemination (rare)

    - *N brasiliensis* (most common)

  * Lymphocutaneous- identical to the lymphocutaneous syndrome caused by Sporothrix schenckii "sporotrichoid nocardiosis"

  * Cutaneous involvement from a disseminated focus

  * Actinomycetoma

    - Initially a nodule, which may progress to a fistula

    - Fistulae tend to come and go

    - Fistulae often contain white granules

    - Systemic symptoms are absent

- **Disseminated infection**

  * Often follows pulmonary nocardiosis

  * 20% cases with no primary pulmonary infection

  * Bacteremia rarely

- **Other less common sites**

  * Bone

* Heart valve

* Joints

* Kidney

* Eye infection– subacute keratitis/endophthalmitis

ID Board Pearls

• CNS involvement by nocardiosis can be asymptomatic.

• A combination of pulmonary and CNS involvement is very common in nocardiosis.

9. Differential Diagnosis

• Fungal infections (Aspergillosis, zygomycosis [mucormycosis], cryptococcosis)

• Mycobacterial infections (*M tuberculosis, M avium intracellulare, M kansasii*)

• Bacterial infections (*Rhodococcus equi* and Gram-negative bacilli such as *Pseudomonas aeruginosa* and *Klebsiella pneumoniae*)

• Malignancy

10. Diagnosis

- A definitive diagnosis requires the isolation and identification of the organism from a clinical specimen

- Recovery of nocardia in the laboratory is difficult because of its fastidious nature and slow growth (up to 2 weeks to appear and up to 4 weeks to become obvious)

- Invasive procedure is often required to obtain an adequate specimen

- Transtracheal aspiration should be avoided as it frequently leads to nocardia cellulitis around the puncture wound

- Polymerase chain reaction provides more accurate and rapid results for the diagnosis, but availability is limited at this point

- CT/MRI of head – some authorities recommend in all cases (at least should do in patients with pulmonary nocardiosis and in immunocompromised patients)

- Nocardia isolates are usually sent to a reference laboratory for precise identification and susceptibility testing

ID Board Pearls

- *Nocardia* spp. can be differentiated from actinomycosis by modified *acid-fast* staining and *aerobic* growth.

- Precise speciation and *susceptibility* testing of clinical isolates is *important* especially if the patient does not respond to initial therapy.

- Suggest in patients with cavitary lung and brain lesions.

11. Treatment

Therapeutic Agents:

1. Oral agents

TMP-SMX – Recommended dose is 5 to 10 mg/kg (TMP) and 25 to 50 mg/kg (SMX) in 2-4 divided doses

- Sulfonamide level is recommended when treating severe difficult cases – Recommended level is 100 to 150 mcg/mL

- If allergic to sulfa – desensitizing is the best option

  * Minocycline

  * Other tetracycline medications are ineffective

Minocycline – dose is 100-200 mg BID

- Can be used as monotherapy or in combination with other agents

Linezolid – found to have *in vitro* activity

2. Parenteral agents

- Preferred as primary therapy for immunocompromised patients with severe and progressive disease

  * Amikacin (10-15 mg/kg/day)

  * Ceftriaxone (6 g/day)

  * Cefotaxime (6 g/day)

  * Imipenum (2 g/day)

- Patients with nocardiosis should be monitored for the response to therapy and possible drug toxicity

ID Board Pearls

- Immunocompromised patients whose immunosuppression cannot be reversed, should receive *indefinite suppressive therapy with TMP-SMX.*

12. Prognostic Factors

- Outcome is dependant on site and extent of the disease and underlying host factors

- **Cure rates with nocardia infection**

    * 100% with skin and soft tissue infection

    * 90% in pleuropulmonary disease

    * 63% in disseminated infection

    * 50% in brain abscess

- Poor prognosis in those patients who are immuno-compromised and elderly patients

- Delayed diagnosis and early cessation of the therapy are poor prognostic factors

13. Overview of Actinomycosis

- *Indolent and slowly progressive* infection

- Classically – formation of the *"sulfur granule " or "grains"*

- One of the most misdiagnosed diseases

14. Microbiology

- Filamentous, Gram-positive

- *Anaerobic* or microaerophilic

- *Non acid-fast*

15. Etiological Agents

- *A israelii* (most common)

- *A naeslundii*

- *A odontolyticus*

- *A viscosus*

- *A meyeri*

- *A gerencseriae*

16. Epidemiology

- Male > female (3:1)

- Peak incidence in middle decades

17. Geographical Distribution

- Worldwide

18. Pathogenesis and Pathology

- Hallmark of actinomycosis → indolent chronic phase appears as single or multiple nodule → contiguous spread → sinus tract to the skin, *adjacent bone/organs*

- Hematogenous spread (very rare)

- *May mimic malignancy*

- Histopathology: central necrosis consisting of neutrophils and *sulfur granules*, *"wooden" fibrotic walls*

19. Clinical Presentations

- **Oral-Cervicofacial Disease**
  - * Most common presentation

  - * Often misdiagnosed as mass or neoplasm

  - * Angle of the jaw most common site

  - * Should be considered if mass lesion or relapsing infection in the head and neck

- **Thoracic Disease**
  - * Lung/pleural space most common site

  - * Mediastinum– most likely from contagious spread, rarely after esophageal perforation, trauma

  - * Involvement of bone and chest wall from lung tissue

  - * Primary endocarditis and isolated disease of breast have been described in the literature

  - * Radiological appearance– central area of low attenuation with ring-like enhancement on CT scan

    - Hilar adenopathy

    - Pleural thickening (50%)

    - Thick-walled cavitary disease

- **Abdominal Disease**

  - * Diagnosis is a challenge

  - * Abscess or mass or mixed lesion

  - * Sinus tracts – may mimic inflammatory bowel disease

- **Pelvic Disease**

  - * Most commonly associated with IUCD

  - * Rarely present months after removal of IUCD

- * Use of *actinomyces-like organism* (ALOs) from cervical or endometrial specimen to screen IUCD-associated disease is not universally accepted

- **CNS Disease**

  - * Rare

  - * Single or multiple brain abscesses

  - * CT scan– ring enhancing lesion with thick wall

    - Irregular or nodular appearance

- **Musculoskeletal/Soft-tissue Disease**

  - * Mostly associated with adjacent tissue infection but can be after trauma and rarely from hematogenous spread

  - * New bone formation and bone destruction seen simultaneously

- **Disseminated Disease**

  - * Rare

  - * Liver and lungs most commonly affected

20. Diagnosis

• **Often missed/delayed**

• Microscopic identification of sulfur granules

• Occasionally sulfur granules can be seen by naked eye from draining sinus tract or pus

• 16S rRNA gene amplification and sequencing can increase diagnostic sensitivity

21. Treatment

• **Penicillin or amoxicillin**, administered over a prolonged period, is the cornerstone of therapy for actinomycosis

• Lack of a clinical response to penicillin usually indicates the presence of other bacteria

• Duration

    * Until cured, often needs 12 months

    * For less extensive disease, shorter duration may be reasonable but should be based on clinical response

• Other active agents based on clinical experience

    * Erythromycin

    * Tetracycline/doxycycline/minocycline

    * Clindamycin

• Agents to be avoided

    * Metronidazole

    * Aminoglycosides

    * Oxacillin/dicloxacillin

    * Cephalexin

• Agents effective based on *in vitro* activity

    * Moxifloxacin

    * Vancomycin

    * Linezolid

    * Quinuprostin-dlafopristin

ID Board Pearls

- Presence of sulfur granules in sinus tract drainage is pathognomonic.

- Unlike nocardia, actinomycosis has a predilection for sinus tract formation.

- Unlike nocardia, actinomycosis commonly affects the lungs and liver, not lungs and CNS.

- Actinomycosis occurs primarily in normal hosts, whereas nocardia occurs mainly in compromised hosts.

- Orofacial actinomycosis resembles squamous cell carcinoma.

- Often misdiagnosed as malignancy, therefore a biopsy is essential.

22. Further Reading

1. Khardori N, Shawar R, Gupta R, Rosenbaum B, Rolston K. In vitro antimicrobial susceptibilities of Nocardia species. *Antimicrob Agents Chemother*. 1993,4:882-884.

2. Saubolle MA, Sussland D. Nocardiosis: Review of clinical and laboratory experience. *J Clin Microbiol*. 2003;41:4497-4501.

Chapter 10: Systemic Mycoses for the ID Boards

Donna C. Sullivan, PhD
Stanley W. Chapman, MD

Contents

1. Classification

Clinical Classification

• Based on the site of infection.

• Includes superficial, cutaneous, subcutaneous and systemic mycoses.

Mycologic Classification

The mycologic classification listed below is useful for treatment decisions. The yeasts and dimorphic fungi are susceptible to both amphotericin B (AmB) and the azoles. In contrast, the molds are generally resistant to the azoles, in particular, ketoconazole and fluconazole, and AmB deoxycholate, or any of the lipid preparations, is the drug of choice when mold forms are seen in tissue. The newer azoles, including itraconazole and voriconazole, have proven successful in the treatment of aspergillosis, and posaconazole appears promising for the treatment of mucormycosis.

Yeasts
• Unicellular organisms that reproduce by budding.

• Clinical examples are *Candida albicans* and *Cryptococcus neoformans.*

Molds
• Filamentous, tubular structures called hyphae.

• Grow by branching and longitudinal extension.

• Clinical examples are *Aspergillus* species and those organisms causing mucormycosis (ie, *Rhizopus, Absidia, Cunninghamella*).

Dimorphic
• Pathogens that grow in the mycelial phase in nature and in culture at 25° C.

• Converts to yeast form after infection and in culture at 37° C.

Opportunistic vs. Nonopportunistic Classification

• Opportunistic fungi are typically associated with a low virulent potential for normal hosts, but can cause invasive disease in immunocompromised hosts (eg, invasive mold disease in transplant patients or disseminated candidiasis in neutropenic patients) and are associated with high morbidity and mortality.

• Nonopportunistic fungi possess innate virulence that allows them to infect and invade host tissues in immunocompetent patients. Clinical examples include the organisms causing the endemic mycoses, *B dermatitidis* and *H capsulatum*.

   * Increased severity of disease, however, is noted to occur when these organisms infect immunocompromised patients, particularly AIDS patients. Disseminated disease is more frequent, as is CNS disease, including meningitis and brain abscess.

Immune Response

• Humoral response is not felt to be important in host defense or establishing immunity. It is the basis of diagnostic testing; in general, complement fixation antibody testing is more sensitive but less specific than precipitin antibodies.

• Cellular response is of major importance in host defense and in immunity against reinfection.

• A positive skin test indicates prior exposure to the organism and is generally not helpful as a diagnostic tool.

Microbiology

• A majority of the endemic mycoses are dimorphic fungi; they occur in nature and in culture at room temperature (eg, 25° C) as filamentous molds, but they grow as unicellular yeast forms in tissue or in culture at 37° C.

• A definitive diagnosis requires culture of the organism from clinically relevant tissue.

• A presumptive diagnosis is made by visualization of the characteristic yeast or hyphae form in sputum, secretions or tissue.

- Assays identifying fungal antigens in serum and urine are commercially available and may have some utility in the diagnosis, monitoring response to therapy and early identification of relapse.

- Several nucleic acid detection assays have been developed for the systemic mycosis.

Candida Species
- Yeast forms, hyphae, and pseudohyphae are easily seen in clinical specimens.

- Cells are 4-6 micrometers in diameter and are thin-walled.

Blastomyces dermatitidis
- Broad-based budding yeast approximately 8-15 micrometers in diameter with multiple nuclei.

- Double refractile cell wall typically with single bud.

Histoplasma capsulatum
- Oval to round budding cells approximately 1-3 micrometers in diameter; often found clustered in histocytes.

- Difficult to detect in small numbers; in disseminated disease, can be seen intracellularly in neutrophils when buffy coat preparations from peripheral blood are examined with Giemsa stain.

Cryptococcus neoformans
- Encapsulated yeast approximately 2-15 micrometers in diameter.

- Buds are single and "pinched off." Capsule is usually easily seen and is useful for diagnosis. In some cases, however, only minimal capsule is present. Pseudohyphae are rarely seen.

Coccidioides immitis
- Spherules vary in size from 10-200 micrometers in diameter; some contain endospores.

- Endospores can be released and form new spherules.

Sporothrix schenckii
- Cells are variable in size ranging from 4-6 micrometers in diameter.

- Classically described as cigar-shaped, but can be round to oval-shaped as well.

Paracoccidioides brasiliensis
- Cells are variable in size ranging from 5-60 micrometers in diameter.

- Larger cells are surrounded by smaller buds and fat globules thus creating the "pilot's wheel" appearance.

Therapy
- AmB is generally used as initial therapy in disseminated or life-threatening disease, with switch to an azole when patient is stabilized.

- Lipid formulations of AmB are commonly used instead of AmB deoxycholate, owing to poor tolerance or disease progression.

- Initial therapy with an azole is generally acceptable in patients with endemic mycoses who have a normal immune function and non-CNS limited disease.

- The echinocandins (caspofungin, anidulafungin and mycafungin) have activity against Candida species, including fluconazole resistant strains.

- The echinocandins have proven utility as primary or salvage therapy for aspergillosis, alone or in combination with itraconazole or voriconazole.

- Posaconazole appears to be promising in the prevention and treatment of mucormycosis in immunocompromised hosts.

- 5-flucytosine is only used in combination therapy for patients with cryptococcal meningitis, and for patients with candidal endocarditis and meningitis. It should never be used as a single agent due to the rapid development of resistance.

2. Candidiasis

Microbiology

- Causative organisms are *Candida albicans, C parapsilosis, C tropicalis, C lusitaniae, C glabrata, C guilliermondii, C kefyr (formerly pseudotropicalis), C krusei* and *C dubliniensis*.

Epidemiology

- *Candida* species are normal commensals in the mouth, GI tract, vagina, and less commonly, on the skin. Opportunistic infection occurs when there is a shift in the balance of normal flora, disruption of normal biologic barriers and when immune status is compromised.

- *Candidiasis* is the most common fungal infection and is characterized by diversity in clinical manifestations, ranging from benign mucocutaneous disease to invasive dissemination, deep-tissue involvement and candidemia.

- *Candida* species are the fourth most common cause of nosocomial bloodstream infections in the United States.

- The majority of disseminated infections appear to be from an endogenous source, usually the gut, and not from exogenous sources, although nosocomial infections have been reported.

- Fungemia with *C parapsilosis* has been strongly associated with catheter-related infections.

- Patients at high risk for development of candidemia include those with hematologic malignancies, solid or bone marrow transplantation, neutropenia, corticosteroid use, treatment with broad-spectrum antibiotics, renal failure, complications of GI surgery, critical care instrumentation and hyperalimentation.

- Although *C albicans* is the most common single species to cause infection, non-*albicans* species are increasing, especially in invasive and vaginal candidiasis, and are associated with azole resistance.

Key Clinical Features

Cutaneous
- Skin lesions are pruritic, erythematous, confluent papules that may progress to pustules or ulcers characteristically associated with satellite lesions. Tend to develop in areas where the skin is moist, such as the perineal area; infection is more extensive and persistent in immunocompromised hosts.

Mucous Membrane
Oral candidiasis
- Raised, creamy white lesions on tongue and buccal mucosa; other forms are atrophic and appear as glossitis and angular cheilitis; risk factors are recent antibiotic or steroid use, cancer and AIDS.

Vulvovaginitis
- Common infection; 75% of women will have at least 1 episode.

- Edema and pruritus of vulva with curd-like discharge.

- Associated with increased estrogen states, diabetes mellitus, antibiotic use, HIV infection, corticosteroid use, IUDs and diaphragm use.

Esophageal candidiasis
- Odynophagia, dysphagia and substernal chest pain.

- May occur in absence of oral candidiasis.

- Primarily seen in setting of AIDS or chemotherapy.

Chronic Mucocutaneous Candidiasis
- Represents a heterogenous group of persistent or recalcitrant *Candida* infections of skin, mucous membranes, hair and nails despite antifungal therapy; typically does not progress to dissemination.

- Typically presents in first 2 years of life.

- Alopecia and disfiguring lesions of the face, scalp and hands.

- Associated with cell-mediated defect against *Candida* antigens; endocrinopathies in 50%.

Genitourinary

- Presence in urine may represent colonization, lower tract disease, upper tract disease or disseminated disease that involves the renal pelvis.

- Ascending infection is the most common route for UTIs; it is unusual for candiduria to result in candidemia

- Lower tract infection is usually asymptomatic and is seen in patients with indwelling catheters.

- Fever, dysuria, hematuria, frequency, suprapubic pain, with or without costovertebral angle tenderness, are seen most commonly with upper tract infection; not distinctive from other urinary pathogens.

- Fungus balls occasionally form and obstruct the GU tract, requiring emergent drainage.

Candidemia and Acute Disseminated Candidiasis

- Most commonly seen in patients with cancer (particularly hematologic malignancies and neutropenia), complicated postoperative courses and burns; multiple organs are usually involved, including kidneys, brain (including meninges), lungs, heart, eye, GI tract, skin, lungs and endocrine glands.

Chronic Disseminated Candidiasis (Hepatosplenic Candidiasis)

- Reported almost exclusively in patients with hematologic malignancies; patients exhibit right upper quadrant pain, nausea, vomiting, anorexia and high spiking fevers; classically occurs after recovery from neutropenia.

Respiratory

- Rare manifestation; occurs usually as a local or diffuse bronchopneumonia or from hematogenous spread; can also involve the larynx and epiglottis.

Gastrointestinal

- Can occur in setting of peritoneal dialysis, complicated GI surgery, or dissemination and contiguous extension from another localized infection; dissemination occurs in only 25% of focal infections and very rarely when associated with peritoneal dialysis.

Bone and joint

- Occurs in disseminated disease or from direct extension from injection drug use, trauma or surgical inoculation; typically requires open drainage for optimal outcome.

Endocarditis

- Usually seen in patients with prosthetic valves, injection drug users or in line-associated candidemia that has been prolonged; typically associated with large vegetations; antifungal and surgical therapy is needed for cure.

Key Laboratory and Radiologic Features

Chronic Mucocutaneous Candidiasis
Labs
- T-cell abnormalities; 50% exhibit anergy.

- Immunoglobulins and B cells are normal.

Genitourinary
Labs
- Pyuria; yeast cells and hyphae.

Radiology
- CT may reveal abscess or masses if renal involvement is via hematogenous spread.

Candidemia and Acute Disseminated Candidiasis
Labs
- Blood cultures positive in 50%.

- Biopsy of skin lesions typically reveals organisms; culture of material usually yields growth of organism.

- Pyuria and positive urine cultures typically occur.

- The sensitivity and specificity of antigen based tests are still being investigated.

Radiology
- CT may or may not reveal abscesses or masses.

Chronic Disseminated Candidiasis (Hepatosplenic Candidiasis)
Labs
- Elevated transaminases.

- Blood cultures are frequently negative (approximately 85%).

- The sensitivity and specificity of antigen based tests are still being investigated.

Radiology
- CT reveals characteristic multiple lucency in liver, spleen, and occasionally kidneys and lung.

Respiratory
Labs
- Yeast is typically present in sputum in many hospitalized patients and causes difficulty in discerning colonization from infection; histopathology may be necessary to diagnose invasion.

Radiology
- CXR reveals bilateral finely nodular diffuse infiltrates.

Gastrointestinal
Labs
- Blood cultures are usually negative.

- Peritoneal or abscess/mass cultures are usually positive.

Radiology
- CT of abdomen may reveal localized abscesses.

Bone and Joint
- Blood cultures are usually negative.

- Material from open drainage or aspirate typically reveals yeast on smear with positive culture.

Radiology
- Similar to other fungal or mycobacterial bone infections.

Endocarditis
- Blood cultures are typically positive with established fungemia.

Radiology
- Echocardiogram reveals large vegetations, which are friable and easily embolize.

Therapeutic Options

Oropharyngeal, Skin and Paronychia
- Topical therapy is first line of therapy, followed by systemic therapy for refractory or recurrent disease; drainage is most important in paronychial infections.

- Topical therapy most frequency involves the azoles such as miconazole, ketoconazole and itraconazole. Polyenes such as amphotericin B can also be used topically.

- Systemic therapy includes oral azoles such as fluconazole, itraconazole or voriconazole. Intravenous AmB and caspofungin are reserved for azole-refractory infections.

- Duration of therapy depends on clinical response, comorbid diseases and underlying immune status.

- AIDS patients are more likely to have more severe disease and usually require prolonged therapy because of the high relapse rates

Esophageal Candidiasis
- Topical therapy is ineffective, so oral azoles (fluconazole, itraconazole solution or voriconazole) are used for initial therapy.

- Intravenous lipid AmB formulation or *echinocandins (caspofungin, anidulafungin or mycafungin) are used for azole refractory or recurrent infections*.

- Duration is for at least 2 weeks; recurrent or refractory infections may require prolonged therapy.

- Suppressive therapy may be used for patients with disabling recurrent infections; itraconazole solution, voriconazole or caspofungin may be used for fluconazole-refractory esophageal candidiasis.

Candidal Onychomycosis
- Topical therapy is ineffective; treat with itraconazole 200 PO BID.

- Treat for 7 days; repeat monthly for 3-4 months.

Table 1

Differential Diagnosis of Candidiasis

Type	Infectious	Noninfectious
Mucocutaneous	Erythrasma	Seborrheic dermatitis Langerhans cell histiocytosis
Chronic mucocutaneous candidiasis	Other chronic fungal infections Dermatophyte infection	Squamous cell carcinoma
Genitourinary	Bacterial UTI Tuberculosis (disseminated or miliary) Acute or chronic urethral syndromes including STDs	Bladder malignancy Renal calculi
Candidemia and acute disseminated candidiasis	Bacterial sepsis Viral hepatitis Other disseminated fungal infections Tuberculosis	Drug fever Graft versus host disease Drug-induced hepatitis
Chronic disseminated candidiasis (hepatosplenic candidiasis)	Tuberculosis Other fungal infections Viral hepatitis	Drug fever Graft versus host disease Drug-induced hepatitis Shock liver
Respiratory	Pneumocystis pneumonia Tuberculosis Other fungal pneumonias Bacterial pneumonia	Congestive heart failure Noninfectious ARDS Graft versus host disease Drug-induced lung injury
Gastrointestinal	Tuberculosis Bacterial peritonitis Cholecystitis	Malignancy
Bone and joint	Tuberculosis Other fungal bone infections	Malignancy
Endocarditis	Bacterial endocarditis	SLE endocarditis Marantic endocarditis

Table 2

Complications of Candidiasis

Type	Clinical outcome	Prognostic factors
Mucocutaneous	Generally good; may be recurrent	Immune status
Chronic mucocutaneous candidiasis	Recurrent candidiasis; bacterial superinfection may occur; disseminated candidiasis is rare	Presence of secondary bacterial infections
Genitourinary	Response to therapy is generally good if involvement is at bladder or below	Presence of urinary catheter Immune status
Candidemia and acute disseminated candidiasis	High attributable mortality	Resolution of risk factors, particularly neutropenia
Chronic disseminated candidiasis (hepatosplenic candidiasis)	Response to therapy may be delayed; high relapse rate	Resolution of risk factors Appropriate antifungal therapy
Respiratory	Similar to disseminated candidemia	Prompt diagnosis Appropriate antifungal therapy
Gastrointestinal	Peritoneal dialysis infection responds well to catheter removal and antifungal therapy Dependent on underlying cause of breach in GI mucosa	Resolution of risk factors Adequate drainage and debridement Appropriate antifungal therapy
Bone and joint	Tends to be chronic and associated with poor functional outcome	Prompt diagnosis Adequate drainage or debridement Appropriate antifungal therapy
Meningitis	High mortality; associated with high relapse rate	Prompt diagnosis Removal of CNS devices if related to neurosurgical procedure
Endocarditis Suppurative phlebitis	Good response with resection of vein	Involvement of peripheral vein; appropriate antifungal therapy
Pericarditis	Generally poor prognosis	Ability to resection pericardium; appropriate antifungal therapy
Endocarditis	Generally poor prognosis; propensity relapse	Ability to perform valve resection; appropriate antifungal therapy

Chronic Mucocutaneous Candidiasis

- For oropharyngeal, topical azoles, oral azoles or polyenes (nystatin, AmB solution).

- For refractory or recurrent infections, fluconazole 100-200 mg/day PO or itraconazole 200 mg/d PO, lipid AmB >0.3 mg/kg/d IV if azole-refractory infection.

- For esophageal candidiasis, PO or IV fluconazole 100-200 mg/day or itraconazole 200 mg/d.

- Chronic suppressive therapy with an azole is the rule.

Urinary Candidiasis

- Important to remove any GU catheter or prosthesis if possible to reduce relapse rates.

- Oral fluconazole 200 mg/day for 7-14 days, lipid AmB (0.7-1.0 mg/kg/d), or flucytosine (in patients with infection due to non-*albicans* species of *Candida*).

- Bladder irrigation with AmB (50-200 µg/ml) may transiently clear funguria but is rarely indicated.

- Treat for at least 2 weeks; if candiduria is persistent despite therapy, evaluate for disseminated disease.

Candidemia and Acute Hematogenously Disseminated Candidiasis

- If feasible, remove all existing central venous catheters.

- Lipid AmB (0.7-1.0 mg/kg/d), fluconazole IV (400 mg/d), or combination of the two.

- Caspofungin 70 mg IV PB first dose, then 50 mg/d.

- For uncomplicated line-associated infection, therapy can be continued for 2 weeks following the first negative blood cultures; otherwise, therapy should continue for at least 4-6 weeks.

- Neutropenic patients should receive recombinant cytokine (GC-, SF- or MC-stimulating factor).

Candidal Endophthalmitis

- AmB (0.7-1.0 mg/kg/d) ± flucytosine.

- Oral or IV fluconazole, 6-12 mg/kg/d.

- Vitrectomy plus antifungal therapy (both intravenous and intravitreal) may improve visual outcome.

- All patients with candidemia should have at least 1 dilated retinal exam by an ophthalmologist.

- Continue antifungal therapy until complete resolution of disease (6-12 weeks).

Endovascular Candidiasis

- AmB (0.7-1.0 mg/kg/d) or lipid AmB (3-6 mg/kg/d) ± flucytosine.

- Oral or IV fluconazole 6-12 mg/kg/d.

- Caspofungin 70 mg IV PB first dose, then 50 mg/d.

- Surgical therapy is essential for successful outcome.

- Suppurative phlebitis of peripheral vein: 2 weeks of antifungal therapy after surgical resection of vein.

- Endocarditis: early removal of infected valves (native and prosthetic) followed by at least 6 weeks of antifungal therapy; if valve replacement not possible, continue lifelong suppressive therapy with fluconazole.

- Pericarditis: resection or debridement of infected pericardial tissue followed by a minimum of 6 weeks of antifungal therapy.

Chronic Disseminated Candidiasis (Hepatosplenic Candidiasis)

- Mild or stable disease: fluconazole 6 mg/kg/d.

- Severely ill or refractory disease: lipid AmB (3-5 mg/kg/d) or AmB (0.6-0.7 mg/kg/d).

- If patient has clinical response and stabilizes with initial course of AmB, may switch to fluconazole for remainder of course; therapy should continue until there is calcification or resolution of lesions.

Respiratory Candidiasis
- Pneumonia: lipid AmB (3-5 mg/kg/d) or AmB (0.7-1.0 mg/kg/d) or fluconazole; caspofungin 70 mg IV PB first dose, then 50 mg/d.

- Laryngeal: lipid AmB (3-5 mg/kg/d) or AmB (0.7-1.0 mg/kg/d) as initial therapy; may change to oral or IV fluconazole when improvement and/or stability have occurred.

- Pneumonia and laryngitis usually secondary to hematogenously disseminated infection and therapy should be directed to primary focus

- Therapy should continue until clearance of local and systemic sites of infection.

Bone and Joint Candidiasis
- Combined surgical debridement and antifungal therapy: lipid AmB (3-5 mg/kg/d) or AmB (0.5-1.0 mg/kg/d) for 6-10 weeks.

- AmB IV for 2-3 weeks followed by oral fluconazole for a total 6-12 months of therapy.

GI Candidiasis
- Biliary tree should be treated by mechanical restoration of functional drainage combined with antifungal therapy: Lipid AmB (3-5 mg/kg/d) or AmB (0.7-1.0 mg/kg/d) or fluconazole (400-800 mg/d IV or PO).

- Treatment for 2-3 weeks generally required; catheter removal is necessary in peritoneal dialysis infection

Candidal Meningitis
- AmB (0.7-1.0 mg/kg/d) + flucytosine (25 mg/kg QID) adjusted to produce serum levels of 40-60 µg/ml.

- Fluconazole has been used as follow-up therapy and long-term suppressive therapy.

- Therapy should continue for a minimum of 4 weeks after resolution of all CSF and radiographic abnormalities and patient is neurologically stable.

Empirical Therapy in Febrile Non-neutropenic Patients
- Lipid AmB (3-5 mg/kg/d) or AmB (0.7-1.0 mg/kg/d) or fluconazole (400-800 mg/d).

- With empirical use, less toxic agents are preferred; selected patients that demonstrate Candida colonization at multiple sites, other risk factors for candidiasis or candidemia, and lack of alternative etiologies of fever.

Empirical Therapy in Febrile Neutropenic Patients
- Lipid formulation AmB (3-6 mg/kg/d), AmB deoxycholate (0.7-1.0 mg/kg/d) or caspofungin 70 mg loading dose followed by 50 mg IV.

- Oral or IV fluconazole if patient is low risk for invasive aspergillosis.

- Treat for duration of febrile neutropenia.

ID Board Pearls

- Host factors that predispose patients to candidiasis include:

    * Physiological (pregnancy, extremes of age)

    * Trauma (maceration, infection, burn wound)

    * Hematological (neutropenia, cellular immunodeficiency)

    * Endocrinological (diabetes mellitus, hypoparathyroidism, Addison's disease)

    * Iatrogenic (chemotherapeutics, corticosteroids, oral contraceptives, antibiotics, catheters, surgery)

    * Other (intravenous drug addiction, malnutrition, malabsorption, thymoma)

- Candida pneumonia occurs only as part of disseminated candidiasis

3. Blastomycosis

Synonyms

• Gilchrist's disease, Chicago disease, North American blastomycosis.

Microbiology

• The causative organism is *Blastomyces dermatitidis*.

Epidemiology

• Endemic areas include the south-central and southeastern states bordering on the Mississippi and Ohio River basins, and states bordering the Great Lakes and the St. Lawrence River.

• In sporadic cases, most patients are male (1.7:1), 30-70 years of age, and are associated with occupational or recreational exposure to soil.

• Epidemics have been reported and noted to exhibit no seasonal pattern or predilection to a particular age, sex or race.

• Infections in immunocompromised hosts are associated with increased severity, more frequent dissemination (especially to the CNS) and higher mortality.

Diagnosis

• Definitive diagnosis is by culture of the organism from clinical specimens. However, slow growth of the organism makes culture impractical for rapid diagnosis.

Table 3

Differential Diagnosis of Blastomycosis

Type	Infectious	Noninfectious
Acute pulmonary infection	Bacterial pneumonia Viral pneumonia	Hypersensitivity pneumonitis
Chronic pulmonary infection	Tuberculosis Other fungal pneumonias	Sarcoidosis Neoplasm
Skin	Bacterial infection Histoplasmosis Sporotrichosis (*Mycobacterium* other than TB)	Carcinoma
Bone	Tuberculosis Other fungal pathogens	Metastatic bone disease
Genitourinary	Bacterial pathogens Tuberculosis Cryptococcosis	BPH Neoplasm
CNS	Tuberculous meningitis Bacterial abscesses Other fungal meningitis CNS toxoplasmosis	Neoplasm

- Direct visualization of characteristic broad-based budding yeast forms in histologic or cytologic specimens allows prompt, presumptive diagnosis of blastomycosis and may serve as the basis for initiation of therapy.

- Antigen testing of urine or other body fluids may also be diagnostic of blastomycosis, and is useful when the organism is suspected but not rapidly demonstrated by other methods.

- Serologic testing lacks sensitivity and specificity and must be interpreted with caution.

- Complement fixation (CF) tests are positive in fewer than 50% of patients; cross reactions with *Histoplasma capsulatum* and *Coccidioides immitis* frequently occur.

- Immunodiffusion tests are highly specific but lack sensitivity, particularly in acute disease.

Table 4

Therapeutic Options for Blastomycosis

Type	Preferred	Alternative
Pulmonary		
Mild-to-moderate	Itraconazole 200-400 mg/d for at least 6 months	Fluconazole 6 months 400-800 mg/d for at least TK
Disseminated		
CNS	AmB deoxycholate at least 2 g total dose Lipid AmB 3-5 mg/kg/d	Fluconazole 800 mg/d can be considered if patient is intolerant of AmB
Non-CNS		
Mild-to-moderate	Itraconazole 200-400 mg/d for at least 6 months; if bone involvement is present, treatment should be for 12 months	Ketoconazole or fluconazole 400-800 mg/d for at least 6 months
Life-threatening	AmB deoxycholate 1.5-2.5 g total dose Lipid AmB 3-5 mg/kg/d	Initial therapy with AmB with switch to itraconazole 200-400 mg/d after clinical stabilization
Immunocompromised host	AmB deoxycholate 1.5-2.5 g total dose Lipid AmB 3-5 mg/kg/d	Initial therapy with AmB with switch to itraconazole 200-400 mg/d after clinical stabilization
Pregnancy	AmB 1.5-2.5 g total dose	Azoles contraindicated in pregnancy

- Radioimmunoassay of WI-I (cell wall antigen) antibody has been shown to have a sensitivity and specificity of 85% and 95%, respectively. This test is under investigation for future clinical use.

- Nucleic acid detection techniques are currently available for the diagnosis of blastomycosis. A commercially available chemiluminescent DNA probe (Gen Probe, San Diego, CA) has been shown to have a sensitivity of 87.4% and 100% specificity when 74 target and 219 nontarget fungi were tested.

Therapy

- Some immunocompetent hosts with limited pulmonary disease may spontaneously resolve the infection without therapy. Patients who are not treated should be followed carefully for progression of disease.

- Treatment is required for all patients with extrapulmonary disease or progressive pulmonary disease. Immunocompromised hosts should be treated, most frequently with amphotericin B (AmB).

- Lipid AmB (3-5 mg/kg/d) or AmB deoxycholate (0.7-1.0 mg/kg per day) for 1-2 weeks is the preferred initial treatment for life-threatening blastomycosis and patients with CNS disease.

- Itraconazole is the drug of choice for treatment of patients with mild-to-moderate pulmonary or non-CNS disseminated disease. Two oral preparations are available. Important differences in bioavailability of the two preparations have clinical significance. Oral capsules require acid for absorption and should be taken with Coca-Cola or food. Treatment failures have been well documented in patients on H2-blockers or proton pump inhibitors. The liquid preparation does not require acid and is taken on an empty stomach.

- Owing to the bioavailability of itraconazole, blood levels should be performed on all patients failing treatment with this drug. Some physicians routinely obtain blood levels on patients treated with the capsules irrespective of clinical response. A serum level >1.0 µg/ml is recommended.

Key Clinical Features

Acute Pulmonary Infection
- 50% of cases may be asymptomatic; after incubation period of 4-6 weeks, a flu-like illness occurs with fever, chills, myalgias, arthralgia, cough and pleuritic chest pain, often with spontaneous recovery; severity of illness is variable and can be mild to fulminant disease.

Chronic Pulmonary Infection (Most Common)
- Weight loss, low-grade fever, fatigue, productive cough, pleuritic chest pain.

Disseminated Non-CNS
Skin
- Most common extrapulmonary site of disseminate infection can occur in isolation, but is most often seen in multiorgan involvement. Lesions are verrucous or ulcerative in appearance; skin involvement can also occur via direct inoculation (eg, dog bite) and is associated with regional lymphadenopathy; subcutaneous nodules or "cold abscesses" that contain numerous organisms occur in the setting of pulmonary or extrapulmonary disease.

Bone and joint
- Second most common site of dissemination; most common sites include the ribs, vertebrae and long bones; usually not associated with pain, but can be painful in setting of contiguous soft tissue abscesses and draining sinuses; arthritis is purulent and occurs via contiguous spread.

Genitourinary
- Prostatitis and epididymo-orchitis are most commonly reported sites; GU disease is involved in less than 10% of cases.

CNS
- Intracranial abscesses or meningitis usually occurs in less than 5% of disseminated disease in normal hosts. CNS disease occurs in 40% of AIDS patients.

Key Laboratory and Radiologic Features

Acute Pulmonary Infection
Labs
- Nonspecific.

Radiology
• Patchy alveolar infiltrates in single or multiple lobes; hilar enlargement, pleural effusions and cavitation are uncommon; in severe fulminant disease, CXR may have diffuse military pattern.

Chronic Pulmonary Infection
Labs
• Nonspecific.

Radiology
• Alveolar infiltrates and mass lesions are most common finding; pleural effusions, hilar adenopathy and cavitation occur as well.

Disseminated Disease Non-CNS
Labs
Skin
• Nonspecific.

Bone
• Nonspecific.

Radiology
• Typically well-circumscribed osteolytic bone lesions are seen.

Genitourinary
Labs
• Pyuria is common.

• KOH/wet prep of urine may be positive.

• Urine cultures are frequently positive after prostatic massage.

• Examination of urine sediment after centrifugation enhances visual and cultural identification.

CNS
Labs
• CSF formula reveals lymphocytic pleocytosis with elevated protein and normal glucose.

• CSF culture is low yield.

Radiology
• Ring-enhancing mass lesions on CT or MRI.

Prognosis

Acute Pulmonary Infection
• Some immunocompetent hosts may resolve spontaneously without therapy; treated patients typically do well.

• Prognosis depends on immune status.

Chronic Pulmonary Infection
• Generally responds well to therapy.

Prognosis depends on timeliness of diagnosis, underlying pulmonary disease and immune status.

Disseminated Pulmonary Infection
• Generally responds well to therapy; CNS has poorer prognosis, especially in immunocompromised patients.

• Prognosis depends on timeliness of diagnosis and immune status.

ID Board Pearls

• Fungus usually occurs with broad based bud, usually single refractile yeast in clinical specimens.

• Blastomycosis may coexist or mimic bronchogenic carcinoma and tuberculosis.

• Skin and mucous membrane lesions may mimic squamous cell carcinoma.

4. Histoplasmosis

Synonyms

- Darling's disease, reticuloendothelial cytomycosis, cave disease, spelunker's disease.

Microbiology

- The causative organism is *Histoplasma capsulatum*, which is typically found in tissue as intracellular yeast in histiocytes.

- Mycelial phase occurs in environment and culture at 37°C.

Epidemiology

- Endemic in the United States throughout the Ohio and Mississippi river valleys; also found in Central and South America.

- Found in the soil; particularly soil contaminated with bird and bat guano.

- Outbreaks have been reported in persons with heavy exposure to chicken houses, blackbird roosts and caves.

- Primary infection is via inhalation of spores with dissemination to the reticuloendothelial system; 90% of cases in normal hosts are subclinical.

- Severe disseminated disease is associated with infants and immunocompromised hosts, particularly HIV-infected patients.

Therapy

- Mild acute pulmonary disease in normal host may not need antifungal therapy.

- All patients with chronic pulmonary histoplasmosis and disseminated disease require therapy.

- Lipid AmB 3 mg/kg per day or AmB deoxycholate 0.7-1.0 mg/kg per day for 1-2 weeks followed by itraconazole 200 mg BID is standard therapy for moderately severe or severe disease.

Table 5

Differential Diagnosis of Histoplasmosis

Type	Infectious	Noninfectious
Acute pulmonary	Blastomycosis Histoplasmosis Coccidioidomycosis Paracoccidioidomycosis Tuberculosis Pneumocystis pneumonia Viral pneumonia Bacterial pneumonia	Neoplasms SLE Sarcoidosis
Chronic pulmonary	Histoplasmosis Blastomycosis	Neoplasms SLE Sarcoidosis
Disseminated	Bacterial sepsis	Lymphoproliferative disorder Inflammatory bowel disease Sarcoidosis Neoplasms

- Itraconazole is the azole of choice. The different formulations of itraconazole, including bioavailability of the two different oral preparations are discussed in the therapy section for blastomycosis.

- Alternative azole therapies include fluconazole and voriconazole.

- AIDS patients require suppressive therapy following the initial treatment course, preferably with itraconazole 200 mg/d indefinitely.

Key Clinical Features

Acute Pulmonary
- May be asymptomatic in normal hosts with mild exposure. Flu-like illness within 10-18 days characterized by fever, chills, malaise, headache, nonproductive cough and chest pain. Disease has a shorter incubation period and is typically milder in a previously exposed person. Immune-mediated granulomatous inflammatory pericarditis, erythema nodosum or erythema multiforme occur in less than 10% of cases.

Chronic Pulmonary
- Occurs in approximately 8% of cases. Seen in older males with underlying chronic, obstructive pulmonary disease. Symptoms are typically progressive and include low-grade fever, productive cough, dyspnea and weight loss.

Progressive Disseminated
- Rare. Seen primarily in immunocompromised host. Clinical course may be acute, subacute or chronic over months to years. Symptoms include fever, malaise and weight loss. Patients typically have hepatosplenomegaly. Mucosal ulcerations throughout the GI tract are seen in 40% of patients. Other sites that may be involved: skin, bone, heart and meninges. AIDS patients with overwhelming disease may present with a sepsis syndrome and ARDS.

Disseminated in Infants
- Uncommon. Onset is acute with fever, lethargy, cough, weight loss and diarrhea. Most patients have hepatosplenomegaly. Less than half of patients are seen with palpable lymphadenopathy and oropharyngeal ulcers.

Table 6

Complications of Histoplasmosis

Type	Clinical outcome	Prognostic factors
Acute pulmonary	Spontaneous recovery without therapy occurs in some normal hosts; response to therapy is generally good	Immune status
Chronic pulmonary	Response to therapy is generally good Blastomycosis	Immune status Underlying lung disease
Disseminated	Response to therapy generally good	Immune status Site of involvement
Granulomatous mediastinitis	May result in significant airway obstruction	Time to diagnosis Extent of inflammatory reaction Response to steroid therapy
Fibrosing mediastinitis	Generally poor despite antifungal or steroid therapy	Time to diagnosis Extent of fibrosis

Granulomatous Mediastinitis

- Represents a hyperimmune response with bulky enlargement of mediastinal lymph nodes due to granulomatous inflammation from active disease. Chest pain, hemoptysis and dyspnea may occur secondarily to nodal compression of the airways, superior vena cava or pulmonary vessels. Symptoms are typically mild and resolve within a few months.

Fibrosing Mediastinitis

- Rare hyperimmune response characterized by a slowly progressive and extensive fibrosis in reaction to prior episode of histoplasmosis. Most patients are between 20 and 40 years of age and exhibit night sweats, cough, dyspnea, chest pain and hemoptysis. Usually progresses to involve structures adjacent to the mediastinal lymph nodes, including the heart and great vessels, upper airways and esophagus.

Key Laboratory and Radiologic Features

Acute Pulmonary
Labs
- WBC is variable.

- Elevated serum alkaline phosphatase.

Radiology
- Hilar adenopathy.

- Patchy infiltrates that evolve to calcification.

- Radiographic findings in histoplasmosis may be similar to sarcoidosis. Histoplasmosis must be excluded before treating patients with immunosuppressive agents.

Chronic Pulmonary
Labs
- Anemia in 50%.

- Elevated alkaline phosphatase in 30%.

- Elevated WBC in 30%.

Radiology
- Cavitary lesions with thin or thick walls are seen in the upper lobes.

- Minimal or no hilar or mediastinal adenopathy.

Disseminated in AIDS
Labs
- Anemia.

- Pancytopenia.

- Elevated alkaline phosphatase.

- Marked LDH elevation.

Radiology
- Reticulonodular infiltrates.

- Mediastinal adenopathy.

- CXR may be normal in 30%.

Disseminated in Infants
Labs
- Severe anemia.

- Pancytopenia.

- Elevated bilirubin.

- Elevated alkaline phosphatase.

Radiology
- Diffuse patchy pneumonitis.

- Hilar and mediastinal adenopathy.

Therapeutic Options

Acute Pulmonary
Mild to moderate
- Treatment is usually unnecessary in immunocompetent hosts.

- Itraconazole loading dose of 200 mg every 8 hours for 3 days followed by 200-400 mg/d for 6-12 weeks.

Severe
- Lipid AmB 3 mg/kg/d or AmB deoxycholate 0.7 mg/kg/d ± prednisone 60 mg/d for 2 weeks followed by itraconazole 200-400 mg/d for 12 weeks.

Chronic Pulmonary

Mild to moderate

- Itraconazole loading dose of 200 mg every 8 hours for 3 days followed by 200-400 mg/d 1-2 years; 75%-85% response rate.

Severe disease or itraconazole failure

- Lipid AmB 3 mg/kg per day or AmB 0.7 deoxycholate mg/kg/d, then itraconazole 200 mg/d for 1-2 years; >95% effective.

Disseminated

CNS meningitis

- Lipid AmB 3 mg/kg /d or AmB deoxycholate 0.7-1.0 mg/kg/d for 3 months followed by fluconazole 200-400 mg/d for 1 year.

Non-CNS

Mild to moderate

- Non-AIDS: Itraconazole 200 mg/d for 6-18 months; >95% effective.

- AIDS: Itraconazole 200 mg/d indefinitely.

Severe

- Non-AIDS: AmB deoxycholate 0.7-1.0 mg/kg/d or lipid AmB 3-5 mg/kg/d initially, followed by itraconazole 200-400 mg/d for 6-18 months.

- AIDS: AmB induction prior to itraconazole 200 mg/d indefinitely.

Granulomatous Mediastinitis

- Treatment is usually unnecessary in immunocompetent hosts.

- Itraconazole loading dose of 200 mg every 8 hours for three days followed by 200-400 mg/d for 6-12 weeks for symptomatic cases.

- Surgical resection of bulky nodes should be considered in patients with persistent obstructive symptoms following antifungal therapy.

Fibrosing Mediastinitis

- Antifungal therapy is generally felt to be of little benefit in late fibrotic stage; if ESR and CF titers are elevated, antifungal therapy (itraconazole 200-400 mg/d for 12 weeks) may be beneficial; corticosteroid therapy is not recommended; surgical and surgical stents to relieve obstruction may be considered in special cases.

ID Board Pearls

- AIDS-defining illness in HIV positive patients.

- Associated with bilateral hilar adenopathy and cavitary lesions (like coccidiomycosis).

- Associated with peripheral eosinophilia (like coccidiomycosis), which distinguishes histoplasmosis from tuberculosis.

- Mouth ulcers frequently present and scrapings usually reveal organisms.

- Mucous membrane and gastrointestinal lesions may present with bleeding in disseminated disease in immunocompromised hosts.

5. Cryptococcosis

Microbiology

- The causative organism, *Cryptococcus neoformans*, is monomorphic yeast in tissue and culture. The mucopolysaccharide capsule plays a key role in pathogenesis in addition to providing a distinctive appearance in clinical specimens.

Epidemiology

- Worldwide distribution; most associated with pigeon debris and feces without causing avian disease.

- Infection follows inhalation of fungi; approximately 60% of patients have an initial subclinical course.

- High predilection to invade the central nervous system.

- Disease is typically more frequent in immunocompromised hosts, but also occurs in patients with no demonstrable underlying immune defects.

Treatment

- Asymptomatic immunocompetent hosts with culture positive pulmonary infection without evidence of CNS involvement can be monitored carefully without antifungal therapy.

- Patients with progressive pulmonary infiltrates can be treated with fluconazole for 3-6 months when disease is mild and there is no evidence of disseminated disease, including any spread to the CNS.

- If flucytosine (5FC) is administered for more than 2 weeks, renal function should be monitored carefully and doses adjusted by nomogram or, preferably, by a serum level obtained 2 hours after administration of a dose. Optimal levels are 30-80 mcg/mL.

- Management of increased intracranial pressure (ICP) is important in reducing morbidity and mortality in HIV-infected patients with cryptococcal meningitis.

- Maintain ICP ≤20 cm H_2O with daily CSF drainage. Persistent elevated pressure may require a lumbar drain or ventriculoperitoneal shunt.

- Corticosteroids are not recommended in HIV-infected patients with increased ICP due to cryptococcal meningitis.

Key Clinical Features

Pulmonary
- May be asymptomatic. Typical symptoms include low-grade fever, weight loss, and dull chest pain with scant productive cough and dyspnea. Severe disease with respiratory failure is more common in immunocompromised patients.

CNS
- May occur in isolation without evidence of prior pulmonary involvement or in a setting of disseminated disease. Clinical presentation may be acute or chronic. Nonspecific symptoms include headache and nausea. Patient may be afebrile with minimal meningeal signs. Papilledema is seen in approximately 30% and cranial nerve palsies are seen in 20% of patients. Altered mental status can range from mild behavioral changes to obtundation.

Disseminated
- Painless, morphologically variable skin lesions are seen in about 10% of cases. Osteolytic bony foci can be seen in about 10% of cases. Unusual reported sites include eye, heart, GI (including liver), GU (including epididymitis, prostatitis and orchitis) and arthritis.

Key Laboratory and Radiologic Features

Pulmonary
Labs
- Routine laboratory studies are nonspecific.

- Sputum culture sensitivity is 10%-30% in active disease. May require lung biopsy to demonstrate tissue invasion.

- Serum cryptococcal antigen may be positive in isolated pulmonary disease.

- If the serum cryptococcal antigen is positive, a lumbar puncture with CSF evaluation should be performed to rule out CNS disease.

Radiology
- Variety of findings, including nonspecific interstitial pattern, solitary nodules or focal infiltrates.

- Pleural effusions and cavitary formation are uncommon.

CNS
Labs
- Routine laboratory studies are nonspecific.

- CSF formula reveals lymphocytic pleocytosis with low glucose and high protein.

- India ink usually demonstrates the encapsulated yeast.

- CSF and serum cryptococcal antigen are usually positive. Serum cryptococcal antigen may be more sensitive than CSF.

- AIDS patients may present with a noninflammatory cellular response. A poor clinical outcome can be predicted by a CSF cell count of less than 20 WBC, greater than 1:2024 antigen titer and an altered mental status.

Radiology
- Hydrocephalus may be seen on head CT.

Disseminated
Labs
- Blood culture and serum cryptococcal antigen may be positive.

- Nonspecific.

- Serum cryptococcal antigen is usually positive.

Radiology
- Depends on organ involvement; can appear as tumors on imaging.

Differential Diagnosis

- **Infectious Pulmonary**
  * Blastomycosis
  * Histoplasmosis
  * Coccidioidomycosis
  * Paracoccidioidomycosis
  * Tuberculosis
  * *Pneumocystis jiroveci (carinii)* pneumonia

- **Noninfectious Pulmonary**
  * Neoplasms
  * SLE
  * Sarcoidosis

- **Infectious CNS**
  * Tuberculous meningitis
  * Viral meningitis
  * Viral meningoencephalitis
  * Histoplasmosis
  * Blastomycosis

- **Noninfectious CNS**
  * Mollaret's meningitis
  * Drug-induced meningitis
  * Vasculitides

- **Infectious Disseminated**
  * Blastomycosis
  * Histoplasmosis
  * Coccidioidomycosis
  * Tuberculosis

- **Noninfectious Disseminated**
  * Neoplasms

Therapeutic Options in HIV-Negative Patients

Pulmonary
Mild to moderate symptoms
- Fluconazole 200-400 mg/d for 6-12 months.

- Itraconazole 200-400 mg/d for 6-12 months.

- Lipid preparation 3-5 mg/kg/d or AmB deoxycholate 0.7 mg/kg/d (total dose 1-2 g) for 6-10 weeks.

Severe symptoms and immunocompromised hosts
- Lipid preparation 3-5 mg/kg/d or AmB deoxycholate 0.7 mg/kg/d plus flucytosine 100 mg/kg/d for 2 weeks, then fluconazole 400 mg/d for at least 10 weeks.

- Lipid preparation 3-5 mg/kg/d or AmB deoxycholate 0.7 mg/kg/d + flucytosine 100/kg/d for 6-10 weeks.

- Lipid preparation 3-5 mg/kg/d or AmB deoxycholate 0.7 mg/kg/d for 6-10 weeks.

Therapeutic Options in HIV-infected Patients

Pulmonary
Mild to moderate
- Fluconazole 200-400 mg/d indefinitely.

- Itraconazole 200-400 mg/d indefinitely.

- Fluconazole 400 mg/d *plus* flucytosine 100-150 mg/kg/d for 10 weeks.

CNS
- Lipid preparation 3-5 mg/kg/d or AmB deoxycholate 0.7-1.0 mg/kg/d *plus* flucytosine 100 mg/kg/d for 2 weeks, then fluconazole 400 mg/d for at least 10 weeks.

- Lipid preparation 3-5 mg/kg/d or AmB deoxycholate 0.7-1.0 mg/kg/d *plus* flucytosine 100 mg/kg/d 6-10 weeks.

- Lipid preparation 3-5 mg/kg/d or AmB deoxycholate 0.7 mg/kg/d for 6-10 weeks.

- Fluconazole 400-800 mg/d for 10-12 weeks.

- Fluconazole 400-800 mg/d *plus* flucytosine 100-150 mg/kg/d for 6 weeks.

Maintenance therapy
- Fluconazole, 200-400 mg PO QD, until CD4+ count ≥300.

- Itraconazole, 200 mg PO BID, until CD4+ count ≥300.

- Lipid AmB 5 mg/kg or AmB deoxycholate 1 mg/kg IV 1-3 times weekly, until CD4+ count ≥300.

ID Board Pearls

- Skin lesions of disseminated disease mimic molluscum contagiosum.

- Cryptococcal pneumonia does not produce cavitary lesions.

- Risk factors for cryptococcal meningitis include HIV/AIDS, organ transplant, cancer, sarcoidosis, corticosteroid therapy, diabetes mellitus, COPD, cirrhosis, rheumatoid arthritis, SLE, pregnancy and splenectomy.

- Intracranial hypertension needs to be monitored and aggressively managed with daily lumbar puncture or shunt, if necessary.

6. Coccidioidomycosis

Synonyms

• Valley fever.

Microbiology

• The causative organism is the dimorphic fungus *Coccidioides immitis*; it exists as a saprophytic mycelium in the environment. Arthroconidia form from the mycelia and break away, either to return to the soil or to become airborne and potentially inhaled. In the tissues, the arthroconidia develop into spherules that contain endospores; each endospore has the potential to form a new spherule.

• Growth occurs rapidly (3-4 days) in the laboratory without special requirements. Laboratory personnel should be informed that coccidioidomycosis is suspected so proper caution can be used when handling cultures of the highly infectious mycelial forms.

Epidemiology

• Endemic in soil of southwestern United States including California, western Texas, New Mexico and Arizona. It is also found in some areas of Mexico and Central and South America.

• Primary infection is via inhalation of arthroconidia.

• Approximately 100,000 cases are reported per year in the United States. Outbreaks have been associated with conditions that disturb the soil and periods when there is rain/drought cycling.

• At-risk populations for disseminated disease include immunocompromised hosts (infants, patients receiving any immunosuppressive therapy, pregnant patients, AIDS patients) and those of African or Filipino ancestry.

Diagnosis

• IgM antibodies can be measured by various methods, are usually positive within 3 weeks of primary infection and disappear within 4 months.

• IgG antibodies are complement-fixing and tend to occur later in illness, correlate more closely with disease activity and persist for 6-8 months.

• IgG titers can be used to determine responsiveness to therapy and to predict relapses.

Therapy

• Although the majority of normal hosts spontaneously resolve early infection without therapy, some patients may benefit from antifungal treatment. The decision to treat may be based on several clinical factors:

  * Greater than 10% body weight loss

  * Night sweats for greater than 3 weeks

  * Infiltrates in more than 50% of one lung or portions of both lungs

  * Persistent or prominent hilar adenopathy

  * Complement-fixation antibody titer greater than 1:16

  * Anergic to coccidioidal antigens

  * Inability to work

  * Persistent symptoms for more than 2 months

• All immunocompromised hosts or patients at risk for dissemination should be treated.

• Relapse following a course of therapy occurs in approximately one-third of all patients and most often at site of initial infection. The decision to treat patients with prolonged or indefinite therapy is based on the precarious location of the initial infection and immune status.

• Coccidioidal meningitis is the most lethal complication of disseminated infection and requires early diagnosis and aggressive treatment. Without therapy, the mortality is greater than 95% within 2 years.

Table 7

Differential Diagnosis for Coccidioidomycosis

Type	Infectious	Noninfectious
Acute pulmonary	Viral upper respiratory infection Viral or bacterial sinusitis Viral or bacterial tracheobronchitis Rickettsial diseases *P jiroveci (carinii) pneumonia*	Asthma Drug-induced hypersensitivity pneumonitis
Solitary pulmonary nodule	Early lung abscess Blastomycosis Histoplasmosis Tuberculosis	Neoplasm
Cavitary lung disease	Early lung abscess Tuberculosis	Sarcoidosis Neoplasm
Chronic fibrocavitary disease	Blastomycosis Histoplasmosis Coccidioidomycosis Paracoccidioidomycosis Tuberculosis	Sarcoidosis Neoplasm
Disseminated CNS	Tuberculous meningitis Viral meningitis Viral meningoencephalitis Other fungal pathogens	Mollaret's meningitis Drug-induced meningitis SLE Granulomatous angiitis
Non-CNS Skin	Syphilis Actinomycosis Tuberculosis	Neoplasm Sarcoidosis
Osteoarticular	Fungal pathogens Mycobacterial pathogens Bacterial pathogen	Trauma Gout Osteoarthritis

Table 8

Key Diagnostic Tests for Coccidioidomycosis

Type	Microbiology	Serology
Acute pulmonary disease	Sputum 40%-70% positive	IgM 90% positive within 3 weeks IgG 50% positive within 3 months
Solitary pulmonary nodule	Sputum culture is typically negative	IgG and IgM may both be negative if primary infection is remote
Cavitary lung disease	Sputum culture may be positive	IgG and IgM may both be negative if primary infection is remote
Chronic fibrocavitary disease	Sputum KOH and culture usually positive	IgM may be positive IgG usually positive
Disseminated disease		Elevated IgG titer is hallmark of disseminated disease
Meningitis	CSF culture 15% positive	CSF IgG 75% positive

Table 9

Complications of Coccidioidomycosis

Type	Clinical outcome	Prognostic factors
Acute pulmonary	Majority of patients resolve primary infection in weeks to months	Immune status Initial spore burden
Solitary pulmonary nodule	Excellent	Immune status
Cavitary lung disease	Generally good	Immune status
Chronic fibrocavitary disease	Progressive pulmonary decline	Early diagnosis and treatment Severity of underlying lung disease Immune status
Disseminated CNS	Significant neurologic sequelae usually occur; associated with high morbidity and mortality	Immune status Early and aggressive therapy Underlying comorbid diseases
Non-CNS Skin	Generally good	Immune status Early diagnosis and treatment
Osteoarticular	Joint infection typically responds well to antifungal therapy; may require surgical debridement of synovial tissue. Vertebral osteomyelitis may require surgical debridement to stabilize neurologic function	Immune status Early diagnosis and treatment

Table 10

Therapeutic Options for Coccidioidomycosis

Type	Preferred	Alternative
Acute pulmonary	Infection usually resolves without therapy	Azole therapy for 3-6 months Itraconazole 200 mg BID Fluconazole 400-800 mg/d Ketoconazole 400 mg/d
Solitary pulmonary nodule	Surgical resection	Adjuvant azole therapy for 3-6 months if resection of nodule is incomplete or reactivation of disease occurs
Cavitary lung disease	Azole therapy for 3-6 months in symptomatic patients	Surgical resection of cavity may be necessary if patient remains symptomatic following multiple courses of azole therapy
Chronic fibrocavitary disease	Azole therapy for 12 months Switch to alternative azole or increase dosage in refractory cases	AmB deoxycholate 0.7-1.0 mg/kg/d for 1-2 grams total or lipid formulation 3-5 mg/kg/day for azole-refractory cases
Disseminated CNS	Azole therapy indefinitely Fluconazole 400 mg/d Itraconazole 400-600 mg/d	Adjuvant intrathecal AmB
Non-CNS	Azole therapy for 12 months; treatment should continue indefinitely in HIV-infected patients Itraconazole 200 mg BID (may be more effective in skeletal infection) Fluconazole 400 mg/d Ketoconazole 400 mg/d	For patients whose disease progresses on azoles, or who are intolerant to azoles, can be treated with AmB

Key Clinical Features

Acute Pulmonary

- Subclinical disease occurs in 60%; remainder develop flu-like illness with fever, malaise, night sweats, cough, dyspnea and pleuritic chest pain 1-3 weeks following exposure ("Valley fever"). Other manifestations include a maculopapular rash and arthralgias ("desert rheumatism"), erythema nodosum or erythema multiforme. The latter usually resolves without therapy in normal hosts.

Solitary Pulmonary Nodule

- May result with 5% of infections; typically is asymptomatic, but may present with chest pain, cough and hemoptysis.

Cavitary Lung Disease

- Occurs in up to 8% of infections; arises in setting of infarcted tissue during primary infection; typically thin-walled, solitary, and peripheral; patients usually asymptomatic, but may present with chest pain, cough and hemoptysis. Cavities can also form after a nodule liquifies and drains into a bronchus.

Chronic Fibrocavitary Disease

- Failure to resolve initial infection; characterized by progressive pulmonary disease, weight loss, fatigue, night sweats, shortness of breath, chest pain, productive cough and hemoptysis. Frequently seen in diabetes.

Disseminated
CNS

- Persistent severe headache and intention tremors. Cerebral infarction can occur late in the disease secondary to arteritis.

Non-CNS
Skin

- Lesions have variable appearance but are typically wart-like and have a predilection for the nasolabial fold.

Osteoarticular

- Bone or joint involvement is seen in approximately 30% of disseminated disease.

- Bone disease is unifocal in 60% of cases, with the skull, metacarpals, metatarsals, spine and tibia being the most frequently involved sites. In contrast, vertebral involvement is typically multifocal with predilection for the ileum and sacrum. Most critical complication results from spread to the meninges.

- Over 90% of joint infections are monarticular. The knee and ankle are the most frequently involved sites. Arthritis is characterized by marked synovitis.

Key Laboratory and Radiographic Features

Acute Pulmonary
Labs

- Nonspecific.

- ESR elevation.

- Eosinophilia >5% in 25% of patients.

Radiology

- Normal in 50% of patients.

- Unilateral infiltrate with ipsilateral adenopathy.

Solitary Pulmonary Nodule
Labs

- Nonspecific.

Radiology

- Nodules are usually peripheral and 2-3 cm in diameter.

Cavitary Lung Disease
Labs

- Nonspecific.

Radiology

- Cavities are very thin-walled with no associated infiltrate; usually 2-3 cm in diameter and are located on the lung periphery.

Chronic Fibrocavitary Disease
Labs

- Nonspecific.

Radiology
• Bilateral nodular densities, cavitation and hilar adenopathy.

Disseminated
CNS
Labs
• Lymphocytic pleocytosis.

• Elevated CSF protein.

• Decreased CSF glucose.

Radiology
• MRI head may show evidence of arteritis or infarct.

Non-CNS
Labs
Skin

• Nonspecific.

Radiology
Osteoarticular
• Bone lesions most commonly osteolytic; bone scans more sensitive than plain films in detecting lesions.

ID Board Pearls

• Coccidioidomycosis may present as erythema nodosa during the early phase of disease.

• Associated with bilateral hilar adenopathy and cavitary lesions (like histoplasmosis).

• Associated with peripheral eosinophilia (like histoplasmosis) which distinguishes coccidiomycosis from tuberculosis.

• CNS disease is difficult to treat and may require long term azole therapy.

7. Sporotrichosis

Microbiology

• The causative organism is *Sporothrix schenckii*.

• Characteristic cigar-shaped yeast form is difficult to identify in clinical specimens.

• The presence of Splendore-Hoeppli bodies, although not diagnostic, is notably associated with sporotrichosis and can provide an important presumptive clue.

• Diagnosis based on recovery of organism from tissue and fluids from infected sites.

Epidemiology

• Worldwide distribution; majority of cases are reported from tropical and subtropical areas.

• Found in the soil, decaying vegetation, plants, and plant products such as commercial sphagnum moss, straw, wood and mulch.

• High-risk activities associated with environmental exposure to fungus include gardening, farming, hay baling and carpentry.

• Cutaneous inoculation has occurred from animals, including cats, armadillos, dogs, birds and insect bites.

• Classically presents as a cutaneous or lymphocutaneous syndrome in immunocompetent hosts with occupational or recreational exposure to fungus.

• Extra cutaneous disease is associated with underlying immunodeficiency; most often seen in patients with AIDS, alcoholism, chronic obstructive pulmonary disease and diabetes.

Key Clinical Features

Fixed Cutaneous
Direct inoculation
• Limited to skin, often on face or trunk; appears as plaque-like or verrucous lesion at site of inoculation; onset after inoculation is days to a few weeks.

Table 11

Complications of Sporotrichosis

Type	Clinical outcome	Prognostic factors
Cutaneous and lymphocutaneous	Spontaneous resolution has been reported; however, it is recommended that all patients receive therapy. Most commonly occurs in immunocompetent hosts with excellent outcome. Dissemination is rare. Potential superinfection of nodular or ulcerative lesions	Immune status Prompt diagnosis and therapy
Osteoarticular	Typically associated with a poor functional outcome due to delays in diagnosis, but is not life-threatening. Characterized by progressive deterioration of joint function despite therapy. Increased risk for disease extension to contiguous structures and beyond in immunocompromised hosts	Early diagnosis with prompt therapy Immune status
Pulmonary	Indolent and progressive pulmonary decline in untreated patients. Response to therapy varies with prognostic factors	Early diagnosis and prompt therapy Extent of disease Underlying lung disease Underlying comorbid diseases Immune status
Disseminated	Rare manifestation; associated with significant morbidity and mortality	Early diagnosis and prompt therapy Immune status Extent of disease
Meningeal	Rare manifestation; associated with significant morbidity and mortality	Early diagnosis and prompt therapy Immune status

Lymphocutaneous
Direct inoculation
- Initial lesion is papular and develops days to weeks after exposure; evolves to erythematous nodules that may ulcerate; lesions are not typically suppurative or tender; similar lesions progress along regional lymphatics proximal to site of inoculation; systemic symptoms are not typically seen.

Pulmonary
Inhalation
- Associated with alcoholism; unusual manifestation; presents as subacute to chronic pneumonia with nonspecific symptoms and signs such as fever, night sweats, weight loss, dyspnea, cough with purulent sputum and hemoptysis. Mimics pulmonary TB and other chronic fungal infections.

Osteoarticular
Hematogenous or direct inoculation
- Arthritis (single or multiple) is the predominant presentation, with or without cutaneous lesions; when osteomyelitis is seen, it usually affects bone contiguous to an infected joint. Commonly affected joints are the knee, elbow, wrist, ankle and hand joints; tenosynovitis and bursitis have been reported.

Disseminated
Direct inoculation or inhalation
- Uncommon, seen primarily in patients with AIDS; fever, night sweats and weight loss; diffuse lymphocutaneous ulcerative lesions; visceral involvement can occur as well.

Meningea
Hematogenous
- Presents as chronic meningitis with fever, altered mental status; usually seen in disseminated disease, but can occur as isolated involvement; seen in severely immunocompromised patients.

Key Laboratory and Radiographic Features

Microbiology
- Fungal stains and culture from infected sites frequently are positive. However, CSF KOH and culture are often negative in meningeal disease.

- Large volumes (20-30 mL) of CSF obtained on three different occasions maximize the yield of organism in culture.

Laboratory
- Routine tests are nonspecific.

- CSF reveals lymphocytic pleocytosis with elevated protein in meningeal disease.

Serology
- Serologic testing is not accessible for routine use.

Radiology
- Chest radiograph findings in pulmonary disease include unilateral or bilateral upper lobe cavitary lesions with degrees of fibrosis and nodular densities.

Differential Diagnosis

Cutaneous/Lymphocutaneous
- *Infectious*

  * Nocardiosis

  * Mycobacterium marinum

  * Leishmaniasis

  * Tularemia

  * Blastomycosis

  * Phaeohyphomycosis

  * Paracoccidioidomycosis

- *Noninfectious*

  * Sarcoidosis

  * Neoplasm

Pulmonary
- *Infectious*
  * Tuberculosis

  * Blastomycosis

* Histoplasmosis

* Coccidioidomycosis

• *Noninfectious*
   * Sarcoidosis

Osteoarticular
• *Infectious*
   * Tuberculosis

   * Blastomycosis

   * Histoplasmosis

   * Candidiasis

• *Noninfectious*
   * Degenerative joint disease

Disseminated
• *Infectious*
   * Tuberculosis

   * Blastomycosis

   * Nocardiosis

• *Noninfectious*
   * Neoplasm

Meningeal
• *Infectious*
   * Tuberculosis

   * Other fungal pathogens

• *Noninfectious*
   * Vasculitides including SLE, GA (granulomatous angiitis)

   * Drug-induced meningitis

Therapeutic Options

Cutaneous and Lymphocutaneous
Preferred
• Itraconazole 100-200 mg/d for 2-4 weeks after all lesions have resolved, usually for 3-6 months total; efficacy is >90%; associated with potential drug interactions.

• Terbinafine, 500 mg BID for patients who do not respond to itraconazole.

Alternative
• 1-SSKI increasing from 5-50 drops/d TID as tolerated for 3-6 months or until 1 month after lesions have resolved.

• Low cost and generally effective.

• Inconvenient dosing frequency and metallic taste; associated with allergic reactions, salivary gland enlargement and GI intolerance.

• Fluconazole 400 mg/d for 6 months; can be used if intolerant of other therapy; less efficacious than itraconazole or SSKI; duration of therapy is longer.

• Local hyperthermia (42-43°C) daily (at least 40 minutes per treatment) for 2-3 months. Low cost with no risk of drug exposure, can be used as adjunctive therapy with itraconazole; dedicated adherence is difficult due to length of time required for treatment response; can be considered when azole therapy is not possible, such as in pregnancy.

• AmB is effective but risk:benefit not justified in a localized non-life-threatening infection.

Pulmonary
Preferred
• Lipid AmB 3-5 mg/kg/d or AmB deoxycholate 0.7-1.0 mg/kg/d for 1-2 g total dose; outcome is generally poor due to underlying lung disease and delay in diagnosis.

• Itraconazole 200 mg orally BID for 12 months after patent has favorable response to AmB.

- In severe life-threatening disease, AmB plus surgical resection appears to be the most effective therapy, if tolerated based on underlying lung disease.

Alternative
- Itraconazole 200 BID if AmB not tolerated or if less severe disease is present; outcome generally poor due to underlying lung disease and delays in diagnosis.

Osteoarticular
Preferred
- Itraconazole 200 BID for 12 months; efficacy is 60%-80%.

Alternative
- Lipid AmB 3-5 mg/kg/d or AmB deoxycholate 0.7-1.0 mg/kg/d for 1-2 g total dose is recommended in extensive disease; efficacy is 60%-80% but is only used if itraconazole fails because of higher intolerance.

Disseminated
- Lipid AmB 3-5 mg/kg/d preferred.

- Itraconazole 200 BID recommended as step-down therapy after patient responds to AmB for 12 months of therapy.

- In AIDS, itraconazole 200 BID for lifelong suppression.

Meningeal
- Lipid AmB 3-5 mg/kg/d preferred but AmB deoxycholate 0.7-1.0 mg/kg/d; in AIDS, itraconazole 200 BID for lifelong suppression.

ID Board Pearls

- Sporotrichosis is generally an indolent infection that requires prolonged therapy.

- Due to the temperature sensitivity of the fungus, local application of hyperthermia can be used in pregnant women for the treatment of cutaneous lesions.

- Pulmonary sporotrichosis may present with thin-walled cavitary lesions (like coccidiomycosis).

8. Paracoccidioidomycosis

Synonyms

- South American blastomycosis, Lutz's mycosis.

Microbiology

- Causative organism is *Paracoccidioides brasiliensis*.

- Yeast forms vary in size and exhibit multiple budding in clinical specimens.

- "Pilot's wheel" appearance is due to the arrangement of the smaller budding cells attached to the larger mother cell with interspersed lipid globules.

Epidemiology

- Endemic to some, but not all areas in Central and South America. Majority of cases (80%) are reported from Brazil, followed by Colombia and Venezuela. All reported cases from outside an endemic area had once lived or visited an endemic area; latency in some cases was as long as 15 years.

- Habitat is elusive, but is presumed to be in the highly humid soil. Inhalation of spores is the primary route of infection.

- No evidence for person-to-person spread; outbreaks have not been reported.

- Most cases occur in men (15:1) between 30-60 years of age. When seen in younger patients (13% of cases), the gender difference diminishes. Estrogens are thought to block conidia from yeast transformation in the infected host.

- Risk factors associated with infection include having a history of agricultural occupation, smoking, alcoholism and malnutrition.

- Infection can result from a primary focus without a latency period or from endogenous reactivation of quiescent foci.

Key Clinical Features

Primary Infection
• Lung.

• Most infections are subclinical.

Acute Juvenile Form
• Extensive infection of liver, spleen, lymph nodes and bone marrow; lung involvement is minimal.

• Clinical course develops in subacute pattern of weeks to months; patients are severely ill with fever, malaise, weight loss and lymphadenopathy. Abdominal pain related to colonic obstruction from enlarged mesenteric nodes can be seen.

Chronic Adult Form
• Lungs involved in 90% of cases; concomitant extrapulmonary involvement is common, including mucous membranes, skin, reticuloendothelial system and adrenals.

• Markedly chronic course of months to years with nonspecific complaints of cough, weight loss, fever; skin and mucous membrane lesions of the face, oral and nasal mucosa may be large, verrucous or ulcerative.

Key Laboratory and Radiographic Features

Microbiology
• KOH smear has 93% sensitivity. Characteristic "Pilot's wheel" morphology of yeast cells from lipid globules.

Laboratory
• Routine tests are nonspecific.

Serology
• Immunodiffusion serology is 95% sensitive and specific, but remains positive for years.

• Complement fixation test is most useful following response to therapy.

Radiology
• CXR reveals bilateral and symmetric disease with patchy infiltrates and nodular densities; cavities can develop, but hilar adenopathy is uncommon.

Differential Diagnosis

Acute Juvenile Form
• *Infectious*
   * Tuberculosis

   * Blastomycosis

   * Leishmaniasis

• *Noninfectious*
   * Lymphoproliferative disease

Chronic adult form
• *Infectious*
   * Tuberculosis

   * Blastomycosis

   * Histoplasmosis

   * MOTT, including *Mycobacterium leprae*

   * Leishmaniasis

   * Syphilis

• *Noninfectious*
   * Neoplasm

   * Sarcoidosis

   * Crohn's disease

Therapeutic Options

Acute Juvenile Form
Preferred
• Itraconazole 100 mg/d for 6 months.

Alternative
• Ketoconazole 200-400 mg/d for 12 months.

• Fluconazole 200-400 mg/d for 12 months.

• Lipid AmB 3-5 mg/kg/d or AmB deoxycholate 0.7 mg/kg/d for 3-4 months ± follow-up therapy with sulfadiazine to decrease relapse rate.

• Sulfadiazine 6 g/d for 3-5 years.

Chronic Adult Form

Preferred

• Itraconazole 200 mg/d for 6 months.

Alternative

• Ketoconazole 200-400 mg/d for 12 months.

• Fluconazole 200-400 mg/d for 12 months.

• Lipid AmB 3-5 mg/kg/d or AmB deoxycholate 0.7 mg/kg/d for 3-4 months ± follow-up therapy with sulfadiazine to decrease relapse rate.

• Sulfadiazine 6 g/d for 3-5 years.

Complications

Acute Juvenile Form

• Behaves as a lymphoproliferative disorder; associated with significant short-term mortality.

• Prognostic factors include early diagnosis, nutritional status and immune status.

Chronic Adult Form

• Chronic course from months to years.

• Relapse rate up to 30% despite therapy.

• Sequelae from fibrotic healing include cor pulmonale, cardiac constriction, and stenosis of glottis and trachea.

• Prognostic factors include early diagnosis, nutritional status, underlying comorbid disease, immune status and development of critical fibrotic sequelae.

ID Board Pearls

• Prognosis of paracoccidioidomycosis is good when treated, however treatment regimens are very long and relapse is frequent.

• Granulomatous inflammation with many giant cells containing organism.

• Focal area of central caseation mixed with pyogenic abscesses are usually present.

• Organism may be seen in clinical specimens with multiple small buds.

9. Emerging Infections

• **Penicilliosis**

  * **Microbiology:** Thermally dimorphic organism Penicillium marneffei

  * **Epidemiology:** Disease of immunocompromised individuals living in or traveling to Southeast Asia.

  * **Diagnosis:** Culture.

  * **Therapy:** AmB for severely ill patients for 2 months, less severe disease or those who have responded to AmB may be treated with itraconazole; HIV/AIDS patients, suppressive therapy with itraconazole.

  * **Clinical manifestations:**

    • Similar to disseminated histoplasmosis.

    • Primary portal of entry is the lungs with hematologic dissemination.

    • Diffuse papular lesions similar to molluscum contagiosum are common in HIV/AIDS patients.

    • Small yeast cells may be seen on histopathologic examination.

• **Fusariosis**

  * **Microbiology:** Invasive mold infection associated with *Fusarium* species, most commonly *F solani*.

  * **Diagnosis:** Blood cultures are positive in up to 50% of cases; presence of a mold in blood cultures obtained from neutropenic patients should be suggestive for fusariosis

  * **Therapy:**

    • Fusarium species are often highly resistant to many antifungal agents.

    • AmB in high doses is most commonly used therapy and has met with limited success.

    • Most clinicians prefer therapy with voriconazole, IV loading dose: 6 mg/kg every 12 hours for 2 doses; followed by maintenance dose of 4 mg/kg every 12 hours successful in a small number of patients.

    • Therapy is continued until the neutropenia has resolved and a clinical response is documented. Prognosis for disseminated infection is related to reversal of the neutropenia.

  * **Clinical manifestations:**

    • Skin and respiratory tract are the primary portals of entry for Fusarium.

    • Localized skin infections may occur at sites of trauma in immunocompetent hosts.

    • Disseminated disease from the skin or gastrointestinal tract occurs in immunocompromised patients.

    • Clinical presentation is generally nonspecific with fever and skin lesions which eventually necrose and appear similar to ecthyma gangrenosum.

    • Radiography and pathology: similar to invasive aspergillosis or zygomycosis.

• **Pseudallescheriasis (Scedosporosis)**

  * **Microbiology:** Pseudoallescheria boydii, Scedosporium apiospermum (the asexual form of P boydii) and S prolificans recognized as emerging pathogens.

  * **Diagnosis:** Hyphal elements seen in the tissues of patients with Pseudoallescheria and Scedosporium infection resemble Aspergillus, including intravascular invasion.

  * **Clinical manifestations:**

- Rare causes of sinopulmonary infections in immunocompetent hosts and may present as fungus balls in the lungs or paranasal sinuses.

- Severe pneumonia, invasive sinusitis and hematogenous dissemination, including brain abscesses, occur in immunosuppressed hosts, especially bone marrow transplant patients.

* **Therapy:**

- Treatment outcome is poor and most patients with disseminated disease die.

- Amphotericin B is not effective in the treatment of pseudallescheriasis or scedosporosis.

- Voriconazole IV loading dose: 6 mg/kg every 12 hours for 2 doses; followed by maintenance dose of 4 mg/kg every 12 hours may be effective.

- Surgical debridement and drainage of abscesses may also be necessary.

10. Further Reading

Books and Book Chapters

Anaissie EJ, McGinnis MR, Pfaller MA. *Clinical Mycology*. New York, NY: Churchill Livingstone; 2003.

Chapman SW. Sullivan, DC. Blastomyces dermatitidis. In: Mandell GL, Gordon DR, Bennett JE, Dolin R, eds. *Principles and Practice of Infectious Diseases*. 7th ed. New York, NY: Churchill Livingstone; in Press.

Chapman SW, Sullivan DC. Diagnosis and treatment of blastomycosis. In: Hospenthal DR, Rinaldi MG, eds. *Diagnosis and Treatment of Human Mycoses*. Totowa, NJ: Humana Press Inc; 2008: 277-293.

Chapman SW, Sullivan DC. Blastomycosis. In: Kasper A, Fauci D, Longo E, et al, eds. *Harrison's Principles of Internal Medicine*. 17th ed. New York, NY: McGraw Hill; 2008: 1249-1251.

Chapman SW, Sullivan DC. Miscellaneous mycoses and algal infections. In: Kasper A, Fauci D, Longo E, et al, eds. *Harrison's Principles of Internal Medicine*. 17th ed., New York, NY: McGraw Hill; 2008: 1263-1267.

Deepe GS. Histoplasma capsulatum. In: Mandell GL, Gordon DR, Bennett JE, Dolin R, eds. *Principles and Practice of Infectious Diseases*. 6th ed. Philadelphia, PA: Churchill Livingstone; 2005: 3012-3026.

Dismukes WE, Pappas PG, Sobel JD. *Clinical Mycology*. Oxford, England: Oxford University Press; 2003.

Edwards JE. Candida species. In: Mandell GL, Gordon DR, Bennett JE, Dolin R, eds. *Principles and Practice of Infectious Diseases*. 6th ed. Philadelphia, PA: Churchill Livingstone; 2005: 2938-2958.

Emmons CW, Binford CH, Utz JP, Kwon-Chung KJ. *Medical Mycology*. 3rd ed. Philadelphia, PA: Lea & Febiger; 1977.

Fleming RV, Anaissie EJ. Emerging fungal infections. In: Wingard JR, Anaissie EJ, eds. *Fungal Infections in the Immunocompromised Patient*. Boca Raton, FL: Taylor & Francis; 2005:311-340.

Frey D, Oldfield RJ, Bridger RC. *Color Atlas of Pathogenic Fungi*. Chicago, IL: Year Book Medical Publishers, Inc; 1979.

Galgiani J. Coccidioides species. In: Mandell GL, Gordon DR, Bennett JE, Dolin R, eds. *Principles and Practice of Infectious Diseases*. 6th ed. Philadelphia, PA: Churchill Livingstone; 2005: 3040-3051.

Larone DH. Medically Important Fungi. 4th ed. Washington, DC: ASM Press; 2002.

Perfect JR. Cryptococcus neoformans. In: Mandell GL, Gordon DR, Bennett JE, Dolin R, eds. *Principles and Practice of Infectious Diseases*. 6th ed. Philadelphia, PA: Churchill Livingstone; 2005: 2997-3012.

Restrepo A. Paracoccidioides brasiliensis. In: Mandell GL, Bennett JE, Gordon DR, Dolin R, eds. *Principles and Practice of Infectious Diseases*. 6th ed. Philadelphia, PA: Churchill Livingstone; 2005: 3062-3068.

Rex JH, Okhuysen PC. Sporothrix schenckii. In: Mandell GL, Gordon DR, Bennett JE, Dolin R, eds. *Principles and Practice of Infectious Diseases*. 6th ed. Philadelphia, PA: Churchill Livingstone; 2005: 2984-2988.

Sarosi GA, Davies SF. *Fungal Diseases of the Lung*. Orlando, FL: Grune & Stratton, Inc; 1986.

Sobel, JD. Candidiasis. In Hospenthal DR, Rinaldi MG, eds. *Diagnosis and Treatment of Human Mycoses*. Totowa, NJ: Humana Press Inc.; 2008: 137-162.

Journal Articles

Benard G, Duarte AJ. Paracoccidioidomycosis: a model for evaluation of the effects of human immunodeficiency virus infection on the natural history of endemic tropical diseases. *Clin Infect Dis*. 2000;31:1032-1039.

Blumberg HM, Jarvis WR, Soucie JM, et al. Risk factors for candidial bloodstream infections in surgical intensive care unit patients: the NEMIS prospective multicenter study. *Clin Infect Dis*. 2001;33:177-186.

Bradsher RW. Clinical features of blastomycosis. *Semin Respir Infect*. 1997;12:229-234.

Brummer E, Castaneda E, Restrepo A. Paracoccidioidomycosis: an update. *Clin Microbiol Rev*. 1993;6:89-136.

Chapman SW, Dismukes WE, Proia LA, et al. Clinical practice guidelines for the management of blastomycosis. *Clin Infect Dis*. 2008;46:1801-1812.

Chapman SW, Lin AC, Hendricks KA, et al. Endemic blastomycosis in Mississippi: epidemiological and clinical studies. *Semin Respir Infect*. 1997;12:219-228.

Chapman SW, Pappas P, Kauffman C, et al. Comparative evaluation of the efficacy and safety of two doses of terbinafine (500 and 1000 mg day(-1)) in the treatment of cutaneous or lymphocutaneous sporotrichosis. *Mycoses*. 2004;47:62-68.

Galgiani JN, Ampel NM, Blair JE, Catanzaro A, Stevens DA, Williams PL. Coccidioidomycosis. *Clin Infect Dis*. 2005;41:1217-1223.

Graybill JR, Sobel J, Saag M, et al. Diagnosis and management of increased intracranial pressure in patients with AIDS and cryptococcal meningitis. *Clin Infect Dis*. 2000;30:47.

Kauffman CA, Bustamante B, Chapman SW, Pappas PG. Clinical practice guidelines for the management of sporotrichosis. *Clin Infect Dis*. 2007;45:1255-1265.

Kauffman CA. Sporotrichosis. *Clin Infect Dis*. 1999;29:231-236.

Kaufmann CA, Vazquez JA, Sobel JD, et al and the National Institute for Allergy and Infectious Diseases (NIAID) Mycoses Study Group. *Clin Infect Dis*. 2000;30:14-18.

Lundstrom T, Sobel J. Nosocomial candiduria: a review. *Clin Infect Dis*. 2001;32:1602-1607.

Ostrosky-Zeichner L. Prophylaxis and treatment of invasive candidiasis in the intensive are setting. *Eur J Clin Microbiol Infect Dis*. 2004;23:739-744.

Pfaller MA, Jones RN, Doern GV, et al. Blood-stream infections due to Candida species: SENTRY antimicrobial surveillance program in North America and Latin America. *Antimicrob Agents Chemother*. 2000;44:747-751.

Pappas PG. Blastomycosis in the immunocompromised patient. *Semin Respir Infect*. 1997;12:243-251.

Pappas PG, Kaufmann CA, Andes D, et al. Clinical Practice Guidelines for the Management of Candidiasis: 2009 Update by the Infectious Diseases Society of America. *Clin Infect Dis*. 2009; 48:503–535.

Powderly WG. Cryptococcal meningitis and AIDS. *Clin Infect Dis*. 1993;5:837-842.

Queiroz-Telles F, McGinnis MR, Salkin I, Graybill JR. Subcutaneous mycoses. *Inf Dis Clin North America*. 2003;17:59-85.

Saag MS, Graybill RJ, Larsen RA, et al. Practice guidelines for the treatment of cryptococcosis. *Clin Infect Dis*. 2000;30:710-718.

Sathapatayavongs B, Batteiger BE, Wheat LJ, et al. Clinical and laboratory features of disseminated histoplasmosis during two large urban outbreaks. *Medicine*. 1983;62:263-270.

Sobel JD for the Mycoses Study Group. Practice guidelines for the treatment of fungal infections. Infectious Diseases Society of America. *Clin Infect Dis*. 2000;30:652.

Stevens D. Coccidioidomycosis. *N Engl J Med*. 1995;332:1077-1082.

Walsh TJ, Anaissie EJ, Denning DW, et al.Treatment of Aspergillosis: Clinical Practice Guidelines of the Infectious Diseases Society of America. *Clin Infect Dis*. 2008; 46:327-360.

Walsh TJ, Rex JH. All catheter-related candidemia is not the same: assessment of the balance between the risks and benefits of removal of vascular catheters. *Clin Infect Dis*. 2002;34:600-602.

Walsh TJ, Pappas P, Winston DJ, et al. Voriconazole compared with liposomal amphotericin B for empirical antifungal therapy in patients with neutropenia and persistent fever. *N Engl J Med*. 2002;346:225-234.

Wheat LJ, Connolly-Stringfield PA, Baker RL, et al. Disseminated histoplasmosis in the acquired immune deficiency syndrome: clinical findings, diagnosis and treatment, and review of the literature. *Medicine*. 1990;69:361-374.

Wheat LJ, Freifeld AG, Kleiman MB, et al . Clinical practice guidelines for the management of patients with histoplasmosis: 2007 update by the Infectious Diseases Society of America. *Clin Infect Dis*. 2007;45:807-825.

Chapter 11: Tuberculosis and Nontuberculous Mycobacterial Infections for the ID Boards

Laurel Preheim, MD
Marvin J. Bittner, MD, MSc

Contents

1. Tuberculosis (TB)

Synonyms

• Consumption (pulmonary TB)

• Pott's disease (TB of the spine)

Causative Organisms

• *Mycobacterium tuberculosis* (common)

• *M bovis* (rare)

• *M africanum, M microti, M ulcerans* (very rare)

Epidemiology

• Currently more than one-third of the world's population is infected with *M tuberculosis*.

• TB causes an estimated 8 million new cases and 2-3 million worldwide deaths annually.

• The incidence of TB in the United States rose in the mid-1980s but has fallen annually since 1992.

• Most current U.S. cases are found in urban and immigrant communities.

  * Among foreign-born persons, TB is largely caused by reactivation of latent infection

  * Among U.S.-born persons, many cases result from recent transmission

  * Substance abuse is frequently encountered, especially among U.S.-born patients

Key Clinical Features

• Person-to-person transmission occurs by inhaled airborne particles 1-5 micrometers in diameter.

• The probability that transmission will occur is related to:

  * Infectiousness of person with TB

  * Environment in which exposure occurred (eg, close quarters)

  * Duration of exposure

  * Virulence of the organism

• Primary TB is usually a self-limited, mild pneumonic illness that often goes undiagnosed.

• Bacillemia and seeding of other organs sets the stage for reactivation in extrapulmonary sites.

• The incidence of progression from latent to active infection is ~5% in the first 5 years, plus an additional 5% lifetime risk thereafter.

• Conditions that increase the risk of progression to TB disease are:

  * HIV infection (risk of TB disease is ~10% each year)

  * Substance abuse

  * Recent infection

  * Chest radiograph findings suggestive of previous TB (untreated)

  * Diabetes mellitus

  * Silicosis

  * Prolonged corticosteroid therapy

  * Other immunosuppressive therapy, including monoclonal antibody against tumor necrosis factor, (TNF) eg, infliximab

  * Cancer of the head and neck

  * Hematologic and reticuloendothelial diseases

  * End-stage renal disease

  * Intestinal bypass or gastrectomy

  * Chronic malabsorption syndromes

  * Low body weight (10% or more below the ideal)

- TB symptoms are nonspecific and may be absent.

- Classic systemic symptoms of TB include:

  * Fever

  * Night sweats

  * Anorexia

  * Weight loss

  * Weakness

- Organ-specific symptoms of pulmonary TB are:

  * Productive, prolonged cough (3 weeks)

  * Pleuritic chest pain

  * Hemoptysis

- Although ordinarily a chronic disease, acute presentations may occur, such as:

  * Miliary TB

  * Acute abdominal TB

- Extrapulmonary TB:

  * More likely in patients with HIV infection or other forms of immunosuppression

  * Most commonly involves lymph nodes, pleura, and bones or joints

  * May involve the genitourinary system, central nervous system, abdomen, pericardium and virtually any other organ

  * May be disseminated (miliary TB)

Differential Diagnoses

Carcinoma of the Lung
- Carcinoma may be present simultaneously with TB.

* Carcinoma diagnosis may be delayed if TB is found first

- Features suggestive of carcinoma include:

  * Isolated involvement of anterior segment of upper lobe

  * Isolated involvement of lower lobe

  * Presence of irregular cavities

  * Lack of acid-fast bacilli in sputum smears

- Fungal infections, especially:

  * Histoplasmosis

  * Coccidioidomycosis

  * Blastomycosis

- Nontuberculous mycobacterial infections, especially:

  * *M avium-intracellulare*

  * *M kansasii*

- Other bacterial pneumonias:

  * Anaerobic lung abscess

  * Melioidosis (caused by *Burkholderia pseudomallei*)

Tuberculin Skin Testing (TST)
- Is used to:

  * Find persons with latent TB infection who would benefit from treatment

  * Find persons with TB disease who would benefit from treatment

- Is not used for routine testing of groups that are not at high risk for TB

- TST is indicated for persons at higher risk for TB exposure or infection:

  * Close contacts of persons known or suspected to have TB (eg, those sharing the same household or other enclosed environment)

  * Foreign-born persons, including children, from areas that have a high TB incidence or prevalence (eg, Asia, Africa, Latin America, eastern Europe, Russia)

  * Residents and employees of high-risk congregate settings (eg, correctional institutions, nursing homes, mental institutions, other long-term residential facilities and shelters for the homeless)

  * Health care workers who serve high-risk clients

  * Some medically underserved, low-income populations as defined locally

  * High-risk racial or ethnic minority populations, defined locally as having an increased prevalence of TB (eg, Asians and Pacific Islanders, Hispanics, African Americans, Native Americans, migrant farm workers or homeless persons)

  * Infants, children and adolescents exposed to adults in high-risk categories

  * Persons who inject illicit drugs, any other locally identified high-risk substance users (eg, crack cocaine users)

- TST is indicated for persons at higher risk for TB disease once infected, including:

  * Persons with HIV infection

  * Persons who were recently infected *with M tuberculosis* (within the past 2 years), particularly infants and very young children

  * Persons who have medical conditions known to increase the risk for disease if infection occurs, eg, diabetes, end-stage renal disease

  * Persons who inject illicit drugs; other groups of high-risk substance users (eg, crack cocaine users)

  * Persons with a history of inadequately treated TB

- Proper TST technique includes:

  * Inject intradermally 0.1 mL of 5 TU PPD tuberculin

  * Produce wheal 6-10 mm in diameter

  * Read reaction 48-72 hours after injection

  * Measure only induration; record reaction in millimeters

- Classification of the tuberculin reaction is as follows:

  * ≥5 mm is positive in:

    - HIV+ persons

    - Recent contacts of TB case

    - Persons with fibrotic changes on chest radiograph consistent with old, healed TB
    - Patients with organ transplants and other immunosuppressed patients

  * ≥10 mm is positive in:

    - Recent arrivals from high-prevalence countries

    - Injection drug users

    - Residents and employees of high-risk congregate settings

    - Mycobacteriology laboratory personnel

    - Persons with clinical conditions that place them at high risk

- Children <4 years of age, or children and adolescents exposed to adults in high-risk categories

* ≥15 mm is positive in:

  - Persons with no known risk factors for TB

  - Factors that may cause false-positive and false-negative reactions include:

* False-positive:

  - Nontuberculous mycobacteria

  - BCG vaccination (note: BCG vaccine efficacy much less than 100%, so some authorities ignore history of BCG vaccination when interpreting tuberculin reaction)

* False-negative:

  - Anergy

  - Recent TB infection

  - Very young age (< 6 months old)

  - Live virus vaccination

  - Overwhelming TB disease

- Rules for use of the two-step TST are:

  * Use for initial testing of adults who will be retested periodically

  * If first test is positive, consider the person infected

  * If first test is negative, give second test 1-3 weeks later

  * If second test is negative, consider person uninfected

Interferon-gamma release assay (such as QuantiFERON®-TB Gold) as an Alternative to TST

- Blood drawn from patient, patient's cells exposed to M tuberculosis antigens, their interferon response measured

  * Advantages

    - No need for repeat visit to read test

    - Results may be available in 24 hours

    - No need for special skills in placing, interpreting TST

    - Specificity of antigens may reduce the risk of false positive TSTs due to nontuberculous mycobacteria or BCG

    - Does not boost response to subsequent tests

  * Disadvantages

    - Requirements for prompt processing may contribute to expense

    - Limited in-the-field experience

    - Subject to errors in collecting and transporting specimen, and in running and interpreting assay

Key Radiology Features

Chest Radiograph
- Patchy or nodular infiltrates are commonly seen in:

  * Apical or posterior segments of upper lobe, or

  * Superior segments of lower lobe

- Early chronic TB is likely if the above findings are:

  * Bilateral

* Associated with cavity formation

• Cavities may be more apparent by computed tomography or magnetic resonance imaging (MRI).

• Pneumonia with hilar adenopathy should always suggest primary TB.

• However, lesions can appear anywhere in the lungs and may differ in size, shape, density and cavitation, especially in HIV+ and other immunosuppressed patients.

• HIV-infected persons with TB disease may present with:

   * Infiltrates without cavities in any lung zone

   * Mediastinal or hilar lymphadenopathy, with or without accompanying infiltrates and/or cavities

   * An entirely normal chest radiograph

• Cannot confirm the diagnosis of TB.

Key Laboratory Features

Diagnostic Microbiology
• *Specimen collection:*

   * Obtain 3 sputum specimens for smear examination and culture.

   * If patient is unable to cough, induce sputum or obtain specimen by bronchoscopy or early morning gastric aspiration (especially in infants and young children).

   * Follow infection control precautions during specimen collection.

   * Other clinical specimens (eg, urine, cerebrospinal fluid, pleural fluid, pus or biopsy specimens) may be submitted when extrapulmonary TB is suspected.

* The typical histopathologic finding is a granuloma with caseous necrosis that resembles cheese.

• *Laboratory examination:*
   * Acid-fast bacilli (AFB) are sought in stained smears.

      • Fluorochrome staining with auraminerhodamine is the preferred method.

   * Smear examination permits only presumptive diagnosis of TB.

      • The AFB in a smear may be nontuberculous mycobacteria.

      • Many TB patients have negative AFB smears.

   * Positive cultures for *M tuberculosis* confirm the diagnosis.

      • Isolation and identification using solid media and conventional biochemical testing takes 6-12 weeks.

      • BACTEC and other liquid media systems allow detection of mycobacterial growth in 4-14 days.

• Nucleic acid probes of positive cultures allow rapid species identification.

   * High-performance liquid chromatography can identify pathogenic mycobacterial species by the spectrum of mycolic acids in the cell wall.

   * Inhibition by p-nitro-α-acetylamido-β-hydroxypropiophenone (NAP test) can identify *M tuberculosis* in 3-4 days.

   * Nucleic acid amplification (NAA) tests are recommended for routine use on at least one respiratory specimen where pulmonary TB is being considered (but not established), and for those where the test result would affect management of that patient or TB control activities

- Value of NAA reflects >95% positive predictive value with AFB smear-positive specimens in settings where nontuberculous mycobacteria are common in addition to rapid confirmation of the presence of *M tuberculosis* in over half of AFB-smear-negative, culture-positive specimens.

  - NAA positive, smear positive: presume TB, start treatment while awaiting culture results

  - NAA positive, smear negative: use clinical judgment. Consider a second NAA specimen; if positive, presume TB, start treatment while awaiting culture results

  - NAA negative, smear positive: test sputum for inhibitors and repeat NAA. If inhibitors present, NAA of no diagnostic use. If no inhibitors, use clinical judgment; if a second AFB smear is positive, presume infection with nontuberculous mycobacteria.

  - NAA negative, smear negative: use clinical judgment. NAA is not sensitive enough to exclude TB in AFB smear-negative patients suspected to have TB.

* Follow-up specimens should be obtained at least monthly until cultures become negative.

* Culture conversion to negative is the most important objective measure of response to treatment.

* The initial *M tuberculosis* isolate should be tested for drug resistance.

* Risk factors for drug-resistant TB include:

  - History of treatment with TB drugs

  - Contacts of persons with drug resistant TB

  - Foreign-born persons from high prevalence drug resistant areas

  - Smears or cultures remain positive despite 2 months of TB treatment

  - Received inadequate treatment regimens for >2 weeks

- Restriction fragment length polymorphism (RFLP):

  * Is a method of DNA fingerprinting

  * Can identify specific TB strains and track transmission during outbreaks

- Other laboratory findings:

  * In advanced disease include:

    - Normocytic, normochromic anemia

    - Hypoalbuminemia

    - Hypergammaglobulinemia

    - Peripheral white blood cell count is usually normal.

  * Hematuria or pyuria should suggest coexisting renal TB.

  * Hyponatremia:

    - With features of inappropriate secretion of antidiuretic hormone can occur with: TB meningitis; isolated pulmonary involvement

    - Can be due to Addison's disease secondary to adrenal involvement

Treatment of Latent TB Infection (LTBI)
- If there is history of TB exposure but the TST is negative:

  * In neonates:

    - Begin isoniazid (INH) 10 mg/kg/d for 3 months

- Repeat TST in 3 months

  - If mother's smear negative and infant's TST negative and chest x-ray normal, stop INH

  * If infant's repeat TST positive and/or chest x-ray abnormal (hilar adenopathy and/or infiltrate) give INH plus rifampin (10-20 mg/kg/d) for total of 6 months

  * Child <5 years of age:

    - Begin INH 10 mg/kg/d for 3 months

    - Repeat TST in 3 months: if negative, stop INH; if positive, continue INH for total of 9 months

  * Older children and adults:

    - No initial therapy

    - Repeat TST in 3 months: if positive, treat with INH for 9 months

- If the TST is positive (organisms likely to be INH susceptible):

  * INH: 5 mg/kg/d, maximum 300 mg/d for adults; 10 mg/kg/d not to exceed 300 mg/d for children

- General guidelines for treatment of LTBI with INH:

  * A 9-month regimen is preferred.

  * Children should receive 9 months of therapy.

  * INH can be given twice weekly if directly observed.

- Rifampin-pyrazinamide regimens no longer recommended for LTBI because of hepatotoxicity.

- An unconfirmed recent study suggests that 4 months of rifampin alone is, compared to INH, associated with better adherence and fewer adverse events.

- Regimens for specific situations:

  * Contacts of INH-resistant TB:

    - 4 months daily RIF if susceptible to RIF

  * Contacts of multidrug-resistant TB:

    - Use 2 drugs to which the infecting organism is shown to be susceptible (potentially useful agents include ethambutol [EMB], PZA and the fluoroquinolones).

    - Treat for 12 months.

    - Follow for 2 years regardless of treatment.

  * Fibrotic lesions on chest radiograph representing old TB (does not include calcified nodes, calcified nodules or apical pleural capping):

    - 9 months of INH, or

    - 2 months of RIF plus PZA, or

    - 4 months of RIF (with or without INH)

  * Pregnancy and breast feeding:

    - Administer INH daily or twice weekly plus pyridoxine supplementation.

    - Breast feeding is not contraindicated.

- Monitoring patients who receive treatment for LTBI:

  * Before treatment is started, clinicians should:

    - Rule out possibility of TB disease

    - Determine history of treatment for LTBI or disease

    - Determine contraindications to treatment

    - Obtain information about current and previous drug therapy

- Recommend HIV testing if risk factors are present.

- Baseline laboratory testing is not routinely indicated.

  * Obtain baseline liver function tests (AST or ALT) for:

    - Patients whose initial evaluation suggests a liver disorder

    - Patients with HIV infection

    - Pregnant women and those in the immediate postpartum period

    - Patients with a history of chronic liver disorder or those at risk for chronic liver disease

    - Patients who use alcohol regularly

- All patients should be monitored at least monthly for:

  * Adherence to prescribed regimen

  * Signs and symptoms of active TB disease

  * Signs and symptoms of hepatitis

- Patient with abnormal baseline liver tests or who are at risk for hepatic disease should be monitored during INH treatment of LTBI with monthly liver tests.

- About 10%-20% of persons taking INH will have mild, asymptomatic elevations of liver enzymes.

  * This tends to resolve even if INH is continued.

  * Consider discontinuing INH if:

    - Any measurements exceed three to five times the upper limit of normal, or

    - The patient reports symptoms of adverse reactions

Treatment of TB Disease

Basic Principles of Treatment
- Provide safest, most effective therapy in shortest time.

- Use multiple drugs to which the organism is susceptible.

- Never add just a single drug to a failing regimen.

- Ensure adherence to therapy with case management and directly observed therapy.

- Directly observed therapy (DOT):

  * Health care worker watches patient swallow each dose.

  * Consider DOT for all patients.

  * DOT should be used with all intermittent regimens.

  * DOT can lead to reductions in relapse and acquired drug resistance.

- Self-administered therapy:

  * Fixed-dose combinations may enhance patient adherence and reduce risk of acquired drug resistance.

  * In the United States, licensed fixed-drug combinations include:

    - INH and RIF (Rifamate)

- INH, RIF and PZA (Rifater)

  * Adherence should be monitored at follow-up visits.

  * Bacteriologic conversion to negative should be monitored closely for all patients.

  * If the patient's sputum remains positive after 2 months of treatment, the patient should be reevaluated and DOT should be considered.

Treatment of Pulmonary TB

- All TB drugs should be given no more frequently than once daily—not in divided doses.

- A 6-month regimen is preferred.

- All regimens of 9 months or less must contain INH and RIF.

- All 6-month regimens must contain INH, RIF, and initially, PZA.

- Ethambutol (EMB) or streptomycin (SM) should be included in the initial regimen until the results of drug susceptibility testing confirms INH and RIF susceptibility.

- The initial use of a 4-drug regimen helps prevent development of multidrug resistant TB in areas where the prevalence of primary INH resistance is 4% or higher.

- If susceptibility to INH and RIF is confirmed, INH and RIF should be continued to complete the 6-month regimen.

- Treatment of TB for HIV- persons:

  * Options for 6-month, intermittent regimens using DOT include:

    - Four-drug therapy, administered daily for 8 weeks, may be followed by therapy with INH and RIF given 2 or 3 times a week for 16 weeks (if susceptibility to INH and RIF is demonstrated).

    - Four-drug therapy, administered daily for 2 weeks and then 2 times a week for 6 weeks, may be followed by therapy with INH and RIF given 2 times a week for 16 weeks (if susceptibility to INH and RIF is demonstrated).

    - Four-drug therapy may be administered 3 times a week throughout the 6-month treatment, continuing all 4 drugs throughout the course of treatment.

  * When INH, PZA, and EMB or SM are given 2 or 3 times a week instead of every day, their dosages must be increased. However, the dose of RIF is the same whether the drug is given daily or intermittently.

  * Alternatively, a 9-month regimen of INH and RIF is acceptable for persons who cannot or should not take PZA (eg, pregnant women).

    - SM (except in pregnant women) or EMB should be included initially unless there is little possibility of drug resistance.

    - If susceptibility to INH and RIF is demonstrated, INH and RIF can be given twice weekly after an initial 4-8 weeks of daily treatment.

  * For adults with smear- and culture-negative pulmonary TB, a 4-month regimen of INH and RIF, combined with PZA for the first 2 months, may be used when drug resistance is unlikely.

- Treatment of TB for HIV+ persons:

  * Whenever possible this care should be provided by or in consultation with experts in the management of both TB and HIV disease.

  * Widely used antiretroviral agents, including most protease inhibitors (PIs) and nonnucleoside reverse transcriptase inhibitors (NNRTIs), interact with rifamycin derivatives, such as rifampin (RIF) and, to a lesser degree, rifabutin (RFB).

  * The nucleoside reverse transcriptase inhibitors are not contraindicated with the use of rifamycins and do not require dose adjustments.

- Treatment of TB in HIV-infected adults is generally the same as in HIV-uninfected adults, but:

  * The continuation regimen of INH-rifapentine weekly is contraindicated.

Table 1

Nontuberculous Mycobacterial Diseases and Etiologic Species

Clinical disease	Etiologic species (Runyon group)[1]	
	Percent (%)	Less common
Pulmonary	*M avium complex* (c) *M kansasii* (a) *M abscessus* (d) *M xenopi* (b)	*M simiae* (a) *M szulgai* (b) *M malmoense* (c) *M fortuitum* (d) *M chelonae* (d)
Lymphadenitis	*M avium complex* (c) *M scrofulaceum* (b)	*M fortuitum* (d) *M chelonae* (d) *M abscessus* (d) *M kansasii* (a)
Cutaneous	*M marinum* (a) *M fortuitum* (d) *M chelonae* (d) *M abscessus* (d) *M ulcerans* (c)	*M avium complex* (c) *M kansasii* (a) *M terrae* (c) *M smegmatis* (d) *M haemophilum* (c)
Disseminated	*M avium complex* (c) *M kansasii* (a) *M chelonae* (d) *M abscessus* (d) *M haemophilum* (c)	*M fortuitum* (d) *M xenopi* (b) *M simiae* (a) *M gordonae* (b) *M terrae complex* (c) *M neoaurum* (b) *M celatum* (c) *M genavense* (c)

1(a), photochromogen (group I); (b), scotochromogen (group II); (c), nonpigmented (group III); (d), rapid grower (group IV).

* In patients with CD4+ counts below 100, therapy must be daily or 3 times a week.

* Particularly in view of rifamycin drug interactions with antiretroviral therapy, dose adjustments may be needed.

* Recovery of the immune system with antiretroviral therapy may lead to a paradoxical worsening of signs of tuberculosis due to immune reconstitution syndrome.

* DOT should be used for all patients with HIV-related TB.

* All HIV+ patients who receive INH should also receive pyridoxine (vitamin B6) to reduce risks of INH-induced neurotoxicity.

Treatment of Extrapulmonary TB

• Regimens that are adequate for treating pulmonary

TB are generally effective for treating extrapulmonary disease.

- Infants and children who have miliary TB, bone and joint TB or TB meningitis should receive a minimum of 12 months of therapy.

- Surgery may be necessary to obtain specimens for diagnosis and to treat constrictive pericarditis and spinal cord compression from Pott's disease.

- Corticosteroids are beneficial in:

    * Preventing cardiac constriction from tuberculous pericarditis.

    * Decreasing the neurologic sequelae of TB meningitis.

- HIV+ patients are more likely to develop extrapulmonary TB, but they usually respond to regimens effective for pulmonary TB.

    * However, for meningitis, bone TB and joint TB a standard rifamycin-based regimen for at least 9 months is recommended.

Treatment of Pregnant or Lactating Women

- A 9-month regimen of INH, RIF and EMB is recommended.

- PZA and SM are contraindicated.

- Breast feeding should not be discouraged, because the small concentrations of TB drugs in breast milk do not harm nursing newborns.

- For HIV+ pregnant women, the benefits of a TB regimen that includes PZA outweigh the potential risks to the fetus.

- Aminoglycosides, capreomycin and fluoroquinolones are contraindicated for all pregnant women because of adverse effects on the fetus.

Treatment of Drug-Resistant TB

TB Resistant Only to INH
- Carefully supervise and manage treatment to avoid development of multidrug-resistant TB.

- In HIV- persons:

    * Discontinue INH and continue RIF, PZA, and EMB or SM for the entire 6 months; or

    * Treat with RIF and EMB for 12 months.

- In HIV+ persons:

    * Treat with a rifamycin, PZA and EMB.

TB Resistant Only to RIF
- Use a 9-month regimen with an initial 2 months of INH, SM, PZA and EMB, followed by INH, SM and PZA for the final 7 months of therapy.

Multidrug-resistant TB (MDR TB)
- Most treatment regimens include an aminoglycoside (eg, SM, kanamycin, amikacin) or capreomycin, and a fluoroquinolone, along with other agents to which the isolate is sensitive.

    * Treat for 24 months after culture conversion.

    * Follow the patient post-treatment every 4 months for 24 months.

    * Always use DOT.

Extensively Drug-resistant TB (XDR TB)
- MDR TB is defined as TB due to isolates resistant to both INH and RIF.

- XDR TB is defined as MDR TB that is also resistant to any fluoroquinolone and at least 1 of 3 injectable second-line drugs (capreomycin, kanamycin, amikacin).

- Treatment of XDR TB requires analysis of susceptibility testing in order to develop a complex, multi-drug regimen.

Monitoring for Adverse Reactions

• Baseline tests are performed to detect any abnormality that would complicate therapy or require a modified regimen.

  * Adults treated for TB should have baseline measurements of hepatic enzymes, bilirubin and serum creatinine, as well as a complete blood and platelet count.

  * Serum uric acid should be measured if PZA is used.

  * Baseline and monthly examination of visual acuity and color vision should be obtained if EMB is prescribed (this applies to children as well).

  * Consider performing audiometry at the beginning of SM therapy.

• Monitoring for adverse reactions must be individualized depending on the drugs used and the patient's risk for adverse reactions.

• At a minimum, patients should be seen monthly during therapy and questioned concerning adverse reactions.

• Patients should be instructed to seek medical attention should symptoms occur.

• If symptoms suggest adverse reactions, appropriate testing should be performed.

Important Adverse Reactions to Anti-TB Drugs
• *Isoniazid (INH)*
  * Rash

  * Hepatic enzyme elevation

  * Hepatitis

  * Peripheral neuropathy

    • Uncommon at doses of 5 mg/kg;

    • Preventable with pyridoxine, 10-50 mg/d

  * Drug interactions:

    • Interaction with phenytoin raises the serum concentration of both drugs

• *Rifampin (RIF)*
  * Gastrointestinal upset

  * Drug interactions:

• May accelerate clearance of drugs metabolized by the liver (eg, methadone, coumarin derivatives, glucocorticoids, estrogens, oral hypoglycemics, digitalis, anticonvulsants, ketoconazole, fluconazole, cyclosporine and PIs)

    • Women using hormonal contraception and taking RIF should supplement the contraception or use barrier methods.

    • Patients taking RIF should be monitored for possible manifestations of thrombocytopenia (bleeding tendency, easy bruising, blood in urine) or flu-like symptoms.

    • Reduces effectiveness of most PI and NNRTI antiretrovirals.

  * Hepatitis

  * Bleeding problems

  * Flu-like symptoms

  * Rash

  * Renal failure

  * Fever

  * Side effect: Colors body fluids orange (may stain soft contact lenses)

• *Rifabutin (RFB)*
  * Rash

  * Hepatitis

  * Fever

* Thrombocytopenia

* Drug interactions:

  • Reduces levels of many drugs (eg, PIs, NNRTIs, methadone, dapsone, ketocona-zole, hormonal contraceptives, etc.)

  • Avoid in persons taking ritonavir or delavirdine

* Side effect: Colors body fluids orange (may stain soft contact lenses)

• *Pyrazinamide (PZA)*
  * Hepatitis

  * Rash

  * Gastrointestinal upset

  * Joint aches

  * Hyperuricemia (treat only if patient has symp-toms)

  * Gout (rare)

• *Ethambutol (EMB)*
  * Optic neuritis

  * Rash

• *Streptomycin (SM)*
  * Ototoxicity (hearing loss or vestibular dys-function)

  * Renal toxicity

2. Overview of Nontuberculous Mycobacterial (NTM) Infections

Synonyms

• Infections due to atypical mycobacteria.

• Infections due to mycobacteria other than tubercle bacilli (MOTT).

Causative Organisms

• The list of NTM pathogens continues to grow as new species are discovered.

• Timpe and Runyon classified NTM based on pig-ment production, growth rate and colonial charac-teristics. Except for Group IV, they grow slowly on culture media (>7 days before growth evident).

• See Table 1 for selected NTM pathogens and infections they cause.

Group I: Photochromogens

• Colonies become yellow or orange after exposure to light.

Group II: Scotochromogens

• Colonies are pigmented in the dark or after light exposure.

Group III: Nonpigmented

• Colonies lack pigment in the dark or the light.

Group IV: Rapid Growers

• May grow slowly on initial culture but grow in 3-5 days on subculture.

• Lack pigment.

Epidemiology

• The rate of isolation of NTM is increasing and has surpassed that for M tuberculosis in some areas.

• Ubiquitous in nature, many have been isolated from ground or tap water, soil, house dust, domes-tic and wild animals, and birds.

- Most infections result from inhalation or direct inoculation from environmental sources.

- Ingestion may be the source of infection for children with NTM cervical adenopathy and for patients with AIDS, whose disseminated infection may begin in the gastrointestinal tract.

- Because person-to-person transmission is extremely rare, infected patients do not require isolation.

Diagnosis

- Approaches to the diagnosis of TB generally apply to NTM infections.

- Standardized, specific skin test antigens for NTM, however, are unavailable.

- Colonization of asymptomatic individuals and environmental contamination of specimens can yield positive cultures in the absence of clinical disease.

- NTM disease can be considered present in patients with a cavitary infiltrate on chest radiogram when:

    * Two or more sputum samples (or sputum and a bronchial washing) are smear-positive for acid-fast bacilli and/or yield moderate to heavy growth on culture

    * Other reasonable causes for the disease process have been excluded (eg, fungal disease, tuberculosis, malignancy, etc.)

- The diagnosis is also established if transbronchial, percutaneous or open lung biopsy tissue reveals mycobacterial histopathologic changes and yields the organism.

- Extrapulmonary or disseminated disease is confirmed by isolation of the organism from normally sterile body fluids, closed sites or lesions, and when environmental contamination of specimens is excluded.

- Liquid culture systems (radiometric and nonradiometric), DNA probes, and nucleic acid amplification assays have increased the speed and accuracy of laboratory diagnosis of pulmonary and extra-pulmonary infections.

Therapy

- Many NTM are resistant to conventional anti-TB agents.

- Choice of treatment regimen should be guided by results of susceptibility testing on the NTM isolate.

- For many NTM pathogens, the optimal treatment regimen remains undefined.

3. *Mycobacterium avium intracellulare* (MAI)

Synonyms

• MAI is also known as *M avium* complex (MAC).

Epidemiology

• MAI is distributed worldwide.

• MAI is the most common cause of NTM infections in the United States.

Key Clinical Features

• MAI causes about 80% of NTM lymphadenitis cases.

Pulmonary Infection

• Usually occurs in individuals with underlying lung disease.

• Generally follows an indolent or slowly progressive course.

Extrapulmonary or Disseminated Disease

• Occurs rarely in immunocompetent patients.

• Is common in HIV-infected patients who have advanced AIDS with CD4+ T-lymphocyte counts <50 cells per microliter.

  * Prophylaxis with clarithromycin (500 mg BID) or azithromycin (1200 mg once weekly) is recommended for these patients.

• Suggestive symptoms of disseminated MAI:

  * Fever and/or weight loss

  * Anorexia, abdominal pain and/or diarrhea

• Findings may include:

  * Hepatosplenomegaly

  * Generalized lymphadenopathy, including mediastinal adenopathy

• Diagnosis of disseminated disease is commonly made by culture of the organism from blood, bone marrow, stool or tissue biopsy.

Treatment

• Current regimens for MAI infections are based on trials involving patients with AIDS who received treatment for disseminated disease.

• These guidelines can be applied to patients with or without AIDS who have either pulmonary or disseminated infections.

• Treatment regimens should include at least 2 agents.

• Every regimen should contain either azithromycin (600 mg QD) or clarithromycin (500 mg BID).

• Many experts prefer EMB (15 mg/kg once daily) as the second drug.

• One or more of the following may be added as second, third or fourth agents:

  * RFB (300-600 mg QD)

  * Ciprofloxacin (750 mg BID)

  * Ofloxacin (400 mg BID)

  * In some situations, amikacin (7.5-15 mg/kg QD)

• INH and PZA are not effective.

• No specific regimen has emerged as being superior for pulmonary or disseminated disease, and the optimal duration of therapy remains unknown.

• Immunocompetent patients probably should receive a minimum of 18-24 months of therapy.

• Immunosuppressed patients should continue lifetime suppression therapy for MAI.

• It may be possible to discontinue chronic suppressive therapy in patients on highly active antiretroviral therapy who have robust CD4+ cell recovery.

• Excisional therapy without chemotherapy is curative in about 95% of cervical adenopathy cases.

4. *Mycobacterium kansasii*

Epidemiology

• *M kansasii*, an important photochromogen, ranks second among NTM in causing human infections in the United States.

• Most disease occurs in the midwestern and southern United States.

Key Clinical Features

• Pulmonary infection is most common and resembles TB and MAI disease.

• Extrapulmonary disease can involve any organ system.

• Risks of dissemination are increased in immunocompromised patients.

Treatment

• INH 300 mg QD, RIF 600 mg QD, and EMB QD (25 mg/kg for 2 months, then 15 mg/kg for 18 months).

• Clarithromycin (500 mg BID) or RFB (150 mg QD) can substitute for RIF in HIV patients receiving PIs.

• Sulfamethoxazole (1 gram TID) may be used in regimens to treat RIF-resistant strains.

• All strains are resistant to PZA.

5. Rapidly Growing Mycobacteria

Epidemiology

• These NTM are ubiquitous in soil and water, including chlorinated municipal water systems.

• Sporadic, community-acquired infections have been reported from most areas of the United States.

• Most infections are acquired by inoculation after accidental trauma, surgery or injection.

• Nosocomial epidemics or clusters have been reported in numerous settings including augmentation mammaplasty, hemodialysis, plastic surgery, long-term venous catheters, cardiac surgery and jet injector use.

• Clustered cases are typically associated with devices contaminated with water from a hospital or municipal water system.

Key Clinical Features

• The spectrum of diseases ranges from localized to disseminated, with cutaneous involvement being most common.

Key Laboratory Features

• Rapidly growing mycobacteria are acid-fast rods that resemble diphtheroids on Gram stain.

• Growth is rapid on subculture to solid media (< 7 days), but primary isolation from clinical specimens may require 2-30 days.

• Unlike other mycobacteria, they grow well on most routine laboratory media.

Treatment

• These NTM are highly resistant to conventional antituberculous drugs, but may be sensitive to traditional or newer antibiotics. Multiple drug therapy is generally recommended for NTM infections.

- Susceptibility testing of individual isolates is important, since resistance patterns vary by and within species subgroups.

- Surgical resection of infected tissue or prostheses is essential for cure.

M chelonae ssp. abscessus Infections
- Clarithromycin 500 mg BID for 6 months is generally part of a regimen.

- Isolates may be susceptible to amikacin, cefoxitin, cefmetazole, clofazimine or linezolid.

M chelonae ssp. chelonae Infections
- Clarithromycin 500 mg BID for 6 months is generally part of a regimen.

- Isolates may be susceptible to amikacin, cefoxitin, cefmetazole, clofazimine or linezolid

M fortuitum Infections
- Amikacin plus cefoxitin plus probenecid for 2 weeks, then oral trimethoprim-sulfamethoxazole or doxycycline for 2-6 months

- Isolates may be susceptible to imipenem, ciprofloxacin, ofloxacin, azithromycin, clarithromycin or linezolid.

6. *Mycobacterium marinum*

Epidemiology

- *M marinum* is a free-living NTM that causes disease in fresh and saltwater fish, and occasionally in humans.

- Currently most infections are acquired from swimming pools and home aquariums.

Key Clinical Features

- Cutaneous infections commonly follow aquatic-related inoculation after a 2-6 week incubation period.

- Painless papules typically are found on an extremity, especially on the elbows, knees, and dorsum of feet and hands.

- Lesions may progress to shallow ulceration and scar formation.

- Spontaneous healing can occur but may take months to years.

- A "sporotrichoid" form occurs in about 20% of cases, with proximal progression up the lymphatics to regional lymph nodes.

- Deep infection is rare but can result in tenosynovitis, osteomyelitis, arthritis, bursitis and carpal tunnel syndrome.

- Disseminated infections have been reported, generally in immunosuppressed hosts.

Treatment

- Approaches have included simple observation or surgical excision for minor lesions.

- Antimicrobial therapy, when indicated, is recommended for 3 months.

- Effective regimens include:

    * Clarithromycin 500 mg BID as a single agent

- Doxycycline (100 mg BID), trimethoprim- sulfamethoxazole (160/800 mg BID) or rifampin (600 mg QD) plus ethambutol (15 mg/kg QD)

- Linezolid and several fluoroquinolones show *in vitro* activity against *M marinum* strains.

7. Other Nontuberculous Mycobacteria

M gordonae

- This scotochromogen is also known as the "tap water bacillus."

- Associated with nosocomial pseudo-outbreaks, its isolation is commonly due to environmental contamination of a clinical specimen.

- It has been reported to cause pulmonary or disseminated infections in patients with AIDS.

    * *M xenopi, M malmoense, M szulgai, M simiae, M haemophilum, M terrae, M neoaurum, M celatum and M genavense*

- These NTM are being reported with increasing frequency as causes of pulmonary or disseminated infections in Europe, England, Canada, and the United States.

- Patients with AIDS appear particularly prone to disseminated disease.

- Initial therapy for severe infections should consist of isoniazid, rifampin, ethambutol with or without clarithromycin, streptomycin or amikacin, pending results of antimicrobial susceptibility testing.

- Optimal duration of therapy is unknown, but at least 18-24 months is recommended.

    * *M shimoidei, M branderi, M asiaticum, M gastri, M phlei, M thermoresistible, M flavescens and M intermedium*

    - These and a growing number of other uncommon NTM are being implicated as rare causes of pulmonary, extrapulmonary or disseminated infections.

    - The clinical significance of these NTM is likely to increase among patients with AIDS or other immunocompromising conditions.

ID Board Pearls

- Record the measurement of induration for every tuberculin skin test in mm, even if the measurement is zero. Deciding whether a subsequent test represents conversion may depend on the number of mm that the test has increased.

- For an individual who reports a history of a positive tuberculin skin test yet lacks documentation and is reluctant to undergo another tuberculin skin test, consider an interferon-gamma release assay for M tuberculosis.

- Predicting adherence to treatment is difficult. Routinely use directly observed therapy for tuberculosis.

- For AIDS patients with CD4+ counts <100, consider starting azithromycin to prevent disseminated Mycobacterium avium-intracellulare infection.

- If you diagnose a nontuberculous mycobacterial infection, tell ancillary staff that this is a condition that is not spread from person to person. Otherwise they may see "Mycobacterium" and confuse it with the infectiousness of M tuberculosis.

8. Further Reading

American Thoracic Society, Centers for Disease Control and Prevention, Infectious Diseases Society of America. Treatment of tuberculosis. *MMWR Recomm Rep*. 2003;52(RR11):1-77.

Brown-Elliott BA, Griffith DE, Wallace RJ. Newly described or emerging human species of nontuberculous mycobacteria. *Infect Dis Clin North Am*. 2002;16:187-220.

Centers for Disease Control and Prevention. Guidelines for preventing the transmission of Mycobacterium tuberculosis in health-care settings, 2005. *MMWR*. 2005;54(RR-17):1-140.

Centers for Disease Control and Prevention. Updated guidelines for the use of nucleic acid amplification tests in the diagnosis of tuberculosis. *MMWR*. 2009;58:7-10.

Geng E, Kreiswirth B, Driver C, et al. Changes in the transmission of tuberculosis in New York City from 1990 to 1999. *N Engl J Med*. 2002;346:1453-1458.

Jacob JT, Mehta AK, Leonard MK. Acute forms of tuberculosis in adults. *Am J Med*. 2009;122:12-17.

Menzies D, Long R, Traiman A, et al. Adverse events with 4 months of rifampin therapy or 9 months of isoniazid therapy for latent tuberculosis infection: A randomized trial. *Ann Intern Med*. 2008;149:689-697.

Oeltmann JE, Kammerer JS, Pevzner ES, Moonan PK. Tuberculosis and substance abuse in the United States, 1997-2006. *Arch Intern Med*. 2009;169:189-197.

Raviglione MC, Smith IM. XDR tuberculosis–implications for global public health. *N Engl J Med*. 2007 (Feb 15);356:656-659.

Schlossberg D, ed. Tuberculosis and Nontuberculous Mycobacterial Infections. 5th ed. New York, NY: McGraw-Hill; 2006.

Chapter 12:
Parasitic Infections for the ID Boards

James H. Maguire, MD

Contents

1. Malaria

Causative Organisms

- *Plasmodium falciparum, P vivax, P malariae P ovale*.

Epidemiology

- Vector: female *Anopheles* mosquitoes.

- 300-500 million cases per year worldwide, nearly all in tropics and subtropics.

- >1500 cases per year in the United States, most imported. Rare cases are transmitted by transfusion, congenitally or introduced (transmitted by local mosquitoes).

Key Clinical Features

All Species
- Fever, rigors, headache, nausea, vomiting, anemia, thrombocytopenia, splenomegaly (spleen palpable only after 7-10 days).

- *Plasmodium falciparum* can produce a variety of syndromes that mimic other diseases, and can be rapidly fatal in nonimmune persons.

Symptoms
- Coma, mental status changes (cerebral malaria), lactic acidosis, hypoglycemia, renal failure, including blackwater fever shock, diarrhea, dysentery, pulmonary edema, tender hepatomegaly, severe anemia, jaundice, placental insufficiency.

- *Plasmodium malariae, vivax* and *ovale* rarely fatal.

- Relapse of *P vivax* and *ovale* from persistent hepatic infection if not treated with primaquine.

Disease Modifiers

Hemoglobinopathies
- Persons with hemoglobin AS (sickle trait) do not develop life-threatening complications when infected with *P falciparum*.

Duffy blood group antigen
- Persons lacking Duffy blood group antigen (West Africans and their descendants) cannot be infected with *P vivax*.

Acquired immunity from repeated infections
- Persons living in highly endemic regions acquire partial immunity that protects against life-threatening complications.

Key Laboratory Features

- Anemia (hemolytic), thrombocytopenia.

- Definitive diagnosis by examination of Giemsa- or Wright-stained thick and thin smears.

Differential Diagnosis

- Blood smears distinguish malaria from other causes of fever.

- Every-other-day or every-third-day fever, when present, suggestive of malaria.

Infectious Diseases
- Enteric fever

- Dengue

- Brucellosis

- East African trypanosomiasis

- Babesiosis

- Influenza

- Hepatitis

Noninfectious Disease Mimics:
- Heat stroke

- Acute hemolytic anemia (drug-induced, sickle crisis)

- Toxic hepatitis

Therapy

- *All plasmodia except chloroquine-resistant P falciparum* and vivax: chloroquine phosphate 1 g PO, then 500 mg at 6, 24, and 48 hours.

- For *P vivax* and *ovale*, add: primaquine phosphate 30 mg (base) PO QD for 14 days (to prevent relapses).

- Primaquine causes hemolysis in G6PD deficiency and is contraindicated in pregnancy.

- Chloroquine-resistant strains of *P vivax* (reported from Papua New Guinea, Indonesia, the Solomon Islands and elsewhere): quinine sulfate 650 mg PO q8h for 3-7 days *plus* doxycycline 100 mg BID for 7 days (or *plus* clindamycin 20 mg/kg/d in 3 doses for 7 days for use in pregnancy)

    *Alternative: mefloquine 750 mg PO followed by 500 mg 12 h later (*note*: high rate of side effects with this dose of mefloquine)

- Chloroquine-resistant strains of *P falciparum* (reported in all endemic areas except Central America, Haiti, the Dominican Republic, North Africa, and parts of the Middle East) or *P falciparum* infections of unknown origin: quinine sulfate 650 mg PO q8h x 3-7 d plus doxycycline 100 mg BID for 7 days (or plus clindamycin 20 mg/kg/d in 3 doses for 7 days for use in pregnancy)

    or

- Combination of atovaquone 1 g and proguanil 400 mg (Malarone®) PO QD for 3 days

- Alternatives: mefloquine 750 mg PO followed by 500 mg 12 h later (note: high rate of side effects with this dose of mefloquine)

    or

- Parenteral therapy for all species: intravenous quinidine followed by doxycycline or clindamycin as above; for severe cases of falciparum malaria or when quinidine is not available: artesunate 4 mg/kg/d IV for 3 days plus atovaquone and

proguanil or mefloquine in doses above (artesunate available from CDC).

Prognostic Factors

- Prognosis excellent for infections with all species except *P falciparum*.

- Prognosis in falciparum malaria related to delay before treatment, level of parasitemia, and presence of severe complications such as cerebral malaria, renal failure and pulmonary edema.

- Pregnant women, spleen-deficient persons and the elderly are at increased risk for severe and complicated falciparum malaria.

ID Board Pearls

- Suspect malaria in any febrile traveler returning from an endemic area.

- Thick and thin blood smears for diagnosis.

- Falciparum malaria can be rapidly fatal and should be treated as a medical emergency.

- Appropriate treatment depends on species of parasites and risk of drug resistance, which varies by geographic origin of infection.

- All travelers to malarious areas should use personal protection measures to avoid mosquito bites and take appropriate antimalarial prophylaxis.

2. Amebiasis

Causative Organism

- *Entamoeba histolytica*

Epidemiology

- Transmission by fecal contamination of food and drink and by person-to-person contact (close contact among institutionalized persons, oral-anal sex).

- Most common in developing areas, but also seen in industrialized countries.

Key Clinical Features

Asymptomatic Infection
- Majority of cases, but cysts shed in stools pose threat to other persons.

Amebic Dysentery and Colitis
- Abdominal pain

- Small ulcers seen on endoscopy

- Blood in stools

- Diarrhea

- Occasionally fever

- Fecal leukocytes usually absent

Ameboma
- Exuberant inflammatory response and granulation tissue

- Mass lesion (pseudotumor)

Liver Abscess
- Fever

- Right upper quadrant pain

- Weight loss

- Hepatomegaly

- Abscess usually single, in right lobe, detected by ultrasound, CT scan or MRI

- Right hemidiaphragm often elevated on chest radiograph

Key Laboratory Features

Colonic Infection
- Microscopic examination of stool for cysts and motile trophozoites (less sensitive than stool antigen test)

- Does not distinguish between *E histolytica* and morphologically identical, nonpathogenic *E dispar* and *E moshkovskii*

- Must distinguish from other nonpathogenic intestinal protozoa: *Entamoeba hartmanni, Entamoeba coli, Iodamoeba butschlii, Endolimax nana;* pathogenicity of *Blastocystis hominis* debated

- Perform endoscopy and microscopic examination of exudates or biopsy for trophozoites: amebas and neutrophils easily confused by the inexperienced observer

- Stool antigen test:

    * More sensitive than microscopy

    * One assay detects *E histolytica* and not *E dispar*

- Serological tests for antibodies to *E histolytica*:

    * Negative in asymptomatic amebiasis

    * Right hemidiaphragm often elevated on chest radiograph

    * Positive in almost 90% of persons with amebic dysentery

    * Right hemidiaphragm often elevated on chest radiograph

Hepatic Infection
- Perform microscopic examination of aspirated abscess fluid:

* Amebas frequently not seen in fluid

* Aspiration not necessary for diagnosis

• Perform microscopic examination of stool; amebas frequently not seen in stool

• Perform serologic test: positive in >90%

Differential Diagnosis

Infectious Diseases
• Bacterial dysentery (fecal leukocytes present)

• Pyogenic liver abscess, infected echinococcal cyst

Noninfectious Disease Mimics:
• Ulcerative colitis

• Colonic carcinoma

• Hepatocellular carcinoma

Therapy

• Invasive disease: metronidazole 500-750 mg PO (or IV) TID for 7-10 days or tinidazole 2 g QD for 3-5 days) *plus* paromomycin or iodoquinol (as below).

• Asymptomatic disease or following metronidazole for invasive disease: Paromomycin 8-12 mg/kg PO TID for 7 days.

   * Alternative: iodoquinol 650 mg PO TID for 20 days

Complications

• Fulminant colonic amebiasis, toxic megacolon, perforation with amebic peritonitis

• Cutaneous amebiasis

• Rupture of liver abscess into peritoneal cavity, pleural space, lungs, pericardium

• Brain abscess (rare)

Prognostic Factors

• Disease more severe in persons taking corticosteroids

ID Board Pearls

• Infection with *Entamoeba histolytica* may be asymptomatic, or cause mild diarrhea, dysentery, fulminant colitis or liver abscess.

• Amebiasis should be ruled out in all persons in whom a diagnosis of inflammatory bowel disease is being considered.

• *Entamoeba histolytica* and *Entamoeba dispar* morphologically identical, cannot be distinguished by microscopy, require stool antigen test or PCR-based assay for differentiation.

• Diagnosis of amoebic liver abscess best confirmed by serology; stool microscopy and microscopic examination of aspirated fluid frequently negative for amoebas.

• All persons with *Entamoeba histolytica* infection should receive a luminal amoebicide (paromomycin, iodoquinol); those with invasive disease required treatment with a tissue amoebicide (metronidazole, tinidazole).

3. Giardiasis

Causative Organism

- *Giardia intestinalis*

Epidemiology

- Most common intestinal parasite and leading cause of water-borne outbreaks of diarrhea in the United States.

- Transmitted via water contaminated with human or animal feces and by person-to-person contact.

- Seen in:

  * Campers who drink water from mountain streams

  * Swimmers

  * Travelers returning from developing countries

  * Children in day-care centers and their families

  * Gay males

Key Clinical Features

- Asymptomatic cyst passage

- Acute self-limited diarrhea

- Persistent diarrhea

- Chronic illness with abdominal cramps, diarrhea, malabsorption, weight loss

- Cramping and gas prominent; no fever

- Diarrhea is watery (no blood or WBCs)

Key Laboratory Features

- Tests for antigen in stool

- Stool examination (multiple specimens may be required)

- String test or duodenal aspiration rarely required

Differential Diagnosis

Infectious Diseases
- Cryptosporidiosis, isosporiasis, cyclosporiasis

- Other secretory infectious diarrheas (viruses, cholera, toxigenic *E coli* infection)

Noninfectious Disease Mimics:

- Sprue, tropical sprue

Therapy

- Tinidazole 2g PO for 1 dose

    or

- Metronidazole 250 mg PO TID for 5 days

    or

- Nitazoxanide 500 mg PO BID for 3 days

  * Alternatives: furazolidone 100 mg or 6 mg/kg PO QID for 7-10 days (less effective, but liquid suspension useful for treatment of children)

    or

  * Paromomycin 25-30 mg/kg/d PO in divided doses for 5-10 days. Not absorbed, may be effective when other agents are contraindicated, such as during early pregnancy

    or

  * Albendazole 400 mg PO QD for 5 days

Complications

- Malabsorption, malnutrition

- Lactase deficiency following treatment

Prognostic Factors

- X-linked agammaglobulinemia and common variable immunodeficiency associated with chronic and recurrent infections.

ID Board Pearls

- Suspect giardiasis in persons with nonbloody diarrhea lasting longer than 7-10 days, abdominal cramping and bloating.

- Risk factors for giardiasis include close contact with an infected person (such as a child in daycare), oral-anal sex, recreational water exposure, consumption of water from potentially contaminated mountain streams and travel to developing countries.

- Multiple microscopic examinations of stool may be necessary to make the diagnosis; stool antigen test as sensitive as free stool examinations.

- Treatment of choice is metronidazole or tinidazole; alternatives include nitazoxanide, parmomycin, albendazole; refractory cases may require multiple courses of treatment or combination treatment.

- In persons with persistent diarrhea after treatment suspect reinfection (eg, from untreated child in daycare), immunoglobulin deficiency or post-infectious lactase deficiency

4. Other Intestinal Protozoan Infections

Causative Organisms

- *Cryptosporidium hominis* (and other species); *Isospora belli; Cyclospora cayetanensis*

Epidemiology

- All are transmitted by ingestion of contaminated water and food in developing countries; cryptosporidiosis also common in industrialized countries.

- *Cryptosporidium* also transmitted directly from person to person and from animals (especially livestock) to persons.

- Contamination of water supply with *Cryptosporidium* the cause of city-wide waterborne outbreaks; most common cause of outbreaks associated with swimming pools and parks.

- Food-borne outbreaks of cyclosporiasis in the United States from contaminated imported produce (raspberries, mesclun lettuce, basil).

Key Clinical Features

Immunocompetent Persons
- Self-limited illness lasting days to several weeks

- Infection limited to small bowel

- Diarrhea, nausea, cramping

- Stool watery, voluminous

- No blood or WBCs in stool

- Fever and flu-like symptoms

Persons with AIDS or Immunosuppression
- Illness may not resolve without treatment

- Infection throughout GI tract, bile ducts, bronchial tree

- Persistent diarrhea with massive fluid loss and malnutrition

- Right upper quadrant pain from sclerosing cholangitis

Key Laboratory Features

- Microscopic examination for oocysts in stool facilitated by acid-fast stain, fluorescence (*Cyclospora*), or immunofluorescence (*Cryptosporidium*).

- Stool antigen test for *Cryptosporidium*.

- *Isospora belli* often associated with peripheral blood eosinophilia.

Differential Diagnosis

Infectious Diseases
- Giardiasis

- Microsporidiosis in persons with AIDS and other immunocompromised persons

- Other secretory infectious diarrheas (cholera, toxigenic *E coli* infection)

Noninfectious Disease Mimics:
- Sprue, tropical sprue

Therapy

- Cryptosporidiosis: nitazoxanide 500 mg PO TID for 3 days (adult dose), moderately effective in persons without AIDS. For persons with AIDS, no consistently effective specific treatment. Some experts recommend trials of nitazoxanide, paromomycin or azithromycin.

- Isosporiasis: 160 mg trimethoprim and 800 sulfamethoxazole PO BID for 10 days. AIDS patients and other immunocompromised persons: 160 mg trimethoprim and 800 mg sulfamethoxazole PO QID for 10 days, then BID for 21 days, followed by suppressive therapy for duration of immunosuppression.

- Cyclosporiasis: 160 mg trimethoprim and 800 mg sulfamethoxazole PO BID for 7-10 days. AIDS patients and other immunocompromised persons

may require longer course followed by suppressive therapy for duration of immunosuppression.

- Reconstitution of immune system by antiretroviral drugs or discontinuation of immunosuppressive therapy often eliminates persistent infection.

Prognostic Factors

- Elderly, infants and debilitated persons may tolerate acute infections poorly.

- AIDS patients and other immunosuppressed persons often unable to clear infection without treatment.

ID Board Pearls

- Prolonged, nonbloody, watery diarrhea lasting greater than 10-14 days should prompt evaluation for infection with *Cryptosporidium*, *Isospora* and *Cyclospora*.

- If diarrhea persists longer than 2-3 weeks, consider HIV infection or other immunosuppression.

- *Isospora* and *Cyclospora* spread by ingestion of contaminated fluids or food; no direct person-to-person transmission; seen in travelers and immigrants except for *Cyclospora* outbreaks within the U.S. due to imported contaminated raspberries, mesclun lettuce and basil.

- *Cryptosporidium* transmitted in the U.S. by person-to-person contact, contact with animals, ingestion of contaminated fluids or food; occasional outbreaks 2o to contamination of recreational water or municipal drinking water.

- *Cyclospora* and *Isospora* infections are treated with trimethoprim-sulfamethoxazole; treatment of cryptosporidiosis unsatisfactory; nitazoxanide effective in healthy children, but not HIV-infected; highly active antiretroviral therapy and immune reconstitution is the best approach in persons with AIDS.

5. Toxoplasmosis

Causative Organism

• *Toxoplasma gondii*

Epidemiology

• Worldwide distribution; as many as 15%-30% of U.S. adults infected.

• Transmission by:

  * Ingestion of tissue cysts in raw or poorly cooked meat, especially lamb and pork

  * Ingestion of food, drink, or soil contaminated with cat feces that contain infective oocysts

  * Transplacental passage of tachyzoites from mother to fetus

  * Transfusion of infected white blood cells or transplantation of an infected organ

Key Clinical Features

• Infection acquired by healthy persons:

  * Usually asymptomatic

  * Painless lymphadenopathy

  * Mononucleosis syndrome

  * Chorioretinitis

  * Serious disease rare

• Infection in persons with depressed cellular immunity (persons with AIDS, transplant recipients, persons receiving immunosuppressants):

  * Focal lesions of the CNS, lethal meningoencephalitis

  * Less commonly myocarditis or pneumonitis

  * Usually due to reactivation of latent infection

  * 40%-50% of AIDS patients with IgG antibodies to *T gondii* develop active toxoplasmosis

  * Headache, seizures, mental status changes, focal neurologic signs, aseptic meningitis

• Congenital infection:

  * Occurs when a previously uninfected mother acquires infection during pregnancy

  * Maternal infection usually unrecognized

  * Infection early in pregnancy results in abortion, stillbirth, live infant with severe neurologic and retinal damage

  * Infections later in pregnancy usually asymptomatic at birth (as are the majority of cases of congenital toxoplasmosis)

  * High rate of recurrent toxoplasmic chorioretinitis in children and young adults with congenital infection that was asymptomatic at birth

• Ocular infection:

  * Necrotizing chorioretinitis results in retinal scars, visual impairment

  * Common sequela of congenital toxoplasmosis; also occurs in acute acquired toxoplasmosis

  * Recurrences frequent

Key Diagnostic Laboratory and Radiologic Features

• Acute Toxoplasmosis in a Healthy Host:

  * Distinctive histology in biopsied lymph node

  * Organisms rarely identified in tissue or isolated by culture

  * Elevated level of serum IgM antibody to *T gondii* (preferred method of diagnosis)

  * Rising level of IgG antibodies to *T gondii* in serum

* Radiographs usually not obtained

- **Toxoplasmosis in AIDS and Other Immunocompromised Persons**
  * Distinctive histology in brain biopsy or at autopsy

  * Organisms identified in tissue sections, occasionally isolated from CSF

  * Specific IgM antibodies usually absent

  * Level of specific IgG antibody elevated in serum

  * PCR-based assays usually not performed; parasite DNA in CSF occasionally detected by PCR

  * Multiple hypodense enhancing lesions by CT or MR presumptive diagnosis based on radiographic findings, positive IgG antibody test and response to anti-toxoplasma therapy (preferred diagnostic approach)

- **Congenital Toxoplasmosis**
  * Distinctive histology in brain biopsy or at autopsy

  * Organisms identified in tissue sections, occasionally isolated from CSF

  * Elevated level of serum IgM antibody to *T gondii* (preferred method of diagnosis)

  * Persistence of specific IgG antibodies in serum during first year of life (preferred method of diagnosis)

  * PCR-based assays usually not performed

  * Cerebral calcifications, areas of cerebral necrosis, hydrocephalus by CT or MRI of head

- **Ocular Toxoplasmosis**
  * Tissue or fluid not usually obtained for culture

  * Specific IgM antibodies usually absent

* Level of specific IgG antibody elevated in serum and in aqueous or vitreous humor

* PCR-based assays limited availability

* Radiographs usually not obtained (preferred method of diagnosis based on funduscopic examination and positive IgG antibody test in serum and/or ocular fluid)

Differential Diagnosis

Infectious Diseases
- Infectious causes of lymphadenopathy (eg, cat-scratch disease)

- Mononucleosis

- Brain abscess

- Congenital infections, such as CMV

- Uveitis or chorioretinitis associated with tuberculosis, syphilis, leprosy, fungal diseases

Noninfectious Disease Mimics:
- Lymphoma, Hodgkin's disease

- Brain tumor

- Sarcoidosis, connective tissue diseases and other causes of noninfectious uveitis

Therapy

- Pyrimethamine 25-100 mg PO QD

  Plus

- Sulfadiazine 1-1.5 g PO QID

  Plus

- Leucovorin (folinic *not* folic acid) 10-25 mg PO QD

- Alternative regimens: pyrimethamine and leucovorin

  Plus

- Clindamycin 600-800 mg IV or PO QID or atovaquone 750 mg PO BID

or

- Spiramycin 3-4 g PO QD in divided doses

- Acute acquired toxoplasmosis usually does not require treatment. The exception is during pregnancy, in which case spiramycin is given during the first trimester and continued throughout pregnancy if there is no evidence of fetal infection (by PCR-based testing of amniotic fluid); if there is evidence of fetal infection, pyrimethamine/sulfadiazine/leucovorin is given until delivery.

- Toxoplasmosis in the immunocompromised host requires treatment for 4-6 weeks followed by suppressive therapy for the duration of immunosuppression. Clindamycin is often substituted for sulfadiazine in AIDS patients who cannot tolerate sulfonamides, and atovaquone substituted for sulfonamides and clindamycin in patients who cannot tolerate these 2 drugs.

- Congenital toxoplasmosis is treated with pyrimethamine, sulfadiazine and leucovorin in pediatric doses (not provided here) for the first year of life.

- Active chorioretinitis is treated with 4 weeks of anti-toxoplasma therapy and corticosteroids to decrease inflammation.

Prognostic Factors

- AIDS and other immunocompromised patients and fetuses in utero (especially during the first trimester) are at risk for severe disease.

- Primary prevention in HIV-infected and other immunocompromised patients with serologic evidence of chronic toxoplasmosis: trimethoprimsulfamethoxazole (or pyrimethamine-dapsone or atovaquone)

ID Board Pearls

- Prevention of acute infection most important in pregnant women, HIV-infected persons and other immunosuppressed persons.

- Acute infection in healthy person usually asymptomatic; may cause isolated, regional or diffuse lymphadenopathy; produce a mononucleosis-like syndrome, and occasionally cause chorioretinitis.

- A positive IgG test for toxoplasma prior to conception virtually guarantees against transplacental transmission unless mother is immunocompromised.

- Toxoplasmosis leading cause of space occupying lesions of CNS in persons with AIDS; a positive IgG test for *Toxoplasma* hypodense, ring-enhancing lesions with surrounding edema on scans should prompt empirical therapy in HIV-infected persons.

- Leucovorin should always be given with pyrimethamine, which in combination with sulfadiazine is the treatment of choice for active toxoplasmosis.

6. American *trypanosomiasis* (Chagas' Disease)

Causative Organism

• *Trypanosoma cruzi*

Epidemiology

• Endemic in 17 countries in Central and South America and in Mexico; as many as 100,000 infected immigrants from impoverished rural areas in Latin America live in the United States.

• Transmission by:

  * Vector triatomine (reduviid) bugs that infest houses of poor construction in rural areas

  * Transfusion of blood from a chronically infected donor

  * Transplacental transfer from infected mother

Key Clinical Features

Acute Stage
• Most persons asymptomatic

• Occasional edematous swelling around eye (Romaña's sign) or other portal of entry (chagoma)

• Occasional mononucleosis-like illness

• Rarely, life-threatening myocarditis or meningoencephalitis, particularly in immunocompromised persons

Chronic Stage
• Most persons asymptomatic for life

• 20%-30% develop chronic heart disease or gastrointestinal disease years to decades later

• *Chronic Chagas' heart cardiomyopathy*
  * Right bundle branch block common

  * Congestive heart failure

  * Arrhythmias and heart block

  * Sudden death

• *Chagas' gastrointestinal disease*
  * Dysphagia and megaesophagus

  * Constipation and megacolon

• Reactivation of chronic Chagas' disease in AIDS and other immunocompromised persons: CNS lesions, myocarditis

Key Laboratory Features

Acute Stage
• Microscopic examination of wet mounts of blood or Giemsa-stained smears shows trypanosomes (motile on wet mounts)

• Isolation of parasites by blood culture or xenodiagnosis

• Detection of specific IgM antibodies or rising titers of IgG antibodies

• PCR-based detection of parasite DNA in blood

Chronic Stage
• Parasites not detectable microscopically

• Parasites isolated by blood culture or xenodiagnosis in up to 70% of persons

• Detection of specific IgG but not IgM antibodies

• PCR-based detection of parasite DNA in blood

Differential Diagnosis

Infectious Diseases
• Orbital cellulitis

• Mononucleosis

• Acute myocarditis

• Acute meningoencephalitis

• Congenital infections such as CMV, toxoplasmosis

• Cerebral toxoplasmosis

Noninfectious Disease Mimics:

• Dilated cardiomyopathy

• Achalasia of the esophagus

• Hirschsprung's disease of the colon

Therapy

• Nifurtimox 8-10 mg/kg/d PO in 3-4 doses for 90 days

• Benznidazole 5-7 mg/kg PO in 2 divided doses for 60 days

• Therapy most likely to eliminate infection when given during the acute stage or early chronic stage

• Treatment indicated for persons with acute or congenital infection; infection in immunocompromised persons; children with chronic infection; effectiveness of treatment in chronically infected adults uncertain, but current guidelines advise consideration of treatment in young and middle-aged adults who do not have advanced cardiac disease.

Prognostic Factors

• Acute stage: infants and immunocompromised at increased risk of severe illness and death

• Chronic stage:

  * Persons who develop evidence of heart disease have a poor prognosis

  * Immunocompromised persons at risk for CNS lesions and acute myocarditis

ID Board Pearls

• Large number of asymptomatic persons with ***Trypanosoma cruzi*** infection in the US; 20%-30% of these will develop chronic heart or gastrointestinal disease.

• Consider Chagas' disease in native of Latin America with congestive heart failure, arrhythmias, right bundle branch block, dysphagia, or prolonged constipation.

• Reactivation of *Trypanosoma cruzi* infection may cause a clinical and radiographic picture identical to that of CNS toxoplasmosis in persons with AIDS or otherwise immunocompromised.

• Diagnosis of chronic *Trypanosoma cruzi* made by detecting specific antibodies and serological tests by at least 2 different methods (IFA, ELISA, IHA, etc.).

• Treatment options include nifurtimox and benznidazole.

7. African *trypanosomiasis*

Synonyms

• African sleeping sickness, West African trypanosomiasis and East African trypanosomiasis.

Causative Organisms

• *Trypanosoma brucei rhodesiense* (East African or Rhodesian trypanosomiasis)

• *Trypanosoma brucei gambiense* (West African or Gambian trypanosomiasis)

Epidemiology

• Vector: tsetse fly (species *Glossina*)

• Limited to sub-Saharan Africa

• West African trypanosomiasis: found in West and central Africa (especially Southern Sudan, Uganda, DR Congo, Angola), anthropronosis, transmission in dark, humid areas near bodies of water; potential for epidemics

• East African sleeping sickness: found in East Africa; zoonosis (cattle and wild game); transmission in savannah areas; acquired by expatriates on safari

Key Clinical Features

• Trypanosomal chancre: inflamed subcutaneous nodule at site of inoculation; seen most commonly in expatriates with East African trypanosomiasis

• Hemolymphatic stage (West African disease): recurrent fever, lymphadenopathy, edematous swellings; illness mild or subclinical and lasts up to 2 or 3 years before CNS invasion occurs

• Hemolymphatic stage (East African disease): acute febrile illness with toxicity, shock, DIC, myocarditis; death may occur before CNS invasion; CNS invasion within several months of infection

• Late stage sleeping sickness: progressive illness with difficulty concentrating, personality changes, daytime somnolence, extrapyramidal and other

motor defects, coma. Death typically in coma from secondary infection, malnutrition and wasting.

Key Diagnostic Laboratory and Radiologic Features

• Nonspecific: anemia; WBC variable, often with a monocytosis (West African disease) or left shift (East Africa disease); elevated serum immunoglobulins, especially IgM.

• West African trypanosomiasis: card agglutination test for screening

• Both: identification of trypanosomes in aspirates of trypanosomal chancre or enlarged lymph node, in peripheral blood and CSF.

• A positive card agglutination test or finding of parasites in the chancre, lymph node or blood requires lumbar puncture to rule out CNS disease.

• Finding of parasites, elevated protein and CSF pleocytosis (>5 cells/cc) indicative of CNS invasion.

Differential Diagnosis

• Malaria

• Typhoid fever

• Acute brucellosis

• Bacterial sepsis

• Mononucleosis

• Acute myocarditis

• Encephalitis

Complications

• 100% fatal if not treated.

Therapy (see The Medical Letter for doses)

• Gambian trypanosomiasis

* Early stage: pentamadine IM or IV

* Late stage: eflornithine IV, combination of eflornithine and oral nifurtimox

* Alternative: IV melarsoprol (*note*: 5%-20% melarsoprol resistance in several countries)

• Rhodesian trypanosomiasis

* Early stage: suramin

* Late stage: melarsoprol

Prognostic Factors

• Fatal without treatment.

• Outcome worse with CNS disease.

• 5%-10% rate of hemorrhagic encephalopathy secondary to melarsoprol with high fatality rate.

ID Board Pearls

• Most cases of African trypanosomiasis seen in the United States are among tourists returning from a safari in wild game parks; they tend to be acutely ill with East African trypanosomiasis.

• Cases of West African trypanosomiasis have been seen in the United States, among African nationals who came to the U.S. to live or study and after a year or so develop signs of CNS disease.

• Definitive diagnosis of African trypanosomiasis requires identification of parasites in smears of aspirates of tissue or lymph nodes, peripheral blood or CSF.

• Anyone suspected of having African trypanosomiasis should have a lumbar puncture. The finding of parasites or greater than 5 cells per cc indicate CNS involvement.

• Treatment of African trypanosomiasis depends on the stage and location of acquisition of the infection (West or central Africa vs. East Africa).

8. *Leishmania* species (visceral leishmaniasis, cutaneous leishmaniasis, mucosal leishmaniasis)

Causative agents

• Visceral leishmaniasis: *Leishmania donovani, infantum, chagasi*

• Cutaneous leishmaniasis: *Leishmania tropica, major, mexicana, braziliensis*, others

• Mucosal leishmaniasis: *Leishmania braziliensis* primarily

Synonyms

• Visceral leishmaniasis: kala-azar

• Cutaneous leishmaniasis: Oriental sore, Delhi button, uta, various others

• Mucosal leishmaniasis: espundia

Epidemiology

• Transmitted by sand flies (*Phlebotomus, Lutzomyia* species).

• Found on all continents, except Antarctica and Australia.

• Some species anthroponotic, others zoonotic (reservoirs include canines, marsupials, rodents, various other species of mammals).

• Leishmaniasis among travelers returning to the U.S. is most commonly cutaneous, associated with visits to nature reserves in Central America or military service in the Middle East.

Key Clinical Features

• Visceral leishmaniasis: prolonged fever, wasting, hepatosplenomegaly, pancytopenia, increased serum immunoglobulins, death after weeks or months from infection and bleeding.

• Cutaneous leishmaniasis: nonhealing papule at site of insect bite that enlarges and ulcerates; typical presentation = nonhealing, painless cutaneous ulcer of weeks or months duration.

- Mucosal leishmaniasis: ulceration of nasal pharynx, usually appearing months to years after healing of cutaneous ulcer; may appear at the same time as cutaneous ulcer or in the absence of cutaneous ulcer; highly disfiguring lesions; found largely in Latin America, where *Leishmania braziliensis* is endemic.

Differential Diagnosis

- Visceral leishmaniasis: disseminated histoplasmosis, miliary tuberculosis, lymphoma

- Cutaneous leishmaniasis: ecthyma, venous stasis ulcer, basal cell carcinoma

- Mucosal leishmaniasis: syphilis, leprosy, midline granuloma

Key Laboratory Features

- All species: intracellular parasites in smears stained by Giemsa; parasites grown on special culture media; PCR-based assays

- Visceral leishmaniasis: parasites in aspirates of bone marrow or spleen; specific IgG antibody test positive

- Cutaneous leishmaniasis: parasites in scrapings of base of lesion, biopsies of leading edge of lesion, aspirates of lesion; serology usually negative; species identification by isoenzymes, monoclonal antibodies or PCR (critical for lesions acquired in the Americas, where multiple different species circulate in the same geographical area)

- Mucosal leishmaniasis: parasites in biopsies of lesions sparse; serology usually positive

Complications

- Visceral leishmaniasis: secondary infections, bleeding, death

- Cutaneous leishmaniasis: infection of open lesions, cutaneous scars; inadequate treatment of *Leishmania braziliensis* can lead to mucosal leishmaniasis

- Mucosal leishmaniasis: destruction of nose, oropharynx; malnutrition; aspiration pneumonia

Therapy (see Medical Letter for specific doses)

- Visceral leishmaniasis: liposomal amphotericin is drug of choice; alternatives include amphotericin B deoxycholate, sodium antimony gluconate (Pentostam® available from CDC); intravenous parmomycin; miltefosine

- Cutaneous leishmaniasis: lesions secondary to *Leishmania major* or *Leishmania mexicana* may heal rapidly and not require therapy; other lesions: sodium antimony gluconate (intramuscular, intravenous or intralesional), liposomal amphotericin

- Mucosal leishmaniasis: liposomal amphotericin, sodium antimony gluconate

Prognostic Factors

- Visceral leishmaniasis: poor outcome with delayed diagnosis and treatment or in severely malnourished individuals. Infection relapses in persons with advanced HIV disease.

- Cutaneous leishmaniasis: depending on species, lesions may heal within months or years or may fail to heal (*Leishmania braziliensis*).

- Mucosal leishmaniasis: may require multiple courses of therapy for healing; may not respond to therapy.

ID Board Pearls

- Consider cutaneous leishmaniasis in travelers returning from developing countries who have nonhealing lesions of the skin.

- In cases of cutaneous leishmaniasis acquired in the Americas, important to obtain a species diagnosis because *Leishmania braziliensis* poses a risk of mucosal leishmaniasis and needs to be treated aggressively.

- Visceral leishmaniasis is rare among travelers, although it has been seen as a cause of febrile illness, pancytopenia and wasting in patients with AIDS who had spent time in endemic areas, even in the remote past.

- Diagnosis of leishmaniasis is made by identifying intracellular parasites on smears, and in microscopic sections of tissue, by culture, by PCR-based assays, and in cases of visceral leishmaniasis, by serological tests

- Liposomal amphotericin B drug of choice for treatment of visceral leishmaniasis. Many experts prefer amphotericin over traditional treatment with sodium antimony gluconate.

9. Schistosomiasis

Synonyms

- Bilharzia, Katayama fever (acute schistosomiasis)

Causative Organisms

- *Schistosoma mansoni, japonicum, hematobium, mekongi, intercalatum*

Epidemiology

- Infection acquired in warm climates by contact with fresh water infested with snail intermediate hosts that shed infective larvae (cercariae).

- Incidence increasing in parts of the world as a consequence of water resource development projects.

Intestinal

- *S mansoni*: Africa, Middle East, Caribbean, South America

- *S japonicum*: China, Philippines, Southeast Asia

- *S mekongi*: Southeast Asia

- *S intercalatum*: Africa

Urinary

- *S hematobium*: Africa, Middle East

Key Clinical Features

Acute Schistosomiasis or Katayama Fever
- Occurs 2-6 weeks after first-time exposure

- Fever

- Headache

- Abdominal pain

- Myalgia, arthralgia

- Dry cough

- Diarrhea

- Lymphadenopathy

- Hepatosplenomegaly

- Urticaria

- Pronounced eosinophilia

Ectopic deposition of eggs
- Lesions in skin and genitalia, transverse myelitis, mass brain lesions

Chronic Intestinal/Hepatic Schistosomiasis
- Usually asymptomatic

- Eosinophilia common

- Intestinal polyps

- Intestinal strictures

- Bloody diarrhea

- Hepatosplenomegaly

- Periportal fibrosis

- Portal hypertension

- Esophageal varices

- Rarely:

    * Transverse myelitis or mass brain lesions from ectopic deposition of eggs in nervous system

Chronic Urinary Schistosomiasis
- Often asymptomatic

- Eosinophilia common

- Hematuria

- Proteinuria

- Dysuria

- Urinary tract infections

- Bladder polyps

- Carcinoma of the bladder

- Hydroureter, hydronephrosis from fibrosis and calcification of bladder and lower ureters

Ectopic deposition of eggs
- Genital lesions common; transverse myelitis rare

Key Laboratory and Radiological Features

Acute Schistosomiasis
Laboratory
- Microscopic examination of urine or stool for eggs often negative until several weeks after onset of symptoms.

- Demonstration of specific antibodies in serum.

Radiologic
- Interstitial infiltrates on chest radiograph

Intestinal Schistosomiasis
Laboratory
- Microscopic examination of stool or urine for eggs

- Examination of snips of rectal mucosa obtained at proctoscopy for eggs

- Demonstration of specific antibodies in serum

Radiologic
- Ultrasound, CT, MR: periportal (pipestem) fibrosis, portal hypertension, and for *S japonicum*, "turtleback" calcification

- Barium swallow: esophageal varices

Urinary Schistosomiasis
Laboratory
- Microscopic examination of stool or urine for eggs

- Examination of snips of bladder mucosa from cystoscopy for eggs

- Demonstration of specific antibodies in serum

Radiologic
- Ultrasound, CT, contrast radiographs: strictures, polyps, masses, hydroureter, hydronephrosis

- Plain radiograph: calcified bladder, distal ureters

Differential Diagnosis

Infectious Diseases
- Malaria, typhoid, other febrile illnesses of travelers

- Visceral larva migrans, trichinellosis

- Chronic hepatitis

- Urinary tract infections, including tuberculosis

Noninfectious Disease Mimics:
- Serum sickness

- Intestinal polyposis

- Bowel tumor

- Cirrhosis of the liver

- Obstructive urinary tract disease

Therapy

- Praziquantel 40 mg/kg PO in 2 doses for 1 day (60 mg/kg for *S japonicum, mekongi*)

- Alternative for *S mansoni*: oxamniquine 15 mg/kg PO for 1 day (40-60 mg/kg over 2-3 days in Africa)

Prognostic Factors

- Persons with heavy infections at risk for severe disease.

- Coinfection with hepatitis B or C worsens prognosis of persons with portal hypertension.

- Treatment may reverse or partially reverse fibrotic lesions.

ID Board Pearls

- A traveler or immigrant with a history of freshwater contact in a schistosomiasis endemic area should be evaluated with serological tests +/- microscopic examination of the stool to rule out infection.

- Expatriate travelers are more likely to present with acute schistosomiasis than immigrants; expatriate travelers with chronic infection usually have lower worm burdens and it may be difficult to find eggs in the stool or urine.

- Acute schistosomiasis develops 2-8 weeks after first-time contact with contaminated water; characterized by fever, headache, myalgia, dry cough, diarrhea, hives and elevated peripheral blood eosinophil counts.

- Most persons with chronic schistosomiasis have no symptoms of infection; eosinophilia common.

- All persons with schistosomiasis (including those with light infections) should receive praziquantel because of the risk of complications, including ectopic egg deposition and neurological catastrophes.

10. Liver Flukes

Synonyms

• Chinese liver fluke (*Clonorchis*), cat liver fluke (*Opisthorchis felineus*)

• Sheep liver fluke (*Fasciola hepatica*), giant liver fluke (*F gigantica*)

Causative Organisms

• *Clonorchis sinensis, Opisthorchis viverrini and O felineus; Fasciola hepatica* and *F gigantica*

Epidemiology

• *Clonorchis* and *Opisthorchis* acquired by ingesting poorly-cooked or raw carp or other fresh-water fish infected with larval stage organisms (metacercariae).

• Distribution of *Clonorchis, Opisthorchis*: East Asia, Southeast Asia, countries of former USSR

• *Fasciola* acquired by ingesting uncooked watercress or other fresh aquatic vegetation in which larval stage organisms (metacercariae) have encysted.

• *F hepatica* endemic in sheep-raising areas throughout the world, especially Bolivia, Peru, Iran, Egypt, Portugal, France; distribution of *F gigantica* more focal.

Key Clinical Features

Clonorchiasis, Opisthorchiasis
• Acute illness (unusual): 2-3 weeks after initial exposure:

  * Fever

  * Abdominal pain

  * Hepatomegaly

  * Urticaria

  * Eosinophilia

• Chronic infection:

  * Usually asymptomatic

  * Eosinophilia occasionally

• Heavy chronic infection causes irritation and inflammation of biliary epithelium:

  * Right upper quadrant discomfort

  * Anorexia

  * Weight loss

  * Hepatomegaly

  * Infrequent: cholangitis, pancreatitis

  * Rare: cholangiocarcinoma

Fascioliasis
• Acute illness due to immature worms migrating through liver:

  * Fever

  * Nausea

  * Tender hepatomegaly

  * Eosinophilia

  * Urticaria

  * Migratory cutaneous nodules from aberrant migration of worms

• Chronic infection:

  * Often asymptomatic

  * Eosinophilia unusual

  * Occasionally symptoms of biliary colic, cholangitis due to inflammation and obstruction of bile ducts

Key Laboratory and Radiological Features

Clonorchiasis, Opisthorchiasis
- Microscopic examination of stool for eggs

- Identification of adult worms or eggs in biliary tree during surgery

- Chronic infection: abnormal gallbladder, cystic dilatations and strictures of bile duct by ultrasound, CT, cholangiogram

- Adult worms seen by cholangiogram, ultrasound

Fascioliasis
- Acute infection: eggs not in stool for several months; acute infection diagnosed by specific antibody tests

- Chronic infection: microscopic examination of stool for eggs; identification of adult worms or eggs in biliary tree during surgery

- Migratory, hypodense lesions in the liver during acute stage by ultrasound, CT

- Chronic stage: ultrasound, cholangiogram demonstrate biliary pathology and adult worms in biliary tree

Differential Diagnosis

Infectious Diseases
- Acute schistosomiasis

- Visceral larva migrans

- Myiasis, other larva migrans syndromes

Noninfectious Disease Mimics:
- Biliary colic, cholecystitis, cholangitis

- Pancreatitis

Therapy

- Clonorchiasis, opisthorchiasis: praziquantel 75 mg/kg/d PO in 3 doses for 1 day

  * Alternative: albendazole 10 mg/kg PO for 7 days

- Fascioliasis: triclabendazole 10 mg/kg PO for 1 day

  * Alternative: nitazoxanide 500 mg BID PO for 3 days

Prognostic Factors

- Severe symptoms associated with heavy infection.

- Prognosis poor with cholangiocarcinoma.

ID Board Pearls

- Suspect infection with liver flukes: history of ingestion of uncooked/poorly cooked fish in Southeast Asia, Far East, or Eastern Europe; raw watercress or other aquatic plants in sheep-raising parts of the world, especially Bolivia, Egypt, parts of the Middle East and elsewhere.

- Symptoms are most pronounced during the first several months of infection, when larvae migrate; at this time fever, abdominal pain, urticaria, markedly elevated peripheral blood eosinophil count and occasionally ectopic lesions are seen.

- In acute *Fasciola* infection, migratory hypodense lesions in the liver by CT or MR scans are characteristic.

- Most chronic infections are asymptomatic; symptoms of biliary tract disease may be present in heavily infected persons; cholangiocarcinoma is associated with chronic opisthorchiasis.

- Diagnosis of acute infections can be made by serological tests; later in the course of infection, identification of characteristic eggs in the stool is diagnostic.

- Praziquantel treatment of choice for clonorchiasis and opisthorchiasis; triclabendazole treatment of choice for fascioliasis.

11. Paragonimiasis

Synonyms

• Lung fluke

Causative Organisms

• *Paragonimus westermani*, other species of *Paragonimus*

Epidemiology

• Ingestion of raw or poorly-cooked freshwater crabs or crayfish infected with larval parasite (metacercaria).

• Most common in East and Southeast Asia and West Africa, but present in many other countries.

Key Clinical Features

Acute Infection
• Usually asymptomatic

• Occasionally (2-15 days after exposure):

  * Diarrhea, abdominal pain

  * Fever, fatigue

  * Chest pain, cough

  * Urticaria, eosinophilia

Pleuropulmonary Infection
• Initially: asymptomatic abnormalities on chest radiograph

• Chronic cough productive of rusty-colored or blood-tinged sputum

• Hemoptysis

• Chest pain, often pleuritic

• Dyspnea on exertion

• Eosinophilia (peripheral blood, pleural fluid)

Extrapulmonary Infection
• Cerebral paragonimiasis:

  * Headache

  * Seizures

  * Focal neurologic deficits

  * Cerebrospinal fluid eosinophilia

• Cutaneous paragonimiasis:

  * Migratory subcutaneous nodules

Key Laboratory and Radiologic Features

• Microscopic expectorated eggs in sputum, swallowed eggs in feces.

• Worms and eggs in biopsy specimens.

• Specific antibody tests positive even in light infections, extrapulmonary infections.

• Chest radiograph: poorly defined infiltrates, cysts, nodules, cavities, calcified lesions, pleural effusions. Plain radiograph of skull shows calcifications ("soap-bubbles").

• CT, MRI of head: hypodense ring-enhancing lesions with surrounding edema in grape-like clusters.

Differential Diagnosis

Infectious Diseases
• Tuberculosis

• Bronchitis, bronchiectasis, lung abscess

• Melioidosis

• Endemic mycoses

• Neurocysticercosis

• Cerebral schistosomiasis

Noninfectious Disease Mimics:

• Chronic bronchitis

• Brain tumor

Therapy

• Praziquantel 25 mg/kg PO TID for 2 days

• Alternative: bithionol 30-50 mg/kg PO QID for 10-15 doses

ID Board Pearls

• Suspect paragonimiasis: history of ingesting uncooked or poorly freshwater crabs or crayfish in Southeast Asia, the Far East, West Africa and elsewhere.

• Acute paragonimiasis associated with fever, abdominal pain, urticaria and eosinophilia.

• In chronic paragonimiasis, adult worms live in cysts in the lungs; about 25% of persons infected have lesions in the brain as well.

• Persons with chronic paragonimiasis present with chronic cough, productive of brown sputum sometimes with blood; picture may resemble cavitary tuberculosis except that there is no fever; eosinophilia common.

• Diagnosis of paragonimiasis: serology in acute stage, finding eggs in sputum and feces in the chronic stage. Praziquantel drug of choice.

12. Tapeworms

Causative organisms/Synonyms

• *Diphyllobothrium latum* (fish)

• *Taenia saginata* (beef tapeworm)

• *Taenia solium* (pork tapeworm)

Epidemiology

• Ingestion of uncooked or poorly cooked fish, beef or pork infected with larval tapeworm.

• Adult tapeworm reaches maturity about one month after infection, lives for years to decades.

• Beef and pork tapeworm is endemic in areas where cattle and swine have access to human feces containing tapeworm segments laden with eggs.

• Fish tapeworm is endemic in areas where human and lower mammalian feces contaminate cold freshwater (especially Scandinavia, mountainous regions of Chile and Argentina).

• No transmission of beef or pork tapeworm in the U.S.; however, pork tapeworm eggs infectious for human beings if ingested, can lead to cysticercosis (see section below).

Key Clinical Features

• Infection with adult tapeworm usually asymptomatic; some persons may complain of vague abdominal discomfort.

• Tapeworm infection not a cause of weight loss; most infected persons harbor a single tapeworm.

• Major symptom with all 3 species is passage of tapeworm segments in stool.

• About 1% of persons infected with the fish tapeworm develop B12 deficiency because the worm absorbs B12 efficiently.

Differential Diagnosis

• Segments passed in stool sometimes mistaken for other helminths.

• Megaloblastic anemia due to folate deficiency or B12 deficiency of other causes.

Key Laboratory and Radiologic Features

• Fish tapeworm eggs readily identified in stool; adult worm sheds approximately 1,000,000 eggs per day.

• Beef and pork tapeworm eggs not found in stool 60%-70% of the time; diagnosis usually made by identification of segment; adhesive tape test (as for pinworm infection) may demonstrate eggs when microscopic examination of stool is negative.

• Adult tapeworms sometimes identified during endoscopy or seen as filling defects in barium contrast studies of the bowel.

Complications

• B12 deficiency and macrocytic anemia in less than 1% of persons with fish tapeworm infection.

• Carrier of pork tapeworm may infect him/herself or others with eggs.

• Other complications such as appendicitis due to obstruction of appendix by adult worm (extremely rare).

Therapy

• Praziquantel 5-10 mg per kilogram PO once or niclosamide 2 g PO (chewed) once.

Prognostic Factors

• In absence of complications (listed above), infection is benign.

• If the entire worm is not eliminated, tapeworm can regenerate. Identification of scolex in feces after treatment will document cure.

ID Board Pearls

• Infection with adult fish, beef, pork tapeworms usually asymptomatic, other than passage of segments in the stool.

• B12 deficiency and macrocytic anemia rare complications of fish tapeworm infection.

• Carrier of pork tapeworm = source of infection with eggs and cysticercosis to him/herself or others.

• Diagnosis of tapeworm infection by speciation of segment passed in stool; fish tapeworm eggs readily found in stool.

• Treatment of adult tapeworms with single oral dose of praziquantel or niclosamide.

13. Cysticercosis

Causative Organism

- Larval stage of pig tapeworm, *Taenia solium*

Epidemiology

- Transmission of cysticercosis by accidental ingestion of tapeworm eggs shed by carrier of adult tapeworm.

- Transmission either by direct person-to-person contact or via food or drink contaminated with tapeworm eggs.

- Cysticercosis is highly endemic in parts of Latin America, Haiti, sub-Saharan Africa, India, and the Far East, where there also is a risk for infection with the adult tapeworm from ingesting cysticerci in pork.

- In the United States, most cysticercosis occurs among immigrants infected abroad. Immigrants may also carry adult tapeworms and thus transmit cysticercosis to other people.

Key Clinical Features

- Asymptomatic infections common.

- Cysticerci in muscle or subcutaneous tissue rarely cause symptoms.

- Neurological symptoms frequently appear for the first time several years after infection occurs.

- In the brain, symptoms result from mass effect, inflammation following degeneration of cysticercus, obstruction of foramina and ventricles:

    * Seizures

    * Focal neurological defects (motor, sensory, visual)

    * Altered mental status

    * Signs of increased intracranial pressure

    * Hydrocephalus

    * Aseptic meningitis

    * Cysticerci may also infect the spinal cord and eye

Key Laboratory and Radiological Features

- Antibody test (immunoblot) highly sensitive and specific for cysticercosis.

- CT scan or MRI: multiple solid nodules or cysts, calcified cysts, ring-enhancing lesions, hydrocephalus.

- Brain biopsy rarely necessary for diagnosis.

- *Taenia solium* eggs found in stool of <30% of patients with cysticercosis.

- Coproantigen test and serological test for antibodies to *Taenia solium* (limited availability).

Differential Diagnosis

Infectious Diseases
- Brain abscess

- Cerebral toxoplasmosis

- Schistosomiasis, paragonimiasis of central nervous system

Noninfectious Disease Mimics:
- Benign cyst

- Brain tumor

Therapy

- There is controversy concerning the need to treat all persons with neurocysticercosis, because of the often-benign course of the disease and the potential adverse sequelae of treatment.

- Symptoms should be treated with anticonvulsants and analgesics.

- Neurocysticercosis can be treated with:

* Albendazole 15 mg/kg/d PO in divided doses for 8-30 days or praziquantel 50 mg/kg/d PO for 15-30 days (more expensive)

• Steroids and anticonvulsants should be given simultaneously to reduce the symptoms due to degenerating cysts.

• Surgery may be indicated to remove intraventricular cysts or place a ventricular shunt.

• All patients and their household contacts should be examined for infection with adult tapeworm.

Prognostic Factors

• Prognosis guarded for persons with large numbers of cysts or subarachnoid cysts.

ID Board Pearls

• People acquire cysticercosis by ingestion of *Taenia solium* eggs shed in feces of an adult tapeworm carrier; people acquire the adult tapeworm through ingestion of uncooked or poorly cooked pork.

• Most persons in the United States with cysticercosis are immigrants from Taenia solium endemic countries, although persons who have close contact to an adult tapeworm carrier can acquire cysticercosis without leaving the U.S. *Taenia solium* not endemic in the United States because of animal husbandry regulations concerning raising of pigs.

• Identification of the cyst containing a scolex by CT scan or MR pathognomonic for cysticercosis. Western blot for antibodies to cysticerci can confirm the diagnosis, but can be positive in persons with inactive cysticercosis or cysts outside of the central nervous system.

• Seizures, the most common complication of neurocysticercosis, occur when cyst begins to degenerate, which may be several years after infection was acquired.

• Treatment of neurocysticercosis is not indicated in all cases; when indicated, high dose albendazole (alternatively, praziquantel) is given along with corticosteroids, because of the inflammatory reaction that develops when cysts are killed.

14. Echinococcosis

Causative organism/Synonyms

- *Echinococcus granulosis*: cystic hydatid disease

- *Echinococcus multilocularis*: alveolar hydatid disease

Epidemiology

- Human beings and the natural mammalian intermediate hosts become infected with larval forms by ingesting eggs shed in the feces of the canid definitive host that harbors the adult tapeworm.

- Cystic hydatid disease occurs most commonly in areas where sheep are raised, including Southern South America, East Africa, the Middle East and China. Domestic dogs are the usual definitive host.

- Alveolar hydatid disease occurs in Northern latitudes, including parts of Alaska, Canada, Northern Europe and Western China. The intermediate hosts are voles, and coyotes and wolves are the natural definitive host.

Key Clinical Features

- Cystic hydatid disease

  * Space-occupying lesions in the liver (75%), lungs (20%), brain, bone and other organs (1%)

  * Cysts are approximately 1 cm per year in the liver; remain viable for years

  * Rupture of cyst can cause anaphylaxis due to release of highly antigenic cyst fluid; development of multiple new cysts from protoscolices and cyst fragments

- Alveolar hydatid disease

  * Slowly progressing destructive lesion that eventually destroys the entire liver

  * Metastatic lesions to CNS

  * High mortality rate

Differential Diagnosis

- Cystic hydatid disease: benign cyst of liver, kidneys, lungs, brain; malignant tumor of bone; anaphylactic shock of various etiologies; carcinomatosis with cyst rupture into peritoneal cavity

- Alveolar hydatid disease: hepatocellular carcinoma, end-stage liver disease, metastatic tumor to brain

Key Laboratory and Radiologic Features

- Cystic hydatid disease: cystic lesions with daughter cysts pathognomonic when seen by ultrasound, CT or MRI; microscopic examination of cyst fluid removed carefully by percutaneous aspiration; confirmatory serology (sensitivity less than 100%)

- Alveolar hydatid disease: appearance by CT or MRI suggestive; serology confirmatory; definitive diagnosis requires biopsy

Complications

- Cystic hydatid disease: anaphylactic shock, disseminated daughter cysts, biliary obstruction from cyst rupture into bile radical; pathological fracture or bone; increased intracranial pressure

- Alveolar hydatid disease: liver failure; brain metastasis: death

Therapy

- Cystic hydatid disease

  * Surgical removal with care to avoid cyst rupture

  * Prolonged courses of high dose albendazole (curative in 25%, causes temporary cyst regression in 25%)

  * PAIR procedure: percutaneous aspiration, instillation of scolicidal fluid, reaspiration for hepatic cyst when appropriate; procedure has a higher rate of the cure and lower risk of complication and surgery; treat with albendazole pre- and post-procedure

- Alveolar hydatid disease

  * Prolonged courses of high dose albendazole

  * Partial or complete resection of liver: liver transplantation

Prognostic Factors

- Improved outcome with early detection and treatment

- Spontaneous death and calcification of lesions without treatment more common with cystic disease, occurs occasionally in alveolar disease

ID Board Pearls

- Rule out cystic hydatid disease before surgical removal of cyst in persons from endemic areas to ensure proper approach and avoid cyst rupture.

- Appearance of hydatid cysts with daughter cysts or detached membranes on ultrasound, CT or MRI pathognomonic; serology age and diagnosis.

- Treatment of cystic hydatid disease with surgery, long courses of albendazole or PAIR procedure.

- Alveolar hydatid disease highly lethal because of liver failure and spread to central nervous system.

- Alveolar hydatid disease may respond to high doses and prolonged courses of albendazole; otherwise, partial or complete hepatectomy with liver transplantation.

15. Strongyloidiasis

Causative Organism

- *Strongyloides stercoralis*

Epidemiology

- In warmer climates, transmission by contact of bare skin with fecally-contaminated soil (developing countries, Southeastern United States).

- Direct person-to-person transmission (developing and industrialized countries in settings of crowding and poor hygiene).

- Because the parasite can complete its life cycle without leaving the host, infection persists for decades, even in the absence of reinfection.

Key Clinical Features

Chronic Infection, Immunocompetent Host
- Asymptomatic infection common

- Eosinophilia in ~75%

- Abdominal pain (resembling peptic ulcer)

- Intermittent nausea

- Intermittent diarrhea

- Rashes ("larva currens" pathognomonic)

- Mild intermittent cough, wheezing

Hyperinfection or Disseminated Infection in an Immunocompromised Host
- Invasion of bowel wall by migrating larvae:

  * Nausea, vomiting, abdominal pain, diarrhea, gastrointestinal bleeding, ileus, bowel obstruction, peritonitis

- Invasion of other organs:

  * Lungs: cough, sputum, dyspnea, hemoptysis, respiratory failure; interstitial infiltrates, consolidation or abscess by radiograph

- Central nervous system:

* Meningitis, focal brain lesions, diffuse encephalitis

• Migrating larvae carry bowel flora:

    * Bacteremia

    * Meningitis

    * Pneumonia

Key Laboratory Features

Chronic Strongyloidiasis
• Identification of larvae in stool (may be difficult), duodenal aspirates

• Demonstration of specific antibodies against *Strongyloides* highly sensitive

Hyperinfection or Disseminated Strongyloidiasis
• Large numbers of larvae (rhabditiform and filari form), sometimes adult worms in stool, gastrointestinal fluid, sputum, bronchial aspirates, urine, cerebrospinal fluid

• Larvae identified in biopsy specimens

Differential Diagnosis

Infectious Diseases
• Infection with other parasites that can cause asymptomatic eosinophilia

• Cutaneous larva migrans

• Bacterial sepsis in immunocompromised persons

• Pneumonia caused by *P carinii*, cytomegalovirus

Noninfectious Disease Mimics:
• Peptic ulcer disease

• Inflammatory bowel disease

Therapy

• Ivermectin 200 mcg/kg PO QD for 2 days

* Alternative: albendazole 400 mg PO BID for 7-10 days (lower efficacy)

or

* Thiabendazole 500 mg/kg PO in 2 divided doses per day for 2 days (maximum 3 g/d) (high rate of side effects)

• Persons with hyperinfection syndrome or disseminated strongyloidiasis require prolonged courses of therapy (minimum of 5 days, usually much longer courses are needed to clear infection); immunocompromised persons with uncomplicated strongyloidiasis may require longer or repeated courses.

• Veterinary preparations of ivermectin for parenteral administration have been used in severely ill patients unable to take PO medication.

• Interruption of hyperinfection syndrome or disseminated strongyloidiasis usually requires reversal of immunosuppression.

Prognostic Factors

• Risk factors for hyperinfection or disseminated strongyloidiasis:

    * Immunosuppressive therapy, especially with corticosteroids

    * HTLV-I infection

    * Impaired cellular immunity from lymphoma, leukemia

    * Malnutrition

    * Achlorhydria

    * Prolonged intestinal transit time

• Heavy infections common in HIV-infected persons, but hyperinfection and disseminated strongyloidiasis syndrome unusual.

- Mortality of untreated hyperinfection or disseminated strongyloidiasis syndrome approaches 100%; mortality with treatment may exceed 50%.

ID Board Pearls

- Strongyloidiasis can complete its life cycle in the human host, and therefore infections acquired even early in life can persist indefinitely.

- Persons with chronic strongyloidiasis who undergo immunosuppressive treatment, especially with corticosteroids, or have HTLV-1 infection, are at risk of *Strongyloides* hyperinfection and disseminated strongyloidiasis.

- Persons with potential exposure to *Strongyloides* should undergo diagnostic evaluation with serology +/- multiple stool examinations, even in the absence of symptoms or eosinophilia.

- Suspect *Strongyloides* hyperinfection or disseminated strongyloidiasis in immunosuppressed persons who presented with diarrhea, abdominal pain, paralytic ileus, pulmonary infiltrates and otherwise unexplained bacteremia or meningitis with enteric flora.

- Uncomplicated chronic strongyloidiasis should be treated with 2 days of oral ivermectin; those with hyperinfection or disseminated disease should receive daily ivermectin until parasites can no longer be detected.

16. Filarial Parasites (lymphatic filariasis, onchocerciasis, loiasis)

Causative Organisms/Synonyms

- Lymphatic filariasis (elephantiasis): *Wuchereria bancrofti, Brugia malayi*

- Onchocerciasis (river blindness): *Onchocerca volvulus*

- Loiasis (eye worm): *Loa loa*

Epidemiology

- Lymphatic filariasis: transmitted by mosquitoes; highly prevalent in India, Africa, Haiti, Guyana; under control or in process of elimination in many other countries in the tropics and subtropics.

- Onchocerciasis: transmitted by black flies (species Glossina); found in Mexico, Guatemala, Columbia, Ecuador, Brazil, Venezuela, sub-Saharan Africa, Yemen.

- Loiasis: transmitted by in deer flies (Chrysops); only in central Africa.

Clinical Features

- Lymphatic filariasis

  * Most infections subclinical (asymptomatic microfilaremia)

  * Recurrent episodes of filarial fever with or without retrograde lymphangitis, lymphadenitis; due to inflammatory reaction worm antigens, degenerating adult worms, Wolbachia (Rickettsia-like endosymbiont) lymphedema progressing to elephantiasis

  * Recurrent episodes of cellulitis, lymphangitis due to bacterial infection of lymphedematous tissue

  * Hydrocele

  * Chyluria

  * Tropical pulmonary eosinophilia: cough, low-grade fever, eosinophilia, migratory pulmonary infiltrates

- Onchocerciasis

  * Dermatitis due to inflammatory reaction directed at degenerating microfilariae: pruritic papules, keratotic papules, hypo- and hyper-pigmentation, loss of elasticity; relentless pruritus and disfiguring skin disease source of major morbidity

  * Ocular disease due to inflammatory reaction directed at degenerating microfilariae: punctate keratitis, corneal scars, uveitis, retinitis, optic nerve atrophy, progressive visual loss, blindness

  * Subcutaneous nodules containing adult worms

  * Hanging groin

- Loiasis

  * Subclinical (asymptomatic eosinophilia in expatriates)

  * Calabar swellings (migratory subcutaneous edema with pruritus due to inflammatory reaction against adult worm)

  * Eye worm: migration of adult worm beneath conjunctiva

Differential Diagnosis

- Lymphatic filariasis: bacterial cellulitis, lymphangitis and lymphadenitis; noninfectious lymphedema; common hydrocele; Loeffler syndrome (pulmonary infiltrates and eosinophilia)

- Onchocerciasis: eczematous dermatitis, vitiligo, trachoma, vitamin A deficiency, ocular trauma, subcutaneous lipomas

- Loiasis: localized angioedema

Key Laboratory and Radiologic Features

- Lymphatic filariasis: microfilariae on wet mount or Giemsa stained smear of peripheral blood (nocturnal periodicity in most parts of the world); anti-filarial antibody test (not species specific); circulating antigen test; lateral worms detectable by high resolution ultrasound

- Onchocerciasis: microfilariae in skin snips; adult worms in excised nodules

- Loiasis: microfilariae on wet mount or Giemsa stained smear of peripheral blood (diurnal periodicity); identification of excised adult worm

Complications

- Lymphatic filariasis: bacterial infection, disability, disfigurement

- Onchocerciasis: disfiguring skin disease and subsequent social isolation; blindness; premature death

- Loiasis: encephalopathy with heavy infection

Therapy

- Lymphatic filariasis: yearly single-dose combination of diethylcarbamazine and either albendazole or ivermectin for 5-6 years to prevent transmission; 12 day course of diethylcarbamazine may kill adult worms; 21 day course of diethylcarbamazine for tropical pulmonary eosinophilia; 4-6 week course of oral doxycycline to kill *Wolbachia* and thus decrease viability of adult worms.

- Onchocerciasis: yearly or twice yearly single-dose ivermectin to prevent transmission and development of complications; 4-6 week course of oral doxycycline to kill *Wolbachia* and thus decrease viability of adult worms. Warning: do not give diethylcarbamazine to persons with onchocerciasis.

- Loiasis: 12 day course of diethylcarbamazine, may need to be repeated multiple times for cure. Warning: do not give diethylcarbamazine to people with high levels of circulating microfilariae; this may provoke a lethal encephalopathy due to inflammation around degenerating microfilariae. Do not use ivermectin in persons with high levels of circulating microfilariae.

Prognostic Factors

- Early treatment prevents complications from developing.

- Advanced lesions not reversible with treatment, eg, elephantiasis, corneal scarring, advanced dermatitis

- Blindness, shortening of life expectancy by approximately 10 years in sub-Saharan Africa

ID Board Pearls

- Diagnosis of all 3 filarial parasites in natives of endemic areas by demonstration of microfilariae in blood (lymphatic filariasis, loiasis) or skin (onchocerciasis).

- Microfilariae usually not detectable in infected expatriates; diagnosis made clinically, supported by high levels of eosinophils in peripheral blood, high levels of IgE antibodies and presence of anti-filarial IgG antibodies.

- Treatment of lymphatic filariasis with diethylcarbamazine may lead to pruritus, localized angioedema; lymphangitis; painful nodules. Treatment of onchocerciasis with ivermectin may lead to exacerbation of dermatitis with pruritus; worsening of ocular disease but unlikely to cause blindness. Treatment of loiasis may lead to appearance of Calabar swelling.

- Ivermectin contraindicated in persons with onchocerciasis, because it kills microfilariae rapidly and may provoke vision-threatening inflammation. Ivermectin and diethylcarbamazine contraindicated in persons with loiasis and high levels of circulating microfilariae because inflammation around degenerating microfilariae in the brain may cause fatal encephalopathy.

- Lymphatic filariasis and onchocerciasis of global elimination programs based on repeated mass chemotherapy and populations at risk of infection.

- Prolonged courses of doxycycline to kill Wolbachia may kill all stages of the agents of lymphatic filariasis and onchocerciasis and AP used as definitive therapy, but not loiasis.

17. Dracunculiasis

Causative Organisms/Synonyms

- Guinea worm disease

- *Dracunculus medinensis*

Epidemiology

- Transmitted by drinking contaminated water infested with infected copepods the intermediate host.

- Persons with emerging adult worm contaminate freshwater bodies by soaking the involved extremity, thus allowing larvae to exit the emerging worm.

- Currently found only in sub-Saharan Africa

- Prevalence reduced from 20 million cases in 1982 to less than 10,000 cases in 2008, as a result of the global Guinea worm eradication program.

Key Clinical Features

- After one year incubation period, 3 foot-long adult female induces painful blister which ruptures upon contact with water.

- Patient incapacitated during emergence of worm, which lasts several weeks.

Differential Diagnosis

- None; clinical picture pathognomonic.

Key Laboratory and Radiologic Features

- Plain x-rays may show calcified worms that died *in situ*

Complications

- Bacterial infection of ulcer; tetanus

- Chronic arthritis due to inflammation around worms dying in situ.

Therapy

- Slow, careful extraction of worm over several days.

- Maintain cleanliness of ulcer.

Prognostic Factors

- Controlled removal of worm shortens period of incapacitation, decrease risk of complications.

ID Board Pearls

- Dracunculiasis will probably be the second infectious disease to be eradicated (after smallpox); target: 2012.

- Transmission prevented by filtering water, provision of clean water, prevention of contamination of water by persons with emerging worms and application of larvacide to contaminated bodies of water.

18. Further Reading

Centers for Disease Control and Prevention. *Health Information for International Travel*, 2008. Atlanta, Georgia: U.S. Department of Health and Human Services, Public Health Service; 2008. Available at http://www.cdc.gov/travel. Accessed on March 25, 2009.

Centers for Disease Control and Prevention and the National Center for Vectorborne and Zoonotic Diseases, Division of Parasitic Diseases. DPDx: *Identification and Diagnosis of Parasites of Public Health Concern 2009*. Available at http://www.dpd.cdc.gov/DPDx/default.htm. Accessed on March 25, 2009.

Drugs for parasitic infections. *The Medical Letter*. 2007; pages 1-15. Available at www.medletter.com. Accessed on March 25, 2009.

Guerrant LR, Walker DH, Weller PF. *Tropical Infectious Diseases: Principles, Practice and Pathogens*. 2nd ed. Philadelphia, PA: Elsevier; 2006.

John DT, Petri WA. *Markell and Voge's Medical Parasitology*. 9th ed. Philadelphia, PA: WB Saunders; 2006.

Chapter: 13
Transplant Infections for the ID Boards

Burke A. Cunha, MD

Contents

1. Overview

- Infectious diseases in organ transplant patients are most commonly due to the *same community-acquired pathogens affecting the normal population*.

- Less often, infections are due to opportunistic pathogens.

- Clinical presentation of opportunistic pathogens in the transplant patient may be protean and range from subtle to severe. Clinicians should be alert to *unusual presentations of common pathogens as well as opportunistic pathogens*.

- Opportunistic infections in transplant patients may be multiple and can be either sequential or simultaneous.

Routine Pathogens

- Transplant patients are subject to the *same* pathogens associated with community exposure that affect normal hosts.

- *Nosocomial exposure* may occur *during* hospitalization:

    * MRSA

    * VRE

    * *C difficile* colitis

    * Non-*albicans Candida* infections

    * *Aspergillus*

    * Legionnaires' disease

- Transplant patients are also subject to the *same postoperative complications* that may occur in immunocompetent hosts:

    * Nosocomial pneumonias

    * IV line infections

    * Wound infections

    * Urinary tract infections

    * Transfusion-associated infections

Opportunistic Pathogens

- Opportunistic infections occur due to new community or healthcare-related exposures, donor-derived infections and from *reactivation* of latent infection harbored by the transplant recipient.

- A transplant recipient may acquire infections via infected donor organs ("donor-derived infections") (Table 1):

    * CMV

    * HIV

    * HBV

    * HCV

    * Lymphocytic choriomeningitis virus (LCMV)

    * Rabies

    * West Nile virus

    * *T cruzi* (Chagas' disease)

- *Reactivation of latent infections* in transplants accounts for a significant number of infections:

    * CMV

    * EBV

    * HSV-1, HSV-2, varicella zoster

    * HHV-6, HSV-7

    * HBV and HCV

    * *Strongyloides*

    * *Toxoplasmosis*

    * Tuberculosis

2. Determinants of Infection

There are 3 major factors that contribute to the risk of infection in transplant recipients: epidemiologic exposures, the net state of immunosuppression and the use of prophylactic or early empiric antibiotic therapy.

Epidemiologic Exposures

• *Environmental* exposures may be community-acquired or nosocomial (surgical and non-surgical) (Table 2). They may be remote (resulting in latent infection) or recent.

Net State of Immunosuppression

Immunosuppression is *additive* and is the result of one or more of the following factors:

* The *status* of the transplant recipient's immune system and underlying disease state(s) prior to transplantation

* The *types, doses and duration* (intensity) of immunosuppressive therapy (Table 3)

* Immunosuppressive effect of immunomodulating viruses (CMV, EBV, VZV, HHV-6/7, HBV, HCV, HIV)

* Overall quality of graft function after the transplant

Prophylactic or Early Empiric Antimicrobial Therapy

• Targeted prophylaxis post-transplant can prevent many infections.

* Antibacterial

* Antifungal

* Antiviral

• Early empiric therapy of suspected infections improves outcomes in this vulnerable population.

Table 1

Pathogens Transmitted by Donor Organs

Viral
CMV
HSV
EBV
HHV-8
HBV/HCV
HIV Lymphocytic choriomeningitis virus (LCMV)
Rabies
West Nile virus

Fungal
Candida albicans
Histoplasma capsulatum
Cryptococcus neoformans

Parasitic
Toxoplasma gondii
Strongyloides stercoralis T cruzi (Chagas' disease)
Malaria

Bacterial
Enteric Gram-negative bacilli
Pseudomonas aeruginosa
Staphylococcus aureus

Mycobacterial
Mycobacterium tuberculosis
Non-tuberculous mycobacteria

Table 2

Infections in Transplant Patients

Infections related to surgical procedures
- Transplantation of a contaminated allograft
- Anastomotic leak or stenosis
- Intravenous line infection
- Biliary, urinary and drainage catheters

Infections related to nosocomial exposure
- *Aspergillus*
- *Legionella*
- *Nocardia asteroides*
- Gram-negative bacilli

Infections related to community exposures
- TB
- Influenza
- Adenoviruses
- Parainfluenza
- *Cryptococcus neoformans*
- *Aspergillus*
- *Nocardia asteroides*
- PCP
- Histoplasma capsulatum
- *Coccidioides immitis*
- *Blastomyces dermatitidis*
- *Strongyloides stercoralis*

Infections related to contaminated food/water
- *Salmonella*
- *Listeria monocytogenes*

Viruses of importance in transplants
- CMV
- HSV
- HIV

From Rubin RH, Young LS, eds. Clinical Approach to Infection in the Compromised Host. 3rd ed. New York, NY: Plenum Medical Book Co; 1994.

3. Solid Organ Transplants

- In solid organ transplant (SOT) recipients, the distribution of pathogens is related to the *net state of immunosuppression* (see previous section), the use of targeted antimicrobial prophylaxis and the *time interval* following transplantation.

- The timetable of infectious complications provides the clinician with a clinical approach to infections in transplant recipients. (Figure 1)

Early Post-transplant (<1 month) Period

- Infections predominantly related to the *surgical procedure*

- Nosocomial infections

- Pre-existing infections in recipient may manifest or reoccur

- Donor-derived infections (Table 1)

Specific problems

Renal transplants
- Urinary tract infections/urosepsis

- Wound infections

Liver transplants
- Cholangitis/liver abscess/bacteremia

- Wound infection

Lung transplants
- Nosocomial pneumonias

- Infection at bronchial suture line

Heart transplants
- Mediastinitis/wound/sternal infections

- Mycotic aneurysm at aortic suture line

- Nosocomial pneumonias

Pancreas or pancreatic/kidney transplants
- Wound infections (more common than in above)

Middle Post-transplant (1-6 months) Period

- *Period of maximal immunosuppression.* Infection risk is substantially decreased by targeted antimicrobial prophylaxis.

- *Peak incidence of primary infection or reactivation of intracellular pathogens.*

  * Viral: CMV, HSV, VZV, HHV-6/7, EBV, HCV, HBV, BK

* Bacterial: *listeria, nocardia*

* Fungal: histoplasmosis, coccidioidomycosis, cryptococcosis

* Parasitic: toxoplasmosis, PCP, Strongyloides, Leishmania

* Mycobacteria: M Tuberculosis, Non-tuberculous mycobacteria

Table 3

Immunosuppressive Drugs Used in Transplants

Agent	Immunosuppressive effects	Side effects
Azathioprine	Inhibits cellular proliferation	Bone marrow suppression
Corticosteroids	Nonspecific inhibition of T lymphocytes	Hypertension, glucose intolerance, osteoporosis, dyslipidemia
ATG/ALG	Inhibits T-lymphocyte activation	Serum sickness, granulocytopenia, thrombocytopenia
OKT3	Binds T-cell CD 3	Fever, aseptic meningitis, pulmonary edema
Sirolimus	Inhibits IL-2	Thrombocytopenia, hyperlipidemia, interstitial pneumonitis
Mycophenolate mofetil	Inhibits T and B lymphocytes	Diarrhea
Basiliximab	Inhibits effector cell response to cytokines	None
Dacliximab	Inhibits effector cell response to cytokines	None
Cyclosporine	Inhibits T-lymphocyte inactivation	Nephrotoxicity
Tacrolimus	10-100 times more potent than cyclosporine	Dyslipidemia

From Simon DM, Levin S. Infectious complications of solid organ transplantations. 2001;15:521-549.

Figure 1

Changing Timeline of Infection after Organ Transplantation

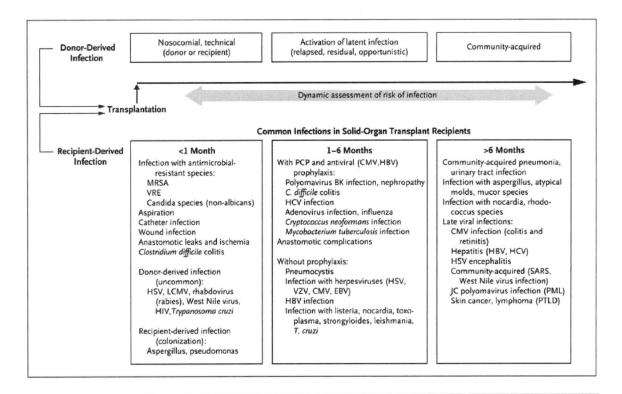

Adapted from Fishman JA. Infection in solid-organ transplant recipients. N Engl J Med. *2007;357(25):2601-2614.*

- Effect of *immunomodulating viruses adds to the net state of immunosuppression*. (CMV, EBV, VZV, HHV-6/7, HBV, HCV, HIV)

Late Post-transplant (>6 months) Period

- *Patients with good allograft function* (baseline immunosuppression) are now at reduced risk for infection compared.

  * Community-acquired respiratory, urinary infections are primary risk

  * Infections with *Nocardia, Aspergillus*, molds and late viral infections can occur

CAVEATS ABOUT TIMELINE
- Patients with poor graft function are more likely to retain the risks in the middle post-transplant period of the timeline.

- Treatment of rejection requires more intense immunosuppression and this effectively "resets the clock" for infection risk, such that the risk of infection are similar to those in the middle post-transplant period, when immunosuppression is maximal.

4. Bone Marrow Transplants

- Infectious complications after bone marrow transplants (BMT) are *similar* to *solid organ* transplants, with some important differences.

- As with solid organ transplantation, BMT patients have a *time-dependent* onset of various pathogens related to the *duration and degree of leukopenia, exogenous immunosuppression and GVHD*.

- Transplant-related infections result from damage to the skin, mouth and gut from preparative regimens, catheters, neutropenia and immunodeficiency.

- Reduced-intensity chemotherapy is associated with lower rates of early infections compared with myeloablative regimens, although the risk of late infection seems to be the same.

- Prolonged neutropenia, GVHD and corticosteroids all independently predispose patients to fungal infection.

- Some patients develop chronic GVHD requiring additional immunosuppression; infections in these patients resemble those of the *early post-engraftment* period.

- Community-acquired viral infections (RSV, parainfluenza, influenza, adenovirus) can be particularly severe in this population.

The Three Phases of Infection after BMT

Pre-engraftment Phase Post-BMT (<1 Month)
- Common infecting bacterial and fungal organisms are those associated with *leukopenia (eg, Candida, Aspergillus)* as well as usual nosocomial infections.

- The length of pre-engraftment phase varies by the type of BMT; thus infection risk varies according to type of BMT.

  * *Fastest neutrophil engraftment*: autologous peripheral blood stem cell transplants (PBSCT)

  * The *next most rapid neutrophil engraftment* is allogenic PBSCT

  * The *next fastest neutrophil engraftment* is with allogenic BMT

  * The *slowest* to engraft are matched unrelated donor PBSCT

  * The *slowest neutrophil engraftment* occurs with matched unrelated donors BMT

- Duration of prophylaxis should relate to the *speed of neutrophil engraftment*.

Early Post-engraftment Phase (31-100 Days)
This phase after BMT is characterized by several of the classic opportunistic infections, as well as standard community-acquired and nosocomial infections. Many infections are similar to those seen 1-6 months after solid organ transplant (Figure 1).

CMV
- The incidence of CMV infection is *highest within the first 100 days* after transplant. Rates of severe, end-organ infection with CMV have been reduced by the increased use of molecular diagnostics. Late-onset CMV is generally only seen in the late post-engraftment period when there is additional immunosuppression to manage GVHD.

PCP
- Mean onset of PCP pneumonia is 9 weeks after BMT. Prophylaxis can mitigate the risk of PCP.

HHV-6
- HHV-6 may reactivate and clinically manifest during this period. HHV-6 occurs in about 22% of patients during the first year post-transplantation. Reactivation of HHV-6 is associated with an increased risk of CMV.

Last Post-engraftment Phase (≥Day 100)

- Patients may acquire the usual community *pathogens of normal hosts* during this period.

- Patients at *the highest* risk of infection during *the late post engraftment phase* are recipients of *allogeneic hematopoietic stem cell transplant* (HSCTs), as well as *those recipients of T-cell depleted marrow* that develop GVHD.

- Two types of infection are *unique* to BMTs in the *late period*: VZV and pneumococcal pneumonia. Approximately 40% of all BMT patients develop VZV (1/3 of which disseminate), usual during the first year, and with a median onset of *5 months* after BMT. Antiviral prophylaxis can mitigate the risk of VZV.

5. Diagnostic Evaluation of Infection in Transplant Recipients

- Immunocompromised hosts need rapid, thoughtful and comprehensive evaluation of potential infections, as they are at risk for rapidly progressive, life-threatening infections. Physical exam findings may range from subtle (due to the reduced inflammatory response) to severe (due to the relative inability to contain infection).

- In pulmonary infections, chest x-rays may underestimate the extent of infection, and chest CT is often necessary for optimal definition of lung abnormalities. Similarly, abdominal examination findings may be blunted, and abdominal CT scan may provide additional information.

- Cultures should include both routine and opportunistic pathogens (such as fungi, mycobacteria, *Nocardia*, etc.)

- *Serological response* in immunosuppressed transplant patients *may be blunted or absent*, thereby limiting the diagnostic usefulness of serology in post-transplant recipients. Molecular diagnostics (ie, nucleic acid or antigen-based assays) are especially useful and potentially more sensitive in this population.

- Specific blood and urine tests can enhance diagnostic ability, as seen with:

  * CMV antigenemia or CMV PCR (note: these are more sensitive than shell vial culture assay)

  * DFA and PCR techniques used in the detection of respiratory pathogens in respiratory secretions and nasal swabs

  * Urinary antigen tests (*Legionella* [serotype O1 only], *S pneumoniae*, *H capsulatum*)

  * Blood PCR for EBV, HHV-6/7/8, HBV, HCV, parvovirus B19, BK, *Ehrlichia*

  * CSF/blood antigen assays for *Cryptococcus neoformans*

* Blood for 1,3-beta-D-glucan and galactomannan antigens for fungi

• Tissue biopsy (skin, brain, lung, etc.) may be necessary to make a diagnosis.

6. Pulmonary Infections in Transplant Patients

• The diagnostic approach to the transplant patient with pulmonary findings involves a careful history of epidemiologic exposures, a detailed physical exam and dedicated imaging studies to characterize the nature of the infection.

• Various patterns can be seen by radiographic imaging and may suggest the etiology of the infection:

* Segmental/lobar pneumonias: typical CAPs, *Pseudomonas*, *Legionella*

* Cavitating and non-cavitating dense infiltrates: *Cryptococcus*, *Aspergillus*, *Nocardia*, tuberculosis

* Diffuse infiltrates: PCP, viruses (CMV, RSV, parainfluenza, adenovirus)

• *Noninfectious* disorders mimicking pneumonia in transplant patients must be excluded.

* Pulmonary drug reactions (sirolimus, azathioprine, various chemotherapeutic agents)

* Pulmonary emboli

* Diffuse alveolar hemorrhage

• A specific etiologic diagnosis in post-transplant patients with pulmonary disease often requires broad sputum and blood cultures, use of specific blood and urine tests (see Diagnostic Evaluation of Infection in Transplant Recipients) and induced sputum samples. BAL may be necessary, sometimes with transbronchial, VATS-guided or open lung tissue biopsy.

7. CNS Lesions in Transplant Patients

- CNS infections are documented in 5%-10% of solid organ transplant recipients, usually occur 2-6 months after transplantation, and are associated with a high mortality rate.

- Clinical syndromes include acute, subacute, or chronic meningitis and encephalitis, and focal deficits because of brain abscesses.

- Magnetic resonance imaging (MRI) is the preferred neuroimaging technique and is one of the key tools in evaluating and enabling early diagnosis of neurologic infections in transplant patients.

- Clinicians should rule out *mimics* of CNS infections, such as *drug-induced* aseptic meningitis/encephalitis due to OKT3, azathioprine, TMP-SMX and ATG/thymoglobulin.

Meningitis in Transplant Patients

- The usual meningeal pathogens include *Listeria*, *S pneumoniae*, *H influenzae*, HSV and *Cryptococcocus*.

Encephalitis in Transplant Patients

- The most common causes of *encephalitis* are viral: HSV, VZV, CMV, HHV-6, enterovirus.

- Other causes include toxoplasmosis, lymphomas (ie, PTLD), *Listeria* and tuberculosis.

Mass Lesions in Transplant Patients

- The most common causes of CNS *mass lesions* include *Nocardia, Aspergillus, Cryptococcocus*, tuberculosis and *Toxoplasma*. JC virus, the cause of progressive multifocal leukoencephalopathy (PML), is less common in transplant recipients.

Diagnostic Approach to CNS Lesions

- Noninvasive tests using serology or PCR as described above (see Diagnostic Evaluation of Infection in Transplant Recipients) may be tried.

- CSF should be sent for cell counts, chemistries, culture, molecular diagnostics and cytology.

- Invasive tests such as brain biopsy may be need for definitive diagnosis.

8. Antimicrobial Prophylaxis, Pre-transplant Evaluation and Early Empiric Antimicrobial Therapy

Antimicrobial Prophylaxis

• *Prophylaxis* is very *effective against predictable organisms* in transplant patients.

• Most solid organ transplant recipients are given prophylaxis with TMP-SMX, an antiviral agent (valganciclovir or an acyclovir product), and an antifungal agent (ranging from oral nystatin to fluconazole to voriconazole for those recipients known to have *Aspergillus*).

• During the leukopenic pre-engraftment phase of BMT, antimicrobial prophylaxis is commonly directed against PCP, HSV/VZV, Gram-negative bacteria and fungi.

• Bacteremias are often secondary to IV line infections; the line should be removed, cultured and specific antibiotic therapy given.

• CMV prophylaxis with ganciclovir or oral valganciclovir is often used when either the solid organ transplant donor or recipient are seropositive for CMV. BMT recipients tend to be monitored for CMV, to avoid the bone marrow suppression seen with ganciclovir.

Pre-transplant Evaluation

• Vaccines should be given both pre- and post-transplant. Live viral vaccines should generally not be given to those that remain on immunosuppressive agents. (Table 4)

  * *Influenza vaccine* should be given to patients pre-transplant.

  * All *nonimmune* solid organ transplant recipients should be considered as candidates for the varicella, measles, mumps and rubella vaccines, assuming they have at least a month after vaccination and before the organ transplant.

  * HAV and HBV vaccine should be given to patients pre-transplant if they are seronegative for these viruses.

• Patients from *Strongyloides*-endemic areas should have serology for *Strongyloides* before transplantation, and if positive, receive an empiric course of ivermectin before transplant.

• Chemoprophylaxis should be considered for all PPD-positive and/or QuantiFERON®-gold positive patients who will undergo immunosuppression. INH is often used, although either agent may be chosen when there is a high suspicion of resistance. Rifampin may have profound drug interactions in transplant recipients.

Early Empiric Antimicrobial Therapy

• *Early* treatment of transplant-associated infections has been essential to survival in transplant patients.

• Empiric therapy is most effective when the clinical presentation suggests a *limited number of diagnostic possibilities* (eg, atypical vs. typical CAP, Gram-negative bacillary UTIs, Gram-positive wound infections), and is *least likely* to be effective when the differential diagnosis involves a *wide number of different pathogens*.

• Specific therapy is preferred if the infecting organism is known (eg, disseminated VZV, HSV, CMV, *Fusarium*, *Aspergillus*). Aggressive diagnostics are indicated in this vulnerable population, until a diagnosis is reached.

• If infected transplant recipients have *not responded* to empiric therapy, then a specific *tissue diagnosis should be attempted* in order to provide specific therapy, if possible.

Table 4

Recommendations for Vaccination for Transplant Recipients

Vaccine Routine	Recommendations for Adult Transplant Recipients
Influenza-parenteral	Yearly
Influenza-intranasal[a]	Contraindicated (unless late after BMT and off immuno suppression)
Pneumococcal polysaccharide	Recommended; booster after 5 years
Tetanus/diphtheria	Recommended; booster every 10 years
Pertussis	Recommended in combination with Tetanus and Diphtheria once
Human papilloma virus	Recommended when indicated
MMR[a]	Contraindicated (unless late after BMT and off immunosuppression)
Varicella[a]	Contraindicated (unless late after BMT and off immunosuppression)
Varicella zoster[a]	Contraindicated (unless late after BMT and off immunosuppression)
Travel-related	
Hepatitis A	Recommended when indicated
Hepatitis B	Recommended when indicated
Meningococcal conjugate	Recommended when indicated
Typhim Vi	Recommended when indicated
Inactivated polio (IPV)	Recommended when indicated
Rabies	Recommended when indicated
Japanese encephalitis	Recommended when indicated
Oral polio (OPV)[a]	Contraindicated in patients/family members (unless late after BMT and off immunosuppression)
S typhi Ty21a[a]	Contraindicated (unless late after BMT and off immunosuppression)

continued

Table 4 *(continued)*

Recommendations for Vaccination for Transplant Recipients

Bacille Calmette Guerin[a]	Contraindicated (unless late after BMT and off immunosuppression)
Yellow fever[a]	Contraindicated (unless late after BMT and off immunosuppression)

[a]*Live, attenuated*

Adapted from the Centers for Disease Control "Recommended Adult Immunization Schedule--United States, 2009"and "Advising Travelers with Specific Needs: The Immunocompromised Traveler" in Centers for Disease Control's "Health Information for International Travel."

Adapted from Kotton CN . Vaccination and immunization against travel-related diseases in immunocompromised hosts. Expert Rev Vaccines. *2008;7(5):663-672.*

ID Board Pearls

- Manifestations of infection in immunosuppressed hosts can be protean.

- The time intervals after solid organ and bone marrow transplant can be helpful at predicting the types of infection seen.

- Infections can be *de novo* (either community-acquired or nosocomial), from donor-derived sources or be reactivation of latent infections.

- CMV is the most common infection after solid organ transplant. Transplant recipients at highest risk are those that were seronegative for CMV prior to transplant and received a seropositive graft.

- Serologic tests may be false negative in transplant recipients; molecular diagnostics may provide additional sensitivity.

- Targeted antimicrobial prophylaxis can prevent or delay many infection complications in transplant recipients.

- Vaccines should be given both before and after transplant. Live viral vaccines should generally be deferred after solid organ transplant and used only late after bone marrow transplant.

9. Further Reading

Books

Mandell GL, Bennett JE, Dolin R, eds. *Mandell, Douglas and Bennett's Principles and Practice of Infectious Disease*. 6th ed. Philadelphia, PA: Elsevier; 2005.

Bowden RA, Ljungman P, Paya CV, eds. *Transplant Infections*. Philadelphia, PA: Lippincott Williams & Wilkins; 2003.

Rubin RH, Young LS, Van Furth R, eds. *Clinical Approach to Infection in the Compromised Host*. 4th ed. New York, NY: Kluwer Academic/Plenum Publishers; 2002.

Wingard RJ, Bowden RA. *Management of Infection in Oncology Patients*. London, England: Martin Dunitz Taylor & Francis Group; 2003.

Journal Articles

Asberg A, Humar A, Rollag H, et al and the VICTOR Study Group. Oral valganciclovir is noninferior to intravenous ganciclovir for the treatment of cytomegalovirus disease in solid organ transplant recipients. *Am J Transplant*. 2007;7:2106-2113.

Avery RK, Michaels M. Update on immunizations in solid organ transplant recipients: what clinicians need to know. *Am J Transplant*. 2008:8: 9-14.

Cunha BA. Central nervous system infections in the compromised host: a diagnostic approach. Infect *Dis Clin North Am*. 2001;15:567-590.

Cunha BA. Pneumonias in the compromised host. *Infect Dis Clin North Am*. 2001;15:591-612.

Fishman JA. Infection in solid-organ transplant recipients. *N Engl J Med*. 2007;357:2601-2614.

Hirsch HH, Brennan DC, Drachenberg CB, et al. Polyomavirus-associated nephropathy in renal transplantation: interdisciplinary analyses and recommendations. *Transplantation*. 2005:79:1277-1286.

Kotton CN. Skin and soft tissue infections in the transplant population. *Curr Infect Dis Rep*. 2008;10(5):387-393.

Kotton CN. Vaccination and immunization against travel-related diseases in immunocompromised hosts. *Expert Rev Vaccines*. 2008;7(5):663-672.

Kotton CN, Fishman JA. Viral infection in the renal transplant recipient. *J Am Soc Nephrol*. 2005;16(6):1758-1774.

Prevention and Treatment of Cancer-related Infections by The National Comprehensive Cancer Network. January 21, 2009. Available at http://www.nccn.org/professionals/physician_gls/PDF/infections.pdf. Accessed on March 26, 2009.

Simon DM, Levin S. Infectious complications of solid organ transplantations. *Infect Dis Clin North Am*. 2001;15(2):521-549.

Zamora MR. Cytomegalovirus and lung transplantation. *Am J Transplant*. 2004;4(8):1219-1226.

Chapter 14: Meningitis and Encephalitis for the ID Boards

Burke A. Cunha, MD

Contents

1. Meningitis Overview

General Concepts

- There are several diagnostic difficulties in patients presenting with the possibility of acute bacterial meningitis (ABM).

- Meningitis may be mimicked by a variety of infectious and noninfectious disorders. The mimics of meningitis are usually easily ruled out on the basis of the history/physical exam and, if any doubt remains, then a lumbar puncture with cerebrospinal fluid (CSF) analysis will include or exclude the diagnosis of ABM.

- ABM may be acquired naturally or as a complication of open head trauma or neurosurgical procedures. Regardless of the pathogen or mode of acquisition, the definitive diagnosis of acute bacterial meningitis rests on analysis of the CSF profile and Gram stain/culture of the CSF.

- The clinical hallmark of ABM is meningeal irritation, ie, nuchal rigidity.

- Nuchal rigidity must be differentiated from other causes of neck stiffness, ie, meningismus associated with the mimics of meningitis.

- It is important to differentiate aseptic or viral meningitis from ABM. Aseptic viral meningitis may be diagnosed by analysis of the CSF profile, as well as specific viral culture/PCR determinations. Patients with mental confusion, ie, encephalopathy, have encephalitis but not nuchal rigidity. Some pathogens, ie, HSV-1, Mycoplasma pneumoniae, Listeria monocytogenes, may present a stiff neck and mental confusion, ie, meningoencephalitis. (Table 1)

ID Board Pearls

- If ABM is suspected, LP should be performed *prior* to head CT/MRI scanning.

- ABM may result from contiguous spread from a local source in close proximity to the brain, ie, sinusitis, mastoiditis or cracks in the cribriform plate.

- ABM may also occur by hematogenous spread of non-respiratory pathogens, eg, *Listeria, E coli, Staphylococcus aureus*, secondary to CNS seeding. MSSA/MRSA ABE is not infrequently complicated by purulent ABM.

- CNS VA/VP shunts for may be complicated by meningitis, reflects either the flora of the skin introduced during the insertion process, or the flora at the distal end of the shunt, ie, a ventricular peritoneal shunt.

- Open head trauma directly introduces the bacteria into the CSF/brain parenchyma.

- Relatively few viruses, eg, enteroviruses, cause aseptic/viral meningitis.

- Partially treated meningitis is bacterial meningitis following initial treatment for meningitis.

- Some viruses, ie, HSV-1 cause a spectrum of CNS infections in normal hosts from aseptic meningitis to meningoencephalitis to encephalitis.

Table 1

Host-Pathogen Associations in Meningitis

Host Factors	Associated Pathogens
Sinopulmonary function	• *S pneumoniae* • *H influenzae* • *N meningitidis*
Elderly	• *H influenzae* • *Listeria monocytogenes* • Brain abscess (2º dental focus)
Sickle cell disease	• *S pneumoniae* • *N meningitidis* • *H influenzae*
Impaired splenic function/splenectomy	• *S pneumoniae* • *H influenzae* • *N meningitidis* • *Klebsiella pneumoniae*
HIV	• HIV • CMV • *Toxoplasma gondii* • *Listeria monocytogenes* • *Nocardia* spp. • *Cryptococcus neoformans* • TB/MAI • Lymphomas
Complement deficiencies	• *S pneumoniae* • *N meningitidis*
CSF leak	• *S pneumoniae*
IVDAs	• *S aureus* • Aerobic GNBs
Alcoholism/cirrhosis	• *S pneumoniae* • *Klebsiella pneumoniae* • TB
Hypogammaglobulinemia	• *S pneumoniae* • *H influenzae* • *N meningitidis* • Enteroviruses

continued

Table 1 *(continued)*

Host-Pathogen Associations in Meningitis

VA shunts	• *S epidermidis (CoNS)* • *S aureus*
VP shunts	• *Aerobic GNBs* • *Group D enterococci*
Recurrent meningitis *(2° to immune/anatomic defects)*	• *S pneumoniae* • *H influenzae* • *N meningitidis*
Recurrent non-infectious meningitis	• SLE • Neuro-sarcoidosis • Neuro-Beçhet's • CNS vasculitis
ABE (emboli)	• *S pneumoniae* • *S aureus*
Brain abscess	• Oral anaerobes • *Citrobacter* (children) • *S aureus* • Aerobic GNBs

IVDAs = IV drug abusers
VA = ventricular aortic
VP = ventricular pulmonary
ABE = acute bacterial endocarditis
GNB = Gram-negative bacilli

2. Mimics of Meningitis

General Concepts

• Acute torticollis, muscle spasm of the head/neck, cervical arthritis or meningismus due to a variety of head and neck disorders can all mimic ABM. But, most of these are *not* associated with fever.

ID Board Pearls

• Fever plus nuchal rigidity is the distinguishing hallmark of ABM. It may be difficult in elderly patients to diagnose on the basis of ABM fever and nuchal rigidity, since fever can be due to a variety of non-CNS infections, patient may have a stiff neck due to cervical arthritis.

3. Non-Infectious Mimics of Acute Bacterial Meningitis (ABM)

General Concepts

• Disorders that commonly mimic ABM include drug-induced meningitis, meningeal carcinomatosis, serum sickness, CNS granulomatous angiitis, Beçhet's disease, SLE and neurosarcoidosis.

ID Board Pearls

• Clues to the diagnosis of systemic disorders that mimic ABM are from the history/physical exam.

4. Drug-Induced Meningitis

General Concepts

• Drug-induced meningitis may present with a stiff neck. The most common drugs associated with drug-induced meningitis are NSIDS, TMP-SMX and, less commonly, azithromycin.

ID Board Pearls

• Leukocytosis in the CSF with a *polymorphonuclear predominance is typical* with drug-induced meningitis, and the clinical clue to the presence of drug-induced meningitis is the presence of *CSF eosinophils.*

• In drug-induced meningitis, the CSF also contains increased protein, but the CSF glucose is not decreased.

• RBCs or increased CSF lactic acid levels are not features of drug-induced meningitis.

5. Serum Sickness

General Concepts

• Serum sickness is a systemic reaction to the injection of serum-derived antitoxin derivatives.

• Since sera are not used much, serum sickness is now most commonly associated with the use of edications, including β-lactam antibiotics, sulfonamides and streptomycin.

• Non-antimicrobials associated with serum sickness include hydralazine, alpha methyldopa, propanolol, procainamide, quinidine, phenylbutazone, naproxen catapril and hydantoin.

• Symptoms typically begin about 2 weeks after the initiation of drug therapy, and are characterized by fever, arthralgias/arthritis and immune complex mediated renal insufficiency.

• Urticaria, abdominal pain or lymphadenopathy may or may not be present.

• Neurologic abnormalities are part of the systemic picture and include a mild meningoencephalitis which occurs early with serum sickness.

• A few patients may have papilledema, seizures, circulatory ataxia, transverse myelitis or cranial nerve palsies.

• The CSF typically shows a mild lymphocytic pleocytosis, protein is usually normal but may be slightly elevated, as is the CSF glucose.

ID Board Pearls

• Clues to serum sickness systemically are an increased ESR, a decreased C^3, microscopic hematuria/RBC casts and hypergammaglobulinemia (SPEP).

6. Collagen Vascular Diseases

General Concepts

- SLE often presents with CNS manifestations ranging from meningitis to cerebritis to encephalitis.

- The most frequent CNS manifestation of SLE is aseptic meningitis.

- CNS manifestations of SLE usually occur in patients who have established multi-system manifestations of SLE.

- CNS SLE is often present as part of a flare of SLE. SLE flare may be manifested by fever, an increase in the signs/symptoms of SLE.

- Laboratory tests suggesting SLE flare include new/SPEP more severe leukopenia, thrombocytopenia, increased ESR, polyclonal gammopathy (SPEP) and proteinuria/microscopic hematuria.

- The CSF in patients with SLE include a lymphocytic predominance (usually <100 WBCs/mm^3). PMNs may predominate early in SLE.

- RBCs are not present in the CSF with SLE and the CSF lactic acid level is also normal.

- Patients with a flare of CNS are predisposed to bacterial meningitis/viral encephalitis.

ID Board Pearls

- The definitive test for diagnosing CNS SLE is to demonstrate a $\downarrow$C$_4$ level in the CSF.

- Be careful to be sure that the patient with an SLE flare with CNS manifestations does not have a superimposed acute bacterial meningitis or acute viral encephalitis.

- Behçet's disease is multisystem disorder of unknown etiology characterized by oral aphthous ulcers, genital ulcers, eye findings and neurological manifestations in ~1/4 of patients.

- CNS presentation of Behçet's may be the presenting finding in about 5% of patients.

- Neuro-Behçet's disease is characterized by fever, headache and meningeal signs closely mimicking ABM, but meningoencephalitis or encephalitis may also be present.

- The CSF profile is indistinguishable from aseptic viral meningitis/encephalitis and there are no distinguishing features on the EEG or head CT/MRI imaging.

- The diagnosis of neuro-Behçet's disease is based on recognizing that the patient has Behçet's disease and has neurologic manifestations not attributable to another or superimposed process.

- Neurosarcoidosis is a common manifestation of sarcoidosis.

- Signs of CNS sarcoid include headaches, mental confusion and cranial nerve palsies sarcoidosis may often presents with polyclonal gammopathy (SPEP), an elevated ESR, leukopenia and mild anemia, and increased ACE levels.

- CXR shows one of the stages of sarcoidosis.

- In neurosarcoid, the CSF is usually abnormal. A lymphocytic pleocytosis (≤ 300 cells/mm) is usual. Protein levels in the CSF are usually elevated, and ~20% of patients have a decreased CSF glucose level.

- Sarcoid meningoencephalitis is more chronic, mimicking the chronic TB or fungal meningitis.

- RBCs are not a feature of neurosarcoidosis.

- Diagnosis of neurosarcoidosis is by demonstrating ↑ CSF ACE levels (Table 2).

Table 2

Mimics of Meningitis

- **Drug-induced aseptic meningitis**

    Toxic/metabolic abnormalities

    NSAIDs

    TMP-SMX

    OKT3

    ATG

    Azathioprine

- **CNS vasculitis**

- **SLE cerebritis**

- **Sarcoid meningitis**

- **Tumor emboli**

    SBE/ABE

    Marantic endocarditis

    Embolic from the heart
    (atrial fibrillation, acute MI)

- **Meningeal carcinomatosis**

- **Primary or metastatic CNS malignancies**

    AML

    ALL

    Hodgkin's lymphoma

    Non-Hodgkin's lymphoma

    Melanoma

continued

Table 2 *(continued)*

Mimics of Meningitis

- **Primary or metastatic CNS malignancies**

    Breast carcinomas

    Bronchogenic carcinomas

    Hypernephromas (renal cell carcinomas)

    Germ cell tumors

- **Legionnaires' disease**

- **Posterier fossa syndrome**

- **Subarachnoid hemorrhage**

    Intracerebral hemorrhage

    CNS leukostasis

    Thrombocytopenia

    DIC

    Abnormal platelet function

    Coagulopathy

    CNS metastases

- **Embolic and thrombotic strokes**

DIC = diffuse intravascular coagulation
CNS = central nervous system
AML = acute myelogenous leukemia;
ALL = acute lymphoblastic leukemia

7. Clinical/Laboratory Features of ABM

General Concepts

- Normal hosts with ABM may or may not have a variety of historical epidemiologic clues as well as physical findings which may suggest a particular organism.

- In compromised hosts, the diagnosis of acute bacterial meningitis depends on correlating the underlying disorder with its host defense defect, which predicts the meningeal pathogen.

- Compromised hosts with impaired cellular-mediated immunity (CMI) usually present with *chronic* rather than bacterial meningitis.

- Compromised hosts are not exempt from the spectrum of infectious diseases that affect immunocompetent hosts (Table 3).

ID Board Pearls

- Compromised hosts with defects in humoral immunity (HI) or those with combined CMI and HI defects, eg, chronic lymphatic leukemia (CLL), are predisposed to meningitis due to encapsulated organisms, *Streptococcus pneumoniae, Haemophilus influenzae* or *Klebsiella pneumoniae*.

8. CSF Profile in ABM

General Concepts

- In ABM the cells in the CSF are nearly all polymorphonuclear neutrophils (PMNs), ie, >90%.

- As ABM is treated, the % of PMNs decreases and there is a parallel rise in the % of CSF lymphocytes.

- ABM begins with a PMN predominance and ends with a lymphocytic predominance.

- With the exception of HSV-1, ≥90% PMNs in the CSF initially always indicates an acute bacterial meningitis.

- In patients with fever and nuchal rigidity, a LP should always be performed before a head CT/MRI scan is obtained.

- Patients with ABM are acutely ill and have a potentially rapidly fatal disorder and it is a waste of valuable time obtaining a head CT/MRI which may result in a fatal outcome.

- Don't get imaging studies done before the LP, unless a mass lesion is suspected (Tables 4 and 5).

ID Board Pearls

- Other CNS infections, eg, tuberculosis, viral infections, fungal infections, syphilis, etc., may all present initially with a pleocytosis with a PMN predominance.

- A PMN predominance of <90% is compatible with a wide variety of CNS pathogens and does not, of itself, indicate a bacterial etiology.

- The typical "purulent profile" in the CSF of bacteria causing acute meningitis includes an early PMN predominance, a decreased CSF glucose, a variably ↑CSF protein, no RBCs and a highly elevated CSF lactic acid level (>6 mmol/L).

- CSF Gram stain positivity depends on the *concentration* and *organism* present.

Table 3

Meningitis: Clinical Summaries

Meningitis	Differential Features and Diagnostic Clues

Enteroviral meningitis	• Seasonal distribution: summer
	• Clinically not as ill as bacterial meningitis
	• Sore throat, facial/maculopapular rash, loose stools/diarrhea
	• CSF:
	  * Gram stain:
	  * Lactic acid: normal (<3 mmol/L)
	• Previous antibiotic therapy
	• Onset: subacute

Partially treated bacterial meningitis (usually 2° to *H.influenzae*)	• CSF: • Gram stain:± • Lactic acid: mildly ↑ (4-6 mmol/L) • Season: non-seasonal • Presentation: dense/prolonged neurologic defects, encephalopathic/coma

HSV-1	• Historical: recent antecedent herpes labialis (not concurrent)
	• EEG unilateral/frontal: temporal lobe focus (early)
	• Head MRI/CT scan: temporal lobe focus (negative early)
	• CSF: Gram stain -
	  * + RBCs (negative early;
	  * ↑ PMNs (may be >90%)
	  * Glucose (may be ↓/normal)
	  * ↑ Lactic acid ~ (RBCs in CSF)

Meningeal carcinomatosis	• History: leukemias, lymphomas, carcinomas, or without known primary neoplasm
	• Onset: subacute/afebrile
	• Mental status changes: ±
	• Nuchal rigidity: ±
	• Multiple cranial nerve abnormality (CNs 3,4,6,7, 8 most common)
	• CSF:
	  * Gram stain: -
	  * RBCs: ±
	  * Rrotein: highly ↑
	  * Lactic acid: variably ↑
	  * Cytology: + (~90%)

---

continued

Table 3 *(continued)*

Meningitis: Clinical Summaries

Meningitis	Differential Features and Diagnostic Clues
Amebic meningoencephalitis (*N fowleri*)	• History: recent swimming in fresh water • Onset: rapid • Olfactory/gustatory abnormalities: (early) • Head MRI/CT: mass lesions

Amebic meningoencephalitis (*N fowleri*)	• CSF:
	  * RBCs: +
	  * Glucose: ↓
	  * Lactic acid: variably ↑
	  * Gram stain: "motile WBCs" on wet prep (ameba)

Brain abscess (with ventricular leak)	• Source usually *suppurative* lung disease (bronchiectasis), *cyanotic* heart disease (R → L shunts), mastoiditis, dental abscess, etc.
	• Head MRI/CT: mass lesions
	• CSF: mimics bacterial meningitis (if ventricular leak)
	  * Protein: highly ↑
	  * Without leak: usually <200 WBCs with leak: ≤100,000 WBCs

Leptospirosis	• Usually with severe leptospirosis (Weil's syndrome)
	
	• Presentation: clinically ill, jaundiced, conjunctival suffusion, ↑ SGOT/SGPT
	• CSF:
	  * CSF: bilirubin ↑
	  * RBCs: +

Tuberculosis/fungal meningitis	• Presentation: subacute, usually with evidence of primary infection. Lung lesions not always apparent in TB (CXR) negative in 50%).
	• Basilar meningitis
	• Fundi: characteristic *choroidal* tubercles
	• CNS: unilateral CN VI) *abducens* palsy,
	• MRI/CT scans: *hydrocephalus/arachnoiditis*
	• CSF:
	  * WBCs: <500
	  * PMNs (early); lymphs (later)
	  * Glucose: ↓ (may be normal)
	  * RBCs: ↑
	  * TB smear/culture + ~80%
	• Serial CSFs: over time ↓ glucose/ ↑ protein
	  * Lactic acid: ↑ (variably elevated)

continued

Table 3 *(continued)*

Meningitis: Clinical Summaries

Meningitis	**Differential Features and Diagnostic Clues**

Neurosarcoidosis	• History/signs of systemic sarcoidosis (bilateral hilar adenopathy /interstitial infiltrates, skin lesions, uveitis, erythema nodosum, arthritis, hypercalciuria,
	• ACE levels
	• Nuchal rigidity: mild
	• Cranial nerves: unilateral/bilateral CN VII (facial nerve palsy characteristic also CN palsies II, VII, VIII, IX, X
	• CSF:
	  * Lymphs:
	  * Glucose :
	  * WBCs: <100
	  * RBCs: none (vs TB or Ca)

SLE cerebritis	• History/signs of SLE (pneumonitis, nephritis, skin lesions, cytoid bodies/cotton wool spots in fundi) eizures/encephalopathy: ±
	
	• CSF:
	  * CSF ANA: +
	  * CSF C4:

Lymphocytic choriomeningitis (LCM)	• Seasonal distribution: fall
	• History: hamster/mouse/rodent contact
	• Presentation: biphasic "flu-like" illness followed by recovery, then headache, fever, mental confusion/meningismus, myalgias
	• CBC:
	  * WBCs: platelets
	  * CSF: resembles aseptic meningitis if glucose normal
	  * Glucose: normal/
	  * WBCs: >1,000 lymphs

RMSF	• Seasonal distribution: spring/fall; woods/animal exposure
	• Onset: sudden with severe headache, myalgias and mild nuchal rigidity conjunctival suffusion, periorbital edema/ edema of dorsum of hands/feet, wrists/ankles rash
	• CSF:
	  * WBCs: <100 lymphs
	  * Lactic acid: normal/slightly
	  * Glucose: normal/
	  * Protein: (variably)

continued

Table 3 *(continued)*

Meningitis: Clinical Summaries

Meningitis	**Differential Features and Diagnostic Clues**
Mycoplasma meningoencephalitis	• History: Mycoplasma CAP • Presentation: non-exudative pharyngitis, otitis/bullous myringitis, loose stools/diarrhea, erythema multiforme • Highly elevated cold agglutinin titers: >1:512 • CSF: 　* Culture for Mycoplasma pneumoniae : ±

- The CSF Gram stain is negative in ~50% with *Listeria monocytogenes* meningitis, but is ~100% culturable from the CSF.

- With ABM due to the meningococcus, *no* organisms may be seen on CSF Gram stain. The CSF may appear turbid or cloudy due to the abundance of WBCs present. The typical CSF TB profile of ABM may also be present with early TB fungal meningitis, or as subacute/chronic meningitis. The various causes of viral/aseptic meningitis are uniformly associated with a normal CSF glucose with a few important exceptions.

- Normal CSF glucose in a patient with suspected meningitis argues strongly against a bacterial ABM TB or fungal and suggests a viral or noninfectious mimic of meningitis.

- The only viruses that are associated with ↓CSF glucose HSV, lymphocytic choriomeningitis (LCM), mumps and, occasionally, enteroviruses.

- A normal CSF glucose virtually excludes a bacterial etiology of acute bacterial meningitis.

- Excluding a traumatic tap, CNS leaking aneuyrism, etc., RBCs in the CSF limit diagnostic possibilities to *L.monocytogenes*, amebic meningoencephalitis, leptospirosis, TB, HSV and anthrax.

- RBCs in the CSF can decrease CSF glucose and increase CSF lactic acid.

- RBCs are not a feature of ABM, and should suggest an alternate explanation.

- The abnormalities in CSF glucose and lactic acid are proportional to the number of RBCs present in the CSF.

- Patients with partially treated meningitis have a mixed picture with both PMNs and lymphocytes as well as a moderately decreased CSF glucose and will have CSF lactic acid levels intermediate between ABM and aseptic/viral meningitis.

Table 4

CSF Gram Stain in Meningitis

Gram-positive bacilli

- *Listeria monocytogenes*
- Pseudomeningitis (*Bacillus*, *Corynebacterium*, etc)

Gram-negative bacilli

- *Haemophilus influenzae*
- Pseudomenigitis (GNBs)

Gram-positive cocci

- Group A, B streptococci
- *S pneumoniae* secondary to ABE
- *S aureus* secondary to ABE (clusters)
- *S epidermidis* VA/VP shunt infections

RMSF = Rocky Mountain spotted fever
SBE = subacute endocarditis
HIV = human immunodeficiency virus
VA= ventriculo-atrial
VP = ventriculo-peritoneal
LCM = lymphocytic choriomeningitis

Table 5

Differential Diagnosis of CSF with a Negative Gram Stain

Purulent CSF/no organisms seen

- *N meningitidis*
- *S.pneumoniae*

Predominantly PMNs/decreased glucose
- Partially treated bacterial meningitis
- Listeria monocytogenes
- HSV-1
- TB (early)
- Syphilis (early)
- Neurosarcoidosis
- Parameningeal infection
- Septic emboli (2° to ABE)
    Amebic meningoencephalitis
    Naegleria fowleri
    Syphilis (early)
    Posterior fossa syndrome

CSF lactic acid
<3 mmol/L
    Aseptic "viral" meningitis
    Parameningeal infections

3-6 mmol/L
    Partially treated meningitis
    RBCs
    TB/fungal meningitis

>6 mmol/L
    Bacterial meningitis

CSF protein (very highly elevated)
- Brain tumor
- TB with subarachnoid block
- Demyelinating CNS disorders

Clear CSF/no organisms seen

- Viral meningitis
- TB/fungal meningitis
- Neurosarcoidosis
- Bacterial meningitis
- Partially treated bacterial meningitis
- Meningitis in leukopenic host
- Meningeal carcinomatosis
- Brain abscess (with ventricular leak)
- Parameningeal infection
- Bland emboli (2° to SBE)
- SLE cerebritis
- Neuroborreliosis
- LCM
- *Listeria monocytogenes*
- HIV
- Syphilis
- Leptospirosis

Gram-negative cocci
- *N meningitidis*

Polymicrobial
- Pseudomeningitis
- Brain abscess (with ventricular leak)
- VA/VP shunt infections
- Disseminated *Strongyloides stercoralis*

RBCs
- Traumatic tap
- Posterior fossa syndrome
- CNS bleed
- CNS tumor
- HSV-1
- Listeria monocytogenes
- Leptospirosis
- TB
- Naegleria fowleri

Predominantly lymphs/normal glucose
- Viral meningitis
- Partially treated bacterial meningitis
- Neurosarcoidosis
- Neuroborreliosis
- HIV
- Leptospirosis
- RMSF

continued

Table 5 (continued)

Differential Diagnosis of CSF with a Negative Gram Stain

Multiple sclerosis
- Leptospirosis
- RMSF

CSF eosinophils
- NSAIDS
- Coccidioidomycosis
- Neurocysticercosis
- CNS lymphomas
- VA/VP shunts
- CNS vasculitis
- Interventional contrast materials
- Bland emboli ($2°$ to SBE)
- Parameningeal infection
- TB
- Fungi
- Meningeal carcinomatosis

9. Other CSF Tests (CRP, PCT, LDH)

General Concepts

• CSF CRP is highly elevated in bacterial meningitis but is not as highly elevated in viral/aseptic meningitis.

• CSF procalcitonin (PCT) levels are highly elevated in ABM and not in aseptic/viral meningitis. Other CSF parameters have been used, ie, LDH to differentiate the various types of meningeal-pathogens, but lack sensitivity and specificity.

• CSF antigen tests, ie, counter immunoelectrophoresis techniques (CIE) of the CSF are generally unhelpful due to a lack of sensitivity/specificity.

• PCR of the CSF is useful to make the diagnosis of enteroviral meningitis, HSV – 1/2, HHV-6 and TB meningitis.

• In ABM, serum CRP levels are higher than in viral/aseptic meningitis.

• Serum PCT levels are more highly elevated than viral/aseptic meningitis vs. ABM.

• Highly elevated serum ferritin levels appear to be a marker for WNE.

• Serum ferritin levels are unelevated/minimally elevated in aseptic/viral meningitis and ABM.

• Neuro-imaging tests are primarily valuable for ruling out the mimics of acute bacterial meningitis.

• EEG is primarily useful in diagnosing encephalitis. The main use for EEG is in the early diagnosis of HSV meningoencephalitis because of the propensity of HSV to localize to the frontal/temporal lobe (Table 6).

ID Board Pearls

• In normal hosts, *HHV-6 encephalitis may localize to the frontal/temporal lobe*.

10. Antimicrobial Therapy of ABM

General Concepts

• Third- and fourth-generation cephalosporins given in "meningeal doses" do not penetrate the CNS well, but penetrate sufficiently with sufficiently high degree of activity that they are effective against common ABM pathogens except *Listeria monocytenges*.

• With *Listeria* meningitis in penicillin, allergic patients chloramphenicol or TMP-SMX may be used.

• If vancomycin is selected to treat MRSA CNS infections, then either 30-60 mg/day of vancomycin is necessary, or the usual dose of vancomycin (15 mg/kg/day [IV]) may be supplemented 20 mg of intrathecal (IT) vancomycin daily.

• Linezolid and minocycline penetrate the CSF well and achieve therapeutic concentrations.

• The use of steroids as an adjunctive measure to treat acute bacterial meningitis remains controversial.

• Steroids have long been used together with TB therapy in TB meningitis.

• Steroids have been shown to be beneficial in the treatment of meningitis in children due to *H influenzae*.

ID Board Pearls

• Steroids affect blood/brain barrier permeability, if used, steroids should be given *after* antimicrobial therapy has been initiated.

Table 6

Meningitis Complications

Complicationis	Associated Organisms
Deafness/hearing loss (acute)	• *H influenzae* • *N meningitidis* • TB • RMSF • Mumps
Seizures (new onset)	• *S pneumoniae (early)* • *H influenzae* • Group B streptococci • HSV-1 • Histoplasmosis • TB • Brain abscess
Subdural effusions (early in course)	• *H influenzae* • *S pneumoniae*
Septic arthritis	• *N meningitidis* • *S aureus*
Hemiplegia	• *S pneumoniae*
Cerebral-vein thrombosis	• *H influenzae* (associated Jacksonian seizures)
Hydrocephalus	• *H influenzae* • TB • Neurosarcoidosis • Neurocysticercosis
Cranial nerve abnormalities	• N meningitidis (CN VI, VII, VIII) • TB (CN VI) • Neurosarcoidosis (CN VII) • Meningeal carcinomatosis (multiple CNs)
Herpes labialis	• *N meningitidis* • *S pneumoniae*
Panophthalmitis	• *N meningitidis* • *S pneumoniae* • *H influenzae*
Purpura/petechiae or shock	• *N meningitidis* • *S pneumoniae* • *Listeria monocytogenes* • *S aureus*

11. Encephalitis Overview

General Concepts

- *Acute* encephalitis is usually caused by *viruses* that invade the *parenchyma*.

- *Acute viral encephalitis is a clinical syndrome* usually accompanied by *fever CSF pleocytosis* and mental Confusion, with or without focal neurologic deficits.

- With few exceptions, it *is not* usually possible to make a specific diagnosis based upon the clinical presentation.

- Seizures, alterations in consciousness, and focal neurologic abnormalities are common, but not nucal rigidity.

- If a patient with acute encephalitis has in addition to a stiff neck the diagnosis is meningoencephalitis.

- The great *majority* of viral infections involving the brain are *subacute or mild* and are manifested only by mild systemic symptoms, including low-grade fever, myalgia and headache.

- *Arboviral encephalitis is* characterized clinically by *extremely rapid onset with prominent headache/myalgias*

- Geographic distribution of arboviral encephalitis can be extremely *helpful* in suggesting a *specific* viral diagnosis.

ID Board Pearls

- Nausea and vomiting *may* reflect *increased intracranial pressure*.

- Diarrhea is unusual *except* in cases of enteroviral encephalitis.

12. Differential Diagnosis of Viral Encephalitis

General Concepts

- The main *problem* clinically is to *differentiate encephalopathy from viral encephalitis from* other infections and non-infections that present with *encephalitic component*.

- The *immediate diagnostic priority* is to establish the diagnosis of *HSV encephalitis*.

- Herpes simplex encephalitis (HSV) remains the most common treatable virus causing *acute* encephalitis in normal hosts.

- Many encephalopathic disorders may mimic that of acute encephalitis, and they should be *ruled out before an infectious cause is considered*.

13. Seasonal Distribution of Acute Viral Encephalitis

General Concepts

• *Seasonal distribution* is also sometimes helpful in suggesting a *specific viral etiology.*

Acute Encephalitis During Summer
• St.LE

• CTF

• WNE

TBE Encephalitis Occurring During Spring/Fall
• Arboviral encephalitis

• Rocky Mountain Spotted Fever (RMSF)

Encephalitis Occurring During the Late Winter/Early Spring
• Measles

• Influenza

• Mumps encephalitis

14. Pathology of Viral Encephalitis

General Concepts

• Acute viral encephalitis is an infection of the brain parenchyma itself, and the meninges are not affected.

• *Many infectious diseases may have an encephalopathic component* but do not actually invade the brain as in *viral encephalitis.*

• Viruses causing acute encephalitis *may also invade the meninges, eg, meningoencephalitis.*

• If the spinal *cord is involved* in addition to the brain, the diagnosis is *encephalomyelitis.*

• In viral encephalitis there are *perivascular infiltrates* that contain histiocytes, lymphocytes and polymorphonuclear neutrophils, and may be associated with hyperemia and hemorrhage.

• Most of the viruses that cause acute encephalitis have no particular anatomic localization.

ID Board Pearls

• In *addition* to the *cortex,* some encephalitic viruses have an *anatomic preference* for specific areas of the nervous system.

• HSV → *temporal lobes*

• VEE → *putamen*

• HHV → *−6 frontal/temporal lobes*

• St.LE → *thalamus, brain stem, basal ganglia*

• WNV → *anterior horn, basal ganglia*

• MVE → *brain stem, basal ganglia, cerebellum*

• JE → *cortex, thalamus, brain stem, basal ganglia*

• Mumps → *choroid plexus*

• EEE → *hippocampus, basal gangli, brain stem,*

• CE (LaCrosse)→ *thalamus, brain stem, pons cerebellum*

15. Post-infectious Viral Encephalitis

• Commonly, acute viral encephalitis may accompany *viral exanthems of childhood*, ie, mumps, rubella, varicella and measles *may directly involve the brain or may represent an immunologic reaction following* infection, eg, measles, postinfectious encephalitis.

ID Board Pearls

• *Demyelination is characteristic of postinfectious encephalitis.*

16. CSF Viral Encephalitis

General Concepts

• CSF usually reveals a mild pleocytosis (usually less than 500 cells/mm^3), with a *lymphocytic* predominance.

• Encephalitis with a pleocytosis of ≥1000 cells/mm^3 should suggest HSV or EEE.

• All *viruses* causing encephalitis or meningoencephalitis are associated with a *lymphocytic predominance*, but the CSF of patients with viral encephalitis *may initially have many polymorphonuclear neutrophils* (PMNs).

• Protein levels in the CSF of patients with viral encephalitis are variably highly elevated.

• The CSF glucose level is usually normal.

• The CSF lactic acid levels are normal in patients with acute viral encephalitis in the absence of hemorrhage, but may be somewhat elevated in the presence of RBCs or HSV-1.

• MRI is very sensitive in diagnosing early abnormalities of the white matter in HIV-infected patients.

• The EEG usually shows diffuse bilateral slow-wave activity in viral encephalitis.

• Any CNS disorder may be associated with a low serum sodium secondary to SIADH, but is particularly *characteristic of St.LE.*

ID Board Pearls

• All CNS viruses *except HSV-1* (which may have 100% PMNs) have ≤90% PMNs in the CSF differential count.

• *Occasionally decreased* CSF glucose may be seen in association with LCM, *mumps, enterovirus or HSV-1 infection.*

• In the absence of bleeding or a traumatic tap, red blood cells *(RBCs) in the CSF of a patient with encephalitis* should suggest *HSV-1* or *Listeria*.

• The CSF may be cloudy with EEE.

• *Early* EEG is useful in diagnosing HSV-1 encephalitis early, *before* abnormalities appear on CT or MRI.

17. HSV Encephalitis

General Concepts

• HSV is the "*great imitator*" of CNS infections. HSV *mimics* many infectious and noninfectious disorders and *vice versa*.

• HSV is the *most common* cause of *non-seasonal* acute viral encephalitis worldwide.

• *Clinical spectrum* includes aseptic meningitis → meningoencephalitis→ *encephalitis* (most *severe* form).

• *Early/mild* HSV encephalitis presents with *mental status changes/confusion*.

• *Late/severe* HSV encephalitis presents with *dense neurologic deficits* (obtundation/stupor).

• *Most sensitive early* diagnostic test is the *EEG*. Shows *frontal temporal lobe focus* of activity.

• *Later* (2-3 days), brain CT/MRI shows *temporal lobe abnormalities*.

• CSF of HSV *variable* and can *mimic* bacterial meningitis. Viral CNS infection in CSF usually present with CSF lymphocytic pleocytosis.

• In HSV encephalitis the CSF protein is *variably elevated* and *unhelpful* diagnostically.

• The *CSF lactic acid level is normal* in HSV encephalitis but may be *slightly* elevated *if* RBCs are present.

• CSF *RBCs are absent* in early/mild HSV encephalitis but are present in *late/severe* HSV encephalitis (*in HSV CSF number of RBCs ~ to temporal lobe damage/hemorrhage*).

• HSV encephalitis is one of the few *treatable causes* of acute viral encephalitis. If HSV is *suspected* as the cause of acute encephalitis, begin *empiric* therapy with acyclovir.

• Presumptive diagnosis of HSV encephalitis based on demonstrating *temporal lobe abnormality* by *EEG* or *CT/MRI*.

- *Definitive* diagnosis of HSV encephalitis is by *CSF PCR*.

- *Prognosis* in *early/mild HSV* encephalitis *good* when *treated early with acyclovir*.

- *Prognosis* in *late/severe* HSV encephalitis *poor even* when treated with acyclovir. *Survivors* often have *severe neurological sequelae*.

ID Board Pearls

- Often there is a *recent* history of *H labialis* (2-3 weeks *before* encephalitis), but in a patient with encephalitis and *H. labialis concurrently* argues *against* HSV as the cause of the encephalitis.

- *Early/acutely* may present with a *PMN predominance (<90% PMNs)*. HSV and EEE may present with a PMN predominance in the CSF, but only with HSV can the PMN% *exceed 90%*.

- The *CSF glucose* is usually *normal* in *viral CNS infections* except mumps, LCM, rarely enteroviral and HSV. HSV is the only cause of viral encephalitis that may present with a *decreased CSF glucose*.

- CSF RBCs (excluding traumatic tap, ICH, leaking aneurysm) should suggest with *Listeria*, anthrax, meningitis, CNS malignancy, TB, *Negleria fowleri or HSV*.

18. Eastern Equine Encephalitis (EEE)

General Concepts

- EEE occurs in *North and South America*, *Cuba*, and along *the Eastern seaboard* from New Orleans to Nova Scotia.

- EEE is one of the *most virulent* arboviral encephalitides.

- EEE presents with rapid and dense *neurologic defects* and carries a fatality rate of up to 70%.

- Infection with EEE *virus frequently results in clinical disease* rather than subclinical infection, as with the other equine encephalitis viruses.

- In *infants and children*, the *onset is typically abrupt*.

- It can be subacute in *elderly patients*.

- EEE neurologic sequelae in children up to 80%.

- EEE mortality is up to 70% in very young/elderly.

ID Board Pearls

- *Very high fever is characteristic* at the onset of EEE.

- A *clue* to EEE in *children* is a peculiar *"brawny edema" of the face and extremities*.

19. California Encephalitis (CE)

General Concepts

- California (LaCrosse) encephalitis (CE) is caused by 10 closely-related viruses.

- *Focal signs* are present in approximately 20%; behavioral changes are common sequelae of CE.

ID Board Pearls

- CE is one of few arboviral causes of encephalitis with *leukocytosis*.

- Unlike other causes of arboviral encephalitis, *gastrointestinal symptoms* are frequent.

20. Western Equine Encephalitis (WEE)

General Concepts

- WEE is *most* common in *children* but may occur in persons of all ages acquired in rural or suburban environments in West Nile encephalitis.

- *Mortality* of WEE is *5%-15%* in both children/adults.

- It is *usually mild*, with recovery occurring in *2 weeks*.

ID Board Pearls

- WEE presents with fever and *seizures*.

21. Venezuelan Equine Encephalitis (VEE)

General Concepts

- VEE common throughout *North and South America*, *Central* America, eastern *Mexico*, southern *Texas* and southern *Florida*.

- Encephalitis caused by VEE is usually *mild*, and recovery without sequelae. Recovery is usually complete in a week.

- Mild/neurologic sequelae in children. Adults usually completely recover.

- VEE mortality is <1%.

ID Board Pearls

- *Conjunctivitis* in *30%* of patients with VEE.

22. St. Louis Encephalitis (St.LE)

General Concepts

- St. Louis encephalitis (St.LE) is most frequent along the Mississippi River. St.LE occurs everywhere, ie, East Coast (urban) and West Coast (rural) *except then northwest quadrant*.

- St.LE is also is *common in Central America and northern South America*.

- St.LE is unique—has a *predilection* for individuals *over 60 years of age*.

- Neurologic sequelae of St.LE in ~25%.

- Mostly in *elderly* with St.LE up to 20%.

- St.LE is the only cause of viral encephalitis associated with *dysuria in 20%*.

ID Board Pearls

- In a patient with encephalitis, tremors of the *tongue and extremities* also suggest St.LE.

- St.LE may present with an influenza-like prodrome and should be thought of during epidemics of "*summer stroke*."

23. Colorado Tick Fever (CTF)

General Concepts

• Colorado *tick* fever (CTF) occurs in the *western half of the United States* and adjacent areas of southern Canada.

• Seizures are distinctly *uncommon*.

• Mortality and neurologic sequelae rare with CTF.

ID Board Pearls

• *"Camel-back fever curve"* is an important clue to CTF.

• Conjunctival suffusion, splenomegaly and a maculopapular rash are also key clues.

24. Japanese Encephalitis (JE)

General Concepts

• Japanese encephalitis (JE) occurs in *Asia* from Japan through southern China, Indochina, and *southeastern India, Malaysia, northern Indonesia and the Philippines*.

• Japanese encephalitis is *primarily a disease of children*.

• Second only to EEE in overall mortality up to 70%.

• *Neurologic sequelae* are common.

ID Board Pearls

• *Extrapyramidal* signs are *prominent*. Generalized *muscle weakness is common*.

• *Unlike* most other *arboviral* encephalitides, Japanese encephalitis is a *protracted illness* that lasts for *weeks*.

• WNV may be transmitted via blood transfusions in organ transplants.

25. West Nile Encephalitis (WNE)

General Concepts

• West Nile Encephalitis (WNE) is caused by a flavivirus (group III).

• Other flaviviruses *antigenically* related to WNE include Murray Valley encephalitis (MVE), Japanese encephalitis (JE) and the St. Louis encephalitis (St.LE).

• WNE is maintained in nature by *Culex mosquitoes and wild birds*.

• Humans, horses, dogs and pigs are *incidental* hosts and are not usually involved in the transmission cycle.

• *Only birds* develop high-grade *WNE viremia* sufficient to perpetuate transmission of WNV.

• *Non*-immune children are common hosts for WNE. WNE produces an acute, nonspecific febrile illness in children.

• The incubation period is from *2-6 days*.

• *Encephalitis plus flaccid paralysis* are the hallmarks of WNE.

• CF and neutralizing antibody *titers rise in 2-5 weeks* (in 4-6 weeks).

• *Common* manifestations include low-grade fevers, myalgias, *weakness* and *tremors*.

• Seizures are *un*common.

• *Thrombocytopenia* is common.

• Serum transaminases are *mildly* elevated.

• The CSF is clear and a lymphocytic pleocytosis (45-450 WBC/mm^3 usual range) is the rule.

• CSF protein is *elevated* (may be highly elevated).

• The CSF glucose is *not* decreased in WNE.

ID Board Pearls

• WNE may be *cultured from blood* during the *first week* in patients.

• *Leukopenia* is the rule and relative *lymphopenia* may be severe and prolonged in WNE.

• Only WNE associated with highly elevated serum ferritin levels.

26. Rabies

General Concepts

- Rabies has a *worldwide distribution*. *Bats* are the *principal rabies reservoir* worldwide.

- Animals infected with rabies include *skunks, raccoons, foxes*, coyotes, bobcats, *cats* and *dogs*.

- Rabies virus may be transmitted by *aerosolization/inhalation* (rabid bats in caves), but most *commonly* via virus-*infected* saliva.

- Rabies has been transmitted via rabies-infected *corneal transplants*.

Clinical presentation of rabies *(5 stages)*
Rabies Stage I

- Usual incubation period (4 days-19 years) is 1-2 months. Patients are asymptomatic.

Rabies Stage II

- *Prodromal period* (1-10 days) characterized by *depression/anxiety with fever/chills* ± GI symptoms.

- *Pain/paresthesias* at bite site *typical. Clinical clue. Myoedema (muscle edema surrounding point of impact* when hit with reflex hammer; disappears in seconds).

Rabies Stage III

- Symptomatic rabies (2-14 days) typically with *agitation/hyperactivity, aggression, bizarre behavior, excessive salivation, sweating, priapisms/ejaculations* and *hysteria*.

- *Clinical clue. Severe muscle spasms* when fanned gently ("fan test").

- *Clinical clue*: "Barking-like" voice secondary to palatal/cord paralysis.

Paralytic Rabies

- *Clinical clue*. Heralded by limb *weakness/paralysis*.

Rabies Stage IV

- *Coma* (14 days after symptoms)

Rabies Stage V

- *Recovery* (with *severe* neurologic sequelae) or *death* (18 days after symptoms)

- *Definitive diagnosis* of rabies by demonstrating *Negri inclusion bodies* in brain biopsy.

ID Board Pearls

- *CSF* in rabies is usually *unremarkable*. CSF abnormalities, if present, include mild lymphocytic pleocytosis/elevated protein.

27. Diagnosis of Viral Encephalitis

General Concepts

• *Direct viral isolation* from the *CSF/blood* is *low yield* in viral encephalitis.

• A diagnosis of viral encephalitis is usually made on the basis of *acute/convalescent serology or PCR*.

• DFA staining of corneal smears, saliva or brain tissue is useful in diagnosing *rabies*.

• DFA techniques are also useful in the diagnosis of *HSV* infection from *brain* biopsy material.

• CSF PCR is the best test for HSV encephalitis.

• HIV infections may be diagnosed by CSF/serum antigen/antibody determinations.

• PCR has been developed for a variety of viruses, but is not always available in clinical laboratories.

ID Board Pearls

• Colorado tick fever (CTF) is best diagnosed by DFA of RBCs in clotted blood.

28. Treatment of Viral Encephalitis

General Concepts

• The most important *treatable* cause of acute viral encephalitis is HSV encephalitis.

• *Optimal* results are obtained when therapy is initiated early in the illness.

• In compromised hosts, CMV encephalitis may be treated with *ganciclovir* or *valgangciclovir*.

ID Board Pearls

• Since HSV and VZV is the only treatable cause of viral encephalitis, empiric acyclovir is frequently used if clinical/laboratory features suggest HSV or VZV encephalitis.

• Supportive therapy and the *avoidance of hypotonic fluids* are important adjunctive measures.

29. Acute Encephalitis in the Compromised Host

General Concepts

• CMV or *T gondii encephalitis* occurs *only* in patients with *severely* impaired *cellular* (T-cell) *immunity.*

• CMV or toxoplasmosis *encephalopathy* encountered most often in *organ transplants* and *advanced HIV* (CD4+ cell count <100)

ID Board Pearls

• The differential diagnosis of encephalitis in *HIV/transplant* patients include: EBV, HIV, CMV and *T gondii.*

30. CMV Encephalitis

General Concepts

• CMV encephalitis *may* have *CN abnormalities* (CN III/VII).

• Patients with CMV encephalitis often have signs of extra-CNS CMV infection, ie, *perivascular retinitis* ("tomato soup" fundi), *esophagitis, colitis,* etc.

• Diagnosis of CMV by tissue specimen with characterized *CMV inclusion bodies* or *CSF PCR.*

ID Board Pearls

• *CMV* encephalitis occurs *only* in hosts with severely *impaired T-cell immunity.*

31. Toxoplasma Encephalitis

General Concepts

- HIV and CMV encephalitis resembles *T gondii* encephalitis.

- Toxoplasma encephalitis may present *with or without* a *mass lesion* on brain CT/MRI.

- Most patients with *T gondii* encephalitis have *concurrent* (*non*-perivascular) *chorioretinitis*.

- Most patients with toxoplasmosis encephalitis have *T gondii* IgG titers (IgM titers are usually *absent*). Conversely, *no T gondii IgG titers argue against* a diagnosis of *T gondii* encephalitis.

- CSF in *T gondii* encephalitis is nondiagnostic. Usual findings include a *mild lymphocytic* pleocytosis/elevated protein.

- Occasionally, toxoplasma tachyzoites may be seen in Giemsa stained (centrifuged) CSF.

- Diagnosis of toxoplasma encephalitis by *CSF PCR* or *brain biopsy*.

ID Board Pearls

- Toxoplasma encephalitis occurs *only* in hosts with severely *impaired T-cell immunity*.

- Toxoplasma mass lesions *resemble CNS lymphoma* or *TB*.

32. Encephalitis: Clinical Vignettes

General Concepts

- Most *vital* encephalatides are *mosquito-borne*.

- Some are *tick-borne*.

- *History of tick exposure* with encephalitis

- Rocky Mountain Spotted Fever (RMSF)

- CTF

ID Board Pearls

- Patients presenting with encephalitis, *especially meningoencephalitis*, from *upper New York State* or southern Canada may have *Powassan encephalitis* (POW).

- The most *common arboviral encephalitides* likely to be encountered in the United States are CE, EE, WEE, VEE, St.LE,CTF, POW and WNE.

- *Travelers returning from Asia* with encephalitis may have Japanese encephalitis (JE), *especially if extrapyramidal signs* are prominent.

33. Further Reading

Arvin AM, Gershon AA. *Varicella-zoster Virus*. United Kingdom: Cambridge University; 2000.

Boos J, Esiri MM. *Viral Encephalitis in Humans*. Washington, DC: ASM Press; 2003.

Halperin J, Encephalitis. New York, NY: Informa; 2008.

Knipe DM, Howley PM. *Fields Virology*. 4th ed. Philadelphia, PA: WB Saunders; 2001.

Scheld WM, Whitley RJ, Marra CM. *Infections of the Central Nervous System*. 3rd ed. Philadelphia, PA: Lippincott Williams & Wilkins; 2004.

Studahl M, Cinque P, Bergstrom T. *Herpes Simples Viruses*. New York, NY: Taylor & Francis; 2006.

Wood M, Anderson M. *Neurologic Infections*. London, England: WB Saunders; 1988.

Chapter 15:
Epstein-Barr Virus (EBV) and Infectious Mononucleosis for the ID Boards

Larry I. Lutwick, MD

Contents

1. **Infectious Mononucleosis**

2. **Heterophile-Positive Infectious Mononucleosis**

3. **Heterophile-Negative Infectious Mononucleosis**

4. **Further Reading**

1. Infectious Mononucleosis

History

- Initially described at the end of the 19th century with fever, malaise, and enlarged liver, spleen and lymph nodes.

- Became referred to as *Drusenfieber* (glandular fever).

- Sprunt and Evans (1921) coined the term *infectious mononucleosis* to describe fever, enlarged lymph nodes and weakness in otherwise healthy young people with abnormal circulating blood mononuclear cells.

- Downey and McKinley (1923) better characterized the atypical lymphocyte.

- Paul and Bunnell (1932) described a sheep red blood cell agglutinating antibody in patients with infectious mononucleosis.

- Epstein, Achong and Barr (1964) characterized a herpes virus in tissue culture from material taken from patients with Burkitt's lymphoma.

- Henle, Henle and coworkers (1968) linked the Epstein-Barr virus (EBV) with infectious mononucleosis.

Clinical Disease

- An evaluation for possible mononucleosis is shown in Table 1.

Symptoms
- Triad of fever, sore throat and lymphadenopathy.

- Other symptoms occurring less uniformly include:
  * Anorexia

  * Nausea and/or vomiting

  * Headache

  * Abdominal discomfort

  * Arthralgias

Table 1

Approach to the Patient with Possible Infectious Mononucleosis

History

Including:
    Exposure to ill children (HHV-6)[a]
    Sexual exposures (HIV)
    Exposure to cats (toxoplasmosis)
    Recent surgery or transfusion (CMV/HIV)
    Dietary history and preferences (toxoplasmosis)
    Travel (toxoplasmosis/HIV)

Physical Examination

Paying close attention to:
    Pharyngeal exudate (EBV)
    Gingival or palatal ulcers (HIV)
    Palatal petechiae (EBV)
    Severe cervical lymphadenopathy
      (toxoplasmosis)
    Splenomegaly (EBV)
    Genital ulcers (HIV)
    Prominent mood changes or confusion (HIV)

Blood Evaluation

CBC with manual differential
    Mononucleosis test
    Liver panel (AST, ALT, ALK-P, bilirubin)
    EBV serologies[b]
    CMV serologies[b]
    Toxoplasmosis serologies[b]
    HIV ELISA, Western blot, viral load, p24 antigen[b]
    HHV-6 antibody[b]

[a] The organism in parentheses is linked to the history or physical exam feature.
[b] These are done selectively based on results of initial testing.

    * Cough

Signs
- *Fever*
  * Can peak each day at as high as 40° C

  * May last for 10-14 days

* 30%-40% have minimal fever

- *Lymph node enlargement*
  * Adenopathy can be generalized

  * Cervical node enlargement most common

  * Posterior cervical involvement frequent

  * Nodes are movable and minimally painful

- *Pharyngitis*
  * ~30% with exudates

  * Tonsillar enlargement can be prominent

- *Splenomegaly*
  * Present in ~50% of cases

  * Peaks in second week

  * Resolves clinically usually over 3-4 weeks

- *Hepatomegaly*
  * In ~10%-20%

  * May be associated with direct tenderness

- *Exanthem/enanthem*

  * Enanthem: 25% with palatal petechiae

  * Exanthem: pleomorphic

- *Icterus*

  * Jaundice is uncommon, 5%-10%

Laboratory Findings

- An assessment of a mononucleosis-type illness is shown in Table 1.

  * Leukocytosis as high as 20,000-30,000/mm^3

  * Lymphocyte percentage increased 60%-70%

  * Atypical lymphocytes (AL) as high as 10% of lymphocytes or more, ~5% of total WBCs. Usually only Epstein-Barr virus and

cytomegalovirus will have AL of >10% of total lymphocytes

* Mild neutropenia, 2000-3000/mm^3

* Mild thrombocytopenia, 100,000-150,000/mm^3

* Cold agglutinins, usually anti-I

* Liver enzyme abnormalities (LFTs): mixed hepatocellular/cholestatic; alkaline phosphatase may be prominent; total bilirubin usually normal

Clinical Course

- Pharyngitis peaks over 3-5 days and resolves over 7-10 days.

- Throat culture necessary to rule out group A streptococcal infection.

- Fever may remain high for 7-10 days and then continue at a lower grade for a similar period.

- Overall feeling of well-being resolves more slowly, beginning in second week and continuing over 3-6 weeks.

- Wellness can wax and wane during convalescence.

- Prolonged fatigue after EBV mononucleosis does not seem to be related to increased viral load or a substantially altered host response.

- Patients should adjust their activities to accommodate their sense of well-being.

Complications

Most individual cases of mononucleosis are without significant complications but can have a slow, prolonged convalescence over a number of weeks. Even with complications, the mortality rate of this disease is quite low. Recognizable complications include:

- **Autoimmune hemolytic anemia**
  - * Usually cold agglutinin, anti-I type

  - * Develops during the second or third week of illness

  - * Lasts 1-2 months

  - * Corticosteroids useful

- **Immune thrombocytopenia**
  - * 50% of patients have counts

  <150,000/mm^3

  - * Severe thrombocytopenia rare

  - * Steroids may be used in severe cases

- **Lymphopenia (rarely occurs)**
  - * Correlates with more severe disease

- **Splenic rupture**
  - * Spleen may be very friable

  - * Peak period during second and third weeks

  - * Avoid over palpation

  - * Avoid contact sports during convalescence

  - * Watch for abdominal pain, dropping hematocrit

- **Obstruction of the upper airway by massive lymphatic tissue enlargement and edema (rarely occurs)**
  - * Airway protection with tracheostomy may be required

  - * Corticosteroids are very effective in this scenario

- **Neurological complications (<1%)**
  - * Aseptic meningitis

  - * Encephalitis

  - * Bell's palsy

  - * Guillain-Barré syndrome

Atypical Lymphocytes

- The Downey cell, a large mononuclear lymphocyte with lobular, eccentrically located nucleus.

- Cytoplasm may be basophilic and vacuolated.

- Larger than the usual (typical) lymphocyte.

- Morphologic differences in atypical lymphocytes may be seen, and in experienced hands can be used to suggest the etiology (type I: cytomegalovirus; type II: Epstein-Barr virus; type III: human herpesvirus-6).

- Seen in diseases other than those associated with infectious mononucleosis (in lower numbers) including:

  - * Measles

  - * Rubella

  - * Mumps

  - * Drug reactions to phenytoin or para-aminosalicylic acid

Table 2

Absorption Effects of Heterophile Antibodies: Agglutination of Sheep Red Blood Cells

Clinical Situation	Unabsorbed	After Absorption With:	
		Beef red cells	Guinea pig kidney
Mononucleosis	++++	0	+++
Serum sickness	+++	0	0
Normal serum	±	±	0

Heterophile Antibody

- Found in ~90% of patients with the EBV form of the disease at some time during the disease.

- Often absent in the first week of illness.

- To be specific for infectious mononucleosis, the Davidsohn exclusion test is used, in which the agglutination of sheep red blood cells persists after absorption with guinea pig kidney cells but not after absorption with beef red blood cells (Table 2).

- False-positive tests are uncommon with either the tube tests or the monospot-type slide tests (uses horse red blood cells and differential absorption).

2. Heterophile-Positive Infectious Mononucleosis

Epstein-Barr Virus (EBV)

Organism
- EBV is a member of the gamma-herpes virus family.

- It replicates primarily in B-lymphocytes and can exist in a latent form in these cells.

- Host range is restricted to humans and some primates.

- It will transform human B lymphocyte cell lines into a permanent cell line, demonstrating its oncogenic potential.

- Asymptomatic reactivation with excretion of EBV in the saliva is common (Table 3).

Epidemiology
- Most people are infected as children by contact with EBV-containing oropharyngeal secretions of asymptomatic people.

- Infection in young children is often asymptomatic or associated with nonspecific illness.

- Infection in older children, adolescents and young adults (~50%) often manifests as infectious mononucleosis.

Table 3

Presence of EBV in Oropharyngeal Secretions

Population Cohort %	EBV Positive
EBV sero-naive (noninfected)	0
EBV mononucleosis	50-100
EBV seropositive (not primary)	15-25
Seropositive transplant patients	50-70
Seropositive lymphoma or leukemia	70-90

- In college students, acquisition of EBV appears to be enhanced by penetrative sexual activity.

- Infection in older adults (>40 years of age) is discussed below.

Diagnostic Methodology
- Heterophile-positive in ~90% of cases during illness.

- Specific EBV antibodies (Table 4) can distinguish primary infection from past infection.

- EBV can be detected in saliva, but such testing is not generally done.

Treatment
- Most people with EBV infectious mononucleosis will recover with only symptomatic interventions.

- Acyclovir and other antivirals can diminish oral viral shedding, but the clinical effects on disease appear minimal and antiviral therapy is not generally advised.

- Corticosteroid use will usually limit the period of fever, decrease the degree of constitutional symptoms and help treat:

  * Hemolytic anemia

  * Significant thrombocytopenia

  * Impending airway obstruction

  * Severe or prolonged constitutional symptoms

- Because of the self-limited nature of this lymphoproliferative disease and corticosteroid-induced immunosuppression, most physicians would not use the medication without clear indications.

EBV in the Older Adult

- The presentation of primary EBV infection in the person greater than 40 years of age is often atypical. The following are common features in these patients:

  * More significant hepatic component with icterus, to the point where the disease may present primarily as a febrile hepatitis

  * Substantially less lymphatic enlargement manifest by less lymphadenopathy (33%) and splenomegaly (15%)

  * More severe disease and higher mortality

  * Less pharyngitis (only ~25%)

  * Heterophile positivity still ~90%

EBV-associated Lymphoproliferative Disorders

- The following disorders reflect the propensity, under certain conditions, for EBV to cause more progressive or frankly malignant diseases. A discussion of these disorders is beyond the scope of this presentation and the reader should consult standard references for more information:

  * X-linked lymphoproliferative syndrome

  * Burkitt's lymphoma

  * Post-transplant B-cell lymphoma

  * AIDS-associated non-Hodgkin's lymphoma

3. Heterophile-Negative Infectious Mononucleosis

Epstein-Barr Virus (EBV)

- In a variety of studies, EBV was found to be the most common cause of heterophile-negative mononucleosis, as well as the only cause of heterophile-positive mononucleosis. Heterophile negativity may occur from:

   * Testing done prior to becoming positive (especially in the first week of symptoms)

   * Testing done late, after clearance

   * ~10% of EBV-associated cases are felt to be negative throughout

- No clear clinical differences occur related to the heterophile reactivity alone.

- Diagnosis made by specific EBV antibody pattern consistent with primary EBV infection (Table 4).

Cytomegalovirus (CMV)

Organism
- Human cytomegalovirus is a member of the beta-herpesvirus family.

- Latency in, and reactivation from, a variety of cells appears to be the case, including neutrophils, T-lymphocytes, renal epithelial cells and salivary acinar cells.

- A significant pathogen usually related to reactivation disease in immunosuppressed individuals.

- The most common congenital infection.

Epidemiology
- Ubiquitous worldwide with 60%-70% of adults in the United States seropositive and higher rates in select groups.

- Often spread from asymptomatic individuals related to excretion in saliva and/or urine.

- Most infections in the normal host are asymptomatic or manifest nonspecific symptomatology.

- Transmission can be associated with blood transfusion, especially fresh whole blood, and is associated with a "postperfusion syndrome."

Clinical Differences From EBV-associated Mononucleosis
- Most common non-EBV cause of heterophile negative mononucleosis.

- Pharyngitis is less common (~25%).

- Prominent lymphatic involvement is less common.

   * Lymphadenopathy ~20%

   * Splenomegaly ~20%

- Liver enzyme abnormalities similar to EBV, but liver biopsy may show granulomas.

Diagnostic Methodology
- Primary cytomegalovirus infection can be diagnosed using CMV antibody by a variety of techniques.

- Specific IgM antibody is useful for primary infection (such as CMV mononucleosis) in nonimmunosuppressed hosts.

   * Some commercial anti-CMV IgM assays may be false-positive.

- IgG anti-CMV antibodies may show a seroconversion or 4-fold titer rise in primary infection.

- CMV culture is readily done using saliva and urine, but will not distinguish between primary infection and reactivation in a patient with another illness.

Treatment
- Specific treatment of CMV infection, including CMV mononucleosis, is almost never indicated in the immunologically normal host.

- Drugs that are active against CMV include ganciclovir, foscarnet and cidofovir.

Toxoplasmosis

Organism

- *Toxoplasma gondii* is a coccidian sporozoan.

- Felines are the definitive hosts in which the sexual reproductive cycle occurs in the intestinal tract.

- Oocysts are excreted only for a limited time in cat stool.

- Humans and other warm-blooded animals are intermediate hosts in whom tissue cysts develop, particularly in muscle and brain.

- Toxoplasmosis is particularly significant in:

    * The cellularly immunosuppressed host (disseminated disease including encephalitis)

    * The pregnant female (congenital infection)

Epidemiology

- May be acquired via ingestion of infectious oocysts in soil or cat litter.

- Also transmitted via the ingestion of undercooked or raw meat (such as pork, lamb, mutton, venison, bear), less commonly beef.

- No person-to-person spread other than vertical transmission and from blood transfusion or organ transplantation (both rare).

Clinical Differences From EBV-associated Mononucleosis

- Pharyngitis less common

- Lymphadenopathy may be very prominent, often nontender and clinically may be confused with lymphoma.

- Atypical lymphocytes (usually less than 10%).

- Causes no more than ~1% of cases of mononucleosis syndrome in most studies.

Diagnostic Methodology
Antibody tests
Indirect fluorescent antibodies

- IgM antibody: should be useful for primary infection, but commercial assays may be positive for years.

- IgA antibody: appears to be a better test for recent infection.

- IgG antibody: elevated in primary infection and persists for lifetime.

Histopathology

- Very characteristic histologic changes are found in the lymph node:

    * Reactive follicular hyperplasia

    * Irregular clusters of epithelioid histiocytes

    * Monocytoid cells distending sinuses

    * Active tissue form (tachyzoite) and cyst rarely seen in the lymph node

Treatment

- Usually no specific treatment is needed for the lymphadenopathy or mononucleosis forms of toxoplasmosis.

- Exceptions: severe or persistent symptoms or visceral involvement.

- Treatment, if needed: pyrimethamine plus sulfadiazine or trimethoprim-sulfamethoxazole or clindamycin (Table 5).

Human Immunodeficiency Virus (HIV)

Organism

- Initially known as human T-lymphotropic virus III (HTLV-III).

- Member of the retroviral group of viruses that contain reverse transcriptase activity.

Table 5

Treatment Modalities in Toxoplasmosis

Preferred treatment for prolonged Toxoplasma mononucleosis

- Pyrimethamine 25-50 mg/d PO for 2-4 weeks
  plus
  Sulfadiazine 1000 mg PO QID

- Trimethoprim 160 mg + sulfamethoxazole 800 mg PO BID for 2-4 weeks

- Clindamycin 300 mg PO QID for 2-4 weeks (for sulfonamide-allergic patients)

Table 6

Clinical Findings in Primary HIV Infection

Suggestive of a mononucleosis-like process
Pyrexia
Sore throat
Enlarged lymph glands
Myalgias and arthralgias
Retro-orbital headache
Loss of appetite
Nausea, vomiting, or diarrhea

Skin and mucosal surface manifestations
Maculopapular rash on face or trunk
Urticaria
Desquamation of palms and soles
Gingival ulcers
Palatal ulcers
Esophageal ulcers
Genital ulcers

Nervous system involvement
Confusion
Depression
Mood changes
Aseptic meningitis
Meningoencephalitis
Polyneuritis
Guillain-Barré syndrome

Epidemiology
- In adult international travelers with a heterophile-negative mononucleosis-like illness, HIV should be especially considered although all non-EBV causes be found.

- Transmitted from person to person by blood contact (transfusion, needlestick, IV drug use), sexually or vertically from infected mother.

- Primary HIV infection, with an incubation period of ~2-4 weeks, can present as a heterophile-negative mononucleosis-like illness (Table 6).

Clinical Differences From EBV-associated Mononucleosis
- Oral (gingival or palatal) ulcers in ~40% of cases.

- Genital ulcers in ~20%.

- Both types of ulcers more common in sexually transmitted cases.

- Lymphocytosis absent.

- Splenomegaly less common.

- Neurologic symptoms more prominent:

  * Depression, irritability, mood changes

  * Less common: aseptic meningitis, meningoencephalitis and polyneuritis

- Patients with neurologic manifestations may be more likely to have more rapidly progressive HIV disease.

Diagnostic Modalities
- Low CD4+ cell count.

- Seroconversion to HIV antibody by ELISA.

- Tests that may be positive before HIV ELISA:

  * HIV antibody by Western blot technique

* HIV RNA viral load

Treatment
- Early infection may be considered for treatment with highly active antiretroviral therapy (HAART).

- A reasonable first-line regimen would be:

    * Two nucleoside reverse transcriptase inhibitors (NRTIs) such as tenofovir or zidovudine (AZT) and emtricitabine (FTC) or lamivudine (3TC).

    Plus

    * An NNRTI such as efavirenz.

    Or

    * A protease inhibitor, such as the fixed combination of lopinavir and ritonavir.

Human Herpesvirus 6 (HHV-6)

Organism
- Described in 1986 as human B-lymphotropic virus.

- Two serotypes recognized, HHV-6A and HHV-6B.

Epidemiology
- Worldwide, most people are infected by the age of 2 years.

- Most infections nonspecific, but HHV-6 causes roseola.

Clinical Differences From EBV-associated Mononucleosis
- Mononucleosis-like illness usually has less fatigue.

- Can have posterior cervical lymphadenopathy like EBV.

- Most cases, however, are mild.

Diagnostic Modalities
- Antibody assays are commercially available.

- One positive titer not helpful given high seroprevalence.

- IgM assays are not currently reliable.

- Seroconversion or 4-fold antibody rise required.

Treatment

- Only anecdotal data available for treatment of any HHV-6 infection.

- Acyclovir inactive; ganciclovir and foscarnet have activity.

- Most primary HHV-6 infections do not require therapy.

Other Agents
- Miscellaneous other pathogens have been linked to one or several cases of heterophile-negative mononucleosis. The significance of these associations is unclear. The infections include:

    * Rubella

    * Adenovirus

    * HTLV-1

    * Scrub typhus

    * Brucella suis

ID Board Pearls

- Almost 100% of patients with mononucleosis will develop a pruritic rash following ampicillin or amoxicillin use (which may be related to the aminobenzyl moiety).

- In mononucleosis, normal liver function tests are distinctly unusual.

- Epstein-Barr virus and Group A streptococcus can cause pharyngitis at the same time.

- The classic atypical lymphocyte population is heterogeneous in appearance, which distinguishes it from the homogeneous population of cells seen in lymphocytic leukemia.

- The atypical lymphocyte is a T-cell reacting to the EBV infection in B cells; it is not infected by EBV.

- The heterophile antibody does not appear to be directed against any specific antigen coded for by EBV itself.

- Because of the high prevalence of previous infection in individuals by young adulthood, most people exposed to the oropharyngeal secretions of a patient with EBV-associated mononucleosis do not develop mononucleosis.

4. Further Reading

Bottieau E, Clerinx J, Van den Enden E, et al. Infectious mononucleosis like syndromes in febrile travelers returning from the tropics. *J Travel Med*. 2006;13:191-197.

Cohen JI, Corey GR. Cytomegalovirus infection in the normal host. *Medicine*. 1985;64:100-114.

Crawford DH, Macsween KF, Higgins CD, et al. A cohort study among university students: identification of risk factors for Epstein-Barr virus seroconversion and infectious mononucleosis. *Clin Infect Dis*. 2006;43:276-282.

Dorfman RF, Remington JS. Value of lymph node biopsy in the diagnosis of acute acquired toxoplasmosis. *N Engl J Med*. 1973;289:878-881.

Horwitz CA, Henle W, Henle G, et al. Infectious mononucleosis in patients aged 40 to 72 years: report of 27 cases, including 3 without heterophilantibody responses. *Medicine*. 1983;62:256-262.

Kinloch-De Loës S, de Saussure P, Saurat JH, et al. Symptomatic primary infection due to human immunodeficiency virus type I: review of 31 cases. *Clin Infect Dis*. 1993;17:59-65.

Schmader K, van der Horst CM, Klotman ME. Epstein-Barr virus and the elderly host. *Rev Infect Dis*. 1989;11:64-73.

Shiftan TA, Mendelsohn J. The circulating "atypical" lymphocyte. *Hum Pathol*. 1978;9:51-61.

Steeper TA, Horwitz CA, Ablashi DV, et al. The spectrum of clinical and laboratory findings resulting from human herpesvirus-6 (HHV-6) in patients with mononucleosis-like illnesses not resulting from Epstein-Barr virus or cytomegalovirus. *Am J Clin Pathol*. 1990;93:776-783.

Thompson SK, Doerr TD, Hengerer AS. Infectious mononucleosis and corticosteroids. Management practices and outcomes. *Arch Otolaryngol Head Neck Surg*. 2005;131:900-904.

Chapter 16:
Acute Pneumonias for the ID Boards

Burke A. Cunha, MD

Contents

Overview of Acute Pneumonia

Acute Pneumonia can be broadly classified into community-acquired pneumonia (CAP), nursing home-acquired pneumonia (NHAP) and nosocomial (hospital-acquired) pneumonia (NP) (Figure 1). The various classifications have implications for the etiologic diagnosis, evaluation, therapy and prognosis. Pneumonia can also be classified by severity of illness, location of treatment, rapidity of onset, pathogen and host immune status.

• *Community-Acquired Pneumonia (CAP).* CAP is usually classified into ambulatory hospitalized pneumonia and typical or atypical pneumonia. Typical CAP presents without extrapulmonary findings, (eg, myringitis, pharyngitis, rash). Atypical CAP presents with extrapulmonary findings and can further be classified into zoonotic or non zoonotic pneumonia based on the presence of a zoonotic vector.

• *Nursing Home-Acquired Pneumonia (NHAP).* NHAP may resemble CAP or HAP and occur sporadically or as part of a nursing home outbreak.

• *Nosocomial (Hospital-Acquired) Pneumonia (NP).* NP is usually classified into ventilator-associated pneumonia (VAP) or non ventilator-associated pneumonia.

Figure 1

Acute pneumonia classification

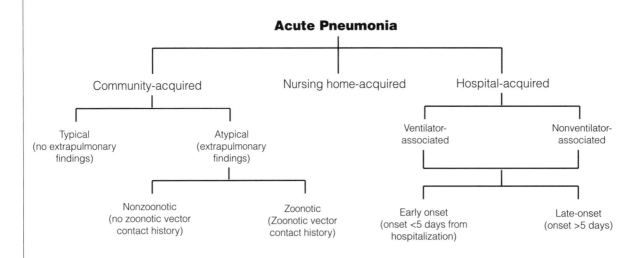

1. Typical Bacterial Community-Acquired Pneumonia (CAP)

General Concepts

A variety of bacteria, viruses, fungi, mycobacteria, chlamydia, parasites and rickettsia can cause pneumonia. *Single pathogens, not copathogens, cause CAP*. (Patients presenting with "multiple bacterial pathogens" occur only with aspiration pneumonia or lung abscess). In normal hosts with CAP, the diagnosis of apparent multiple/copathogens (*except* for MSSA/MRSA with viral influenza) is almost always based on combined serologic. In compromised hosts, pulmonary pathogens usually are present sequentially, not simultaneously, as copathogens. Specific patient subsets are predisposed to certain pathogens and types of pneumonia, as suggested by the history, physical examination, laboratory testing, chest x-ray and sputum Gram stain.

Noninfectious Mimics
Several noninfectious medical conditions can present with pulmonary symptoms, fever and chest x-ray opacities/infiltrates that mimic pneumonia. Pulmonary symptoms in the absence of an opacity/infiltrate on chest x-ray are usually due to acute bronchitis/acute exacerbation of chronic bronchitis (AECB), tracheobronchitis or asthma.

- The most common causes of CAP (85%) are *Streptococcus pneumoniae, Haemophilus influenzae and Moraxella catarrhalis*.

- Other organisms cause CAP only under special circumstances (eg, *Klebsiella pneumoniae, Staphylococcus aureus, MSSA/MRSA, Pseudomonas aeruginosa*).

ID Board Pearls

- *K pneumoniae* CAP occurs almost exclusively in chronic alcoholics.

- *S aureus* may occur with viral influenza pneumonia or an ILI but otherwise rarely, if ever, causes CAP.

- *P aeruginosa* rarely causes CAP and only occurs in the subset of patients with chronic *bronchiectasis* or *cystic fibrosis*.

General Concepts

- If a specific microbiologic diagnosis cannot be determined in CAP, it can be assumed that these patients have the *same pathogen* distribution as the pathogens determined by the usual diagnostic methods (85% typical and 15% atypical pathogens).

- In normal *and* immunocompromised hosts, the causes of CAP are the *same*:

    * Approximately 85% of the cases are caused by *S pneumoniae, H influenzae* or *M catarrhalis*.

    * 15% are distributed among *Legionella, Mycoplasma pneumoniae* and *Chlamydia pneumoniae*.

ID Board Pearls

- *Early* moderately advanced AIDS with CAP also has the *same* pathogen distribution as in *normal hosts*.

- CAP is caused by single pathogens, *not copathogens*.

- Patients presenting with *multiple* bacterial pathogens are seen *with aspiration pneumonia*.

- *Typical* bacterial pneumonias, except for fever and chills, have findings *confined* to the lungs.

- CAP *with extrapulmonary* findings should suggest CAP due to an *atypical* pathogen.

- Atypical pathogens are *systemic* infectious diseases that have a pulmonary *component*.

- *Each atypical pulmonary pathogen has its own characteristic pattern of extrapulmonary organ involvement*.

- Individual symptoms and signs are *not pathognomonic* of any particular pathogen; but is the *characteristic pattern of organ involvement and permits a presumptive clinical diagnosis*.

2. Mimics of CAP

General Concepts

- CAP must be differentiated from other pulmonary conditions mimicking pneumonia as well as systemic disorders with pulmonary manifestations.

- Mild CAP seen in the ambulatory setting may be confused with tracheobronchitis, acute bronchitis or exacerbation of chronic bronchitis (AECB).

- The differential diagnosis of CAP in hospitalized patients includes:

  * Congestive heart failure

  * Systemic lupus erythematosus (SLE)

  * Pulmonary embolism or infarction

  * Pneumonitis

  * Pulmonary drug reactions

  * Bronchogenic carcinomas

  * Asthma

- PHM, and the findings of extrapulmonary manifestations of systemic diseases mentioned, are usually sufficient to differentiate the mimics of pneumonia from CAP.

3. Severe CAP

General Concepts

- Relatively *avirulent* pulmonary pathogens (eg, *M catarrhalis*) are capable of causing severe pneumonia when infecting damaged lungs of patients with advanced chronic bronchitis.

- A variety of indices of severity have been devised to quantitate the severity of CAP, are useful as prognostic indicators and predict a prolonged clinical course, duration of hospital stay and potential complications.

- Severity indicators should not influence in the selection of an antibiotic for CAP. Empiric antibiotic selection is primarily based on spectrum and antimicrobial activity.

ID Board Pearls

- The *severity* of CAP depends on the *extent of pre-existing lung disease and cardiac function, and on the degree of impaired splenic function* (ie, decreased β-lymphocyte function).

- *Host factors, not pathogen virulence* per se, singly or in combination, are the *primary determinants of severity in CAP* in normal hosts.

4. Mycoplasma pneumoniae Pneumonia

Organism

- *Mycoplasma pneumoniae*

Microbiology

- Cell-wall-deficient organism with sterol plasma membrane

- Facultatively microaerophilic

Epidemiology

- Increased incidence in fall and winter

- Highest incidence in young adults, but not uncommon in the elderly

Geographic Distribution

- Worldwide

ID Board Pearls

Clinical Presentation

General
- Fever (usually ≤102° F)

- Headache, myalgias, sore throat

Neurologic (Rare)
- Meningoencephalitis

- Transverse myelitis

- Guillain-Barré syndrome

- Cerebellar ataxia

Respiratory
- Dry, nonproductive cough

- Nonexudative pharyngitis

- Otitis more often than bullous myringitis

Cardiac (Rare)
- Myocarditis

- Pericarditis

- Heart block

Gastrointestinal
- Loose stools/watery diarrhea

Renal
- Glomerulonephritis

- Nephrotic syndrome

Skin
- Erythema multiforme

Laboratory Abnormalities
- Hemolytic anemia (rare)

- ↑ Cold agglutinins (early/transient) ≥1:64

- Thrombocytopenia (rare)

- Normal LFTs

CXR
- Patchy infiltrates

- Small pleural effusion (uncommon)

ID Board Pearls

- Large pleural effusion argues against a Mycoplasma etiology

Differential Diagnostics of *M pneumoniae* CAP

Legionella
- No ↑ cold agglutinins

- ↑ LFTs

- Relative bradycardia

C pneumoniae
- Little or no response to erythromycin

- Hoarseness

Presumptive Diagnosis

• CAP with:

  * Dry, nonproductive cough

  * Loose stools/diarrhea

  * Temp (<102 °F)

  * No relative bradycardia

  * ↑ Cold agglutinin titer >1:64

  * Normal LFTs

  * ↑ Early/↓ rapidly

Definitive Diagnosis

• ↑ IgM ELISA titer (↑ >1 week, ↓<1 year)

• Cultures of throat and respiratory secretions (growth 2-3 weeks)

• ↑IgG CF titer indicates past exposure and is *not* diagnostic of acute infection

• Cell-free media supplement with: horse serum; fresh yeast extract

• ≥4x↑ in IgG CF between acute and convalescent titers (4-8 weeks)

• PCR of nasopharyngeal secretions, sputum, bronchial washings for *M pneumoniae*

Therapy

• Doxycycline

• Quinolones

• Macrolides

Prognosis

• Good in normal hosts

Figure 2

Algorithm of suspected community-acquired pneumonia

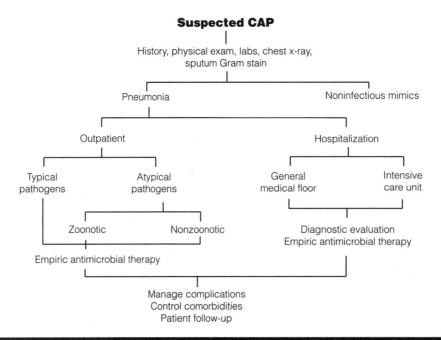

Table 1

Common Respiratory Pathogens in Community-acquired Pneumonia

Typical bacterial pathogens in community-acquired pneumonia (~85%)
   Streptococcus pneumoniae
      Penicillin-sensitive *S pneumoniae*
      Penicillin-resistant *S pneumoniae*
   Haemophilus influenzae
      Ampicillin-sensitive *H influenzae*
      Ampicillin-resistant *H influenzae*
   Moraxella catarrhalis
      All strains penicillin resistant
   Oral anaerobes (aspiration CAP)

Atypical respiratory pathogens in community-acquired pneumonia (~15%)
   Legionella
   Mycoplasma
   Chlamydia pneumoniae

Other bacterial pathogens in community-acquired pneumonia and nursing home-acquired pneumonia (NHAP)
   Klebsiella pneumoniae
      only in chronic alcoholics
   Staphylococcus aureus
      only in postviral influenza setting
   C pneumoniae only in NHAP outbreaks

• Dry cough persists despite early and adequate treatment

• Respiratory secretions contagious for duration of cough

ID Board Pearls

• May be severe in immunoglobulin deficiency/compromised hosts

• Post-*Mycoplasma* asthma

5. Chlamydophilia (Chlamydia) pneumoniae Pneumonia

Organism

• *C pneumoniae*

Microbiology

• Obligate *intracellular* Gram-negative coccobacillus

Epidemiology

• Increased incidence in fall and winter

• Highest incidence in young adults, but not uncommon in the elderly

• Cause of outbreaks in nursing homes (NHAP)

Geographic Distribution

• Worldwide

Clinical Presentation

• Resembles *Mycoplasma pneumoniae* but with *hoarseness*

• Less gastrointestinal complaints

• Cardiac or neurologic involvement

Laboratory Abnormalities

• Patchy infiltrates

• No ↑cold agglutinins

• No pleural effusion

• Normal LFTs

Definitive Diagnosis

• ↑IgM MIF titer (≥1:16)

• ↑IgM MIF titer (≥1:512)

• ↑≥4x in IgG MIF titer between acute and convalescent titers (4-8 weeks)

Table 2

Diagnostic Clues for Pneumonia from the History

Clues	Infectious causes	Noninfectious causes
Painful swelling of lower extremities (erythema nodosum)	Tuberculosis Coccidioidomycosis Histoplasmosis Blastomycosis	Sarcoidosis
Recent cough	Mycoplasma Influenza SARS Adenovirus Pertussis	Bronchogenic carcinoma Heart failure
Night sweats	Tuberculosis	Lymphoma
Abdominal pain	*Legionella*	ARDS-pancreatitis
Severe headache	Aspiration pneumonia (leads to lung or brain abscess) Q fever Psittacosis Plague AIDS (cryptococcosis, nocardiosis)	Metastatic carcinoma Lymphoma
Pleuritic chest pain	Influenza SARS *S pneumoniae* *H influenzae* *Legionella* Group A streptococci Psittacosis *H influenzae*	SLE Bronchogenic carcinoma
Chronic obstructive pulmonary disease	*H influenzae* *S pneumoniae* *M catarrhalis* *Legionella*	
Lymphoreticular malignancy	Cryptococcosis Nocardiosis	Radiation pneumonitis Drug reaction
Sarcoidosis	Tuberculosis	
Pulmonary alveolar proteinosis	Nocardiosis	
Diarrhea	*Legionella* *Mycoplasma*	
Rheumatoid arthritis		Rheumatoid nodules
Periodontal disease	Actinomycosis	
Diabetes mellitus	*S pneumoniae*	
Urinary tract infection	*Escherichia coli* *Klebsiella*	
Alcoholism	*S pneumoniae* *Klebsiella* Tuberculosis Aspiration pneumonia	

(continued)

Table 2 *(continued)*

Diagnostic Clues for Pneumonia from the History

Clues	Infectious causes	Noninfectious causes
Residence in chronic care facility	*H influenzae* *Klebsiella*	
Mental confusion	*Legionella* AIDS (cryptococcosis, nocardiosis) Miliary tuberculosis	Lymphoma Metastatic carcinoma Sarcoidosis
Altered consciousness or swallowing problems	Aspiration pneumonia	Bronchogenic carcinoma
Inactivated measles vaccination		Atypical measles
Tuberculosis contact	Miliary tuberculosis	
Herpes zoster or chickenpox contact	Varicella SARS	
Poultry contact	Psittacosis Histoplasmosis	
Bird contact	Psittacosis	
Animal contact	Plague Tularemia Q fever Anthrax	
Soil contact (gardening)	Sporotrichosis	
Recent construction or excavation contact	Legionnaires' disease Histoplasmosis Blastomycosis	
Coal contact (mining)	Tuberculosis	Silicosis
Foreign travel	Tuberculosis Atypical tuberculosis Coccidioidomycosis Q fever Melioidosis Paragonimiasis	

Seasonal occurrences
  Winter
  Fall
	SARS
	Influenza
	Legionella	

Sexual promiscuity	*Pneumocystis carinii* (AIDS)	
Blood transfusion	*P carinii* (AIDS)	
IV drug abuse	Septic pulmonary embolism *P carinii* (AIDS)	
Drug reaction		

From Cunha BA. Pneumonias acquired from others. 1. History, examination, laboratory findings.
Postgrad Med. *1987;82:126-128,130-132,134-140.*

Table 3

Diagnostic Clues for Pneumonia from the Physical Examination

Physical findings	Infectious causes	Noninfectious causes
Heart		
Relative bradycardia	*Legionella* Psittacosis Q fever	Drug reaction
S3 gallop or cardiomegaly	Influenza *Mycoplasma* Psittacosis	Heart failure
Skin		
Yellow or purple papules		Sarcoidosis
Butterfly rash		SLE
Severe seborrheic dermatitis	*Pneumocystis carinii* (AIDS)	
Vesicles	Varicella	
Urticaria	Atypical measles	
Folliculitis of lower legs	*P. carinii* (AIDS)	
Erythema multiforme (Stevens-Johnson syndrome)	*Mycoplasma*	Drug reaction
Erythema nodosum	Tuberculosis Histoplasmosis Coccidioidomycosis	Sarcoidosis
Facial macules (Horder's spots)	Psittacosis	
Ecthyma gangrenosum	*Pseudomonas aeruginosa* *Serratia*	
Ulcerative lymphangitis	Sporotrichosis	
Eschar	Tularemia	
Skin ulcer	Blastomycosis	
Eyes, ears, nose, throat Choroidal tubercles	Miliary tuberculosis	
Cotton-wool spots		SLE
Tongue ulcer	Disseminated histoplasmosis	
Sinusitis	*S pneumoniae* *H influenzae* Group A streptococci	Wegener's granulomatosis
Otitis or myringitis	*Mycoplasma*	
Herpes simplex	*S pneumoniae*	

(continued)

Table 3 *(continued)*

Diagnostic Clues for Pneumonia from the Physical Examination

Physical findings	Infectious causes	Noninfectious causes
Periodontal disease	Aspiration pneumonia	
Conjunctivitis	Adenovirus Pertussis Chlamydia	
Oral thrush	*P carinii* (AIDS)	
Pharyngitis	*Mycoplasma* Chlamydia Influenza SARS Adenovirus Group A streptococci	
Chest Sinus tracts	Tuberculosis Actinomycosis	Bronchogenic carcinoma
Abdomen Hepatosplenomegaly	Miliary tuberculosis Disseminated histoplasmosis Psittacosis Q fever	Lymphoma SLE
Genitourinary system Epididymo-orchitis	Tuberculosis Blastomycosis	Vasculitis Lymphoma
Extremities Phlebitis	Psittacosis	Bronchogenic carcinoma
Generalized adenopathy	Miliary tuberculosis Human immunodeficiency virus (AIDS) Group A streptococci	Lymphoma SLE
Proximal interphalangeal joint or subcutaneous nodules		Rheumatoid arthritis

AIDS, acquired immunodeficiency syndrome; SLE, systemic lupus erythematosus.
From Cunha BA. Pneumonias acquired from others. 1. History, examination, laboratory findings.
Postgrad Med. 1987;82:126-128,130-132,134-140.

Table 4

Diagnostic Clues for Pneumonia from Sputum

Clues	Infectious causes	Noninfectious causes
Foul smell	Oral anaerobes (aspiration)	
Creamy yellow or salmon color	Staphylococcus aureus	
Currant-jelly color	Pneumococcus *Klebsiella*	
Raspberry-syrup color	Pneumonic plague	
Red color (pseudohemoptysis)	*Serratia*	
Blood streaked (hemoptysis)	*Klebsiella* Influenza Meningococcus Pneumonic plague	Mitral stenosis Pulmonary embolism Chronic obstructive pulmonary disease (COPD) Bronchogenic carcinoma
No polymorphonuclear neutrophils	Q fever	
Eosinophils		Bronchopulmonary aspergillosis Drug reaction
Polymorphonuclear neutrophils	Bacterial pneumonia	
Mononuclear cells	*Legionella* *Mycoplasma*	
Mixed flora	Aspiration pneumonia	COPD

From Cunha BA. Pneumonias acquired from others. 1. History, examination, laboratory findings. Postgrad Med. *1987;82:126-128,130-132,134-140.*

Table 5

Diagnostic Clues for Pneumonia from Laboratory Testing

Clues	Infectious causes	Noninfectious causes
Leukopenia	Influenza SARS *Pneumocystis carinii* (AIDS) Miliary tuberculosis	Drug reaction SLE Carcinoma (bone marrow invasion)
Eosinophilia	Coccidioidomycosis *Chlamydia* Pulmonary migration of parasites	Lymphoma Drug reaction Pulmonary infiltrates with eosinophilia syndrome Atypical measles Sarcoidosis
Basophilia	*Varicella*	Lymphoma
Abnormal results on renal function tests	*Legionella* SARS	SLE Drug reactions Vasculitis
Abnormal results on liver function tests	*Legionella* Psittacosis Q fever	Drug reactions Lymphoma Metastatic carcinoma Sarcoidosis
Hypergammaglobulinemia	HIV	Sarcoidosis
Hypogammaglobulinemia	*H influenzae* *S pneumoniae* *H meningitidis*	

Organisms growing in blood
  culture medium
	Community-acquired
	  Streptococcus pneumoniae
	    (about 30%)
	  H influenzae (about 75%)
	  Klebsiella
	  Group A streptococci (about 15%)
	  Aspiration
	  Acinetobacter
	Nosocomial[a]
	  S pneumoniae
	  Escherichia coli
	  Pseudomonas aeruginosa	

AIDS, acquired immunodeficiency syndrome; SLE, systemic lupus erythematosus.
[a] Positive blood culture is rare with nosocomial pneumonia due to Proteus (Morganella), Providencia, Acinetobacter or Serratia.

From Cunha BA. Pneumonias acquired from others. 1. History, examination, laboratory findings. Postgrad Med. 1987;82:126-128, 130-132, 134-140.

Table 6

Diagnostic Clues to Community-Acquired Pneumonia Seen on Chest Film

Clues	Infectious causes	Noninfectious causes
Bulging-fissure sign	Klebsiella *S pneumoniae* *H influenzae* Plague	Bronchogenic carcinoma
Shaggy-heart sign	Pertussis	
Miliary pattern	Miliary tuberculosis Histoplasmosis Coccidioidomycosis	Sarcoidosis Eosinophilic granuloma Hypersensitivity pneumonitis Carcinoma with lymphangitic spread Lymphoma Alveolar cell carcinoma
Peripheral infiltrates	Actinomycosis Nocardiosis	Loeffler's syndrome Drug reaction Adenocarcinoma Large cell anaplastic carcinoma Adenocarcinoma Vasculitis SLE

Very rapidly progressing pulmonary infiltrates	Unilateral
	  Legionella
	  Aspiration
	Bilateral (asymmetric)
	  Legionella
	Bilateral (symmetric)
	  Hematogenous gram-negative pneumonia
	  Pneumocystis carinii
	  Massive aspiration
	  ARDS
	  Pneumonic plague
		Heart failure
		Noncardiac pulmonary edema

Perihilar infiltrates	Influenza SARS Measles *P carinii* *Varicella* Adenovirus *Chlamydia* Pertussis	Heart failure Pulmonary alveolar proteinosis Bronchogenic carcinoma Sarcoidosis Silicosis
Perihilar calcification	Tuberculosis Histoplasmosis	Silicosis

AIDS, acquired immunodeficiency syndrome; ARDS, adult respiratory distress syndrome;
SLE, systemic lupus erythematosus.
Reproduced with permission from Cunha BA. Pneumonias acquired from others. 2. Radiographic findings, treatment.
Postgrad Med. *1987;82:149-156.*

Table 7

Differential Diagnosis of Severe CAP with Shock

- In normal hosts, community-acquired bacterial pneumonia does not present with shock.

- If CAP presents with shock, look for a cardiopulmonary etiology or decreased splenic function.

- Disorders associated with impaired splenic function include:

hyposplenism of the elderly	congenital asplenia
chronic alcoholism	sickle cell trait or disease
amyloidosis	splenic infarcts
chronic active hepatitis	splenic malignancies
Fanconi's syndrome	systemic mastocytosis
IgA deficiency	rheumatoid arthritis
intestinal lymphangiectasia	systemic necrotizing vasculitis
myeloproliferative disorders	thyroiditis
Waldenström's macroglobulinemia	steroid therapy
non-Hodgkin's lymphoma	gamma globulin therapy
celiac disease	splenectomy
regional enteritis	ulcerative colitis
Sézary syndrome	

- If CAP presents with **shock in the absence of conditions associated with hyposplenism, look for mimics of pneumonia** that present with pulmonary infiltrates, fever, leukocytosis and hypotension, such as **acute myocardial infarction or acute pulmonary embolism.**

- If CAP presents with shock, and without evidence of hyposplenia, acute myocardial infarction or acute pulmonary embolism, then **consider an exacerbation of pre-existing cardiopulmonary disease** that may present with hypotension (eg, coronary insufficiency hypoxemia with emphysema)

- CAP severity is not related to microbial virulence factors or unusual Gram-negative organisms. **CAP, if severe, is related to the severity of pre-existing, pulmonary or splenic function of the host.**

From Cunha BA. Community-acquired pneumonia. Med Clin North Am. *2001;85:43-77.*

Table 8

Possible Causes of Cavitary Lesions Found on Chest Film

Infectious causes	Noninfectious causes
Thick-walled lesions	**Thick-walled lesions**
Staphylococcus aureus	Squamous cell
Klebsiella	carcinoma
Escherichia coli	Pulmonary infarction
Pseudomonas[a]	Silicosis
Tuberculosis	Wegener's
Histoplasmosis[b]	granulomatosis
Blastomycosis	Rheumatoid nodules
Aspergillus	Lymphoma[b]
Melioidosis	Sarcoidosis
Anaerobic lung abscess	Metastatic carcinoma
Septic pulmonary emboli	Metastatic sarcoma
Nocardiosis	
Thin-walled lesions	
Atypical tuberculosis	
Sporotrichosis	
Coccidioidomycosis	
Paragonimiasis	

[a] *Cavitation not a characteristic of Serratia pneumonia.*
[b] *May become thin-walled in advanced disease.*
From Cunha BA. Pneumonias acquired from others.
2. *Radiographic findings, treatment.* Postgrad Med. *1987; 82:149-156.*

Table 9

Possible Causes of Bilateral Hilar Adenopathy Found on Chest Film

Infectious causes	Noninfectious causes
Tularemia	Lymphoma (asymmetric)
Histoplasmosis	Sarcoidosis
Coccidioidomycosis	Silicosis
Anthrax[a]	Bronchogenic carcinoma
Mycoplasma	
Varicella	

[a] *Widened mediastinum also suggests tuberculosis, histoplasmosis, or mediastinitis.*
From Cunha BA. Pneumonias acquired from others.
[b] *Radiographic findings, treatment.* Postgrad Med. *1987;82:149-156.*

Table 10

**Possible Causes of Pleural Effusions[a]
Found on Chest Film**

Infectious causes	Noninfectious causes
None or very small	**Small to moderate**
Streptococcus pneumoniae	Primary tuberculosis
Mycoplasma	Pancreatitis
	Pulmonary infarct
	Meigs' syndrome
Moderate	Drugs
Haemophilus influenzae	Nitrofurantoin
Tularemia[b]	Methysergide
	Drug-induced SLE
Large	SLE
Group A streptococci[c]	Rheumatoid arthritis
	Cirrhosis or ascites[c]
	Congestive heart failure[c]
	Nephrosis or hypoalbuminemia[c]
	Large
	Malignancy[d]

SLE, systemic lupus erythematosus
[a] *Empyema caused by Staphylococcus aureus, anaerobic lung abscess, Escherichia coli, Klebsiella.*
[b] *Bloody pleural effusion is characteristic*
[c] *Serosanguineous pleural effusion is characteristic*
[d] *Pleural fluid is a transudate*
[e] *Trachea is not deviated to opposite side in malignant pleural effusion. (Bilateral pleural effusions are almost never infectious in origin.)*
*From Cunha BA. Pneumonias acquired from others.
2. Radiographic findings, treatment.* Postgrad Med. *1987;82:149-156.*

- Culture from oropharynx (HL, Hep-2, BCMK cell lines)

- PCR of peripheral mononuclear WBCs for *C pneumoniae*

Therapy

- Doxycycline

- Telithromycin

- Quinolones

- Macrolides (except erythromycin)

Complications

Asthma
- May trigger asthma attacks in children

- May cause new-onset asthma in adults

Coronary Artery Disease (CAD)
- May be implicated in acute coronary syndromes

- May be a factor in atherosclerosis or CAD

Prognosis
- Good in normal hosts

- May be severe in compromised hosts

ID Board Pearls

- Mycoplasma, like CAP with hoarseness, is *C pneumoniae* CAP until proven otherwise

- LFTs normal in Mycoplasma and *C pneumoniae*

6. Legionella Pneumonia

Organism

- *Legionella* species

- 42 species

- *Legionella pneumophila* (serogroup 01) most common

- 64 serogroups

Microbiology

- Intracellular Gram-negative coccobacillus

Epidemiology

- Increased incidence in fall and winter

- Highest incidence in elderly

- Nosocomial *Legionella* from contaminated water (showers)

- Nosocomial *Legionella* from TEE probes

- Nosocomial *Legionella* from aerosolized water/soil exposure related to new facility construction

- Community-acquired *Legionella* from fresh water/flower exposure

- Hot tub exposure

Geographic Distribution

- Worldwide

Clinical Presentation

- Fever (≥102° F) with relative bradycardia

- Myalgias

Neurologic
- Mental confusion

- Headache

Table 11

Possible Causes of Pulmonary Nodules Found on Chest Film

Legionella micdadei[a]
Melioidosis
Coccidioidomycosis[b]
Paragonimiasis[a]
Histoplasmosis
Adenovirus
Rheumatoid nodules
Metastatic carcinoma
Wegener's granulomatosis
Bronchogenic carcinoma

[a] *Usually lower lobe*
[b] *Usually upper lobe*
*From Cunha BA. Pneumonias acquired from others.
2. Radiographic findings, treatment. Postgrad Med. 1987;
82:149-156.*

- Encephalopathy

Pulmonary
- *Rapidly* progressive *asymmetric* infiltrates characteristic

- Cavitation (rare)

- Pleural effusions (common)

- Consolidation (common)

Cardiac
- Myocarditis

- Endocarditis (rare)

Gastrointestinal
- Loose stools/*watery diarrhea*

- May have *abdominal pain mimicking an acute abdomen*

Laboratory Abnormalities
• No ↑ cold agglutinins

• ↓ PO$_4$

• ↑ WBC

• ↓ CPK

• ↑ ESR, mildly

• ↑ ESR/CRP

• ↑ LFTs (early/transient)

• ↑ high ferritin levels

Differential Diagnosis

Mycoplasma
• Protracted non-dry cough

• No ↑ LFTs

• No relative bradycardia

• Cold agglutinins (>1:64)

Chlamydia pneumoniae
• No hoarseness

• No ↑ LFTs

• No relative bradycardia

• No ↑ cold agglutinins

Diagnosis

Presumptive
• CAP with *L pneumophila* (serogroup 1) most common (~ 80%) species and serogroup

• Relative bradycardia

• No ↑ cold agglutinins

• LFTs

• Hypophosphatemia

Definitive

• DFA

• ↑ IgM IFA titers

• Positive early in respiratory secretions

• ↑ IgG IFA (≥1:512)

• Sputum DFA rapidly becomes negative

• ≥4x↑ IgG IFA between acute

• *Legionella* urinary antigen

• Convalescent titers with antibiotic therapy (≤24 hours for 4-8 weeks)

ID Board Pearls

• Useful only for *L pneumophila (serotype 01)*

• L-cysteine

• *Initially may be negative* early in infection, but when positive, *persists for weeks after infection*

• Intracellular growth in amoeba

• Cultures of lung/pleural fluid/respiratory secretions

• Extracellular growth requires:

   * Iron

   * CYE (charcoal yeast extract agar) contains both iron and L-cysteine

Antibiotic Therapy

• Doxycycline

• Quinolones

• Macrolides

Complications

• Culture-negative PVE

Prognosis

• Good in normal hosts

• Poor in compromised hosts

• Poor in those with severe cardiopulmonary disease

7. Tularemia Pneumonia

Organism

• *Francisella tularensis*

Microbiology

• *Pleomorphic Gram-negative coccobacilli*

• *Aerobic, Gram-stains poorly*

• Nonmotile

• Requires special media with cysteine

Zoonotic Vector

Nontick-borne Tularemia
• *Deer or rabbit*

• Mosquito bites

• *Deerfly bites*

Tick-borne Tularemia
• Tick bites

Geographic Distribution
• Worldwide

Clinical Presentation
• Extremely *rapid onset*

Clinical Manifestations
• Ulceroglandular tularemia (70%)

• Oropharyngeal tularemia

• Glandular tularemia (10%)

• Gastrointestinal tularemia

• Oculoglandular tularemia

• Typhoidal tularemia (10%)

ID Board Pearls

• Pulmonary tularemia (*may complicate* any of the above 6 clinical varieties)

Differential Diagnosis

Pulmonary Tularemia
Clinical presentation
• Bilateral/unilateral *hilar adenopathy* (BHA)

• *Bloody* pleural effusion

Differential diagnosis
• Q Fever

• *Legionella*

• Plague

• Anthrax

Diagnosis

Presumptive
• Recent/close vector contact history

• WBC normal or slightly ↓

• Normal LFTs

Definitive
• Serology

• TA

• HI

• ELISA

Biohazard
• *Do not send specimen to lab without calling to notify laboratory of biohazard*

ID Board Pearls

• Tularemia serology *cross-reacts with Brucella*

• The only cause of CAP with hilar adenopathy/pleural effusion

Therapy

• Streptomycin

• Doxycycline

• Gentamicin

• Chloramphenicol

• Quinolones

Prognosis

• Good with prompt and appropriate antibiotic treatment

8. Psittacosis Pneumonia

Organism

- *Chlamydophilia (chlamydia) psittaci*

Microbiology

- Obligate *intracellular* coccobacillary organism

Zoonotic Vector

- *Psittacine* birds

Geographic Distribution

- Worldwide

Clinical Presentation

- Zoonotic CAP with:

    * Horder's spot

    * ± Relative bradycardia

    * Severe headache/myalgias

    * ↑ LFTs

    * Blood-streaked sputum

    * ± Splenomegaly

Complications

- *Epistaxis*

- Culture-negative endocarditis (SBE)

- *Obscure phlebitis*

Differential Diagnosis

- Tularemia

- *Legionella*

- Q fever

Presumptive Diagnosis

- CAP with extrapulmonary findings

- Rash (Horder's spots) on face

- **psittacine** bird contact

- ↑ LFTs

Definitive
- ↑ IgM IFA titers (1 month)

- ↑ IgG IFA titers positive (6 months)

Therapy
- Doxycycline

- Quinolones

ID Board Pearls

- Dense infiltrates may mimic typical/bacterial CAP

- In the DDx of CAP with relative bradycardia/splenomegaly, consider psittacosis

- *Erythromycin often fails*

Prognosis
- Good if treated early

9. Q Fever Pneumonia

Organism

- *Coxiella burnetii*

Microbiology

- *Obligate intracellular* (rickettsia-like) Gram-negative coccobacillus

Zoonotic Vector

- *Parturient cats, sheep*, cattle

- Airborne transmission to humans

Geographic Distribution

- Worldwide

Clinical Presentation

- *Dense infiltrates resembles typical CAP*

- Thrombocytosis

- ± Relative bradycardia

- ↑ anti-smooth muscle antibody titers (20%)

Complications

- Culture-negative SBE

- *Large-vessel emboli*

- Chronic SBE

Differential Diagnosis

- *Legionella*

- Tularemic pneumonia

- Psittacosis

Diagnosis

Presumptive
- CAP contact with extrapulmonary findings and recent/close contact with cats, cattle, sheep

- Relative bradycardia

- Splenomegaly

- Mildly ↑ LFTs

Definitive
- ≥4 x ↑ between acute and convalescent IgG, CF, IFA, ELISA titers

Biohazard
- *Do not try to isolate*

Therapy

- Doxycycline

- Quinolones

- Chloramphenicol

ID Board Pearls

- Splenomegaly with CAP should suggest Q fever > psittacosis

- Mildly ↑ LFTs

- May present as FUO/SBE

Prognosis

- Good *except for chronic Q fever SBE*

10. Antibiotic Therapy of CAP

General Concepts

• Empiric therapy of CAP is based on providing *coverage against the most likely typical and atypical CAP pathogens* responsible for CAP.

• *Most* antibiotics with anti-*Legionella* spectrum are also effective against *M pneumoniae* and *C pneumoniae*.

• Because the *zoonotic* atypical pathogens causing tularemia, psittacosis, and Q fever are *geographically limited or require specific* vector contact, routine empiric coverage need *not* include activity against these organisms.

ID Board Pearls

• Aspiration pneumonia presenting as CAP does *not require special therapeutic consideration.*

• *All anaerobes above the waist are sensitive to penicillin, β -lactams and all antibiotics that would be used to treat respiratory tract infections* (ie, *no need* to add anaerobic coverage for aspiration CAP).

11. Nursing Home-Acquired Pneumonias (NHAP)

General Concepts

• Nursing home patients are predisposed to NHAP because of the high frequency of strokes/swallowing disorders in the elderly in chronic care facilities.

12. Mimics of NHAP

- Most nursing home patients admitted to acute care facilities have pre-existing lung disease, AECB, pulmonary emboli, CHF, MI, pulmonary hemorrhage or pulmonary drug reactions.

- NHAP more closely resembles CAP than HAP in pathogen distribution (*P aeruginosa* is extremely rare in CAP and NHAP, but important in HAP) and length of stay (LOS). (LOS: CAP = 7 days, NHAP = 7 days, HAP = 14 days).

ID Board Pearls

- NHAP may occur sporadically

- Nursing home outbreaks are most often due to Legionella, *C pneumoniae* or influenza.

13. Overview of Nosocomial Pneumonia (NP)

- Many factors *predispose* to acquiring bacterial pneumonia in the hospital, but the primary factors are *aspiration* and *intubation*.

- The underlying *status of the cardiopulmonary system* is an *important determinant of severity* and prognosis in NP.

- Many patients who develop NP are elderly, secondary to aspiration, prolonged intubation and impaired cardiopulmonary function.

14. Non-Nosocomial Pneumonia Pathogens

General Concepts

• Such *aerobic nonfermentative GNBs organisms rapidly colonize the patient's respiratory secretions* in the hospital.

• Aerobic GNB that are *common colonizers* of respiratory secretions include:

  * *Enterobacter*

  * *Flavobacterium*

  * *Citrobacter*

ID Board Pearls

• Non-aeruginosa pseudomonads (ie, *Burkholderia [Pseudomonas] cepacia* and *Stenotrophomonas [Pseudomonas] maltophilia) Burkholderia* and *Stenotrophomonas* are potentially pathogenic only for patients with chronic IDP *bronchiectasis* or *cystic fibrosis*.

• Anaerobic organisms aspirated along with the aerobic bacillary flora in hospitalized patients have been shown to be *insignificant* as a cause of nosocomial pneumonias.

15. NP Mimics of Nosocomial Pneumonia

• The disorders *most likely to resemble* nosocomial pneumonia on chest radiograph include:

  * Interstitial lung disease

  * Pulmonary hemorrhage

  * Primary or metastatic lung carcinomas

  * Collagen vascular disease affecting the lungs

  * Pulmonary emboli or infarction

  * Acute respiratory distress syndrome

  * Pulmonary drug reactions

  * Congestive heart failure

16. Nosocomial Pneumonia

• Presumptive diagnosis of NP may be defined as a pulmonary *infiltrate occurring in a patient who has been hospitalized for 1 week or more that is compatible in appearance with a bacterial pneumonia.*

• Fever and leukocytosis, with or without a left shift, are *not diagnostic* of nosocomial pneumonia, and are nonspecific and seen in a variety of noninfectious disorders.

• Infiltrates on CXR are not diagnostic of nosocomial pneumonia *even* with fever and leukocytosis.

• It is important to *rule out* other conditions that may mimic nosocomial pneumonia that *present* with *pulmonary infiltrates, with or without fever* or *leukocytosis.*

17. Necrotizing Nosocomial Pneumonia

• Necrotizing pneumonia with rapid cavitation within 72 hours is the hallmark of *S aureus* or *Pseudomonas aeruginosa* pneumonias.

• Aside from CXR/CT appearance, the next best indirect way to make the diagnosis of necrotizing pneumonia is by demonstrating *elastin fibers* in respiratory tract secretion specimens (KOH stained).

• *Klebsiella pneumoniae also* caus a *necrotizing* pneumonia. The *cavitation* occurs 3-5 days after onset.

• The difference in *cavitation rates* is a diagnostic clue to the presence of *K pneumoniae* vs. *S aureus* or *P aeruginosa*, *if* microbiologic data are *not* available.

ID Board Pearls

• *P aeruginosa commonly colonizes* the secretions of the respiratory tract and *infrequently causes nosocomial pneumonia.*

• The frequency of *P aeruginosa* as a causative pathogen in hospital-acquired pneumonia is probably *overestimated.*

• *P aeruginosa* adheres to respiratory tract cells more avidly than other aerobic Gram-negative bacilli. Although *P aeruginosa* is *not* the *most common* cause of nosocomial pneumonia, it *is the most virulent* pulmonary pathogen and *coverage should be directed primarily against P aeruginosa.*

18. Outbreaks of Nosocomial Pneumonia

General Concepts

• *Acinetobacter* almost always is an intermittent *colonizer* in ICUs and may cause outbreaks or clusters of NP.

ID Board Pearls

• *Acinetobacter outbreaks* are associated with *contaminated respiratory support equipment*.

• *Acinetobacter* may be transferred from patient to patient from *contaminated respiratory secretions* on the hands of medical personnel. *Acinetobacter* recovered from specimens of respiratory secretions *usually* represents colonization. *Acinetobacter pneumonia* outbreaks are *uncommon*.

• *Legionella NP usually occurs in outbreaks and the source of Legionella is usually Legionella-contaminated water.*

• *Legionella* in *hospital outbreaks* has been cultured from a variety of locations, including ice cubes and showerheads.

19. Antibiotic Therapy of Nosocomial Pneumonia

General Concepts

• Combination therapy has been the approach for many years.

• In terms of outcome, empiric combination regimens are no better than monotherapy regimens.

• Combination therapy evolved because of the lack of activity of single agents in the past against *Klebsiella* or *P aeruginosa*.

• Newer potent antibiotics (ie, third-generation cephalosporins, fluoroquinolones, carbapenems) are available that have anti-*Klebsiella* and anti-*P aeruginosa* activity, permitting effective monotherapy.

• Proven *P aeruginosa* in hospital-acquired pneumonia is usually treated with double-drug therapy.

Persistent Fever, Leukocytes and Pulmonary Infiltrates

General Concepts

• If there has been *no change in the pulmonary infiltrates*, despite persistent low-grade fevers and leukocytosis for *2 weeks*, the patient has a nonantibiotic responsive process caused by a *virus* or a *noninfectious disease entity*.

• Such patients should have a *diagnostic procedure* (ie, transbronchial biopsy, percutaneous needle biopsy or open lung biopsy) *to determine the cause of the persistent pulmonary infiltrates*.

• Patients should *not* receive *prolonged* courses of empiric antimicrobial therapy or undergo *changes* in antibiotic therapy.

• Patients who have shown improvement initially in pulmonary infiltrates but become failure-to-wean problems require a different approach.

20. Further Reading

ID Board Pearls

• HSV-1 pneumonitis is a common problem in the ICU, in *failure-to-wean patients* with few or no infiltrates on the CXR.

• *If* HSV-1 is shown in the secretions and a failure-to-wean intubated patient occurs, a 10-day course of acyclovir is indicated.

Cunha BA. *Pneumonia Essentials*. 3rd ed. Sudbury, MA: Jones & Bartlett; 2009.

Gorbach SL, Bartlett JG, Blacklow N, eds. Infectious Diseases. 3rd ed. Philadelphia, PA: Lippincott Williams & Wilkins; 2004.

Jarvis WR, ed. *Nosocomial Pneumonia*. New York, NY: Marcel Dekker; 2000.

Karetzky M, Cunha BA, Brandstetter RD, eds. *The Pneumonias*. New York, NY: Springer-Verlag; 1993.

Levison ME, ed. *The Pneumonias*. Boston, MA: John Wright-PSG, Inc; 1984.

Mandell GL, Bennet JE, Dolin R. *Mandell, Douglas, and Bennett's Principles and Practice of Infectious Diseases*. 6th ed. New York, NY: Elsevier; 2005.

Marrie TJ, ed. *Community-Acquired Pneumonia*. New York, NY: Kluwer Academic/Plenum Publishers; 2001.

Pennington JE. *Respiratory Infections: Diagnosis and Management*. 2nd ed. New York, NY: Raven Press; 1994.

Chapter 17:
Chronic Pneumonias for the ID Boards

Stephen M. Smith, MD
Leon G. Smith, MD

Contents

1. Overview

Chronic pneumonia is loosely defined as the presence of lung infiltrates with pulmonary symptoms for a period of more than a few weeks. Many infectious and noninfectious etiologies cause syndromes which meet this definition. In the evaluation of a patient with chronic pneumonia, epidemiologic and host factors are extremely important. Table 1 lists the infectious etiologies of chronic pneumonia. In the U.S., the most common cause is *Mycobacterium tuberculosis*. Non-tuberculosis mycobacteria (NTM), especially *M avium* complex (MAI), *M kansasii* and *M abscessus* also cause chronic pneumonia. Fungal infections are the next most common. The endemic mycoses, histoplasmosis, blastomycosis and coccidioidomycosis, can and often do present as chronic pneumonia. Less frequently, *Cryptococcus neoformans*, *Sporothrix schenkii* and *Paracoccidioides brasilensis* cause chronic pneumonia. Bacterial causes are few. Both *Nocardia* spp. and *Actinomyces* spp. can cause chronic *pneumonia*. Melioidosis, caused by *Burkholderia pseudomallei*, can be seen in immigrants from southeast Asia. Lung abscess, which causes fairly unique changes on chest x-ray, is caused by mixed, oral flora.

Table 1

Infectious Causes of Chronic Pneumonia

Mycobacterial
M tuberculosis
M avium-intracellulare
M kansasii
M abscessus
M chelonae
M fortuitum

Fungal
Histoplasma capsulatum var. capsulatum
Coccidioides spp.
Blastomyces dermatitidis
Sporothrix shenckii
Cryptococcus neoformans
Paracoccidioides brasilensis

Bacterial
Actinomyces spp.
Nocardia spp.
Burkholderia pseudomallei
Oral flora

2. Tuberculosis

One third of the world's population is infected with M tuberculosis, the causative agent of tuberculosis (TB). M tuberculosis is the most frequent cause of chronic pneumonia. In 2007, over 13,000 were reported in the U.S. 58% of these cases occurred in foreign-born persons. Additionally, rates of infection are higher in non-white Americans, with Asians having the highest rate. TB is associated with alcoholism, intravenous drug use, poverty and incarceration. HIV infection, of course, greatly increases the likelihood that a person will develop clinical, active tuberculosis. TB can affect any organ, but usually presents with pulmonary disease. Most cases of pulmonary TB represent re-activation of latent infection, while some are primary infections. Symptoms are non-specific. Fever, weight loss, night sweats and cough are common. Physical examination is usually unrevealing. Lab studies may show a mild anemia and neutrophilia with a white blood cell count ~15,000 cells/mm^3. Occasionally, hyponatremia and hypercalcemia are found. Chest radiographs show a patchy infiltrate in the apical or subapical posterior areas. Cavitation is common.

The diagnosis is made by examination sputum specimens. Historically, 3 sputum samples on successive days were sent for acid-fast staining. This approach has a sensitivity of 45%-80%. The sputum samples are cultured for M tuberculosis, but cultures become positive only after 1-4 weeks. Recently, the Centers for Disease Control (CDC) has revised its recommendations for the use of nucleic acid amplification testing (NAA) in the diagnosis of TB. Formerly, NAA testing was recommended only for smear positive sputum samples. In this setting, NAA testing is used to determine if the bacilli observed on the smear are M tuberculosis or NTM. The CDC now recommends that "NAA testing should be performed on at least one respiratory specimen from each patient with signs and symptoms of pulmonary TB for whom a diagnosis of TB is being considered but has not yet been established." This approach will hopefully reduce the delay in diagnosis in smear negative TB cases. Culture is still required to confirm NAA(+), smear(-) cases and to determine the antimicrobial sensitivities of the isolate. Fortunately, the rates of TB and the percentage of multi-drug resistant cases (resistance to isoniazid and rifampin) both decreased from 1993 to 2007. Extensively drug resistant TB,

3. Mycobacterium avium intracellulare (MAI)

XDR TB, is defined as resistance to isoniazid, rifampin, a fluoroquinolone and any injectable second-line drug (ie, amikacin, kanamycin and capreomycin). XDR TB is seen rarely in the U.S.; only 17 total cases occurred from 2000-2006. Treatment for TB is beyond the scope of this review.

MAI includes *M avium* and *M intracellulare*. Both organisms are found in water and soil and also in animals. MAI is found more frequently in the southeastern U.S. Skin testing with MAI antigens of army recruits showed a positive rate of 10% in those from the North and West, but >70% in those from the Southeast. MAI frequently colonizes hosts with structural lung disease, such as chronic obstructive pulmonary disease, bronchiectasis, cystic fibrosis and pneumoconiosis. The importance of MAI in worsening symptoms in patients with underlying lung disease is not fully understood. MAI is being found increasingly as a cause of chronic pneumonia in elderly, Caucasian females who do not have underlying lung pathology. MAI typically causes disseminated disease in AIDS patients, but can cause chronic pneumonia.

In middle aged men with pre-existing lung disease, MAI can cause upper lobe fibrocavitary disease. Most patients have a long history of tobacco use and heavy ethanol intake. Patients present with weight loss and fatigue and, rarely, with fever and night sweats. Radiographs typically show thin walled cavities that are often bilateral. Pleural effusions are not common. This infection is not contagious. This disease is progressive and can result in respiratory failure in over 10% of patients within 2 years. In thin, elderly Caucasian women with no history of smoking, MAI can cause reticular nodular infiltrates, which involve the lingula and the right middle lobe. Bronchiectasis often develops. This form of MAI infection has been referred to as "Lady Windermere syndrome." High resolution CT scans reveals multiple, small peripheral nodules. The disease progresses more slowly, but does cause respiratory failure. The diagnosis is made clinically and confirmed by sputum culture. Unlike TB, a positive culture alone is not sufficient to establish the diagnosis.

Treatment is recommended for both forms of MAI pulmonary infection. Clarithromycin has excellent activity against MAI isolates. Monotherapy can lead to high level macrolide resistance. Consequently, rifampin and ethambutol are given with clarithromycin. For severe cases, amikacin or streptomycin is added for the first 2-3 months. For women with mild nodular disease, rifampin, ethambutol and clarithromycin can be given 3 times per week, as opposed to daily. The goal of therapy is sputum culture reversion. Sputum cultures should be performed monthly. Patients typically show clinical improvement within 3 months. Sputum cultures are usually negative after the first 12 months of therapy. Once the sputum culture is negative, therapy should be continued for another 12 months. Each patient must be closely monitored for adherence and the development of adverse effects. Clarithromycin causes significant gastrointestinal side effects in many patients. Monthly eye exams are necessary to detect ethambutol ocular toxicity. Rifampin's potential side effects include hepatitis, flu-like syndrome, rash and thrombocytopenia.

4. M kansasii

M kansasii is the second most frequent NTM infection. M kansasii can be found in tap water. The most common form of infection is pneumonia. Most patients have pre-existing lung disease, such as COPD or bronchiectasis. The clinical presentation of M kansasii infection is indistinguishable from pulmonary TB. Radiographically, *M kansasii* pneumonia and TB are also very similar. Nodular disease as seen with MAI infection has recently been reported. The diagnosis of *M kansasii* currently rests on isolation from sputum. Nucleic acid testing is not yet available. The recommended treatment regimen for *M kansasii* is isoniazid, rifampin and ethambutol. Pyrazinamide should not be used, as *M kansasii* is usually resistant to this drug. Treatment is continued for at least 18 months, with at least 12 months after sputum culture reversion. As above with MAI treatment, patients being treated for *M kansasii* need to be closely monitored and sputum cultures repeated monthly.

5. M abscessus

M.abscessus is another NTM, which can be isolated from patients with underlying lung disease. *M abscessus* is isolated in approximately 10% of patients with sputum cultures positive for MAI. It is unclear if *M abscessus* plays a role in pathogenesis in these co-infections. *M abscessus* can also be isolated from patients with nodular, bronchiectatic disease. In this setting, *M abscessus* probably is pathogenic, albeit progression is very slow. Diagnosis of *M abscessus* rests on sputum culture. Treatment for *M abscessus* lung infection is not well defined. While skin infections with *M abscessus* respond to combination therapy of clarithromycin and other agents, regimens studied to date rarely result in sputum culture reversion. In rare cases, surgical therapy for localized disease may be appropriate.

ID Board Pearls

• Most cases of tuberculosis in the U.S. occur in foreign born persons.

• XDR tuberculosis is very rare in the U.S.

• NAA testing of sputum samples is now recommended on any patient with a likelihood of tuberculosis, and no longer smear positive patients only.

• In elderly Caucasian women with no history of smoking, MAI can cause reticular nodular infiltrates, which involve the lingula and the right middle lobe. This is called "Lady Windermere Syndrome."

• *M kansasii* is resistant to pyrazinamide.

• *M abscessus* is isolated in approximately 10% of patients with sputum cultures positive for MAI.

6. *Histoplasma capsulatum*

Histoplasma capsulatum var. *capsulatum* is found in the Ohio and Mississippi River valleys. This fungus grows well in excrement from birds and bats, and is found in soil rich in nitrogen. Most people from these areas are infected with this organism, as determined by skin testing with histoplasmin antigen. Histoplasmosis encompasses several types of infection, including primary pneumonitis, fibrosing mediastinitis, progressive disseminated histoplasmosis, ocular histoplasmosis and chronic pulmonary histoplasmosis (CPH). In immunocompetent hosts, primary infection is well tolerated and self-limited. In rare cases, primary infection or infection from reactivation can result in serious pneumonia, referred to as acute pulmonary histoplasmosis. This disease typically resolves without therapy, although in severe cases itraconazole (200 mg daily) for 6 weeks has been used.

CPH is a form of chronic pneumonia. As with other forms of histoplasmosis, there is a male predominance. Patients are typically men, older than 50 with pre-existing COPD. The clinical presentation and radiographic findings are very similar to those of pulmonary TB. Patients experience weight loss, fatigue, cough, shortness of breath and fever. Some develop hemoptysis. Chest x-rays show patchy infiltrates and upper lobe cavitary disease. The diagnosis is usually made by sputum culture. Cultures usually take 3 weeks before becoming positive. The histoplasma antigen assay tests for the cell wall polysaccharide and can used on urine and serum. The assay has decreased sensitivity (~ 40%) in CPH compared with disseminated disease. Histopathology can be helpful and the findings can be strongly suggestive of histoplasmosis. Other organisms share histoplasma's morphology. Treatment for CPH is recommended by most experts, although some cases appear to resolve without therapy. Severely ill patients should first receive induction therapy with amphotericin B (0.7 mg/kg/d) for 2 weeks and follow with itraconazole therapy (200-400 mg daily) for 12-24 months. Moderate-mild cases can be treated with itraconazole alone.

Progressive disseminated histoplasmosis (PDH) is usually seen in immunocompromised hosts, such as AIDS patients (see below). Occasionally, patients with no clear immunologic deficiency develop PDH. This disease is systemic and presents with fever, malaise and weight loss. Hepatosplenomegaly and oropharyngeal ulcers are common. Patients with PDH frequently (2/3 of cases) have infiltrates on chest radiograph. The infiltrates can be diffuse interstitial or reticulonodular. While the adrenal gland is often infected by yeast in PDH, adrenal insufficiency is rare. The urine histoplasma antigen assay is useful in establishing this diagnosis, but may be negative in some cases. The organism can be grown from blood, bone marrow, sputum and mucosal ulcer biopsies. Bone marrow cultures are positive in ~50% of cases. The recommended treatment of PDH in non-AIDS or non-immunosuppressed patients is itraconazole (400 mg daily) for at least 6 months.

7. Blastomycosis

Blastomyces dermatitidis is a dimorphic fungus and is seen in certain states, such as Kentucky, North Carolina, South Carolina, Mississippi, Wisconsin and Illinois. Infection occurs after inhalation of the canidia of the mold form. The conidia convert into the yeast form, which replicate by budding, within the lung. Primary pulmonary infection is most often asymptomatic. Chronic infection is felt to occur after reactivation of latent infection. Patients present with typical complaints of chronic pneumonia-fever, weight loss, cough and chills. Chest radiographs may show mass-like infiltrates, which can be confused with bronchogenic carcinoma, or nodular lesions with or without cavity formation. Most patients with pulmonary disease have extrapulmonary manifestations. Skin involvement is frequently seen with pulmonary disease, although skin infection may occur alone. Bone and the genitourinary system (especially the prostate gland) are often infected as well. CNS is infrequently involved. The diagnosis is usually made by sputum inspection. Respiratory secretions can be examined by wet mount or after being treated with potassium hydroxide or calcofluor white. In the appropriate setting, the morphology of the budding yeast is enough to establish the diagnosis and the sensitivity sputum examination is 50%-90%. Sputum cultures are almost always positive, but require several weeks incubation. Itraconazole (200 mg BID) is the recommended therapy for mild to moderate disease. For severe infection, amphotericin B (0.7 mg/kg/d) or liposomal amphotericin (3-5 mg/kg/d) for 1-2 weeks is recommended as induction therapy, followed by itraconazole therapy. After 2 weeks of therapy, patients should be tested to ensure appropriate absorption of itraconazole. The serum level of itraconazole should be greater than 1 µg/ml. The recommended duration of therapy is 6-12 months. Relapses after completion of therapy are rare.

8. Coccidiomycosis

Coccidioides spp. are endemic in the southwestern U.S., including Arizona, New Mexico, west Texas and central California. *Coccidioides immitis* and *Coccidioides posadasii* are the 2 species which infect humans. These fungi are dimorphic and exist as a mycelium or a spherule. The latter structure is unique. Primary infection occurs after inhalation of athroconidia forms of the fungus. Arthroconidia forms are easily aerosolized by small disturbances. Consequently, the prevalence in hyperendemic areas, such as the San Joaquin Valley in California, exceeds 50%. In the lung, arthroconidia transform into spherules, which rupture and release endospores, which in turn form more spherules. Patients then develop acute pneumonia with fever, shortness of breath and cough. Most primary cases present similarly to other causes of acute pneumonia and the chest radiographs show lobar infiltrates, often with pleural effusions. Extrapulmonary manifestations are common. 3 skin rashes, including erythema nodosum, erythema multiforme and maculopapular eruption, occur frequently. Also, many patients develop polyarthralgias and polyarthritis. Most cases resolve without therapy. AIDS patients may develop a severe, bilateral pneumonitis with diffuse reticulonodular infiltrates. Lung nodules and cavities are common and asymptomatic. Most cavities close within a few years. Lung nodules are often confused with malignancy, but are not clinically significant otherwise.

Chronic pulmonary coccidioidomycosis develops in ~5%. This form of chronic pneumonia is indolent and characterized by cavities, fibrosis and surrounding infiltrates involving 1 lobe. Fever is uncommon and the pulmonary findings may wax and wane over a period of years. The diagnosis of chronic pulmonary coccidioidomycosis can be made by direct examination of the sputum for the presence of spherules. The addition of potassium hydroxide may improve detection of the spherules. While *Coccidioides* spp. grow well on many types of media, the spherules during the process revert to mycelia, which easily shed the arthroconidia. The cultured mold is extremely contagious. Therefore, cultures should not be sent from patients suspected of having coocidioidomycosis, since these cultures endanger laboratory workers. Therapy with either fluconazole (400-800 mg/d) or itraconazole (200 mg BID) for one year is recommended. Unlike disseminated histoplasmosis, disseminated coccidioidomycosis usually occurs in the absence of pulmonary disease. People at risk for disseminated disease include pregnant women and those of Filipino or African American descent.

9. Sporotrichosis

Sporothrix shenckii is another dimorphic fungus which can cause chronic pneumonia. The most common form of sporotrichosis is cutaneous disease, which occurs after the mold is inoculated into the subcutaneous tissues. Rarely, *S shenckii* causes pneumonia. Patients typically have underlying lung disease and a history of ethanol abuse. The organism enters the lungs via inhalation. Patients present with fever, productive cough, malaise and weight loss. Radiographs reveal nodular and cavitary disease. The diagnosis is made by culture of the fungus from sputum or bronchoalveolar lavage. There are little data on treatment and response rates are low (~30%). Experts recommend amphotericin B therapy (1-2 gm total) or itraconazole (200 mg BID) for several months. Adjunctive surgical resection may be helpful in selected cases.

ID Board Pearls

• The urine histoplasma antigen assay has relatively low sensitivity (40%) in chronic pulmonary histoplasmosis, but a high sensitivity in disseminated disease.

• Most patients with disseminated histoplasmosis have lung infiltrates.

• The diagnosis of pulmonary blastomycosis is usually made by sputum inspection.

• In coccidioidomycosis, extra-pulmonary manifestations are common. 3 skin rashes, including erythema nodosum, erythema multiforme and maculopapular eruption, occur frequently.

• Groups at risk for disseminated coccidioidomycosis include people of Filipino or African American descent and pregnant women.

• Sputum cultures should not be sent from patients suspected of having coccidioidomycosis, since these cultures endanger laboratory workers.

10. Nocardiosis

Nocardia spp. are filamentous Gram-positive rods. These aerobic organisms are ubiquitous and found in water and soil. Over 30 species exist, of which only handful are responsible for the vast majority of human infections. *Nocardia asteroides* complex, *N brasiliensis*, *N farcinica*, *N nova*, *N ititidiscavirarum* and *N transvalensis* are the species most often seen in humans. *Nocardia asteroides* complex causes pneumonia in most cases (85%), while other species tend to cause skin disease. Most commonly, *Nocardia* infects immunocompromised hosts, such as solid organ transplant recipients and patients with hematologic malignancies. Nocardiosis is occasionally seen in AIDS patients. Long-term corticosteroid use also predisposes patients to nocardiosis. Most patients with *Nocardia* pneumonia do have at least chronic obstructive pulmonary disease. 20%-40% of patients with pulmonary nocardiosis have no known health problems.

Pulmonary nocardiosis begins with inhalation of the organism. The clinical presentation of pulmonary nocardiosis is non-specific. Patients present with evidence of chronic disease and complain of fatigue and cough. Laboratory studies show a moderate leukocytosis in some, but not all patients. Chests radiographs have varied findings, including bilateral lobar infiltrates, cavitary disease and multiple abscesses. Pleural effusions are seen in 10%-30%. Pleural-cutaneous fistulas may be present. The diagnosis is established by culture of the organism from sputum, bronchoalveolar lavage or pleural fluid. Although *Nocardia* frequently metastasize via the bloodstream, blood cultures are not useful. Gram stain of sputum is often highly suggestive of Nocardia, which appear as beaded, Gram-positive rods. *Nocardia* spp. cannot be differentiated from *Actinomyces* spp. on Gram stain. However, *Nocardia* spp. are weakly acid-fast, while *Actinomyces* spp. are not. Cultures may take several days to weeks before becoming positive. Clinicians need to alert the microbiology laboratory, so that the specimens will be handled appropriately. Any patient diagnosed with pulmonary nocardiosis should undergo evaluation for concomitant CNS disease. Approximately 35% of cases will have metastatic disease in the brain. Unlike *Actinomyces* spp., *Nocardia* spp. rarely colonize humans and their isolation is strong evidence of infection. Sulfonamides are the backbone of treatment for nocardiosis and have been used since the 1940s. Trimethoprim-sulfamethoxazole (TMP-SMX) is used most often. The typical dose in patients with normal renal function is 10 mg/kg (based on TMP) 2-4 divided doses per day. Higher daily doses, 15 mg/kg/day (based on TMP), should be used in patients with brain abscesses. While *N asteroides* complex is usually sensitive to sulfonamides, isolates should be tested for antimicrobial sensitivities. *N farcinica* is often sulfonamide resistant. Many other antibiotics, including imipenem, ceftriaxone, minocycline and amoxicillin/clavulanic acid, have been used successfully in the treatment of nocardiosis. Patients with pulmonary nocardiosis should be treated for at least 6 months. Therapy should be given for a total of 12 months if CNS disease is also present. Patients with necrotic, large lung abscesses may benefit from adjunctive surgery.

ID Board Pearls

• *Nocardia asteroides* complex causes pneumonia in most cases (85%).

• 20%-40% of patients with pulmonary nocardiosis have no known health problems.

• 35% of pulmonary nocardiosis cases will have metastatic disease in the brain.

• Trimethoprim-sulfamethoxazole (TMP-SMX) is the drug of choice for pulmonary nocardiosis.

11. Actinomycosis

Actinomyces spp. are anaerobic, Gram-positive rods. Many species exist and many colonize the human mouth, vagina and colon. Actinomycosis is a rare infection and can affect many different organs. The species most often associated with disease is *Actinomyces israelii*. Cervico-facial disease is the most common. Abdominal and pelvic disease also occur, and have been associated with intrauterine devices in women. Pulmonary or thoracic disease occurs in 15% of cases. Presumably the bacteria enter the lungs via aspiration. Actinomyces spp. cause a characteristic histopathology with acute inflammation, surrounding fibrosis and the formation of "sulfur granules." Containing no sulfur, these particles, usually macroscopic, are aggregates of the organism. Further, sinus tract formation is common in all forms of actinomycosis. There are no clear risk factors for this disease, although most patients have some underlying disease such as alcoholism or COPD. The presentation of pulmonary actinomycosis is non-specific and patients report weight loss, fatigue, cough and chest pain. Radiographs typically show a mass-like infiltrate, with or without a cavity. Pulmonary actinomycosis is often confused with malignancy. The diagnosis is consequently delayed. Detection of sulfur granules aids in the diagnosis. Sulfur granules can be found in sputum samples or lung biopsies. Some fungi may produce sulfur granules. However, these organisms do not cause pneumonia. The diagnosis of pulmonary actinomycosis can be made by Gram stain of sulfur granules. If the Gram stain shows branching bacteria, the diagnosis is established. *Actinomyces* spp. can be cultured from sputum samples or pleural fluid. However, the cultures must be performed under anaerobic conditions. Penicillin is the mainstay of therapy. Intravenous penicillin (18-24 million units per day) is given for 2-6 weeks, followed by oral amoxicillin for 6-12 months. Tetracyclines, clindamycin and erythromycin have been used with success.

ID Board Pearls

• Pulmonary or thoracic disease occurs in 15% of cases of actinomycosis.

• Pulmonary actinomycosis is often confused with malignancy.

- The diagnosis of pulmonary actinomycosis can be made by Gram stain of sulfur granules. If the Gram stain shows branching bacteria, the diagnosis is established.

12. Melioidosis

Burkholderia pseudomallei is a small Gram-negative rod found in the soil and water of southeast Asia and northern Australia. In these areas *B pseudomallei* is endemic. Most infections are asymptomatic. However, *B pseudomallei* can cause a variety of clinical syndromes, referred to as melioidosis. Patients may present with septicemia with or without pneumonia. While most cases are acute, *B pseudomallei* may also reactivate decades after initial infection to cause chronic pneumonia. Reactivation, seen in 3% of cases, has occurred as many as 29 years after exposure. Chronic pneumonia form of melioidosis is similar to pulmonary tuberculosis. Over 300 hundred cases of melioidosis occurred in US troops during the Vietnam War. Serology studies suggested that over 100,000 armed forces personnel were infected with *B pseudomallei*. Melioidosis did not result in the "Vietnam time bomb", as some had predicted. While cases of melioidosis continue to occur occasionally in Vietnam veterans, the number of total cases is small compared with number exposed. The diagnosis of melioidosis is made by isolation of the organism from culture of sputum or blood. The recommended treatment is 2 weeks of intravenous ceftazidime or carbapenem, followed by oral TMP-SMX for 3 months.

ID Board Pearls

- Reactivation of *Burkholderia pseudomallei*, seen in 3% of cases, has occurred as many as 29 years after exposure.

- Chronic pneumonia form of melioidosis is similar to pulmonary tuberculosis.

13. Lung Abscess

More common in the pre-antibiotic era, lung abscess is a unique form of chronic pneumonia. The risk factors for lung abscess include alcoholism, seizure disorder and poor dentition. The disease is caused by aspirated oral flora, including mouth anaerobes. Patients typically present with weight loss, fever and productive cough. Patients produce copious amounts of foul-smelling sputum. The diagnosis is easily made by chest radiograph and Gram stain. The chest radiograph shows lower lobe cavity or cavities with an air fluid level. The Gram stain reveals multiple organisms. Anaerobic cultures are not usually performed, but if done, grow several mouth anaerobes. Treatment is 6-8 weeks of oral clindamycin, amoxicillin/clavulanic acid or penicillin.

Section II: Chronic Pneumonia in AIDS Patients

14. Histoplasmosis

15. Tuberculosis in AIDS Patients

16. Rhodococcus equi

14. Histoplasmosis

Several agents which cause chronic pneumonia do so with greater frequency in patients with AIDS. *Histoplasma* and *M tuberculosis* each cause chronic pneumonia in immunocompetent hosts. However, each has a much increased frequency in HIV-infected individuals.

In endemic states such as Missouri, Indiana, Ohio and Tennessee, the rates of histoplasmosis in AIDS patients are up to 25%. For all AIDS patients in the U.S., the rate is only 2%-5%. Histoplasmosis pneumonia may represent recrudescent or primary infection. Consequently, histoplasmosis can be seen in AIDS patients who once lived in an endemic area. Typically, AIDS patients with histoplasmosis have lung infiltrates and 90% have CD4+ T–cell count <200 cells/μl. However, in most AIDS patients the disease is disseminated throughout the reticuloendothelial system. Chest x-ray findings may mimic those found in PCP, and the infiltrates are diffuse and reticulonodular. Concurrent involvement of the central nervous system, the skin and the gastrointestinal tract can be seen. The diagnosis of histoplasmosis can be made by culture (bone marrow positive in 70%-90% and bronchoalveolar lavage in ~50%). Cultures may take several weeks before becoming positive. The histoplasma antigen test has excellent sensitivity in AIDS patients (95% in urine and 85% in serum). Liposomal amphotericin (Ambisome) performed well in AIDS patients with histoplasmosis. Itraconazole is used for suppressive therapy, and in mild cases may be used for induction therapy as well. Maintenance therapy is continued for life or 12 months, if the CD4+ cell count increases through highly active antiretroviral therapy.

ID Board Pearls

• Typically, AIDS patients with histoplasmosis have lung infiltrates and 90% have CD4+ T–cell count <200 cells/μl.

• Histoplasmosis pneumonia may represent recrudescent or primary infection.

• The histoplasma antigen test has excellent sensitivity in AIDS patients (95% in urine and 85% in serum).

• Itraconazole is used for suppressive therapy, and in mild cases may be used for induction therapy as well.

• Maintenance therapy is continued for life or 12 months, if the CD4+ cell count increases through highly active antiretroviral therapy.

15. Tuberculosis in AIDS Patients

In the U.S., 13% of active tuberculosis cases are infected with HIV, while less than 0.5% of the population is HIV+. The risk of clinical tuberculosis increases with worsening immunosuppression, and overall is 6-60 times higher in HIV-infected individuals than in those without HIV infection. The clinical presentation is changed by HIV co-infection. Patients with lower CD4+ T-cell counts tend to have lower and middle lobe disease. Cavitation is less frequent, while adenopathy is more pronounced. Their sputa are more often smear-negative. Extrapulmonary disease is also more common with HIV co-infection. The diagnosis of TB in HIV patients can be difficult. Several autopsy studies revealed undiagnosed TB in a high proportion of AIDS patients. Heightened awareness and persistence are helpful. Examination of sputum samples is still important. As above, nucleic acid amplification testing may detection in smear negative cases and should be used routinely. Skin testing with purified protein derivative is complicated, because it does not discriminate between clinically active and latent disease, and is unreliable in HIV patients with low CD4+ cell counts. Treatment of TB in HIV patients is the same as for those without HIV, with some minor exceptions. Twice weekly therapy should not be used in patients with CD4+ cell counts less than 100 cells/μl. Most HIV-infected TB patients are advanced and meet criteria for the initiation of HIV therapy. The current guidelines recommend that HIV therapy be withheld for the first 4-8 weeks of TB therapy. HIV patients more frequently have paradoxical reactions, characterized by fever, increased shortness of breath and worsening of chest radiographs. These reactions are thought to be secondary to improved immune system function. HIV therapy is felt to increase the chance of these reactions.

Additionally, the rifamycins interact with protease inhibitors and with efavirenz. Rifampin causes a slight decrease in efavirenz levels, but can be coadministered at normal doses. Standard doses of rifampin, which lowers the trough level by greater than 90%, cannot be given with protease inhibitors. Rifabutin does not have this effect. Rifabutin levels are increased by ritonavir, but can be safely used at a decreased dose.

ID Board Pearls

- The risk of clinical tuberculosis increases with worsening immunosuppression, and overall is 6-60 times higher in HIV-infected individuals.

- Patients with lower CD4+ T-cell counts tend to have lower and middle lobe disease. Cavitation is less frequent, while adenopathy is more pronounced.

- The current guidelines recommend that HIV therapy be withheld for the first 4-8 weeks of TB therapy.

- HIV patients more frequently have paradoxical reactions, characterized by fever, increased shortness of breath and worsening of chest radiographs.

16. Rhodococcus equi

Rhodococcus equi causes granulomatous pneumonia in foals. It was first recognized as a human pathogen in 1967. Since then, several cases of chronic, often cavitary pneumonia have been reported, primarily in AIDS patients. The mean CD4+ T–cell count in 1 study was 35 cells/µl. Cavities were seen in 67% of cases. The organism is easily cultured and can be grown from blood and sputum samples. *R equi* is sensitive to several antibiotics, including vancomycin, rifampin and quinolones. However, the mortality rate is high (>30%). Concomitant antiretroviral therapy is associated with better outcomes.

Section III: Non-infectious Mimics of Chronic Pneumonia

17. **Chronic Eosinophilic Pneumonia**

18. **Cryptogenic Organizing Pneumonia**

19. **Hypersensitivity Pneumonitis (HP)**

20. **Further Reading**

17. Chronic Eosinophilic Pneumonia

Chronic eosinophilic pneumonia (CEP) is a rare disorder of unknown etiology. Patients usually develop this disease in early to mid-adulthood (20s-50s). Patients present with cough, shortness of breath, fever and wheezing. The mean duration of symptoms is 7.7 months. Chest x-rays characteristically show peripheral alveolar infiltrates with central clearing. The radiographic findings are nearly unique for CEP. Peripheral eosinophilia is found in 80%. IgE levels are usually elevated as well. Lung biopsy reveals mature eosinophils and histiocytes in the alveolar spaces. Charcot-Leyden crystals are often seen. The disease responds well to corticosteroids, but spontaneous remissions are rare.

18. Cryptogenic Organizing Pneumonia

Cryptogenic organizing pneumonia (formerly known as bronchiolitis obliterans organizing pneumonia or BOOP) is an uncommon disease, which presents with fever, cough, shortness of breath and patchy alveolar infiltrates. COP has been linked to many diseases and medications. For instance, it has been seen more frequently in transplant patients on sirolimus and tacrolimus. However, as the name implies, the etiology is unknown and the link between some medications is not understood. COP typically presents in the fourth to sixth decades of life. The rates are the same for women and men. Symptoms are present for 1-12 weeks before presentation. Laboratory findings are non-specific, although an elevated erythrocyte sedimentation rate is often greater than 100 mm/h. Chest radiographs reveal patchy alveolar infiltrates, most often in the lower lobes. The diagnosis is established by lung biopsy, usually via video-assisted thorascopic approach. The histology shows plugs of granulation tissue called Masson bodies, which block the bronchiolar lumens and extend into the alveolar spaces. COP responds very well to prednisone therapy, which is usually continued for at least 1 year. Relapses can occur, especially after shorter courses therapy.

19. Hypersensitivity Pneumonitis (HP)

In some hosts, repeated inhalation of certain antigens leads to hypersensitivity pneumonitis (HP). The antigens which can cause HP are varied and can be from animals, plants or chemicals. Some more common forms of HP include Farmer's lung from thermophilic actinomyces and pigeon breeder's lung from avian proteins. Acute HP presents with fever, cough and shortness of breath within 4-6 hours of exposure. Repeated exposures lead to chronic HP, which is associated with fibrosis and scarring. Removal of the offending antigen prevents further deterioration.

20. Further Reading

Barnes PF, Lakey DL, Burman WJ. Tuberculosis in patients with HIV infection. *Infect Dis Clin North Am*. 2002;16:107-126.

Chapman SW, Dismukes WE, Proia LA, et al. Clinical practice guidelines for the management of blastomycosis: 2008 update by the Infectious Diseases Society of America. *Clin Infect Dis*. 2008;46:1801-1812.

Currie BJ. Melioidosis: an important cause of pneumonia in residents of and travellers returned from endemic regions. *Eur Respir J*. 2003;22:542-550.

Galgiani JN, Ampel NM, Blair JE, et al. Coccidioidomycosis. *Clin Infect Dis*. 2005;41:1217-1223.

Griffith DE, Aksamit T, Brown-Elliott BA, et al. An official ATS/IDSA statement: diagnosis, treatment, and prevention of nontuberculous mycobacterial diseases. *Am J Respir Crit Care Med*. 2007;175:367-416.

Jederlinic PJ, Sicilian L, Gaensler EA. Chronic eosinophilic pneumonia. A report of 19 cases and a review of the literature. *Medicine* (Baltimore). 1988;67:154-162.

Kauffman CA, Bustamante B, Chapman SW, Pappas PG and the Infectious Diseases Society of America. Clinical practice guidelines for the management of sporotrichosis: 2007 update by the Infectious Diseases Society of America. *Clin Infect Dis*. 2007;45:1255-1265.

Lederman ER, Crum NF. A case series and focused review of nocardiosis: clinical and microbiologic aspects. *Medicine* (Baltimore). 2004;83:300-313.

Lynch JP 3rd, Sitrin RG. Noninfectious mimics of community-acquired pneumonia. *Semin Respir Infect*. 1993;8:14-45.

Peacock SJ. Melioidosis. *Curr Opin Infect Dis*. 2006;19:421-428.

Schlesinger C, Koss MN. The organizing pneumonias: an update and review. *Curr Opin Pulm Med*. 2005;11:422-430.

Torres-Tortosa M, Arrizabalaga J, Villanueva JL, et al. Prognosis and clinical evaluation of infection caused by Rhodococcus equi in HIV-infected patients: a multicenter study of 67 cases. *Chest*. 2003;123:1970-1976.

Wheat J. Endemic mycoses in AIDS: a clinical review. *Clin Microbiol Rev*. 1995;8:146-159.

Wheat LJ, Freifeld AG, Kleiman MB, et al. Clinical practice guidelines for the management of patients with histoplasmosis: 2007 update by the Infectious Diseases Society of America. *Clin Infect Dis*. 2007;45:807-825.

Yildiz O, Doganay M. Actinomycoses and Nocardia pulmonary infections. *Curr Opin Pulm Med*. 2006;12:228-234.

Chapter 18:
Infective Endocarditis
for the ID Boards

John L. Brusch, MD

Contents

1. Synonyms

Infective endocarditis (IE), subacute bacterial endocarditis, acute bacterial endocarditis, fungal endocarditis, nosocomial infective endocarditis (NIE), health care-associated infective endocarditis (HCIE), intravenous drug abuser infective endocarditis (IVDAIE), native valve infective endocarditis (NVE) and prosthetic valve infective endocarditis (PVE); pacemaker infective endocarditis (PMIE), endocardial infection, bloodstream infection (BSI).

2. Causative Organisms

- There is a close association between the infecting organism and the type of IE that it produces (Tables 1 and 2).

- *S aureus* (MSSA and MRSA) is the #1 cause of both NVE and PVE (32%-50% of cases overall). Prevalence of MRSA HCIE approximates that of MSSA HCIE.

- Coagulase-negative staphylococci (CoNS) cause 10.5% of cases, usually PVE with a growing involvement in NVE (7.5% of cases).

- Not all CoNS represent *S epidermidis*. *S lugdunensis* is much more aggressive clinically than other types of CoNS, with a mortality rate of 70%. Difficult to differentiate *S lugdunensis* because it produces a clumping factor and its colonies have a golden hue resembling that of *S aureus*.

- The *S viridans* group is the second most common cause of IE. It remains the classic pathogen of subacute IE. Many isolates have developed various degrees of resistance to penicillin.

- *S viridans* strains are commensals of the respiratory and gastrointestinal tracts. With the exception of the *S angiosus* group, *S viridans* has little tissue-invasive potential. This group produces both the myocardial and valvular abscesses, and is becoming a more frequent cause of health care-associated BSI, especially among neutropenic patients.

- *Abiotrophia* spp. (formerly nutritionally-variant streptococci) require the presence of cystine or pyridoxine for growth. Many isolates are relatively resistant to penicillin.

- *S pneumoniae* cause less than 5% of cases. Follows an acute course and is usually a complication of pneumonia in alcoholics.

- Enterococci are currently categorized as members of the genus Enterococcus (*E faecalis* and *E faecium*). They produce 20% total cases of IE, of which *E faecalis* produces 90%. Enterococcal BSI/IE is due to UTIs, abdominal/wound/biliary tract infections. Many are polymicrobial. Enterococcal BSI, due to infection of intravascular catheters, are an increasing cause of HCIE. Antibiotic therapy of enterococcal IE requires a synergistic combination. VRE BSI is an increasing problem, usually caused by *E faecium*.

• Gram-negative IE accounts for 5% of cases, most commonly IVDA IE and HCIE. Cirrhotics are at particular risk.

• Less than 1% of disseminated gonoccocal disease is complicated by IE. It usually follows the onset of genital infection by 3 weeks. Its clinical course is acute. The cervical, rectal and pharyngeal cultures often are negative.

• Fungal IE has increased by 270% over the last 30 years; primarily in 5% of IVDA IE and 13% and 5%, respectively, of early and late PVE.

• *T whippelii* is a Gram-positive bacterium that produces Whipple's disease, which is characterized by arthritis, abdominal pain, malabsorption syndrome and central nervous system manifestations. Myocarditis, endocarditis and pericarditis occur in 33% of cases. Valvular infection may occur without any of the other associated symptoms during diagnosis and is based on the histologic findings of PAS positive macrophages (foamy macrophages) in resected valves. The clinical course is quite indolent.

• Culture negative IE constitutes 5% of all cases (Table 3).

Table 1

Microbiology of Infective Endocarditis in Different Risk Groups

Microorganism Recovered (% of cases)	Native Valve Endocarditis	Intravenous Drug Users	Prosthetic Valve Endocarditis	
			Early	Late
Viridans-group streptococci	50	20	7	30
Staphylococcus aureus	35a/42b	67	17	12
Coagulase-negative staphylococci	4	9	33	26
Enterococci	8	7	2	6
Miscellaneous	19	7	44	26

a Community acquired
b Healthcare acquired

Table 2

Causative Organisms of IE

Organism	Comments
S aureus	The most common cause of acute IE including PVE. IVDA and IE are related to intravascular infections. Approximately 35% of cases of S aureus bacteremia are complicated by IE.
Coagulase-negative *S aureus* (CoNS)	30% of PVE; currently causes <5% of IE of native valves but increasing frequency; subacute course that is more indolent than that of S viridans.
S viridans (S mitior, S sanguis, S mutans, S salivarius)	70% of cases of subacute IE. Signs and symptoms are immunologically mediated with a very low rate of suppurative complications. Penicillin resistance is a growing problem, especially in patients receivin chemotherapy or bone marrow transplants.
S milleri group (S anginosus, *S intermedius, S constellatus*)	Up to 20% of streptococcal IE. Unlike other streptococci they can invade tissue and produce suppurative complications.
Abiotrophia spp. (Nutritionally variant streptococci)	5% of subacute IE. Examples require nutritionally variant streptococci active forms of vitamin B6 for growth. Characteristically produce large valvular vegetations with a high rate of embolization and relapse.
Group D streptococci	Third most common cause of IE. They may produce alpha, beta or gammahemolysis. Source is GI or GU tracts; associated with a high rate of relapse. Growing problem of antimicrobial resistance. Most cases are subacute.
Non-enteroccocal group D streptoccoci (*S bovis*)	50% of group D IE; associated with lesions of large bowel.
Group B streptococci	Increasing cause of acute IE in alcoholics, cancer patients, and diabetics as well as in pregnancy. 40% mortality rate. Complications include CHF, thrombi, and metastatic infection. Surgery often required for cure.
Groups A, C, G streptococci	More frequently seen in the elderly (nursing homes) and diabetics. 30%-70% death rate. Commonly cause myocardial abscesses.
Bartonella spp.	*B quintana* is the most common isolate. Culture negative subacute IE in a homeless male should suggest the diagnosis. Usually treated with a combination of a beta-lactam antibiodic and an aminoglyside.

(continued)

Table 2

Causative Organisms of IE

Organism	Comments
HACEK organisms	Most common Gram-negative organisms in IE (5% of all cases). Presents as subacute IE. They are part of the normal flora of the GI tract. Intravenous drug abuse is a major risk factor. Complications are arterial macroemboli and congestive heart failure. Cases usually require the combination of ampicillin and gentamicin, with or without surgery, for cure.
P aeruginosa	Most commonly acutely seen in IVDA IE (right-sided disease is subacute) and in PVE.
Serratia marcescens	NIE (acute IE), often requires surgery for cure.
Fungal IE	An increasing problem in the CrCU and among IVDA. C albicans most common example (especially in PVE) as compared to IVDA IE, in which C parapsilosis or C tropicalis predominate. Aspergillus species recovered in 33% of fungal IE. Most cases of fungal IE follow a subacute course.
Polymicrobial IE	Most common organisms are Pseudomonas and enterococci. It occurs frequently in IVDA and cardiac surgery. It may present acutely or subacutely. Mortality is greater than that of single-agent IE.

Abbreviations: GI, gastrointestinal; GU, genitourinary; CrCU, Critical Care Unit;
IE, Infective Endocarditis; PVE, Prosthetic Valve Endocarditis

Table 3

Causes of Culture Negative Infective Endocarditis

Causes	Comments
Prior antibiotic use	Most frequent cause, at least 35%-79% of cases
Sequestration of infection within the thrombus	Surface sterilization phenomena
Fastidious organisms	*Bartonella* spp are the most common. Fungi, Q-fever, *T whipplei, Brucella* spp., Rickettsiae, Chlamydiae, Legionella
Right-sided endocarditis	Non-virulent organisms are filtered out by the lungs
Bacteria free stage	Untreated infection for >3 months
Mural infective endocarditis in VSD	-
Infection related to pacemaker wires	-

3. Epidemiology

- The incidence of IE is 4/100,000 patient years.

- It has become a disease of the older population. 50% of cases occur in those greater than 60 years of age. The major exception to this trend is IVDA IE (mean age 30 years).

- There has been marked a marked increase in HCIE, IVDA IE and PVE. Currently, they respectively account for 22%, 36% and 16%. These figures are due both to a increase in *S aureus* HCBSI coupled with a significant decrease in *S viridans* IE.

- 75% of cases of IVDAIE have underlying normal valves. 60% involve the tricuspid valve.

- Over their lifetimes, 5% of prosthetic valves become infected. Mechanical valves more commonly in the first 3 months after placement and bioprosthetic after 1 year.

- Analogous to PVE are PMIE and infective endocarditis of ICDs. Usually these devices become infected within a few months of their implantation.

- *The pathogenesis, shared by all varieties of IE, is infection of a sterile platelet/fibrin thrombus or nonbacterial thrombotic endocarditis (NBTE) that is due to a BSI with an appropriate organism.*

- NBTE may be the result of pre-existing valvular or other intracardiac abnormalities (VSD) or be produced by *S aureus* infection of a previously normal valve.

- *S aureus* uniquely may invade the valvular endothelial cells (endotheliosis). Once inside, this organism can turn off anticoagulant factors of these cells. Microthrombi then form on their surfaces.

- The responsible BSI may be spontaneous (transient BSI of a normal bowel movement) or caused by invasive procedures or an intravascular catheter.

- 78% of *S aureus* BSI in the U.S. is associated with vascular catheters. At least 30% of these bacteremias progress to IE.

- The 3 major determinants of catheter infections are the type of catheter; the insertion site and how long the catheter has been in place.

- The risk of line infection markedly increases after 4 days of placement.

- Catheters inserted in the internal jugular are at greater risk of becoming infected than those positioned in the subclavian vein. Femoral lines are the most prone to become infected.

- The major risk factors for complications of CR-BSI are hemodialysis dependence, MRSA involvement and length of symptoms prior to diagnosis.

- IE results in at least 30% of *S aureus* BSI.

- The term NIE has been superseded by the term HCIE, since intravascular devices of all types are used outside the hospital (dialysis center, infusion center, home care). Formerly, 57% of BSI were acquired in the hospital. Currently, they arise equally in the community and in the hospital. 20% of *S aureus* BSI currently develops outside the hospital and is related to intravascular devices.

- Mortality from HCIE ranges from 35%-56%.

- A previous episode of IE is the most important risk factor for development of valvular infection (Tables 4-6).

Table 4

Changing Patterns of Infective Endocarditis Since 1966

Marked Increase in the Incidence of Acute IE

Rise of HCIE, IVDA and Prosthetic Valve IE
  a) Change in the Underlying Valvular Pathology: Rheumatic heart disease <20% of cases as compared to 50% prior to the antibiotic era. 6% of these will develop IE during their lifetime.
  b) Mitral valve prolapse 30% of cases
  c) Prosthetic valve endocarditis 10%-20% of cases
  d) 50% of elderly patients have calcific aortic stenosis
  e) 15% of cases are due to congenital heart disease. Bicuspid aortic valve is the most common abnormality; 20% of cases in those over 60.

These changes are due to :
  a) The "Graying" of patients (excluding cases of IVDA IE, 55% of patients >60 years of age)
  a) The increased numbers of vascular procedures

Abbreviations: IE, Infective Endocarditis; HCIE, Health Care Associated IE; IVDA, Intravenous Drug User

Table 5

Risk of Bacteremia Associated with Various Procedures

Low (0%-20%)	Moderate (20-40%)	High (40%-100%)	Organism
	Tonsillectomy		
Bronchoscopy (rigid)			
Bronchoscopy (flexible)			Streptococcal spp. or *S epidermidis*
Endoscopy			*S epidermidis*, streptococci and diphtheroids
Colonoscopy			*E coli* and Bacteroides spp. *S epidermidis*
Barium enema			Enterococci; and aerobic Gram-negative rods

(continued)

Table 5

Risk of Bacteremia Associated with Various Procedures

Low (0%-20%)	Moderate (20-40%)	High (40%-100%)	Organism
	Transurethral resection of the prostate		Coliforms, enterococci, *S aureus*
Cystoscopy			Coliforms and Gram-negative rods
		Traumatic dental procedures	*S viridans*
Liver biopsy (in setting of cholangitis)			Coliforms and enterococci
Sclerotherapy of esophageal varices			*S viridans*, Gram-negative rods, *S aureus*
Esophageal dilatation			*S aureus, S viridans*
	Suction abortion		*S viridans* and anaerobes
Transesophageal echocardiography			Streptococcal spp.

Table 6

Risk and Rates of Bloodstream Infections Produced by Intravascular Catheters

Types Of Vascular Catheters	% Risk For BSI[a]/Catheter	Rates Of Catheter BSI/1000 Catheter Days
Standard CVC[b]	3.3%	2.3-2.7
Antibiotic coated CVC[b]	0.2%	0.2
Picc[c]	1.2%	0.4-1.1
Tunnel and cuffed CVC[b]	20.9%	1.2
Swan-Ganz CVC[b]	1.9%	3.7-5.5
Hemodialysis catheters	-	2.8
Arterial catheters	-	1.7

[a] Bloodstream infection
[b] Central venous catheter
[c] Peripherally inserted central venous catheter

4. Key Clinical Features

- ABE is a rapidly progressive disease that often involves normal valves due to the pathogenic properties of the common causative pathogens. Untreated, it may cause death within a few days.

- SBE inevitably involves previously damaged valves because of the indolent pathogenic nature of the causative organisms. Untreated, its clinical course may extend past 1 year.

- Complications of IE are due to embolization, valvular destruction and deposition of immune complexes.

- Congestive heart failure is most frequent complication of SBE and ABE (15%-54%); usually due to aortic insufficiency. In SBE, it rarely occurs earlier than 1 month into the disease, but often develops after microbiological cure has been achieved. In ABE, it can occur within a few days of infection.

- Other types of suppurative intracardiac complications are seen in ABE. These include: intraventricular, myocardial, ring abscesses; intracardiac fistulas; mycotic aneurysms; septic coronary artery emboli and pericarditis.

- Arterial emboli are the second most common complication of ABE and SBE (35% of cases). The prevalence is the same for ABE and SBE.

- The most common organisms producing emboli are *Candida aspergillus*, *S aureus*, members of the HACEK group, *Abiotrophia* spp. and Group B streptococci. These involve the brain (33%, middle cerebral artery most commonly involved), kidney, spleen and coronary arteries.

- Stroke that occurs in a younger patient should always raise the possibility of IE. The mortality rate is 2-4 greater for those patients with IE who suffer a stroke.

- In SBE, emboli usually cause infarcts. Emboli to the vasa vasorum lead to sterile aneurysms of the involved vessel.

- In ABE (*S aureus*), emboli produce abscesses at the point of deposition.

- In SBE, circulating immune complexes produce many of the extracardiac forms of the disease. These include glomerulonephritis, Osler nodes, Roth spots, subungual hemorrhages and a variety of musculoskeletal symptoms (back pain). Janeway lesions are usually due to septic emboli (Tables 7,8).

Table 7

The Early Nonspecific Signs and Symptoms of Subacute IE[a]

Low-grade fever (absent in 3%-15% of patients)
Anorexia
Weight loss
Influenza-like syndromes
Polymyalgia-like syndromes with arthralgias, dull sensorium and headaches resembling typhoid fever
Pleuritic pain
Right upper quadrant pain and right lower quadrant pain
85% of patients present with a detectable murmur; all will eventually develop one

a The manifestations of SBE are caused by emboli and/or progressive valvular destruction and/or immunologic phenomena.

Table 8

Organ Involvement in NVE

Peripheral Stigmata (20% of patients)	Musculoskeletal (40%-50% of patients)	Intracardiac
Janeway lesions	Low back pain (presenting symptom)	Valvular vegetations in 15% of patients
Osler nodes	Diffuse myalgias, especially of legs	CHF
Roth spots	Disc space infection	Myocardial abscess
	Hypertrophic osteoarthropathy	Septal abscess (leading to heart block)
	Splenomegaly	Vascular necrosis
	Arthritis (ankle, knee, wrist)	Aortocardiac fistula
		Suppurative pericarditis
		Rupture of papillary muscles, chordae tendinae
		Annular abscess
		Mycotic aneurysm of sinus of Valsalva
		Destruction of valvular leaflets
		S aureus responsible for 55%-70% of congestive heart failure

(continued)

Table 8

Organ Involvement in NVE

Neurological System	Renal	Mycotic Aneurysms	Metastatic infections
Neurological complications are the presenting symptoms in 50%-70% of patients.	Congestive heart failure and antibiotic toxicity are currently the most common causes of renal failure.	Life-threatening in 2.5% of patients.	Metastatic infections are produced by septic emboli (usually in Acute IE) to liver, spleen, gallbladder, coronary arteries (myocardial infarction occurs in 50% of patients), myocardium, lung and retina.
Hemorrhage	Renal abscesses due to highly invasive organisms (ie, *S aureus*).	Usually produced by organisms of low invasive capacity (ie, *S viridans*).	
Toxic manifestations (headache, irritability).	Renal infarction (cortical necrosis) occurs in two-thirds of infected patients.	Silent until they leak; seen most commonly in brain.	
Psychiatric effects (neurosis).	Focal glomerulonephritis occurs in 50% of untreated cases and is associated withrenal failure and nephrotic syndrome.	Sinus of Valsalva, abdominal aorta and its branches, mesenteric, splenic, coronary and pulmonary arteries.	
Psychoses, disorientation, delirium (hallucinations) and stroke.	"Flea bitten" kidney, multiple emboli and hemorrhages.		
Meningoencephalitis			
Dyskinesia			
Spinal cord and small nerves (girdle pain,paraplegia, weakness, myalgias and perhipheral neuropathy).			

5. IVDA IE

- 5%-8% of febrile IVDA have IE.

- Left-sided IVDA IE is caused by the same types of pathogens as non-IVDA NVE, with the exception of increased preponderance of *Pseudomonas* and *Serratia* spp.

- 5% of IVDA IE are polymicrobial.

- 6.2% of patients have underlying valvular disease.

- CHF and intracardiac complications are rare in right-sided IVDA, since infection does not usually spread beyond the cusps of the valve.

- 50% of right-sided IVDA IE present with respiratory symptoms (cough and pleurisy) that are due to septic pulmonary emboli. 12% of these will develop empyema.

- Patients will often defervesce within hours after admission without antibiotic therapy. This is seen in those whose fever is caused by adulterants in the injected drugs (cotton wool fever).

6. PVE

- PVE may be divided into early, intermediate or late stages. Early PVE extends through the first 3 months past the time of valve implantation; intermediate 3-12 months and late after 12 months.

- Within the first 6 months of implantation, mechanical prosthetic valves have a higher rate of infection than bioprosthetic ones. After 5 years, PVE occurs much more frequently in the latter because of wear and tear on the valvular leaflets.

- CoNS is the chief pathogen in the early and immediate stages (30% of cases overall). *S aureus* (17% and 12% of early and late cases, respectively), JK corynebacteria, nonenterococcal streptococci, Fungi (*C albicans, C stellatoidea* and *Aspergillus* spp.), Legionella and the HACEK group; each produce 2%-4% of all cases.

- Early infection is usually due to contamination of the field during surgery or to infected intravascular lines or other medical equipment.

- Early PVE is similar clinically to NVE. However, if due to *S aureus*, PVE may present with the complications of a paravalvular abscess that may result in valvular insufficiency with CHF, conduction disturbances and septic emboli.

- There is a high rate of embolic stroke in the first 3 days of PVE.

- The pathogens of late PVE closely resemble those found in NVE. The profile of the organisms found in intermediate cases is a mixture of those found in the early and late stages.

- Late PVE usually follows a subacute course, with a 20% rate of peripheral stigmata (Osler nodes, subungual hemorrhages).

- Prosthetic valves are quite susceptible to becoming infected during HCBSI or health care-associated fungemia. 60% of these cases are due to CRB-SIs (55% are due to *S aureus* and 33% to Gram-negatives).

7. HCIE

- HCIE differs from community-acquired IE. It more frequently presents as a nonspecific picture sepsis associated with hypotension and multiple organ failure, especially CHF. Fever/chills and leukocytosis are less common in HCIE. The dermatological manifestations of IE are rarely seen.

8. IE in the Immunosuppressed Hosts

- The outcomes of IE in immunosuppressed patients are inversely proportional to the degree of immunosuppression. For example, those with advanced age had a significantly high mortality rate compared to those who have not yet developed clinical AIDS.

9. Key Differential Diagnostic Features

- Tables 9-11 present the differential diagnosis of IE, as well as the major mimics of IE.

- The presence of a continuous bacteremia differentiates IE from its infectious and noninfectious mimics.

- PMIE may be classified as primary, in which the pacemaker or its pocket is the source of infection, or secondary in which the leads are seeded from a BSI.

- Early PMIE may be acute or subacute clinically. It is due to infection of the pulse-generator pocket quiet during implantation. There may be associated bacteremia. 33% of patients are febrile.

- Late PMIE are due to erosion of the skin overlying pocket, which leads to infection of at least the generator and possibly of the leads.

- Late PMIE presents with more systemic signs and symptoms then do infections of the pacemaker pocket alone. *S aureus* and CoNS are the most frequent organisms. At least 84% of patients are febrile. 45% of cases of PMIE have signs and symptoms of septic pulmonary emboli.

Table 9

Differential Diagnoses of IE

Noninfectious Entities
      Marantic endocarditis
      Antiphospholipid syndrome
      Atrial myxoma
      Cardiac neoplasms
      Polymyalgia rheumatica
      Reactive arthritis and Reiter's syndrome
      Systemic lupus erythematosus
      Thrombotic nonbacterial endocarditis
      Temporal arteritis and other forms vasculitis
      Cholesterol emboli syndrome

Infectious Entities
      Lyme disease
      Viral hepatitis
      Disseminated gonococcal infection / gonococcal arthritis

The presence of a continuous bacteremia differentiates IE from its infectious and noninfectious mimics.

Table 10

Mimics of IE

Disease	Type of Valvular Involvement	Comments
Antiphospholipid Syndrome	Stenosis or regurgitation	Patients have thrombotic events and/or recurrent spontaneous abortions. Antibody titers have no direct correlation with disease activity.
Systemic Lupus Erythematosus	Stenosis or regurgitation occurs in 46% of patients (usually of the mitral valve)	4% of cases of Libman-Sacks endocarditis become secondarily infected usually early in the course of the disease.
Rheumatoid Arthritis	Regurgitation occurs in 2% of patients	Valvular infection usually occurs later in the course of the disease.
Atrial Myxoma	Primarily obstruction of the mitral valve due to its "ball valve" effect	It is the most effective mimic due to its valvular involvement, embolic events and constitutional signs and symptoms.

Table 11

Mimics of Infective Endocarditis: Clinical and Laboratory Features

Mimics of Endocarditis	Bacteremia	Cardiac Vegetation	Fever	Splenomegaly	Emboli	↑ESR	Abnormal SPEP[a]
Marantic endocarditis	-	+	-	-	±	-	-
Viral myocarditis	-	-	+	-	±	+	-
SLE (Libman-Sacks endocarditis)	-	+	+	±	-	+	+
Atrial myxoma	-	±	+	-	+	+	+
Infective endocarditis	+	+	+	±	±	+	-

[a] *Polyclonal gammopathy on SPEP*

Abbreviations: ESR, erythrocyte sedimentation rate; SLE, systemic lupus erythematosus; SPEP, serum protein electrophoresis

10. Key Laboratory/Radiology Features

• The diagnostic hallmark of all types of IE is the presence of a continuous BSI. This is defined as 2 sets of blood cultures, drawn at 12 hours apart, that grow out of the same organism, or 3 out of 4 sets of blood cultures, positive for the same organism, the first and last sets separated by at least 1 hour.

• The skin should be prepped with 70% isopropyl alcohol, followed by application of an iodophor or tincture of iodine. The skin should then be allowed to dry. Blood should be drawn at separate sites to lower the risk of contamination. Samples should not be drawn from an intravascular line, except for the purpose of determining line infection.

• A 10 ml aliquot should be added to each bottle, to produce a ratio 1/10 of blood to broth. This dilution inhibits the suppressive effect of both antibiotics and the patient's own antibodies.

• For *S aureus* BSI, the shorter the time to positivity of the blood culture, the greater the likelihood that the BSI represents valvular infection.

• 3 sets of blood cultures will detect the pathogen in approximately 99% of cases.

• Up to 10% of cases of PVE do not have a continuous BSI. 5 sets of blood cultures should be drawn when PVE is suspected.

• 64% of patients with SBE, who have received prior antibiotics, will have false negative blood cultures.

• Modern automated blood culture systems make it unnecessary for cultures to be incubated for multiple weeks in order to recover most fastidious organisms (HACEK group members, *Brucella* spp and *F tularensis*). Pyridoxine supplementation is also present in these systems to allow ready retrieval of *Abiotrophia* spp.

• In Candida IE, only 50% of blood cultures are positive. Aspergillus and histoplasma are rarely recovered from the bloodstream.

• The diagnosis of IE, produced by truly fastidious organisms (*Bartonella* spp., *C burnetti*, *Legionella* spp.) depends on serologic studies and DNA amplification techniques. PCR techniques have been directly applied to valvular tissue obtained at surgery. They appear more sensitive and more specific than standard culture methods.

• Cardiac conduction abnormalities are seen in 9% of cases. They are the result of septal abscesses or myocarditis. During the first 2 weeks of treatment of acute IE, electrocardiography should be performed every 48-72 hours to rule out these complications.

• Rheumatoid factor develops in 50% of patients with subacute IE. It disappears with successful treatment.

• The use of radionuclide scans (gallium-67, indium-111 tagged white cells and platelets) are of marginal benefit in diagnosing IE because of the high rate of false negative studies.

• A CT scan of the brain should be obtained in patients who exhibit central nervous system symptoms or findings consistent with a mass effect.

• TTEs can image vegetations down to 3-6 mm in diameter. TEEs have a resolution down to 1 mm in diameter.

• The sensitivity of a TTE in detecting NVE is 68% as compared to 95% for TEE. TTE has a 20%-35% sensitivity for detecting PVE is compared to >75% for TEE.

• 15% of patients have no detectable vegetations at a given time on TTE.

• The negative predictive value of TEE for IE approaches 100% in some series.

• Neither technique should be used in screening in those with a low clinical probability of IE. Up to 50% of vegetations detected on echocardiography are sterile.

• There is good deal of interobserver variability in reading echocardiograms. 15% of "vegetations" are, in reality, nodules, valvular calcifications or benign thickening of a valve leaflet.

- Echocardiography is most useful as a primary diagnostic tool in those patients with persistent BSI of unknown etiology; in BSI in the presence of prosthetic valves; in diagnosing HCIE and those with a high pretest probability of IE, but whose blood cultures remain negative (Table 12).

- Certain findings on echocardiography may be predictive of the risk for embolization. Among these are: vegetations >10 mm in diameter, multiple vegetations, mobile pedunculated vegetations, prolapsing vegetations and vegetations that increase in size during the first 2 weeks of appropriate antimicrobial treatment. Size and growth appear to be the significant parameters.

- The risk for embolization is greatest during the initial 2 weeks of infection.

- Definitive pathologic diagnosis is made by demonstrating microorganisms by culture or histology and vegetations removed by surgery, embolectomy or by drainage of intracardiac abscess.

- The Duke criteria codify the characteristics of blood cultures and the findings of echocardiography into a clinical guideline for the diagnosis of IE.

- The major blood culture criteria of this guideline are: 2 sets of blood culture positive organisms typically found in patients with IE. The blood cultures must be drawn at least 12 hours apart or in 3 or more separate sets of blood cultures drawn at least 1 hour apart.

- The major echocardiographic criteria are: oscillating intracardiac mass on the valve or on supporting structures, in the path of a regurgitant jet or on implanted material in the absence of an alternative anatomic explanation; myocardial abscess; development of a partial dehiscence of a prosthetic valve and new onset of valvular regurgitation.

- Minor criteria consist of predisposing heart condition or intravenous drug abuse.

- Fever of >38° C, vascular phenomena including: major arterial emboli, septic pulmonary infarcts, mycotic aneurysms, intracranial hemorrhage, conjunctival hemorrhage or Janeway lesions; immunologic phenomena, such as glomerulonephritis, Osler nodes, Roth spots and rheumatoid factor positivity; blood culture not meeting major criteria or serological evidence of active infection with organism consistent with IE (*Brucella* spp., *C burnetti*, *Legionella*) and echocardiographic results consistent with IE but not meeting major echocardiographic criteria.

- According to these criteria, the definite diagnosis of IE can be made by pathological criteria (see above) or

- A definite diagnosis of IE can be made by the presence of 2 major criteria or 1 major criterion and 3 minor criteria or by 5 minor criteria.

- Possible IE is defined as findings consistent with infective endocarditis that fall short of definite but do not fit the rejected category.

- The rejected category includes cases with a firm alternate diagnosis explaining the evidence of IE or resolution of IE syndrome with antibiotic therapy for 4 days or less, or no pathological evidence of IE at surgery or autopsy, with antibiotic therapy for 4 days or less.

- The sensitivity of these guidelines is at least 80%. Specificity is somewhat less. Use of these criteria probably over-diagnose IE.

- The proposed modifications to the changes to the Duke criteria by JS Li et al would include all *S aureus* positive blood cultures and Q fever serology as major criteria. These changes would also define the Possible IE category as 1 major and 1 minor or 3 minor criteria.

Complications (refer to Clinical Features)

- CT scans of the brain should be performed in those who show symptoms consistent with a mass effect (macroscopic brain abscess in 0.5% of cases of ABE).

Table 12

American College of Cardiology/American Heart Association

Guidelines for Echocardiography in Native Valve and Prosthetic Valve Endocarditits

1. Indication	Class[a] (native/prosthetic valve)
2. Detection and characterization of valvular lesions and their hemodynamic severity or degree of ventricular decompensation[b]	I/I
3. Detection of associated abnormalities (eg, abscesses, shunts, etc.)[b]	I/I
4. Re-evaluation of complicated endocarditis (eg, virulent organisms, severe hemodynamic lesion, aortic valve involvement, persistent fever or bacteremia clinical change or deterioration)	I/I
4. Evaluation of patients with high clinical suspicion of culture-negative endocarditis[b]	I/I
5. Evaluation of persistent bacteremia or fungemia without a known source[b]	Ia/I
6. Risk stratification in established endocarditis[b]	IIa/-
7. Routine re-evaluation in uncomplicated endocarditis during antibiotic therapy	IIb/IIb
8. Evaluation of fever and non-pathalogical murmur without evidence of bacteremia[c]	III/IIa

[a] *Class I: evidence and/or general agreement that an echocardiography is useful; IIa: conflicting evidence or divergence of opinion about usefulness, but weight of evidence/opinion favor it; Iib:usefulness is less well established; III: evidence or general opinion that echocardiography is not useful.*

[b] *Transesophegeal echocardiography (TEE) may provide incremental value in addition to information obtained by transthoracic echocardiography (TTE). The role of TEE in first-line examination awaits further study.*

[c] *Prosthetic valves-IIa:for persistent bacteremia; III: for transient bacteremia.*

Adapted from Cheitlin MD, Armstrong WF, Aurigemma GP, et al. ACC/AHA/ASE 2003 guideline update for the clinical application of echocardiography: summary article: a report of the American College of Cardiology/American Heart Association Task Force on Practice Guidelines (ACC/AHA/ASE Committee to Update the 1997 Guidelines for the Clinical Application of Echocardiography).Circulation. 2003;108:1146-1162.

- MRI may reveal multiple microabscesses in the brain (4% of cases of ABE). Many of these have negative CT scans.

- Mycotic aneurysms of the cerebral arteries occur in 2%-10% of SBE; probably less in ABE where abscesses predominate. The most common presentation is headache and visual field defects. An arteriogram or MRA should be performed. 65% rupture; 30% without warning.

- Prior to valvular surgery, a search for a mycotic aneurysm should be performed because the requirement for anticoagulation may produce a massive cerebral bleed.

- In suspected ABE, 3-5 sets of blood cultures should be obtained within 60 minutes, and antibiotic therapy begun immediately thereafter to minimize intracardiac complications (Table 13).

- In SBE, treatment may be delayed safely until culture and sensitivity results are available. Such a delay does not increase the risk of complications in this setting.

- The Gram-positive organisms have become the major challenge to successful antibiotic therapy of IE. *S viridans* has become progressively resistant to penicillin.

- A maximum daily temperature after 10 days of apparently appropriate antibiotic therapy greater than 37° C degrees indicates the possibility of a relatively resistant pathogen, extracardiac infection, pulmonary and systemic emboli, drug fever, a large/difficult to sterilize vegetation, *C difficile* colitis or an infected intravenous site.

- However, complete defervescence in a case of uncomplicated IE may require 2-3 weeks of therapy

- 30% of patients will have a return of fever during therapy, which is usually due to metastatic infection

Table 13

Basic Principles of Antibiotic Therapy of the Infective Endocarditis

The necessity of using bactericidal antibiotics because of the "hostile" environment of the infected vegetation.[a]

The MIC and MBC of the administered antibiotic against the isolated pathogen needs to be determined in order to insure adequate dosing of the agent.

Generally, intermittent dosing of an antibiotic provides superior penetration of the thrombus as compared to a continuous infusion. Its penetration into tissue is directly related to its peak level in serum.

All patients with infective endocarditis should be treated in a health care facility for the first 1-2 weeks to monitor their hemodynamic stability.

In cases of potential acute infective endocarditis, antibiotic therapy should be started immediately after 3-5 sets blood cultures have been drawn. Preferably all of them should be obtained within 1 to 2 hours so as to allow the expeditious commencement of antibiotic therapy. The selection of antibiotic/antibiotics to needs to be made empirically on the basis of physical examination and clinical history.

In cases of potential subacute infective endocarditis, antibiotic treatment should not be started until the final culture and sensitivity data are available. A delay of 1 to 2 weeks in doing so does not adversely affect the final outcome.

The usual duration of therapy ranges from 4-6 weeks. A 4 week course is appropriate for an uncomplicated case of native valve endocarditis. A shorter course of 2 weeks may be appropriate in certain cases (see text). 6 weeks required for the treatment of prosthetic valve endocarditis and in those infections with large vegetations such as associated with infection by members of the HACEK family.

[a] Linezolid and quintristin/dalfopristin appear to be exceptions to this principle.

12. Antibiotic Therapy of Streptococci and Enterococci

- The MIC of sensitive *S viridans* is less than 0.12 mcg/ml. The MIC of relatively resistant *S viridans* ranges from 0.12 mcg/ml to 0.5 mcg/ml. The MIC of highly resistant *S viridans* is >0.5 mcg/ml (Tables 14,15).

- 13.4% of *S viridans* retrieved from BSIs have MIC >1.0 mcg/ml; 17% of these are also highly resistant to ceftriaxone (MIC >2.0 mcg/ml).

- 2 weeks therapy (short course therapy) of *S viridans* NVE may be appropriate if the isolate is sensitive to penicillin; the disease is of less than 3 months duration; vegetation size is less than 10 mm in diameter; there are no cardiac or extracardiac complications; there is a low risk for developing after aminoglycoside nephrotoxicity and there is a good clinical response during the first week of therapy.

- All *Abiotrophia* spp. have some degree of resistance to penicillin.

- Penicillin, ampicillin and vancomycin are only inhibitory to the enterococci. Synergism with an aminoglycoside is required for their killing by these agents.

- Enterococci are resistant to all the cephalosporins and other beta-lactam compounds, except penicillin and ampicillin.

- Because of the potential for multiple mechanisms of resistance, enterococcal isolates from cases of IE need to be tested for high-level resistance to streptomycin and gentamicin, beta-lactamase production and sensitivity to penicillin, ampicillin and vancomycin.

- When there is resistance to both gentamicin and streptomycin, ampicillin continuously infused to achieve a serum level of 60 mcg/ml has had some success.

- In the setting of gentamicin resistant/ampicillin sensitive enterococci, the addition of ceftriaxone (2 gms IV every 12 hours) for 12 weeks has had some success (67%).

- The use of quinpristin/dalfopristin, linezolid and daptomycin should be considered in treating resistant enterococci.

- Quinpristin/alpha person is only active against *E faecium*, but not against *E faecalis* (the most commonly isolated enterococcus).

- Linezolid is bacteriostatic. The addition of an aminoglycoside may have an additive effect against some isolates of enterococci.

- Daptomycin is bactericidal against enterococci, however, there is little experience with the use of this compound against these organisms (Table 16).

Table 14

Guidelines for Antimicrobial Therapy of Nonenterococcal Streptococcal Native Value IE[b]

Antibiotic	Dosage Regimen
A. Penicillin-sensitive S viridans and S bovis[d]	
Penicillin G[a]	Penicillin G 20,000,000 U IV in 4 divided doses for 4 weeks
Penicillin G[a] and Gentamicin[c]	Penicillin 20,000,000 U IV in 4 divided doses for 2 weeks gentamicin 3 mg/kg given QD as a single dose or in divided doses TID for 2 weeks (Ceftriaxone 2 g IV/1M for 4 weeks may be used in patients with mild reactions to penicillin).
or Ceftriaxone	Ceftriaxone 2 g IV/1M for 4 weeks (may be used in patients with mild reactions to penicillin)
B. Penicillin- relatively resistant or tolerant S viridans and S bovis for[d,e]	
Penicillin G[a] or Ceftriaxone	Penicillin G 24,000,000 U IV in 4 divided doses for 4 weeks and Ceftriaxone 2 g IV/IM for 4 weeks
Gentamicin	Gentamicin 3 mg/kg given QD as a single dose or in divided doses TID for 2 weeks
Resistant S viridans Abiotrophia spp. and Group B streptococci[d,f]	
Penicillin G[a] and	Penicillin G 24,000,000 U IV in 4 divided doses for 6 weeks
Gentamicin	Gentamicin 3 mg/kg given QD as a single dose or in divided doses q8h for 2 weeks

Drug dosages:
[a] Vancomycin 30 mg/kg IV BID in patients highly allergic to penicillin.
[b] For patients with normal renal function.
[c] Short course therapy (see text)
[d] See text for definition
[e] Regimen is appropriate for treatment of prosthetic valve endocarditis with penicillin sensitive S viridans or S bovis
[f] For relatively resistant S viridans PVE treatment

Table 15

Treatment of Enterococcal Native Valve Infective Endocarditis

Type of Resistance	Regimen[c]
1) None	Penicillin G (18-30 million units/24hrs IV)[a] Or Ampicillin (12 gms/24hrs IV) Or Vancomycin (30 mg/kg/24hrs IV) Plus Gentamicin (3 mg/kg/24hrs IV/IM)
2) Resistant to Penicillins due to beta-lactamase Production	Ampicillin-sulbactam (12 gms/24hrs IV)[a] Or Vancomycin (30 mg/kg/24hrs)
3) Intrinsic Penicillin Resistance[d,e]	Vancomycin (30 mg/kg/24hrs) Plus Gentamicin (3 mg/kg/24hrs) of the
4) Resistance to Penicillins	Aminoglycosides and Vancomycin[d,e]
a) *E faecium*	Linezolid (1200 mg/24hrsIV/PO)[b,d] Or Quinupristin-dalfopristin (22.5 mg/kg/24hrsIV)[b,d]
b) *E faecalis*	Imipenem (2 gm/24hrs)[b,d] Plus Ampicillin (12 gm/24hrs IV)

[a] *4 weeks duration in symptoms <3 months; 6 weeks if symptoms >3 months*
[b] *Treatment should extend for at least 8 weeks*
[c] *For adults with normal renal function*
[d] *For both native and prosthetic valve endocarditis*
[e] *May require emergent valve surgery for cure*

13. Antibiotic Therapy of *S aureus*

- The penicillinase-resistant penicillins are the drugs of choice in treating MSSA IE; vancomycin is significantly less effective (35% failure rate). Part of this failure is due to increasing prevalence of high sets of *S aureus* with an MIC >4.0 mcg/ml. In addition, penetration of vancomycin into target tissues is decreased, especially in diabetics. Accordingly, a target trough level of 15 mcg /ml is advocated (Table 17).

- Because of the high failure rate in treating MSSA and MRSA IE with vancomycin, other therapies should be considered (Table 16).

- Abbreviated therapy (2 weeks for IVDAIE) cannot be used in patients with advanced AIDS, left-sided disease or evidence of metastatic infection.

- The addition of 5 days of gentamicin (1 mg/kg TID) to vancomycin to the penicillinase-resistant penicillin should generally be avoided because of a significant increase in renal failure with this combination.

- A growing clinical challenge is the management of *S aureus* BSI and the presence of an intravascular catheter. More than 25% of these BSIs represent IE. Short-term catheters always need to be removed in the setting of an *S aureus* BSI.

- It is essential to differentiate cases of uncomplicated staphylococcal BSI from IE, not only for deciding the length of antibiotic therapy but whether the long-term catheter needs to be removed (Table 18).

- *S aureus* bacteria and hematuria may be indicative of a sustained *S aureus* BSI.

- TEE is the most specific approach for separating an uncomplicated continuous BSI from IE. At least 23% of *S aureus* CRBSI with negative TTEs have significant evidence of valvular infection by TEE. Table 13 presents an approach to the management of long-term intravascular catheter-associated *S aureus* continuous BSI.

- Surgically implanted long-term catheters (Brophy act, Hickman) do not need to be automatically removed, except: in the presence of IE, infection of the past in the tunnel, separative thrombophlebitis or infection by certain pathogens (corynebacteria JK, *Pseudomonas* spp., fungi, *S aureus* or mycobacteria). Intraluminal infusions of antibiotic achieve a cure rate of 30%-50% against the other pathogens.

Table 16

Alternative Treatment Regimens for Endocarditis Caused by Highly Resistant

Gram-Positive Organisms[a]

Antibiotic and Dosage	Undesired Effects
Linezolid 600 mg every 12 hours IV or PO[b]	Peripheral Neuropathy Optic Neuritis Hematological Effects Development of Resistance
Quipristin/Dalfopristin 7.5 mg/kg Every 8 Hours	Thrombophlebitis Myalgias
Daptomycin 6 mg Or 12 mg/kg Every 24 Hours[c]	Myositis Increasing Resistance;Cross Resistance with Vancomycin
Tigecycline initial dose 100 mg IV; 50 mg IV every 12 hours	Gastrointestinal Intolerance

[a] *See Text For Discussion*
[b] *Excellent Po Absorption Is Useful For Transition Therapy*
[c] *Higher Dosage Has Been Used In Relatively Resistant Organisms*

Table 17

Antibiotic Therapy of *S aureus* Infective Endocarditis[a]

Valve type (IE type)	Antibiotic	Dosage
Native (MSSA)	Oxacillin[d] ± Gentamicin	Oxacillin 2 g IV q4h for 4-6 weeks ± gentamicin 3 mg/kg q gentamicin 3 mg/kg q 24h as a single dose or in divided doses TID for 5 days in
	Or	
	Vancomycin[b,c] ± Gentamicin	Vancomycin 15 mg/kg IV BID for 4-6 weeks ± Gentamicin 3 mg/kg QD as a single dose or in divided doses TID for 5 days
	Or	
	Cefazolin ± Gentamicin	Cefazolin 1.5 g IV TID for 4-6 weeks (in patients with mild allergies to penicillin) ± Gentamicin 3 mg/kg QD as a single dose or in divided doses TID for 5 days
Prosthetic (MSSA)	Oxacillin[d]	Oxacillin 2 g IV q4h for 4-6 weeks or Vancomycin 15 mg/kg IV BID for 4-6 weeks or Cefazolin 1.5 g IV TID for 4-6 weeks in patients with mild allergies to penicillin
	Or	
	Vancomycin	
	Or	
	Cefazolin	
	And	
	Rifampin	Rifampin 300 mg PO TID for 6 weeks
	And	
	Gentamicin	Gentamicin 3 mg/kg QD as a single dose or in divided doses TID for 2 weeks
Native (MRSA)	Vancomycin[c]	Vancomycin 15 mg/kg IV BID for 4-6 weeks
Prosthetic (MRSA)[e]	Vancomycin[c]	Vancomycin 15 mg/kg IV BID for 4-6 weeks
	And	
	Rifampin	Rifampin 300 mg PO TID for 6 weeks
	And	
	Gentamicin	Gentamicin 3 mg/kg QD as a single dose or in divided doses TID for 2 weeks

[a] For patients with normal renal function.
[b] For patients with severe penicillin allergy
[c] Substitute linezolid in critically ill patients or those with significant renal failure (refer to discussion in text and Table 7)
[d] May substitute nafcillin at equal doses for patients in significant renal failure
[e] If the isolate is resistant to the aminoglycosides, a quinolone to which it is proven sensitive may be substituted

Table 18

Management of *S aureus*, Noncontinuous Bacteremia in the Presence of a Short-term Intravascular Catheter

1. Prompt removal of the catheter
2. Institution of appropriate antibiotic therapy
3. Follow-up blood cultures within 24-48 hours
    A. If follow-up blood cultures are negative and :
        1. The TEE shows no signs of infective endocarditis
        2. There is no evidence of metastatic infection

            Then 2 weeks of antibiotic therapy would be appropriate

    B. If follow-up blood cultures are positive and:
        1. The TEE shows signs of infective endocarditis

            Then 4 weeks of intravenous therapy is appropriate

    C. If follow-up blood cultures are positive and:
        1. The TEE shows no signs of infective endocarditis,

    Further imaging studies should be performed to rule out other sources of bacteremia
        (osteomyelitis, mediastinitis, splenic abscess)

14. Antibiotic Treatment of CoNS IE

- Rifampin is the key component of treatment of PVE, whether it is caused by CoNS or *S aureus*, because is able to kill both within the adherent biofilm. The other 2 components are to prevent development of rifampin-resistant organisms. In those strains that are resistant to gentamicin, a fluoroquinolone may substitute (Table 19).

15. Antibiotic Treatment of Assorted Organisms and of Fungal IE

- A combined medical and surgical approach is usually necessary for the cure of fungal IE (Tables 20-24).

- Capsofungin and voriconazole appear to be less toxic alternatives to amphotericin B.

16. Surgical Treatment of IE

- Overall, surgery is required in 25% of cases of IE. 25% of these are performed during the early stage of the disease.

- In both NVE and PVE, CHF, refractory to standard medical therapy, is the most common cause for surgery.

- Other clinical indications include: fungal IE; BSI that persist past 7 days of appropriate antibiotic therapy and which is determined to originate from an extracardiac source (especially splenic abscess); recurrent septic emboli after 2 weeks of appropriate antibiotic therapy; rupture of an aneurysm of the sinus of Valsalva; conduction disturbances secondary to septal abscesses and "kissing" infection of the anterior mitral valve leaflet occurring in cases of aortic valve IE.

- The echocardiographic findings that are most predictive of the need for surgery are: detectable vegetations following a large embolus; anterior mitral valve vegetations >1 cm in diameter; continued growth of vegetation after 4 weeks of anabolic therapy; development of acute mitral insufficiency; rupture or perforation of the valve leaflet and perivalvular extension of the valvular infection.

- Splenic abscess is a significant mimic of unresponsive IE, since it is clinically occult and may produce a continuous BSI.

- Surgery is often needed to eradicate a variety of metastatic infections, including mycotic aneurysms and cerebral abscesses.

- Cure of PMIE requires that the entire system be removed. Pacemaker leads that have been in place for more than 18 months are actually difficult to remove. Excimer laser sheaths successfully dissolve the fibrotic bands that encase the electrodes and free up the wires in more than 90% of cases.

Table 19

Therapy for Coagulase-Negative Staphylococcal Infection of PVE[a,b]

Antibiotic	Dosage Regimen
Vancomycin	15 mg/kg BID for 6 weeks
And	
Rifampin	300 mg PO TID for 6 weeks
And	
Gentamicin	3 mg/kg QD IV as a single dose or in divided doses BID for 2 weeks

[a] 80% of isolates recovered within the first year after valve replacement are resistant to the beta-lactam antibiotics. After this period, 30% are resistant. Sensitivity to the penicillins must be confirmed because standard sensitivity testing may not detect resistance. If the isolate is sensitive, oxacillin or cefazolin may be substituted.

[b] If the organism is resistant to the aminoglycosides, a quinolone, to which it is proven sensitive, should be substituted.

Table 20

Suggested Representative Antibiotic Therapy of IE Caused by Enterobacteriaceae

Organism	Antibiotic	Dosage Regimen[a,b,c]
E coli and Proteus mirabilis	Ampicillin	12 grams/day
	±	
	Gentamicin	5 mg/kg/day
	Or	
	Ceftriaxone	1-2 g/day
	Or	
	Ciprofloxacin	400 mg IV BID
Enterobacter spp. Klebsiella spp.	Ticarcillin/Clavulanic acid	6 gm (ticarcillin) IV QID
Citrobacter spp.[d], Providencia spp.	Meropenem	2 g IV TID
	Or	
	Ceftriaxone	2 g IV BID
	Or	
	Cefipime	2 g BID
	Plus	
	Gentamicin	5 mg/kg/day

(continued)

Table 20

Suggested Representative Antibiotic Therapy of IE Caused by Enterobacteriaceae

Organism	Antibiotic	Dosage Regimen[a,b,c]
S marcescens[e]	Cefipime	2 g IV TID
	Or	
	Imipenem	1g IV QID
	Or	
	Ciprofloxacin	400 mg IV BID
	Plus	
	Amikacin	7.5 mg/kg IV BID
Salmonella spp.	Ceftriaxone	2 gm IV BID
	Or	
	Ciprofloxacin	400 mg IV BID

[a] For patients with normal renal function.

[b] Duration of therapy at least 6 weeks.

[c] Final selection must be based on sensitivity testing.

[d] C freundi most resistant species of Citrobacter.

[e] High frequency of multidrug resistance. Amikacin sensitivity usually preserved. Plasmid-mediated resistant to third and fourth generation cephalosporins and carbapenems. Extended spectrum beta-lactamases encountered. Quinolone resistance occurs.

Table 21

Antibiotic Therapy of Various Types of IE[a]

Organism	Antibiotic Regimen	Alternative Regimen
Culture-negative	Ampicillin 2 g IV q4h for 4 weeks[b] And Gentamicin 5 mg/kg QD IV given in a single dose or in divided doses TID for the first 2 weeks And Oxacillin 2 g IV q4h for 4 weeks Or If MRSA is suspected or prosthetic material is present, vancomycin 30 mg/kg BID for 4 weeks	
Ps. aeruginosa	Ticarcillin 3 g IV q4h for 6 weeks[b] And Tobramycin 5 mg/kg QD IV given in a single dose or in divided doses TID	Ceftazidime[c] 2 g IV TID for 6 weeks Or Aztreonam[d] 2 g IV q6h for 6 weeks And Tobramycin 5 mg/kg IV QD given in a single dose or in divided doses TID
HACEK group	Ampicillin 2 g IV q4h for 4-6 weeks[b] And Gentamicin 5 mg/kg QD as a single dose or in divided doses TID	Ceftazidimec 2 g IV TID for 4-6 weeks And Gentamicin 5 mg/kg QD given in a single dose or in divided doses

[a] For patients with normal renal function.
[b] Preferred regimen (see text).
[c] 1n patients with mild penicillin allergy.
[d] 1n patients with severe penicillin allergy.

Table 22

Antibiotic Therapy of Various Forms of Infective Endocarditis[a,b]

Organism	Dosage Regimen
C jeikium	Vancomycin 1 g BID IV Plus Gentamicin 1 mg/kg TID
L monocytogenes	Ampicillin 12 g/day Plus Gentamicin 1.7 mg/kg TID
C burnetii	Doxycycline 100 mg IV/PO BID Plus Chloroquine 200 mg TID[c]
Brucella spp.	Doxycycline 100 mg BID PO Plus Rifampin 900 mg/day PO Plus Trimethoprim - Sulfamethoxazole 160/800 mg PO TID
Bartonella spp.	Ceftriaxone 2 g/day for 6 weeks, gentamicin 1 mg/kg TID for 14 days Plus Doxycycline 100 mg IV for 6 weeks

[a] For patients with normal renal function
[b] Given for at least 6 weeks
[c] See text for duration of therapy

Table 23

Resistance Patterns of Candida Species

Candida Species	Sensitivity to Antifungals[a]
C albicans	Sensitive to all classes of antifungals
C glabrata	Potentially resistant to all azole antifungals and relatively resistant to amphotericin
C parapsilosis	Sensitive to all classes of antifungals but may be relativel resistant to caspofungin
C krusei	Resistant to fluconazole. May be relatively resistant to amphotericin
C lusitaniae	Resistant to amphotericin

[a] Standardization of testing has not been established for echinocandins

Table 24

Approach to the Patient at Risk for Candidal Endocarditis

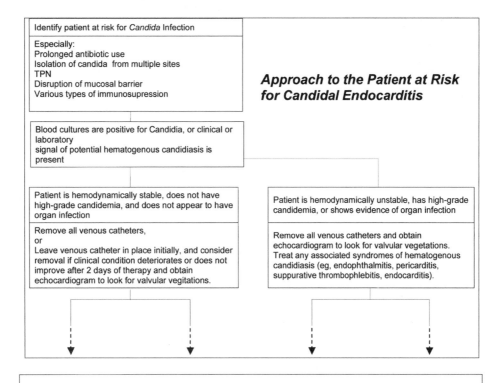

Identify patient at risk for *Candida* Infection

Especially:
Prolonged antibiotic use
Isolation of candida from multiple sites
TPN
Disruption of mucosal barrier
Various types of immunosupression

Approach to the Patient at Risk for Candidal Endocarditis

Blood cultures are positive for Candidia, or clinical or laboratory
signal of potential hematogenous candidiasis is present

Patient is hemodynamically stable, does not have high-grade candidemia, and does not appear to have organ infection

Remove all venous catheters,
or
Leave venous catheter in place initially, and consider removal if clinical condition deteriorates or does not improve after 2 days of therapy and obtain echocardiogram to look for valvular vegitations.

Patient is hemodynamically unstable, has high-grade candidemia, or shows evidence of organ infection

Remove all venous catheters and obtain echocardiogram to look for valvular vegetations. Treat any associated syndromes of hematogenous candidiasis (eg, endophthalmitis, pericarditis, suppurative thrombophlebitis, endocarditis).

Patient is infected or colonized by *C albicans, C tropicalis, C parapsiolsis.*

Give fluconazole, 600-800 mg/day IV for 2-3 days, then, if possible, lower dosage to 400 mg/day PO
Treat for 7-10 days (patient should be free of signs and symptoms of infection for 5 days before treatment is ended).

Patient is infected or colonized by *C krusei, C glabrata,* or *C lusitaniae*

Capsofungin or Voriconazole preferred to the older regimin of Amphoterecin ± flucytosine.
Treat for 5-7 days (patient should be free of signs and symptoms of infection for 5 days before treatment is ended).

Patient is infected or colonized by *C albicans, C tropicalis , C parapsiolsis.*

Give amphotericin B at full dosage. Consider adding flucytosine, 25 mg/day PO in 2 divided doses. Also consider adding G-CSF, 300 g/day).
Capsofungin or Voriconazole may be preferable.
Treat for 10-14 days and then evaluate for need of valvular replacement.

Patient is infected or colonized by *C krusei, C glabrata* or *C lusitaniae*

Capsofungin or Voriconazole may be preferable to the older regimen of Amphoterecin B +/- flucytosine. Consider adding G-CSF, 300 g/day.
Treat for 10-14 days and then evaluate for need of valvular replacement.

Adapted from Anaisse EJ, Bishara AB, Solomkin JS. Fungal Infection. In: ACS Surgery 2005. Souba WW, Fink Mp, Jurkovich GJ,et al. New York, NY: Web Professional Publishing; 2005: 1486-1487.

17. Anticoagulation in IE

- Because of the risk of cerebral bleed in IE, anticoagulation should generally be avoided. There is no therapeutic effect on the course of IE itself by anticoagulation.

- A major exception is those patients already with prosthetic valves in place.

- When thrombi occur in extracardiac sites, anticoagulation may be used as ordinarily indicated. Other approaches such as interrupting the vena cava must also be considered.

18. Outcome of Treated IE

- Relapse of IE usually occurs within 2 months of the end of apparently successful anabolic therapy (Table 25).

- *S aureus*, enterococci and Gram-negative organisms, especially P aeruginosa, have the highest rates of relapse (8%-20%).

- Those with symptoms of IE for more than 3 months prior to the beginning of treatment have a higher incidence of relapse.

- Enterococcal IE of the mitral valve has the greatest chance of relapse.

- Recurrent IE is seen most often in IVDA IE. Other risk factors for recurrence are a previous episode of IE, the presence of a prosthetic valve and congenital heart disease.

19. Antimicrobial Prophylaxis

- Antimicrobial prophylaxis is recommended only in those conditions which have the greatest potential for developing a severe outcome if valvular infection was to occur. In sharp contrast to previous recommendations, abnormalities of native valves, except those that have suffered a previous case of IE, are not felt to be candidates for antimicrobial prophylaxis (Table 26).

- These revisions are predicated on the following principles: 1.) IE results much more frequently from BSI associated with daily living (eg, brushing one's teeth) than from the BSIs due to dental, GI or GU invasive procedures; 2.) Since the administration of antibiotics prevent an extremely small amount of cases of IE, serious adverse reactions to these agents exceeds the benefit of prophylaxis; and 3.) Adherence to establish guidelines for the establishment of good oral hygiene that limits the amount of spontaneous BSIs is probably more effective and far safer than antibiotics.

- Cardiac conditions with the highest risk for adverse outcomes from IE:

  * Previous IE.

  * Prosthetic cardiac valve.

  * Congenital heart disease, specifically unrepaired cyanotic disease, including palliative shunts in conduits and completely repaired congenital heart defects with prosthetic material during the first 6 months after procedure, and repaired congenital heart disease residual defects of the site adjacent to the site of a prosthetic patch or device which inhibits endothelialization.

  * Cardiac transplant recipients who develop valvulopathy.

- Dental procedures that require prophylaxis are all procedures that involve manipulation of gingival tissue, the periapical region of teeth or perforation of the oral mucosa.

Table 25

Mortality Rates of Left-sided Native Valve Infective Endocarditis Due to Various Organisms

Organism	Mortality Rates
S viridans and *S bovis*	4%-6%
Enterococci	15%-25%
S aureus	25%-47%
Groups B, C, G streptococci	13%-50%
C burnetti	5%-37%
P aeruginosa, Enterobacteriaceae, fungi	>50%

Table 26

Antibiotic Regimens for Prophylaxis of IE

Situation	Agent and dosage given 30 to 60 minutes before procedure
Oral	Amoxicillin 2 g PO
Unable to take oral medication	Ampicillin or cefazolin / ceftriaxone, 1 g IM or IV
Allergic to penicillin or ampicillin - oral	Cephalexin 2 g or clindamycin 600 mg or azithromycin / clarithromycin 500 mg
Allergic to penicillins or ampicillin and unable to take oral medication	Cefazolin/ceftriaxone 1 g IM or IV or Clindamycin 600 mg IM or IV

- Recommendations for respiratory tract procedures are to cover for *S viridans*, as in dental procedures. Add vancomycin if the likelihood of *S aureus* is high.

- Recommendations for GI/GU tract procedures are generally to not give prophylaxis because of lack of evidence that it is necessary. Consider antimicrobial prophylaxis for a GU procedure in the presence of enterococci in the urine.

- Recommendations for procedures on uninfected skin, skin structure or musculoskeletal tissue are to use prophylaxis aimed at staphylococci/beta-hemolytic streptococci.

- Antibiotic prophylaxis may be considered for patients at highest risk for adverse outcomes who undergo an incision or biopsy of the respiratory mucosa (tonsillectomy, adenoidectomy). As in dental procedures, the targeted organism would primarily be *S viridans*.

20. Prevention of Intravascular Catheter Infections

- Because of its significant role in HCIE, prevention of CRBSI must be considered another form of prophylaxis (Table 27).

ID Board Pearls

- There is an association of vancomycin and daptomycin resistance in *S aureus*. This may be seen especially in patients previously exposed to vancomycin. 1 possible mechanism is decreased penetration of daptomycin into the staphylococcus in patients previously exposed to vancomycin. Therefore, consider an increased dosage of daptomycin (12 mg/kg per day) in patients with *S aureus* IE.

- *T whipplei* IE often present as an indolent infection with arthralgias, CHF and emboli with mild-to-absent GI symptoms.

  * Often there is no fever. Blood cultures are negative. Echocardiogram shows large vegetations with pericardial abscess and valvular incompetence. Blood cultures are negative. Vegetations are PCR positive. PSA stains show foamy macrophages with bacteria on silver stain. Treatment consists of surgery plus ceftriaxone, followed by 1-3 years of cotrimoxazole.

- The most common cause of culture-negative IE due to fastidious pathogens is Bartonella. *B quintana* is seen in homeless alcoholics associated with lice. B henselae is associated with cats. Diagnosis is made primarily by PCR testing of blood cultures with extended incubation in isolator tubes. Serologic testing with ELISA or PVE immunofluorescence absent is available. Pathology shows pleomorphic intracellular bacteria on silver stains. Treatment: doxycycline for 6 weeks plus gentamicin for 2 weeks.

- *S aureus* is most common cause of NVE and PVE. Primary risk factors: exposure to health care facilities and IVDA.

- Always use 2 synergistic antibiotics for treatment of enterococcal IE. When sensitivities allow, ampicillin is preferable to penicillin, which is markedly preferable to vancomycin/daptomycin. In gentamicin resistance, always test for streptomycin, as about 25% of such strains will be sensitive to the latter.

- *S lugdunensis* IE is a coagulase-negative staphylococcus that is community-acquired. It is usually susceptible to oxacillin. It is quite damaging to valves, leading to a high rate of surgery. Mortality is 50%.

- *C burnetti* causes 3%-5% of IE in France, Israel and the UK. Involves previously abnormal valves. Transmitted from farm animals. It is chronic in nature. Examination shows hepatosplenomegaly and a purpuric rash. Diagnosis is PCR test of excised valves or IgG ab >800. Treatment is doxycycline plus hydrocortisone for 18 months. Usually valves surgery is required.

- Under the 2007 guidelines, the only indication for antibiotic prophylaxis of a native valve is a previous bout of endocarditis.

- Treatment of penicillin-resistant (M. IC >0.5 mcg/ml) *S viridans* and *S bovis* NVE.

- Treat as if they have enterococci with synergistic combination of ampicillin/penicillin plus gentamicin or vancomycin plus gentamicin; each for 4-6 weeks.

- *S bovis* IE always should trigger a bowel work-up because of its association with colonic disease (neoplasia).

- 15% of cases of SBE present with low back pain. Etiology is not clear, but the pain disappears with successful treatment of the valvular infection.

- Currently the most common causes of renal failure in IE are congestive heart failure and antibiotic nephrotoxicity.

- The major risk factors for development of PMIE are: manipulation of the pacemaker system; prior temporary transvenous pacer, inexperienced interventionist with a history of doing less than 100 procedures and presence of a hematoma in the pacemaker pocket.

- IE that develops past 2 weeks following an invasive dental procedure is highly unlikely to be caused by that procedure.

- Noninfectious anatomic abnormalities sitting in the IE on echocardiography include: sterile thrombus, capillary fibroma, aortic valve Lambl's excrescence (a short filamentous projection off a valve leaflet), beam-width artifact from a calcified valve, marantic endocarditis and myxomatous mitral valve.

- An infected thrombus of the anterior leaflet of the mitral valve has the highest incidence of embolization.

- Recovery in blood cultures of a coagulase negative staphylococcus from a case of rapidly progressive valvular infection should not be discounted as a contaminant (eg, *S epidermidis*). It must be assumed to be *S lugdunensis* until proven otherwise.

- Currently, about 5% of cases of NVE are now caused by non-*S lugdunensis* coagulase-negative staphylococci.

- In the diagnosis of IE, the chance of obtaining positive blood cultures has no relationship to the course of the patient's fever, since the bacteremia is continuous. The blood cultures can be drawn at any time.

- In adults, bicuspid aortic valves are the most common underlying congenital cardiac abnormality in IE.

Table 27

The Most Effective Strategies for the Prevention of Infection of Intravascular Catheters

Development of a comprehensive prevention strategy.

100% compliance with hand washing.

Insertion of central catheters under strict sterile conditions

Use of chlorhexidine as skin disinfectant.

Avoidance of inserting femoral catheters.

No routine replacement of intravenous catheters.

Removal of catheters as soon as medically feasible.

Use of antibiotic impregnated catheters[a]

[a] *Use only under special circumstances (refer to text)*

21. Further Reading

Baddour LM, Wilson WR, Bayer AS, et al. Infective endocarditis: diagnosis, antimicrobial therapy and management of complications: a statement for health care professionals From the Committee on Rheumatic Fever, Endocarditis and on Clinical Cardiology, Stroke and Cardiovascular Surgery and Anesthesia, American Heart Association: endorsed by the Infectious Diseases Society of America. *Circulation*. 2005;111:e394-434.

Brusch JL, ed. *Infective Endocarditis: Management in the Era of Intravascular Devices*. New York, NY: Informa; 2007.

Fang G, Keys TF, Gentry LO, et al. Prosthetic valve endocarditis resulting from nosocomial bacteremia: a prospective multicenter study. *Ann Intern Med*. 1993;119:560-567.

Fowler VJ JR, Miro JM, Hoen B, et al. Staphylococcus aureus endocarditis: a consequence of medical progress. *JAMA*. 2005;293:3012-3021.

Houpikian P, Raoult D. Blood culture-negative endocarditis in a reference center. *Medicine*. 2005;84:162-173.

Maki DG, Kluger DM, Cnrich CJ. The risk of bloodstream infections and adults with different intravascular devices: a systemic review of 200 published prospective studies. *Mayo Clin Proc*. 2006;81:1159-1171.

Mylonakis E, Calderwood SB. Infective endocarditis in adults. *N Engl J Med*. 2001;345:1318-1330.

Pronovost P, Needham D, Berenholtz S, et al. Intervention to decrease catheter-related bloodstream infections in the ICU. *N Engl J Med*. 2006;355:2725-2732.

Roe MT, Abramson MA, Li J, et al. Clinical information determines the impact of transesophageal echocardiography on the diagnosis of infective endocarditis by the Duke criteria. *Am Heart J*. 2000;139:945-953.

Safar N, Kluger D, Maki D. A review of risk factors for catheter related bloodstream infection caused by percutaneously inserted noncuffed central venous catheters. *Medicine*. 2002;81:466-474.

Sambola A, Miro JM, Tornos MP, et al. Streptococcus agalactiae infective endocarditis: analysis of 30 cases in review of the literature, 1962-1998. *Clin Infect Dis*. 2002;34(12):1576-1584.

Sheagren J. Staphylococcus aureus, the persistent pathogen. *N Engl J Med*. 1984;310:1368-1374.

Towns ML, Reller LB. Diagnostic methods: current practices guidelines for isolation of bacteria and fungi in infective endocarditis. *Infect Dis Clin NA*. 2002;16:363-376.

Wilson W, Taubert KA, Gewitz M, et al. Prevention of infective endocarditis: guidelines for the American Heart Association: a guideline for the American Heart Association Rheumatic Fever, Endocarditis and Kawasaki Disease Committee, Council on Cardiovascular Disease in the Young and the Council on Clinical Cardiology, Council on Cardiovascular Surgery and Anesthesia, and the Quality of Care and Outcomes Research Interdisciplinary Working Group. *Circulation*. 2007;116:1736-1754

Chapter 19:
Viral Hepatitis
for the ID Boards

Raymond S. Koff, MD

Contents

1. Acute Viral Hepatitis

- Viral hepatitis is the most common cause of liver disease in the world; its sequelae are responsible for 1-2 million deaths annually.

- Subclinical or anicteric infections are more common than symptomatic infections with jaundice.

- The blood-borne hepatitis viruses (hepatitis B, D, and C) are globally the most common causes of persistent viremia.

The Agents of Viral Hepatitis

Overview
The responsible agents can be classified into 3 major groups:

- The enterically transmitted viruses: hepatitis A virus (HAV) and hepatitis E virus (HEV).

- The blood-borne viruses: hepatitis B virus (HBV), hepatitis D virus (HDV) and hepatitis C virus (HCV).

- Agents producing a liver injury that is usually overshadowed by involvement of extrahepatic organs: herpes simplex virus, CMV, Epstein-Barr virus and others.

The Enterically Transmitted Hepatitis Viruses

- Are nonenveloped.

- Survive exposure to bile.

- Are shed in feces.

- Are usually spread via fecal-oral routes.

- Do not cause chronic liver disease (rare reports of chronic HEV infection in organ-transplant recipients).

- Do not cause persistent viremia or intestinal carriage.

- Generally cause self-limited infections, which may be severe.

The Blood-borne Hepatitis Viruses
- Are enveloped.

- Can be disrupted by contact with bile or detergents.

- Are not shed in feces.

- Can cause chronic liver disease.

- Can cause persistent viremia.

The Nonhepatitis Viruses That Cause Liver Injury
- Include members of the *Herpesviridae, Parvoviridae, Togaviridae, Flaviviridae, Filoviridae, Bunyaviridae, Arenaviridae* and *Picornaviridae*.

- Should be considered in immunocompromised individuals and infants in whom tests for conventional hepatitis virus infections are negative.

- Should be considered when evidence of liver injury occurs in hemorrhagic fevers.

Characteristics of Hepatitis A Virus (HAV)

- Classified as a member of the *Picornaviridae*, the sole member of the *Hepatovirus* genus.

- A 27-32 nm, spherical particle.

- Single-stranded, linear RNA genome, 7.5 kb.

- Has 1 open reading frame.

- Has 4 virion polypeptides in capsomere.

- 1 human serotype, 4 genotypes.

- Replication is limited to cytoplasm of the infected hepatocyte.

- Is propagated in nonhuman and human cell lines.

- Noncytopathic; injury is immunologically mediated.

- Host range: human, chimpanzees, marmosets.

- High level of thermal and chemical resistance.

Hepatitis E Virus (HEV)

- Classified as a member of the *Hepeviridae*, sole member of the Hepevirus genus.

- 27-34 nm spherical particle.

- Linear RNA genome, 7.2 kb.

- 3 overlapping reading frames.

- 1 serotype, 4-9 genotypes: genotypes 1 and 2 in human cases and waterborne outbreaks; genotypes 3 and 4 in swine, other animals, foodborne outbreaks (pork, shellfish, venison).

- *In vivo* replication is limited to hepatocyte cytoplasm.

- Low-level propagation in primate cell lines; cytopathic only in some.

- Host range: humans, nonhuman primates, swine, other mammals; zoonotic transmission suspected.

- Relatively stable in mild acid or alkaline conditions.

Hepatitis B Virus (HBV)

- A member of the hepatotropic DNA-containing viruses (the *Hepadnaviridae*).

- 42 nm spherical particle with a 27-nm electron-dense nucleocapsid core and a 7-nm thick outer lipoprotein-containing envelope (the hepatitis B surface antigen [HBsAg]).

- HBsAg contains 3 envelope proteins, minor lipid and carbohydrate components, and is present both on the intact virion and in 22-nm spherical or tubular, noninfectious but immunogenic particles in excess of HBV particles.

- Nucleocapsid core contains circular, partially double-stranded 3.2-kb DNA, DNA polymerase with reverse transcriptase activity and the hepatitis B core antigen (HBcAg).

- 4 overlapping reading frames.

- The hepatitis B e antigen (HBeAg), a nonstructural derivative of HBcAg, is correlated with active wild-type HBV replication; a precore/core promoter mutant, replicating HBV virus does not express HBeAg (HBeAg-negative).

- Hepatitis B x protein: transactivator, induces apoptosis.

- 8 HBV genotypes (A to H) recognized.

- *In vivo* replication, predominantly but not exclusively in hepatocyte.

- Host range: humans and chimpanzees.

- Limited replication *in vitro* in primary adult and fetal human hepatocytes.

Hepatitis D Virus (HDV)

- Defective, single-stranded, covalently closed circular, 1.7 kb RNA satellite virus (viroid-like) requiring helper functions of HBV for assembly and release.

- Genome complementary HDV antigenome in infected hepatocyte.

- 35-37 nm spherical particle enveloped by HBsAg.

- 1 serotype, at least 3 genotypes.

- Replication limited to hepatocyte (humans and chimpanzees).

- HDV antigen: 2 phosphoprotein isoforms, 1 (the larger) is prenylated and inhibits RNA synthesis; the smaller is a transactivator of RNA replication.

- HBV presence is essential for HDV replication and pathogenicity.

• Primary chimpanzee and woodchuck hepatocytes and human hepatocellular carcinoma cells have been transfected with HDV RNA.

Hepatitis C Virus (HCV)

• Member of *Flaviviridae*, separate genus: *Hepacivirus*

• Lipid, carbohydrate, and protein enveloped spherical virus, 55-60 nm in diameter.

• 33 nm nucleocapsid or core.

• 2 glycosylated envelope proteins.

• Genome is positive-sense, 9.4 kb RNA.

• 1 open reading frame.

• 5 nonstructural proteins include:

    * Metalloproteinase

* Serine protease

* Nucleoside triphosphate-binding helicase

* RNA-dependent RNA polymerase

* Interferon sensitivity determinant region

• 6 major genotypes (nucleotide homology of 65%-70%), more than 80 subtypes (nucleotide homology of 75%-80%).

• Variable geographic distribution (genotypes 1a and 1b represent 70% of all US infections; see Figure 1).

• No relationship of genotype to disease severity, but affects responsiveness to antiviral therapy.

• Closely related genomes called quasispecies with nucleotide homology of 90%-99% in infected patients.

Figure 1

Geographic distribution of HCV genotypes

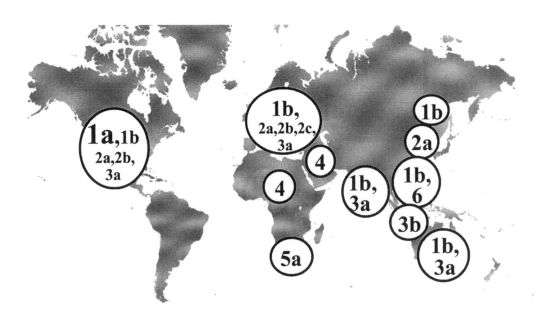

Growth in Tissue Culture

- High level HCV replication by transfection of subgenomic replicons into human hepatocellular cell lines.

Epidemiology

Hepatitis A
- Incubation period: 15-45 days (mean about 30 days).

- Widely distributed globally; high endemicity in developing countries.

- Diminishing incidence in the United States; overall U.S. seroprevalence <30% and declining.

- Accounts for <45% of reported acute viral hepatitis in the United States.

- Excretion of HAV in stool begins during late incubation period and continues for at least 1 week after onset of illness, longer in children.

- Peak fecal HAV shedding and the period of maximal communicability occur at the onset of illness in the majority of affected patients.

- Prolonged fecal excretion (detected by PCR) for months in some but uncertain importance (no long-term intestinal carriers).

- Viremia averages about 30-90 days; viremic carriers are unknown.

- Fecal-oral transmission via person-to-person spread, usually involving children or contaminated water or food; outbreaks in day-care centers, institutions for the developmentally disabled, among men who have sex with men, injection drug users, travelers to endemic regions; community-wide outbreaks.

- Contamination of clotting factor concentrates: rare outbreaks in hemophilia patients.

- Secondary household attack rates average 20%-50%.

- Prevalence correlates with sanitary standards and large household size.

- No identified risk factors in 50% of US cases.

- No evidence for maternal-neonatal infection; transfusion-associated HAV extremely rare.

Hepatitis E
- Incubation period: 40 day average, range 15-60 days.

- Widely distributed: epidemic and endemic forms in Southeast and Central Asia, North Africa, the Middle East, and Mexico, Brazil, Venezuela, and Cuba; rare cases in U.S. usually from travelers from endemic regions, but zoonotic transmission may occur.

- The most common form of sporadic hepatitis in young adults in developing countries (hepatitis A is more common in young children); peak attack rates approach 30%.

- HEV excretion in stools begins during the latter half of the incubation period, or at the onset of illness or 2-3 weeks later.

- Maximal duration of fecal excretion of HEV: 30 days after onset of symptoms.

- HEV may appear in blood before stool but is short-lived; maximal duration of about 45 days after onset of symptoms.

- Waterborne outbreaks common, vary in length, may last months.

- Household transmission infrequent.

- Maternal-neonatal transmission reported, uncertain importance.

Hepatitis B
- Mean incubation period 60-70 days, range 30-180 days.

- HBV DNA detected as early as 1 week after exposure but generally at 30 days.

- HBsAg in serum as early as 1 week after exposure but generally by day 50.

- Viremia lasts for weeks to months in self-limited infections; for decades in persistent infection.

- Persistent infection in 90% of infected neonates, 50% of infants, 10% of immunocompromised adults and <2% of immunocompetent adults.

- Persistent infection linked to chronic hepatitis, cirrhosis, hepatocellular carcinoma and premature death in 25%.

- Widely distributed worldwide (350 million actively infected persons); prevalence of HBV carrier (HBsAg-positive) in the United States is <0.5% (1.25 million); in Asia, sub-Saharan Africa prevalence of HBV carrier is >5%.

- Incidence declining in the United States; greatest decline in Taiwan associated with universal vaccination program.

- HBV present in descending concentrations in blood, semen, cervicovaginal secretions, saliva and other body fluids (Figure 2).

Modes of transmission
- Sexual spread (heterosexual and homosexual) in 50% of cases in Western countries.

- Maternal-neonatal, maternal-infant and child-to-child spread in Asian and African countries.

- Use of shared injection equipment by illicit drug users.

- Hemodialysis patients (intra-unit spread).

- Needlestick or splash accidents in unvaccinated individuals.

- Recipients of multiple blood products (now rare in the United States).

- Tissue penetration via tattoos, body piercing, acupuncture; shared razorblades, toothbrushes.

Figure 2

Estimates of HBV infectivity in body fluids

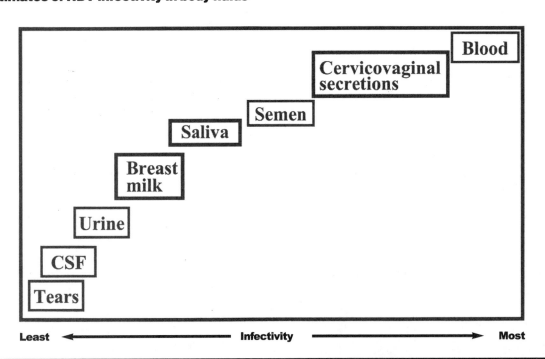

      * Contamination of multidose vials, re-use of syringes or needles

- No evidence for fecal-oral spread.

- No risk factor identified in 25% of cases.

Hepatitis D
- Incubation period: 4-8 weeks.

- Viremia usually short-lived in coinfection with HBV; may be prolonged in superinfection of HBV carriers.

- Declining incidence worldwide; 5 million HBsAg carriers are HDV-infected.

- Modes of transmission are similar to those of HBV.

- Endemic in the Mediterranean littoral, the Balkans, in Africa, the Middle East and the Amazon basin.

- In endemic regions, spread by person-to-person contact, involving children, intrafamilial and sexual contact.

- In non-endemic regions, users of illicit injection drugs are the high-risk group.

- Maternal-neonatal infection reported but importance uncertain.

- No evidence of fecal-oral spread.

Hepatitis C
- Incubation period: average 40-60 days, range 15-130 days.

- Viremia detectable 7-20 days after exposure.

- Persistent viremia in 55%-85% of infections leading to chronic hepatitis, cirrhosis, hepatocellular carcinoma.

- Worldwide distribution, with about 200 million chronic HCV infections; seroprevalence in the United States: 1.6% or 4-5 million people with past or present infection; active infections in the United States: 3-4 million.

- Declining incidence of new infections in the United States.

- Seroprevalence higher in African Americans, highest in age group 39-50 years.

- Modes of transmission include:

    * Shared contaminated equipment for injection drug use

    * In some geographic regions, reuse of unsterilized medical or dental equipment

    * Receipt of multiple blood products (now rare in the United States)

    * Hemodialysis patients (intraunit spread)

    * Sexual contact (3%-5% in monogamous couples over decades)

    * Maternal-neonatal spread (1%-5% if mother is infected)

    * Cocaine snorting, tattooing, body piercing

    * Accidental needle sticks, splash accidents

    * No evidence for fecal-oral spread

    * 10%-40% without identifiable risk factor

Key Clinical Features

Typical acute viral hepatitis (mild to moderate hepatic inflammation and necrosis).

Subclinical Infections
- Recognized only by serologic or biochemical studies undertaken in individuals without symptoms.

Anicteric Infections
- Transient gastrointestinal or upper respiratory symptoms.

- Short-lived anorexia and fatigue.

• Fever for 1-2 days.

Hepatitis with Jaundice
Generally similar clinical syndromes for all agents but:

• Fever more common in HAV and HEV than blood-borne hepatitis.

• Onset usually more abrupt for HAV and HEV infections.

• Serum sickness-like syndrome (immune-complex mediated) in as many as 10% of patients with HBV infection:

  * Fever

  * Arthralgias/migratory polyarthritis

  * Rash (maculopapular or urticarial)

  * Glomerulonephritis (hematuria, nephrotic syndrome)

  * Angioedema

• Nonspecific prodromal constitutional and gastrointestinal symptoms:

  * Malaise, anorexia, nausea, vomiting

  * Flu-like symptoms of pharyngitis, cough, coryza, photophobia, headache and myalgias

• Prodromal symptoms abate or disappear with onset of jaundice, although the anorexia, malaise, and weakness may persist for days.

• Jaundice preceded by the appearance of dark urine, followed by lightening of stool color.

• Pruritus (usually mild, transient) may accompany jaundice.

• Distaste or aversion to cigarettes and cigarette smoke.

• Mild enlargement and slight tenderness of the liver.

• Mild splenomegaly and cervical lymphadenopathy in <20%.

• Jaundice peaks during second week after onset and disappears during the next 2-8 weeks in 85% of cases.

• Symptomatic improvement occurs with resolution of biochemical abnormalities in most cases.

Acute Liver Failure (Severe, Massive Hepatic Necrosis)
• Most common in those >40 years of age.

• Increased risk in patients with pre-existing liver disease.

• Defined by changes in mental status and coagulopathy.

• Shrinking liver size.

Complications
• Cerebral edema.

• Sepsis.

• ARDS and cardiac arrhythmias.

• Renal failure, ascites, anasarca.

• Gastrointestinal bleeding.

• Incidence in icteric hepatitis: generally <1% except among pregnant women with hepatitis E during third trimester, in whom there is a 10%-20% incidence.

• Case fatality rates: 70%-95% if stage 4 encephalopathy (coma) in absence of liver transplantation.

Cholestatic Hepatitis (Intrahepatic Cholestasis)
• Most commonly seen in hepatitis A.

• Persistent jaundice, usually with pruritus, for several months.

• High serum bilirubin and alkaline phosphatase levels.

• Prognosis excellent: full recovery anticipated.

Relapsing Hepatitis (Mild to Moderate Necro-inflammatory Changes)
• Most common in hepatitis A (reappearance of HAV in stool during relapse).

• Symptoms and biochemical abnormalities reappear weeks after apparent recovery.

• Multiple relapses most common in children.

• Infrequently arthritis, vasculitis, cryoglobulinemia.

• Prognosis for full recovery excellent.

Key Laboratory Features
Typical viral hepatitis (self-limited disease).

• Peak alkaline aminotransferase and aspartate aminotransferase: 400-4000 U/mL.

• Peak serum bilirubin: usually <10 mg/dL.

• Peak serum alkaline phosphatase: usually less than twice upper limits of normal.

• Prothrombin time: normal or 1-2 seconds prolonged.

• Serum albumin: normal or minimally reduced.

• Peripheral blood: normal or mild leucopenia with or without mild lymphocytosis.

Acute Liver Failure
• Coagulopathy with striking elevation of prothrombin time (>6 seconds prolongation).

• Low level of factor VII.

• Leukocytosis.

• Hyponatremia, hypokalemia, hypoglycemia.

• Marked elevation of serum bilirubin.

• Elevated aminotransferase levels decline toward normal despite disease progression.

Cholestatic Hepatitis
• Serum bilirubin: may be >20 mg/dL.

• Serum aminotransferases may decline toward normal despite persistent jaundice.

• Variable elevation of serum alkaline phosphatase: 2-6 times upper limit of normal.

• Prothrombin time: normal or near-normal.

Relapsing Hepatitis
• Serum bilirubin and/or serum aminotransferases rise after apparent normalization or near normalization.

• Peak bilirubin and aminotransferase levels in relapse may be higher or lower than in initial episode.

Serologic and Virologic Diagnosis

Hepatitis A
• Circulating IgM antibody to HAV (IgM anti-HAV) detected during acute phase and for 3-6 months thereafter.

• IgG antibody to HAV without IgM anti-HAV: past infection.

Hepatitis E
• An IgM anti-HEV may be present in serum; persists for 6 weeks or more.

• IgG anti-HEV develops later and may persist for a variable period (20 months or longer) after convalescence.

Hepatitis B
• Hepatitis B surface antigen (HBsAg) generally detected about 10-50 days after infection.

 * May persist for weeks to months in self-limited infections

 * Disappears before loss of IgM antibody to hepatitis B core antigen (IgM anti-HBc)

• IgM antibody to hepatitis B core antigen (IgM anti-HBc) detected about 60 days after infection.

- In 10% of patients with acute hepatitis B, IgM anti-HBc present but HBsAg absent (cleared).

- IgG antibody to hepatitis B core antigen (IgG anti-HBc): replaces IgM anti-HBc.

  * IgG anti-HBc:

  * Indicative of past or continuing infection

  * Persists for decades

  * Not elicited by HBV vaccines

- HBV DNA and HBeAg appear in serum early (about 10-30 days after infection) but not routinely measured in acute cases.

  * HBV DNA may persist for weeks to months in self-limited infections

  * HBeAg declines and disappears before HBsAg in self-limited infections

  * HBeAg is detected only in HBsAg positive sera

  * HBV DNA may be present without HBeAg (the pre-core or core promotor HBV variant)

- Antibody to HBsAg (anti-HBs).

  * Neutralizing, protective antibody (correlated with immunity)

  * Last serologic marker to appear (as HBsAg disappears or thereafter)

  * Persists for decades

  * Elicited by HBV vaccines

Hepatitis D
- HBsAg-positive.

- IgM anti-hepatitis D virus (IgM anti-HDV) in acute phase.

- HDV/HBV coinfection:

  * IgM anti-HDV and IgM anti-HBc

- HDV superinfection of HBV chronically infected individual:

  * IgM anti-HDV and IgG anti-HBc

- Anti-HDV declines and disappears over time unless chronic HDV infection.

- HDV RNA present in serum but not routinely measured.

Hepatitis C
- HCV RNA:

  * Earliest marker of HCV infection (within days to weeks of infection)

  * Appears before antibodies

  * Disappears in self-limited infection usually by 16 weeks after exposure

  * Marker of chronic HCV infection

- Antibodies to HCV (anti-HCV):

  * Appear in serum in 60% of patients during acute phase

  * Anti-HCV appears (weeks to several months later) in remainder

- <5% of infected patients without anti-HCV (immunosuppressed patients)

- Anti-HCV persists for prolonged periods both in self-limited and chronic infection

Differential Diagnosis

Infectious Diseases Associated With Hepatic Injury (Inflammation)
- Herpes simplex

- CMV infection

- Epstein-Barr virus infection

- Parvovirus B19

- Others

Noninfectious Disorders
- Drug- and toxin-induced acute hepatitis

- Ischemic hepatitis (shock liver)

- Autoimmune hepatitis

- Alcoholic hepatitis

- Acute biliary tract obstruction

Empiric Therapy

Typical Acute Viral Hepatitis
- Managed at home.

- Prolonged, vigorous exercise best avoided.

- Hospitalization for persistent vomiting or dehydration.

- Maintain calories and fluid intake with multiple small meals.

- Bed rest only if desired by patient.

- No alcohol or nonessential medications but oral contraceptives may be continued.

- In acute hepatitis C, pegylated interferon injections may reduce the risk of chronic infection in those who remain viremic after week 16.

- Treatment of acute hepatitis B with lamivudine is ineffective; use of other drugs remains experimental.

Acute Liver Failure
- Hospitalization required, preferably in an ICU in a liver transplant center.

- Early recognition, treatment of hypoglycemia, infection, electrolyte, acid-base disturbances and renal failure.

- Intracranial pressure monitoring to control cerebral edema.

- Factor VII and fresh frozen plasma for bleeding.

- Anecdotal treatment success with oral antivirals for HBV-induced disease but single controlled trial with lamivudine was negative.

Early administration of intravenous N-acetylcysteine appears benefical.

- Early listing for liver transplantation.

- Survival rates of about 70% achieved by transplantation if liver failure complications (renal failure cerebral edema) are minimal.

Cholestatic Hepatitis
- Cholestyramine, ursodeoxycholic acid for severe pruritus.

- Course may be shortened by short-term treatment with ursodeoxycholic acid or prednisone, but no randomized, controlled trials available.

Relapsing Hepatitis
- Manage as in typical acute hepatitis.

Prevention

Hepatitis A
Hepatitis A virus vaccine for pre-exposure immunoprophylaxis

- Inactivated whole-virus vaccine induces antibody in nearly 100% of recipients of two-dose regimen (0-6, or 0-12 months).

- Antibody appears by day 15 after first dose in about 90%.

- Protective efficacy approaches 100%.

- Duration of protection estimated to be at least 10, probably >25 years.

- Major adverse event: transient pain at deltoid injection site.

Indications

• All children beginning at >12 months of age; children in regions with high attack rates.

• Travelers to endemic regions (may also receive immune globulin concurrently).

• Military and peacekeeping personnel.

• Injecting drug users.

• Men who have sex with men.

• Recipients of clotting factor concentrates.

• Patients with chronic liver disease.

• Laboratory workers exposed to HAV.

• Workers in daycare centers.

• Food handlers where infection rates are high.

• Control of community-wide outbreaks.

Hepatitis A virus vaccine for post-exposure immunoprophylaxis

• Approved for use within 2 weeks post-exposure for healthy persons aged 12 months to 40 years.

• Can be used for older healthy individuals if immune globulin unavailable.

• In children aged <12 months, immunocompromised persons, persons with chronic liver disease and persons for whom vaccine is contraindicated, IG should be used.

Immune globulin for postexposure immunoprophylaxis

• Protective efficacy approaches 75%-90%.

• Effective if given within 2 weeks of exposure.

• Duration of protection with dose of 0.02 mL/kg body weight: 2-3 months; higher doses (0.06 mg/kg) afford protection for 4-5 months.

• Transient pain at deltoid injection site.

Indications

• Infants, immunocompromised persons, and persons with chronic liver disease who are household and intimate contacts of acutely infected patients.

• Not for casual contacts.

• For travelers leaving immediately for endemic regions, it may be given concurrently with HAV vaccine.

Hepatitis E

• No effective immune globulin preparation is available.

• A recombinant vaccine with 95% protective efficacy awaits approval in United States.

Hepatitis B

Recombinant HBV vaccine for preexposure immunoprophylaxis.

• HBsAg is the immunogen in the vaccines.

• Seroprotective levels of anti-HBs (≥10 mIU/mL) induced in >95% of recipients of full (3-dose) regimen.

• 90%-95% effective in prevention of clinical HBV infection.

• Given intramuscularly (deltoid in children and adults, anterolateral muscle of thigh in infants).

• No relationship to multiple sclerosis, autism, mercury poisoning, Guillain-Barré syndrome, systemic lupus erythematosus.

  * Impaired response to vaccination (may require booster doses) in:

  * Immunosuppressed individuals

  * Chronic renal failure or chronic cardiac or pulmonary disease

  * Individuals over age 40 years

* Obesity

* Smokers

* Advanced chronic liver disease

• Adverse events: transient pain at deltoid injection site.

Indications
• Newborn children of HBsAg-negative mothers.

• Catch-up vaccination through age 18 years.

• Targeted high-risk groups:

* Health care workers and health care students likely to have exposure to blood or body fluids

* Household and sexual contacts of HBV carriers

* Alaskan natives, Pacific islanders (endemic regions)

* Injecting illicit drug users

* Men who have sex with men

* Individuals with multiple sexual partners

* First responders (public safety personnel)

* Staff in institutions for the developmentally disadvantaged

* Recipients of high-risk blood products

* Maintenance hemodialysis patients

* Prisoners

Hepatitis B Immune Globulin for Postexposure Immunoprophylaxis

• Contains high titers of anti-HBs.

• Given intramuscularly (deltoid in children and adults, anterolateral muscle of thigh in infants).

• Transient pain at injection site is major adverse event.

Indications
• Susceptible sexual contacts of acute hepatitis B patients together with HBV vaccine.

• Following needlestick or splash accident in non-vaccinated individual, together with HBV vaccine.

• Given with hepatitis B immune globulin within 12 hours of birth to neonate of HBsAg-positive mother: protective efficacy is 95%.

Hepatitis D
• No vaccine or immune globulin available for HBsAg-positive patients.

• HBV vaccine will prevent HBV infection and, thereby, HDV infection in susceptible individuals.

Hepatitis C
• Anti-HCV and HCV RNA screening of blood donors has reduced risk of transfusion-associated hepatitis C.

• Needle exchange programs and clean needle programs: possibly effective.

• Avoidance of unprotected sex, tattoos, body-piercing.

• Prototype vaccine in trials.

• Hyperimmune globulin preparations: under study.

Combined Vaccine for Hepatitis A and B
• Approved for individuals 18 years of age or older.

• Administered in a 3-dose regimen (0, 1 and 6 months).

Accelerated schedule (0, 1, 4 and 52 weeks) available: provides more rapid appearance of antibody.

• Highly immunogenic, well-tolerated.

2. Chronic Viral Hepatitis

- Necro-inflammatory disorders associated with viral persistence.

- May be asymptomatic or may present with fatigue or symptoms of advanced liver disease.

- Characterized histopathologically by hepatocyte necrosis, mononuclear and plasma cell infiltration of the portal triads and adjacent parenchyma (interface hepatitis), with or without fibrosis.

- Progression of fibrosis may lead to cirrhosis.

- Outcomes for progressive disease are cirrhosis, end-stage liver disease, hepatocellular carcinoma and death.

  * Hepatocellular carcinoma develops in HBV infection in those with or without cirrhosis

  * Hepatocellular carcinoma develops in HCV infection in those with cirrhosis or advanced bridging fibrosis

- 50% of patients with chronic hepatitis B may ultimately develop cirrhosis or hepatocellular carcinoma; 2%-20% of those with chronic hepatitis C develop cirrhosis within 20 years of infection.

Host factors (age, gender, immune status, etc) and viral factors (replication) contribute to disease progression.

- The goals of treatment are:

  * Eradication or suppression of viral replication

  * Improvement of liver histopathology

  * Reduction of sequelae of infection

Treatment, when effective, improves liver function, reverses hepatic decompensation, delays progression and reduces the risk of hepatocellular carcinoma.

Chronic Hepatitis B

Prevalence
- 1-1.25 million chronically infected individuals in the United States; 350 million worldwide.

- Age-dependent risk of chronic infection: 90% for neonates, <5% for adults.

- Serologic marker of chronic HBV infection: persistence of HBsAg.

Spectrum of Disease
- Asymptomatic, inactive carrier with normal aminotransferases.

- Chronic hepatitis with elevated aminotransferases.

- Chronic hepatitis with cirrhosis.

- Chronic hepatitis with cirrhosis and hepatocellular carcinoma.

- Chronic hepatitis with hepatocellular carcinoma.

- Extrahepatic manifestations of chronic HBV infection (<2% of infections).

- Glomerulonephritis.

- Necrotizing vasculitis (polyarteritis nodosa).

- Cryoglobulinemia (uncommon).

- Weak association with porphyria cutanea tarda.

Diagnosis
- Detection of HBsAg, IgG anti-HBc and elevated aminotransferases in chronic hepatitis B; normal aminotransferases in carriers with low-level or undetectable HBV DNA.

- HBV DNA detected in serum.

- HBeAg present (except in patients with precore or core promoter HBV variant).

Candidates for Treatment
- Presence of HBV DNA >10,000 copies/mL (>2000 IU/mL) with elevated aminotransferase

levels, regardless of HBeAg status; if aminotransferases are normal, treat if liver biopsy shows moderate/severe inflammation or fibrosis.

• HBeAg-positive and HBeAg-negative patients; the latter generally require long-term oral treatment.

• Detectable HBV DNA in compensated cirrhosis; in decompensated cirrhosis refer for live transplant.

• No treatment for inactive carriers with normal aminotransferases and low-level HBV DNA (<2000 IU/mL).

Treatment

Interferon alfa-2b
• Treatment for patients with elevated aminotransferases for 4-6 months.

• HBV DNA clearance, loss of HBeAg and appearance of anti-HBe with normal aminotransferases: achieved in 35%; durability of response 85%.

• Risk of flare with disease exacerbation; hence, interferon contraindicated in decompensated disease.

• Route of administration: subcutaneous injection.

• Adverse events: common, poorly tolerated in many patients: infrequently used.

Pegylated Interferon alfa-2a
• Long-acting interferon given subcutaneously once a week for 48 weeks.

• HBeAg seroconversion achieved in about 30%; loss of HBV DNA in 34%.

• Better-tolerated than conventional interferon, but more adverse events than with oral antivirals.

• Contraindicated in decompensated disease.

Lamivudine
• Oral nucleoside analogue.

• Terminates HBV nascent proviral DNA chain.

• No mitochondrial toxicity; nearly no side effects.

• Improves hepatic pathology in 50%.

• HBV clearance, loss of HBeAg, development of anti-HBe and normal aminotransferases in about 20% of patients treated for 1 year.

• No flares during treatment: may be given to decompensated patients.

• Lamivudine resistance (YMDD variant) develops in as many as 70% of patients after 4 years of treatment: variable course but breakthroughs leading to disease exacerbation or progression may occur.

  * No longer first-line drug in U.S.

Adefovir
• Orally administered nucleotide inhibits reverse transcriptase and DNA polymerase.

• Approved dose of 10 mg may be suboptimal; higher doses nephrotoxic.

• Loss of HBV DNA, HBeAg seroconversion: 21% and 12%, respectively, at 1 year of treatment.

• Genotypic resistance >20% after 2 years of treatment.

• Adefovir resistance seen in patients with lamivudine resistance switched to adefovir.

• Well-tolerated.

• Slow-acting agent.

  * No longer first-line drug in U.S.

Entecavir
• Nucleoside inhibits HBV replication at 3 separate steps.

• High antiviral potency and low risk of emergence of resistance after 4-5 years of treatment.

- Loss of HBV DNA and HBeAg seroconversion: 67% and 21%, respectively, at 1 year of treatment.

- Not studied in decompensated patients.

- Well-tolerated.

- Less effective for patients with lamivudine resistance.

Telbivudine
- Potent nucleoside in naïve patients, but emergence of resistance common by 2 years of treatment.

- Loss of HBV DNA and HBeAg seroconversion: 60% and 22%, respectively.

- Cross-resistant with lamivudine.

- Durability of response about 80%.

- Well-tolerated.

    * No longer first-line drug in U.S.

Tenofovir

- Potent, rapid-acting nucleoside in naïve and lamivudine-resistant patients.

- Loss of HBV DNA in 80%; HBeAg seroconversion in 21%.

- Histologic improvement in 75%.

- HBsAg loss in 3% at 1 year.

- Viral resistance: none at 1 year.

- Equally effective in naïve and lamivudine-resistant patients.

Drugs in Development
- Pegylated interferon and oral antivirals simultaneously: under study, but combination with lamivudine did not increase virologic response rates.

- Combinations of tenofovir with emtricitabine.

- Other nucleoside/nucleotides alone or in combination.

- Immunomodulatory agents, including a therapeutic vaccine.

- Immunoprophylaxis against HAV and HBV infection, by use of HAV and HBV vaccines in susceptible patients.

Chronic Hepatitis D
- Declining prevalence in the United States; worldwide <5 million individuals affected.

- Serologic diagnosis: circulating HBsAg and anti-HDV.

- Wide spectrum of disease, similar to chronic hepatitis B.

Treatment
- Long-term (years) interferon alfa-2b effective in few.

- Immunoprophylaxis against HAV infection by use of HAV vaccine in susceptible patients.

Chronic Hepatitis C

Prevalence
- 3-4 million chronically infected individuals in United States; 200 million worldwide.

- Risk of chronic infection: 55%-85% (children with lower rate).

- Spectrum of histological disease:

    * Chronic hepatitis with persistently normal, fluctuating, or elevated aminotransferases

    * Chronic hepatitis with cirrhosis

    * Chronic hepatitis with cirrhosis and hepatocellular carcinoma

- Progression to cirrhosis related to alcohol consumption, older age, immunosuppression, hepatic steatosis, insulin resistance.

- Extrahepatic manifestations of chronic HCV infection (<2% of patients):

    * Glomerulonephritis

    * Cutaneous vasculitis

    * Cryoglobulinemia (more often than in chronic HBV infection)

    * Association with porphyria cutanea tarda, diabetes mellitus, thyroiditis, lichen planus

Candidates for Treatment
- HCV RNA-positive with or without elevated serum aminotransferase levels.

- Absence of severe depression, suicidal ideation, active immunologic disorders (eg, systemic lupus erythematosis, rheumatoid arthritis, inflammatory bowel disease, etc.).

Treatment

Interferon alfa-2a, 2b, and alfacon-1
- Nonpegylated interferons no longer first-line option.

- High frequency of adverse reactions due to high doses utilized.

- Replaced by pegylated interferons.

Pegylated Interferon Plus Ribavirin
- Treatment of choice for chronic hepatitis C, including patients coinfected with HIV.

- Pegylated interferon given once weekly by subcutaneous injection for 48 weeks in genotypes 1 and 4 and for 24 weeks in genotypes 2 and 3.

- Ribivirin given daily in weight-based dose in genotypes 1 and 4 (1000 if body weight <75 kg or 1200 mg if more) or 800 mg in genotypes 2 and 3.

- Sustained virologic response rate: defined as HCV RNA-negative 6 months after completing therapy (relapse rate about 5%, <1% at 2 years).

- Sustained virologic response rate: genotype dependent, affected by viral load, rapidity of viral decline, race, insulin resistance, hepatic steatosis, body weight and adherence to therapy.

- Sustained virologic response in genotype 1: about 50%.

- Sustained virologic response in genotypes 2 and 3: about 80%.

- Higher sustained response rates in genotype 1, if adherence to treatment is high and if loss of HCV RNA is rapid (HCV RNA negative at week 4 of treatment), approaching 80%-90%

- Adverse events develop in most patients:

    * Interferon-associated flu-like illness, depression, thyroid dysfunction, granulocytopenia, thrombocytopenia

    * Ribavirin-associated hemolytic anemia, bronchospasm, rash

- HCV/HIV coinfected patients with stable HIV and adequate CD4+ cell counts may be treated if they have compensated liver disease and are not receiving didanosine.

- Immunoprophylaxis against HAV and HBV is recommended for susceptible patients.

Drugs in Development

- HCV RNA-dependent RNA polymerase inhibitor.

- HCV serine protease inhibitor.

- HCV helicase inhibitor.

- Albumin-linked interferon.

- Nitazoxanide.

- Immunomodulators.

4. Further Reading

ID Board Pearls

- When acute hepatitis B is suspected on clinical and epidemiologic grounds, but testing is delayed for several weeks and HBsAg is absent, the presence of IgM anti-HBc confirms the diagnosis.

- In a pregnant woman in the third trimester with acute viral hepatitis who has just returned from a trip to India, the risk of acute liver failure is greatest if the causative agent is the hepatitis E virus.

- Inactive HBV carriers who are HBsAg-positive but have normal serum aminotransferase levels and HBV DNA levels of <2000 IU/mL are not currently candidates for pegylated interferon or oral antiviral therapy.

- The 2 most potent, and rapidly-acting oral antivirals for the treatment of chronic hepatitis B are also the least likely to induce resistance: entecavir and tenofovir.

- The most important factors affecting the efficacy of pegylated-interferon and ribavirin in chronic hepatitis C are viral genotype, viral load, the rapidity of viral decline, and host factors which include race, insulin resistance, hepatic steatosis and adherence to treatment.

Armstrong GL, Wasley A, Simard EP, et al. The prevalence of hepatitis C virus infection in the United States, 1999 through 2002. *Ann Intern Med.* 2006;144:705-714.

Centers for Disease Control and Prevention. Prevention of hepatitis A through active or passive immunization: recommendations of the Advisory Committee on Immunization Practices (ACIP). *MMWR.* 2006;55(RR07):1-23.

Centers for Disease Control and Prevention. A comprehensive immunization strategy to eliminate transmission of hepatitis B virus infection in the United States: recommendations of the Advisory Committee on Immunization Practices (ACIP) Part II: Immunization of Adults. *MMWR.* 2006;55(RR16):1-25.

Dienstag Jl. Hepatitis B virus infection. *N Engl J Med.* 2008;359:1486-1500.

Farci P, Roskams T, Chessa L, et al. Long-term benefit of interferon alfa therapy of chronic hepatitis D : regression of advanced hepatic fibrosis. *Gastroenterol.* 2004;126:1740-1749.

Hoofnagle JH, Seeff LB. Peginterferon and ribavirin for chronic hepatitis C. *N Engl J Med.* 2006;355:2444-2451.

Koziel MJ, Peters MG. Viral hepatitis in HIV infection. *N Engl J Med.* 2007;356:1445-1454.

Khuroo MS, Khuroo MS. Hepatitis E virus. *Curr Opin Infect Dis.* 2008;21:539-543.

Kumar M, Satapathy R, Monga R, et al. A randomized controlled trial of lamivudine to treat acute hepatitis B. *Hepatology.* 2007;45:97-101.

Lok ASF, McMahon BJ. Chronic hepatitis B. *Hepatology.* 2007;45:507-539.

Chapter 20: Infectious Diarrhea for the ID Boards

Davidson H. Hamer, MD
Sherwood L. Gorbach, MD

Contents

Definitions

Diarrhea
Increase in the volume or change in the consistency of stool. Usually defined as 3 or more loose or watery bowel movements in a 24-hour period.

Persistent Diarrhea
Diarrhea lasting 14 days or more.

Toxigenic Diarrhea
Watery diarrhea caused by strains of bacteria, which produce toxins that cause fluid secretion without any damage to the epithelial surface.

Invasive Diarrhea
Diarrhea characterized by the visible presence of blood or mucus. This is usually caused by direct invasion of the gastrointestinal mucosa by the pathogen or via the production of cytotoxins, which cause injury to the mucosa and induce fluid secretion.

Traveler's Diarrhea
Diarrhea occurring in travelers, usually when visiting a less developed area of the world.

1. Toxigenic Diarrhea

Causative Organisms

- *Vibrio cholerae* O1

- *V cholerae* 0139 Bengal

- Enterotoxigenic *Escherichia coli* (ETEC)

- Enteroaggregative *E coli* (EAggEC)

Epidemiology

Cholera
- Seventh pandemic of cholera started in 1961 in Southeast Asia, spread to the Middle East and Africa, and then reached South America in 1991. Cholera is now endemic in several countries in South America and remains endemic in many countries in Asia and Africa.

- An epidemic due to *V cholerae* 0139 Bengal began in southern India and Bangladesh in late 1992. *V cholerae* 0139 is now endemic on the Indian subcontinent.

- Sporadic endemic cases of *V cholerae* 01 diarrhea occur along the Gulf Coast of the United States, primarily in Texas and Louisiana.

- Contaminated water and food are the major vehicles for the spread of cholera.

ETEC
- Contaminated food and beverages are the major vehicles of infection.

- The highest incidence occurs in the tropics especially in children.

- ETEC is the most common cause of diarrhea in travelers from North America and Northern Europe to the developing world.

EAggEC
- EAggEC has been implicated as a cause of traveler's diarrhea and HIV+ patients with persistent diarrhea.

- The vehicles of infection are unknown, but are likely to be contaminated food and beverages based on the epidemiology of the disease.

Key Clinical Features

Cholera
- A spectrum of clinical manifestations may occur, ranging from an asymptomatic carrier state to severe watery diarrhea.

- Early symptoms of vomiting and abdominal distention are soon followed by diarrhea, which may quickly progress to large volumes of rice water stools.

- Low-grade fever may be present.

- Patients present with severe dehydration and hypovolemic shock, with an associated hypokalemic acidosis, which may lead to renal failure.

ETEC
- After an incubation period of 1-2 days, infected persons develop abdominal cramping, which is shortly followed by watery diarrhea.

- Infection may be mild, with only a few loose bowel movements, or severe, cholera-like watery diarrhea with severe dehydration.

- Associated symptoms may include abdominal pain, nausea and vomiting.

EAggEC
- Infection varies in severity from relatively mild with frequent, small volume mucoid bowel movements to bloody diarrhea.

- Children in developed countries and AIDS patients often develop persistent diarrhea.

Key Differential Diagnostic Features

Infectious Diarrheal Diseases
- One approach to diagnosing diarrheal disease on clinical grounds is to separate pathogens that target the upper small intestine from those that attack the large bowel (Table 1). Toxigenic bacteria

(ETEC, *V cholerae*), viruses, *G lamblia* and *Cryptosporidium* spp. are examples of small bowel pathogens which produce watery diarrhea, dehydration and abdominal pain (often periumbilical).

- Clinically, there is no way to distinguish among enteropathogens that cause watery diarrhea.

Noninfectious Diseases
- Carcinoid syndrome (flushing may be present; 5hydroxyindole acetic acid level elevated).

- Zollinger-Ellison syndrome (symptoms of peptic ulcer disease refractory to therapy are usually present; elevated fasting serum gastrin level).

- Vasoactive intestinal peptide-secreting pancreatic adenoma (flushing and hypotension may be present; VIP level elevated).

- Medullary carcinoma of thyroid (thyroid mass or enlarging nodule).

- Villous adenoma of rectum (diagnose and treat with colonoscopy).

Key Laboratory Findings

Cholera
- WBC and RBC are not visible in the stool on microscopy.

- Hyponatremia or hypokalemia may be present.

- Darkfield microscopy can provide a rapid presumptive diagnosis if motile bacteria are seen.

- Definitive diagnosis depends on isolation of the organism in stool culture. May be isolated on selective media such as MacConkey's or TCBS.

- Confirmation of serotype is done with specific antisera.

- An immunodiagnostic test has been developed which allows for the rapid detection of both *V cholerae* 01 and 0139 in stool samples.

Table 1

Clinical Features of Diarrheal Diseases

	Location of Infection	
	Small Intestine	**Large Intestine**
Pathogens	*E coli* (enterotoxigenic and, enteropathogenic), *V cholerae*, viruses, *Giardia, Cryptosporidium, Cyclospora*	*Shigella*, enteroinvasive and enterohemorrhagic *E coli*, *Campylobacter, E histolytica*
Location of pain	Midabdomen	Lower abdomen, rectum
Volume of stool	Large	Small
Type of stool	Watery	Mucoid
Blood in stool	Rare	Common
Leukocytes in stool	Rare	Common (except in amebiasis)
Proctoscopy	Normal	Mucosal ulcers; hemorrhage; friable mucosa

ETEC

• WBC and RBC are not visible in the stool on microscopy.

• Specialized diagnostic tools needed to diagnose ETEC (eg, PCR or DNA probes for detection of toxin).

EAggEC

• Isolation of *E coli* from stool specimens and specialized cell culture techniques demonstrating an adherence-aggregation pattern is required for diagnosis.

Empiric Therapy

• The major goal of treatment is the replacement of fluid and electrolytes. Although administration of fluids by the intravenous route has long been the standard approach, oral rehydration solutions (ORS) have been shown to be equally effective physiologically, and less costly. Even in the United States, ORS is the treatment of choice for mild to moderate diarrhea in both children and adults, and it can be used in severe diarrhea after some initial parenteral rehydration.

• Although dietary abstinence has been the traditional approach to acute diarrhea, it is better to eat judiciously during an attack of diarrhea than to severely restrict oral intake. In children, it is especially important to restart feeding as soon as the child is able to accept oral intake.

• Foods or fluids that may increase intestinal motility or potentiate abdominal cramps and diarrhea, such as dairy products, alcohol, coffee, tea, cocoa and soft drinks should be avoided.

• Since most patients with infectious diarrhea have a mild, self-limited course, neither a stool culture nor specific treatment is required for many cases. Empiric antimicrobial therapy should be instituted for more severe cases, pending results of culture of stool and blood. A fluoroquinolone antibiotic is a good choice for empiric treatment, since these drugs have broad spectrum activity against all bacteria responsible for acute infectious diarrhea (except *C difficile*) and resistance remains limited.

- The choice of antibiotic, when indicated, is based on *in vitro* sensitivity patterns, however, these data are often not available when treatment is initiated. Therefore, empiric therapy with a fluoroquinolone is advised.

- The duration of antimicrobial therapy has not been clearly defined. There are several studies that suggest a single dose is as effective as more prolonged therapy for bacterial diarrhea. The combination of an antibiotic with an antimotility drug may provide more rapid relief of diarrhea than either agent alone, especially in the treatment of traveler's diarrhea.

- Antimotility drugs are useful in controlling moderate to severe diarrhea. Loperamide, as opposed to opiate derivatives, is the best agent, because it is not likely to be habit-forming and is unlikely to cause depression of the respiratory center. Treatment with loperamide produces rapid improvement, often within the first 24 hours of therapy.

- Bismuth subsalicylate is effective in treating mild to moderate diarrhea. The drug possesses antimicrobial properties, on the basis of the bismuth and antisecretory properties related to the salicylate moiety.

Definitive Therapy

See Table 2 for specific therapies.

Complications

Cholera
- Moderate to severe dehydration.

- Hypoglycemia.

- Severe dehydration may lead to circulatory collapse and death.

ID Board Pearls

- Contaminated food and water are the major sources of infection with toxigenic enteropathogens.

- *V cholerae* is endemic in many parts of Asia, Africa, Latin America and US states along the Gulf Coast.

- EAggEC is a cause of persistent diarrhea in children and patients with AIDS, and is a common cause of traveler's diarrhea.

- Oral rehydration therapy is the mainstay of therapy for most toxigenic diarrhea-causing bacteria.

- Short courses (1-3 days) of azithromycin or fluoroquinolones may be required for more severe episodes of diarrhea or community-acquired diarrhea lasting 4 days or more.

Table 2

Antimicrobial Drug Therapy of Infectious Diarrhea

Recommended in symptomatic cases	Antibiotic of choice	Dose, route and duration	Alternative drugs
Shigella	Ampicillin	500 mg PO QID or 1 g IV QID for 5 days; 50-100 mg/kg/d for children	Nalidixic acid
	Ampicillin-resistant strains: TMP-SMX; Fluoroquinolones	10 mg/kg/d TMP and 50 mg/kg/d SMX for 5 days; 500 mg PO BID for 5-7 days	
C difficile	Metronidazole or vancomycin	500 mg PO TID for 10 days; 125-500 mg PO QID for 10 days	
Travelers' diarrhea	Ciprofloxacin 500 mg PO BID for 3 days; Levofloxacin 500 mg PO QD; Azithromycin 500 mg PO BID; Rifaximin 200 mg PO TID		TMP-SMX, other fluoroquinolones
EPEC, EAggEC, and DAEC in infants; EIEC	TMP-SMX	500 mg PO or IV QID for 14 days	
Typhoid fever	Chloramphenicol	40 mg/kg/d in 4 doses (max: 4 g/d) for 2 days; 100 mg PO BID for 2 days	Amoxicillin 1 g PO QID for 14 days; ciprofloxacin 500 mg PO BID for 7 days; TMP-SMX; third-generation cephalosporins
Cholera	Tetracycline; Doxycycline		TMP-SMX, norfloxacin, furazolidone
Salmonella (complicated cases)	Ampicillin; Ampicillin-resistant strains: TMP-SMX	50-100 mg/kg/d in 4 doses for 10-14 days; 8 mg/kg/d TMP and 40 mg/kg/d SMX (max: 320 mg+1600 mg/d) for 14 days	Ciprofloxacin 500 mg PO BID for 14 days; third generation cephalosporins
Not generally recommended due to inconclusive findings or no studies			
Campylobacter	Erythromycin; Ciprofloxacin	250-500 mg PO QID for 7 days; 500 mg PO BID for 5-7 days	
Yersinia	Fluoroquinolones, TMP-SMX, chloramphenicol		Aminoglycosides, tetracycline
Aeromonas	TMP-SMX, third generation cephalosporins, fluoroquinolones		Tetracycline, chloramphenicol
Vibrio, noncholera species	Tetracycline		
EPEC, EAggEC, or DAEC in adults, EHEC	TMP-SMX		

Not recommended except in unusual cases: Nontyphoidal *Salmonella*; ETEC; viral diarrhea

2. Invasive Diarrhea

Causative Organisms

- *Shigella* spp. including *S sonnei* (responsible for 60%-80% of bacillary dysentery in the United States), *S dysenteriae*, *S flexneri* and *S boydii*.

- Nontyphoidal *Salmonella* spp.

- Enterohemorrhagic *E coli* (EHEC).

- Enteroinvasive *E coli*.

- *Campylobacter jejuni*.

- *Vibrio parahaemolyticus*.

- *Yersinia enterocolitica*.

Epidemiology

- Approximately 100,000 infections caused by *Campylobacter jejuni*, *E.coli* O157, *Salmonella* and *Shigella* are reported annually to local health departments in the U.S.

Shigellosis

- Dysentery is most common in children 6 months to 5 years old.

- *Shigellae* are usually transmitted from person to person, although epidemics related to milk, ice cream, other foods and recreational water exposure may occur.

- Low infective dose accounts for the rapid spread of *Shigella* in daycare centers and among people living in conditions of poor hygiene.

Nontyphoidal salmonellosis

- Modes of transmission include contaminated food, person to person, flies and fomites. *Salmonella* spp. can cause large, common source outbreaks.

- Nonhuman reservoirs including poultry, pigs, cattle and household pets (especially turtles and lizards) play an important role in the transmission of disease.

- Poultry, meats, eggs, dairy products and a variety of commercially prepared foods including peanut butter have been implicated in disease outbreaks.

- Children <1 year of age have the highest attack rates.

- There is also a high attack rate and increased mortality in elderly persons.

- *Salmonella* infections have been increasing during the last 3 decades in the United States, with approximately 25,000 cases reported annually during the 1970s, with an increase to 45,000 cases by the mid-1980s. As under reporting is believed to be common, it is estimated that about 1.4 million cases of *Salmonella* food poisoning occur each year.

- Associated diseases that increase the risk of salmonellosis include sickle cell anemia (especially *Salmonella* osteomyelitis), malaria, bartonellosis, louse-borne relapsing fever, schistosomiasis, leukemia, lymphoma, disseminated malignancy, AIDS, corticosteroid use, chemotherapy, radiation therapy and gastric surgery.

EHEC

- More common in northern locations such as Canada, Great Britain, and, within the United States, Massachusetts, Minnesota and the Pacific Northwest.

- The leading vehicle of infection is hamburger meat, although precooked meat patties, roast beef, salami, fresh-pressed apple cider, lettuce, alfalfa sprouts, unpasteurized milk and recreational water exposure have also been implicated.

- Person-to-person transmission may be responsible for outbreaks in daycare centers and nursing homes.

- Peak incidence is from June to September.

Enteroinvasive *E coli*

- Rare cause of dysentery in Asia.

- In 1971, contaminated imported cheese was responsible for an outbreak in the United States.

Campylobacter jejuni

- Responsible for 4%-11% of all diarrhea episodes in the United States (an estimated 2 million cases each year).

- Reservoir animals include cattle, sheep, swine, birds and dogs.

- Consumption of improperly cooked or contaminated foodstuffs is the cause of most human infections.

- Chickens account for 50%-70% of infections.

Vibrio parahaemolyticus

- Responsible for many outbreaks in Japan, especially in warm months.

- In the United States, most cases occur in coastal states.

- Usually associated with the consumption of seafood or vegetables contaminated with sea water, especially if improperly refrigerated.

Yersinia enterocolitica

- Reported more frequently in Scandinavian and other European countries than in the United States.

- Epidemics related to the consumption of contaminated milk and ice cream have been described.

- The organism can be found in stream and lake water as well as many animals, including puppies, cats, cows, chickens and horses.

Key Clinical Features

- Large bowel pathogens such as Shigella, C jejuni, EHEC and enteroinvasive E coli are invasive organisms that cause dysentery.

- Characteristic rectal pain, known as tenesmus, strongly suggests colonic involvement.

- Although initially the fecal effluent may be watery, by the second or third day of illness it becomes a relatively small volume stool, often bloody and mucoid.

Shigellosis

- Lower abdominal pain and diarrhea are present in most patients, fever in about 40%, and bloody mucoid stool in only one-third.

- The illness may be biphasic with initial symptoms of fever, abdominal pain and watery, non-bloody diarrhea, followed in 3-5 days by tenesmus and small volume bloody stools.

- Bacteremia is uncommon.

- Malnutrition, especially in young children, and infection with S dysenteriae type 1 are associated with a more severe course.

- Most infections will resolve in 1-3 days in children or up to a week in adults, although symptoms may persist for 3-4 weeks in severe cases.

Nontyphoidal Salmonellosis

Clinical syndromes seen with Salmonella include:

- Gastroenteritis (~75%).

- Bacteremia (~10%).

- Typhoidal or "enteric fever" (~8%).

- Localized infections (eg, bones, joints and meninges) (~5%).

- Asymptomatic carriage (usually in the gallbladder).

- Usual incubation period for gastroenteritis is 6-48 hours.

- Nausea and vomiting are followed by abdominal cramps and diarrhea which usually lasts 3-4 days.

- Fever is present in about 50%.

- Diarrhea can vary from loose stools to grossly bloody and purulent feces to a cholera-like syndrome (more common in achlorhydric patients).

- Chronic carriage (defined as persistence for more than 1 year) of nontyphoidal-Salmonella develops in 0.2%-0.6% of infections.

- Younger age (<3 months), advanced age (>60 years), cholelithiasis and nephrolithiasis predispose to the carrier state.

EHEC
- Median incubation period of 3-4 days (range, 1-14).

- Initially symptoms include watery, non-bloody diarrhea and severe abdominal cramping. Diarrhea may progress to visibly bloody stools.

- Related symptoms include nausea, vomiting, low-grade fever and chills.

- Median duration of diarrhea is 3-8 days.

- Leukocytosis with a left shift is usually present but anemia is uncommon unless infection is complicated by hemolytic uremic syndrome or thrombotic thrombocytopenic purpura.

Enteroinvasive *E coli*
- Symptoms include diarrhea, tenesmus, fever and intestinal cramps.

Campylobacter jejuni
- Usual incubation period is 24-72 hours (range 1 hour to 10 days).

- Spectrum of clinical illness ranges from frank dysentery to watery diarrhea to asymptomatic excretion.

- Symptoms include diarrhea and fever (90%), abdominal pain (70%) and bloody stools (50%).

- Constitutional symptoms such as headache, myalgias, backache, malaise, anorexia and vomiting may be present.

- Duration of illness usually is <1 week, although symptoms can persist for longer. Relapses occur in as many as 25% of patients.

Vibrio parahaemolyticus
- Explosive, watery diarrhea is present in >90% of cases with associated symptoms including abdominal cramps, nausea, vomiting and headache.

- Fever and chills occur in ~25%.

- Clinical manifestations resemble that produced by nontyphoidal-*Salmonella*.

- Median duration of illness is 3 days (range, 2 hours to 10 days).

Yersinia enterocolitica
- Enterocolitis occurs in ~65% of patients, is most common in children <5 years old.

- Clinical manifestations include fever, abdominal cramps and diarrhea, which usually lasts 1-3 weeks.

- In children >5 years of age, mesenteric adenitis and associated ileitis may develop with symptoms including nausea, vomiting and aphthous oral ulcers.

- Yersinia is less likely to cause disease in adults; in this age group it is associated with acute diarrhea.

Key Differential Diagnostic Features

Infectious Diseases
- CMV colitis (usually present in severely immunocompromised patients such as those with AIDS or S/P transplant; intranuclear inclusions on biopsy help confirm the diagnosis).

- Intestinal Kaposi's sarcoma (diagnosed by biopsy; most likely to occur in the setting of HIV).

Noninfectious Diseases
- Ulcerative colitis (chronic diarrhea associated with extraintestinal manifestations plus characteristic histopathologic findings).

- Crohn's disease (chronic diarrhea associated with extraintestinal manifestations plus characteristic histopathologic findings).

- Radiation enterocolitis (history of radiation therapy; colonoscopy may show luminal narrowing, ulceration and diffuse inflammatory changes).

- Eosinophilic gastroenteritis (diarrhea often associated with nausea, vomiting, abdominal pain and weight loss; peripheral eosinophilia present in 75%).

- Ischemic colitis (history of atherosclerotic vascular disease; usually presents with abdominal pain and bloody stools).

Key Laboratory Findings

- Microscopy usually reveals abundant erythrocytes and leukocytes.

- A diffusely ulcerated, hemorrhagic, and friable colonic mucosa will be visible on proctoscopy.

- Certain pathogens, *Salmonella* and *Yersinia*, mainly involve the lower small bowel but may invade the colon as well. Although watery diarrhea is the usual presentation, depending on the focus of infection, the spectrum extends from dehydrating diarrhea to a frank colitis.

Shigellosis
- Diagnosis should be suspected when the triad of lower abdominal pain, rectal burning and diarrhea is present.

- Microscopic examination of the stool will reveal many polymorphonuclear leukocytes (PMN) and red blood cells (RBC).

- Culture is needed for the identification of the specific bacterial pathogen.

- As *Shigella* spp. are very fastidious, stool specimens or rectal swabs should be rapidly inoculated into selective media.

- Cytotoxins may be detected using cell culture, animal models, DNA probes or PCR.

Nontyphoidal salmonellosis
- *Salmonella* species grow on several types of artificial media. They can be separated on differential media by the inclusion of certain chemicals that favor their growth and suppress other coliforms.

- For convenience in the laboratory, a series of Kauffmann-White serogroups containing several serotypes have been developed which are based on shared antigens among the most common *Salmonella* types.

- Recent molecular techniques have shown that all commonly encountered nontyphoidal *Salmonella* are members of the same species, *S enterica*. Consequently, species are named as subspecies of S enterica. For example, Salmonella enteritidis is now classified as S enterica serovar Enteriditis or *S enteriditis*.

EHEC
- Microscopic examination of the stool reveals RBCs, whereas PMNs are present in lower quantity.

- Tissue culture (using Vero or HeLa cells), DNA probes, PCR and enzyme immunoassays can directly detect verotoxins in stool specimens.

- Some EHEC strains produce only SLT I or II whereas others produce both toxins.

- As most isolates of *E coli* 0157:H7 do not ferment D sorbitol, screening for this organism can be done with sorbitol-MacConkey agar.

- Serotyping and toxin testing must be done for confirmation.

- Specimens should be cultured as early as possible after the onset of symptoms. Within 2 days after onset, nearly all stool specimens are positive for EHEC, whereas only one-third are positive after 7 days.

Enteroinvasive *E coli*
- Examination of the stool shows many PMNs.

- An enterotoxin has been identified in enteroinvasive *E coli* strains but diagnosis in a routine bacteriologic laboratory is generally impractical.

C jejuni
- Stool examination usually reveals fecal leukocytes and occult blood.

- Endoscopy may reveal an inflammatory colitis.

- Stool culture is the most reliable way to diagnose

- Selective isolation medium containing antibiotics must be used because *Campylobacters* grow more slowly than other enteric bacteria; plates are grown at 42°C under CO_2 and reduced oxygen.

- Darkfield or phase contrast microscopy of fresh diarrhea shows the organism as a curved, highly motile rod, with darting, corkscrew movements.

V parahaemolyticus

- Few PMNs are present on stool examination.

- Culture on TCBS medium and biochemical tests is used to identify this facultative anaerobe.

Yersinia
- Diagnosis is established by culture of stool or body fluids. Since the organism is slow growing and overgrowth of normal fecal flora may make it difficult to isolate from stool, the laboratory should be advised to watch out for this pathogen.

- When antisera are appropriately absorbed, serological tests are useful in diagnosing recent infection. Agglutinating antibodies appear shortly after symptom onset and usually disappear in 2-6 months.

Empiric Therapy
- See Empiric Therapy in the toxigenic diarrhea section.

- Concerns about potentially exacerbating a case of dysentery with an antimotility drug have been largely eliminated by clinical experience. Nevertheless, antimotility agents generally should not be used in patients with acute, severe colitis.

- Since the use of antibiotics has not been shown to decrease morbidity due to EHEC and appears to increase the risk of HUS, *antimicrobial therapy should be avoided if E coli O157:H7 is suspected or conclusively identified*.

Definitive Therapy
See Table 2 for specific therapies.

Complications

Shigellosis
- Intestinal perforation.

- Intestinal protein loss.

- Meningismus.

- Seizures.

- Hypoglycemia.

- Leukemoid reaction.

- Thrombocytopenia.

- Hemolytic uremic syndrome (HUS). Most of these complications are more common in children.

- A postdysenteric, asymmetric arthritis, usually associated with histocompatibility type HLA B27, may develop 2-3 weeks after the onset of diarrhea.

Nontyphoidal salmonellosis
Salmonella gastroenteritis may be complicated by:

- Bacteremia.

- Meningitis.

- Arteritis.

- Endocarditis.

- Osteomyelitis.

- Wound infections.

- Septic arthritis.

- Focal abscesses.

EHEC
- HUS.

- Thrombotic thrombocytopenic purpura.

- Risk factors for HUS include age under 5 years, attendance at a large daycare center, presence of bloody diarrhea and high white blood cell count.

Campylobacter jejuni
Rare complications include:

- * Gastrointestinal hemorrhage

- * Toxic megacolon

- * Pancreatitis

- * Cholecystitis

- * HUS

- * Bacteremia

- * Meningitis

- * Purulent arthritis

- Postinfectious complications include reactive arthritis (usually occurs in individuals with the HLA-B27 phenotype) and Guillain-Barré syndrome.

Yersinia enterocolitica
- 2-3 weeks after an episode, reactive polyarthritis may develop (~2% of patients, especially those who are HLA B27 positive).

- *Yersinia* bacteremia, a rare complication, is seen in patients with underlying diseases, such as malignancy, diabetes mellitus, anemia and liver disease.

- Metastatic foci can occur in bones, joints and lungs.

ID Board Pearls

- Invasive diarrheal pathogens are the most common reportable enteric infections in the U.S.

- A extensive range of foods, exposure to recreational water and close contact with an infected individual are the major modes of transmission.

- A broad array of clinical syndromes can be seen with *Salmonella*, including acute gastroenteritis, bacteremia, a typhoid fever-like syndrome, and localized infections in bones, joints and meninges.

- Inflammatory cells are usually present in fecal samples.

- Shigellosis should be suspected when the triad of lower abdominal pain, rectal burning and diarrhea is present.

- Although clinical experience has shown that antimotility drugs are unlikely to exacerbate a case of dysentery, nevertheless antimotility agents generally should not be used in patients with acute, severe colitis.

- Antibiotics should be avoided in patients in whom *E coli* O157 is suspected or confirmed.

3. Additional Bacterial Causes of Diarrhea

Causative Organisms

- Noncholera vibrios including *V cholerae* non-01, *V vulnificus*, *V mimicus*, *V hollisae*, *V furnissii* and *V fluvialis*

- *Aeromonas hydrophila, A caviae* and *A sobria*.

- Enteropathogenic *E coli*.

- Diffusely adherent *E coli*.

- *Plesiomonas shigelloides*.

Epidemiology

Noncholera Vibrios
- Non-01 cholera vibrios can be isolated from salty coastal waters of the United States, most commonly in the summer and fall when the temperature rises.

- Mollusks, particularly oysters (reported contamination rate of 10%-15%), are the major source; clams, mussels and crabs have also been implicated.

- *V vulnificus* may be the most important noncholera vibrio in the United States, based on its severity of illness, especially in patients with underlying liver disease.

- *V vulnificus* infection can result from a wound infection, by contact with seawater or seafood or through direct consumption of seafood, usually raw oysters.

- *V mimicus*, *V hollisae*, *V furnissii* and *V fluvialis* are all rare causes of gastroenteritis; the latter 2 have been more frequently described in Southeast Asia.

Aeromonas spp.
- Ubiquitous environmental organisms found principally in fresh and brackish water, especially during the summer.

- Frequently mistaken for coliforms in the laboratory, leading to falsely low reported rates. *Aeromonas* infections are often associated with

drinking untreated water such as well water or spring water.

Plesiomonas shigelloides
- Isolated less frequently in the United States than *Aeromonas*.

- Infections associated with consumption of raw oysters or recent travel to Mexico or the Orient.

Enteropathogenic *E coli*
- Common cause of childhood diarrhea in the developing world, especially in children less than 1 year old.

Enteroaggregative *E coli*
- Inconsistently implicated as a cause of acute and persistent diarrhea in children in developing countries.

Diffusely Adherent *E coli*
- Has been associated with diarrhea in children in some developing countries.

- Some strains may be more pathogenic for older children.

- May also be a rare cause of nosocomial diarrhea in developed countries.

Key Clinical Features

Noncholera Vibrios
- Non-01 cholera vibrios may cause severe, dehydrating diarrhea, wound and ear infections, septicemia, pneumonia and infections of the biliary tract.

- Incubation period is usually 3 days.

- Duration is usually <1 week.

- *V vulnificus* may cause gastroenteritis (characterized by abdominal pain, vomiting and watery diarrhea), wound infections or septicemia.

- *V mimicus* causes diarrhea or ear infections.

- *V hollisae* may cause gastroenteritis or bacteremia.

- *V furnissii* and *V fluvialis* may cause severe watery diarrhea.

Aeromonas spp.

- Clinical syndromes include wound infections, bacteremia or deep organ infections (especially in immunocompromised hosts), and gastroenteritis, which ranges from mild to severe diarrhea.

- Most cases resolve within 1 week, although adults may rarely develop chronic diarrhea.

Plesiomonas shigelloides

- Usually causes diarrhea with prominent abdominal pain.

Enteropathogenic and Diffusely Adherent *E coli*

- Both cause acute, non-bloody diarrhea.

Key Laboratory Findings

- Vibrios produce different clinical presentations, apparently related to the virulence factors in each infecting strain.

- Potentially infected sites, ie, stool, wounds and blood should be cultured on appropriate media with biochemical tests used to differentiate the species.

Noncholera Vibrios

- Best isolated with TCBS agar.

Aeromonas spp. and *P shigelloides*

- Aeromonas spp. and P shigelloides both grow well on primary, nonselective agar, such as Salmonella-Shigella or MacConkey agars.

Enteropathogenic and Diffusely Adherent *E coli*

- Enteropathogenic and diffusely adhering strains of *E coli* are characterized by their adherence patterns to certain cell lines *in vitro*.

- Slide agglutination test using specific antisera is used to identify serogroups of enteropathogenic *E coli*.

- DNA probes or PCR are used to identify the presence of virulence factors for these *E coli* strains and EAggEC.

Empiric Therapy

See Empiric Therapy in the toxigenic diarrhea section.

Definitive Therapy

See Table 2 for specific therapies.

ID Board Pearls

- Non-01 cholera vibrios can be isolated from ocean waters of the U.S., most commonly in the summer and fall when the temperature rises.

- *V vulnificus* can cause diarrhea, severe wound infections and bacteremia, with more severe cases occurring in individuals with underlying liver disease.

- *Aeromonas* spp. may be responsible for a range of clinical syndromes including wound infections, bacteremia or deep organ infections (especially in immunocompromised hosts), and gastroenteritis.

4. Viral Diarrhea

Causative Organisms

- Rotavirus.

- Caliciviruses, including the noroviruses (previously known as Norwalk-like viruses).

- Astrovirus.

- Enteric adenovirus.

- Toroviruses.

Epidemiology

Rotavirus
- Responsible for 35% of diarrhea in hospitalized children and 10% of cases in the community.

- Probably is spread by the fecal oral route.

- In temperate zones, the disease is more common in wintertime, but in the tropics it is endemic year round.

- Within a family grouping, the young child is often afflicted with the clinical illness, while older siblings and adults may be asymptomatic carriers.

Caliciviruses Including the Noroviruses
- Caliciviruses cause disease mainly in infants and young children, particularly in daycare centers.

- Noroviruses are recognized as the cause of approximately 50% of all food-borne epidemics of gastroenteritis in the United States.

- Noroviruses most commonly cause outbreaks in the fall and winter months in temperate climates.

- Diarrhea outbreaks caused by noroviruses occur in camps, cruise ships, hotels, nursing homes and hospitals, and are characterized by a high attack rate, with all age groups affected except infants.

- Transmission occurs by person-to-person contact, primarily by the fecal oral route.

- Raw shellfish and contaminated drinking water supplies are additional sources.

Astrovirus
- A major cause of diarrheal illness in children, responsible for outbreaks of diarrhea in daycare centers and in communities with children <1 year old.

Enteric Adenovirus
- Approximately 5%-10% of childhood diarrhea is associated with enteric adenovirus, without any seasonal occurrence.

- Children <2 years of age are most commonly infected.

- Nosocomial and daycare center outbreaks are common, although high rates of asymptomatic infections occur.

Toroviruses
- Diarrhea due to toroviruses usually occurs in children under the age of 2 years.

- Older children are at risk for symptomatic infections, especially those who are immunocompromised.

Key Clinical Features

Rotavirus
- Average incubation period is 1-3 days.

- Clinical illness ranges from asymptomatic carriage to severe dehydration, with rare fatalities.

- Children aged 3-15 months have the highest infection rates.

- Adults rarely may develop mild infections, usually from contact with a sick child in the household.

- Acute onset of vomiting is followed shortly by watery diarrhea, which can lead to moderate dehydration.

- The mean duration of illness is 5-7 days.

Caliciviruses

- Typical caliciviruses cause disease, mainly in infants and young children, that is generally mild and indistinguishable from rotavirus.

- In outbreaks caused by noroviruses, nausea, vomiting, diarrhea, abdominal cramps and myalgias are common symptoms.

- The mean duration is 24-48 hours.

Astrovirus

- Asymptomatic infections are more common in adults than children.

- Illness is characterized by watery or mucoid stools, nausea, vomiting, and occasionally, fever, but it tends to be milder than rotavirus diarrhea as dehydration is rare.

Enteric Adenovirus

- The mean incubation period is 8-10 days, and symptoms may last as long as 2 weeks.

- Clinical manifestations are similar to those seen with astrovirus.

Toroviruses

- Associated with both acute and persistent (lasting greater than 14 days) diarrhea in children.

- When compared to rotavirus, children infected with torovirus have less vomiting and more bloody diarrhea–however, this only occurs in 11%.

Key Laboratory Findings

- Since none of the enteropathogenic viruses can be grown in the laboratory, the diagnosis can only be established by identifying virus particles or antigen in stool specimens. Several commercial immunoassays allow the rapid detection of rotavirus antigen in the feces.

- Polymerase chain reaction, electron microscopy and nucleic acid probes are also available to detect rotavirus and identify its serogroups.

- Immune electron microscopy, enzyme linked immunoabsorbent assay (ELISA), PCR, and DNA or RNA hybridization assays are used to identify noroviruses, enteric adenovirus and astrovirus in stool specimens, but these tests currently are available only in research laboratories.

- Reverse transcriptase (real time) PCR for the detection of noroviruses is available in most state public health laboratories.

- Toroviruses can be detected in stool specimens by electron microscopy or ELISA.

Empiric Therapy

- Treatment is supportive with an emphasis on oral rehydration. (See empiric therapy in the toxigenic diarrhea section.)

Definitive Therapy

- No definitive, antiviral antimicrobial agent is currently available for any of the viral etiologies of diarrhea.

- Antirotavirus immunoglobulin of bovine colostral origin has been found to be effective in reducing the duration of rotavirus duration and the amount of oral rehydration therapy required.

- Rotarix, a vaccine composed of a live attenuated rotavirus strain, and RotaTeq, a live oral pentavalent vaccine, are both FDA-approved for prevention of rotavirus diarrhea in infants in the U.S. Both vaccines have >80% protective efficacy against severe rotavirus disease. Neither vaccine has been associated with intussusception or shown to interfere with responses to other routine immunizations.

Complications

- Rotavirus can result in moderate to severe dehydration, requiring hospitalization and parenteral rehydration.

5. Traveler's Diarrhea

ID Board Pearls

- Most causes of viral diarrhea are transmitted by the fecal-oral route.

- Rotavirus is a common cause of moderate to severe dehydrating diarrhea in children aged 3-15 months.

- Noroviruses are responsible for large scale outbreaks in daycare centers, camps, cruise ships, hotels, nursing homes and healthcare facilities.

- Oral rehydration therapy should be the main focus of treatment.

- 2 effective live attenuated rotavirus vaccines are now licensed in the U.S. for prevention of disease in infants.

Causative Organisms

- No pathogen identified (22%-83%)

- ETEC (0%-70%)

- EaggEC (0%-30%)

- *Campylobacter* spp. (0%-41%)

- *Shigella* spp. (0%-30%)

- *Salmonella* spp. (0%-15%)

- Enteroadherent *E coli* (0%-15%)

- Enteroinvasive *E coli* (0%-5%)

- *Vibrio* spp. (0%-30%)

- *Aeromonas* spp. (0%-30%)

- Rotavirus (0%-36%)

- *Giardia lamblia* (0%-6%)

- *Entamoeba histolytica* (0%-6%)

- *Cryptosporidium parvum* (rare)

- *Cyclospora cayetanensis* (rare)

- *Hafnia alvei* (rare)

Epidemiology

- At least 16 million persons from industrialized countries travel to developing countries each year, where they are at increased risk for traveler's diarrhea.

- Prospective studies have found median traveler's diarrhea rates of slightly >50% in Latin America (range, 21%-100%), in Asia (21%-100%) and in Africa (36%-62%).

- Intermediate-risk destinations, with an incidence of 10%-20%, include Southern European countries, Israel and a few Caribbean islands.

- Low-risk areas, where the incidence is <8%, include Canada, the United States, Northern Europe, Australia, New Zealand, Japan and most Caribbean islands.

- Travelers who go from one less developed country to another are at a lower risk for the acquisition of traveler's diarrhea. Longer residence in a high-risk country may lead to increased resistance to traveler's diarrhea, but previous short-term travel to areas of high risk does not necessarily produce protection.

- The greatest frequency of diarrhea occurs in students or itinerant tourists, the lowest risk in those visiting relatives and an intermediate risk in business travelers.

- Additional risk factors include younger age and a failure to adhere to dietary precautions. Traveler's diarrhea is acquired through the ingestion of fecally contaminated food or beverages.

- Risky foods include tap water, ice, undercooked or raw vegetables, meat, seafood, unpasteurized milk and dairy products, open salsas and unpeeled fruits.

Key Clinical Features

- Watery, loose stools (usually 3-5/day) are the primary manifestation.

- Associated symptoms may include (in relative order of occurrence): gas, fatigue, cramps, nausea, fever, abdominal pain, anorexia, headache, chills, vomiting, malaise and arthralgias.

- Approximately 2%-10% of patients have fever, bloody stools or both; they are more likely to have shigellosis.

- Average duration of illness in untreated subjects is 3-5 days, although symptoms may last weeks to months in a minority of patients (~1%-3% of travelers will develop persistent diarrhea).

Key Laboratory Findings

- The diagnosis should be suspected in recent travelers to less developed regions of the world who present with characteristic symptoms.

- Specific etiologic diagnosis can be performed as described above for specific pathogens. Since most episodes will be self-limited, making a specific diagnosis is generally unnecessary.

- Travelers with persistent diarrhea should be evaluated for parasitic and enteric bacterial pathogens, which are more likely to cause prolonged diarrhea such as *Campylobacter*.

Empiric Therapy

- A fluoroquinolone or azithromycin are good choices for empiric treatment, since these drugs have broad spectrum activity against all bacteria responsible for acute infectious diarrhea in travelers and resistance remains limited.

- Due to rising fluoroquinolone resistance in Asia, empiric therapy with azithromycin should be considered for travelers to this area of the world.

- Rifaximin, a nonabsorbable oral antibiotic, is effective for the treatment of mild to moderate traveler's diarrhea but should be avoided in patients with invasive diarrhea.

- The duration of antimicrobial therapy has not been clearly defined.

- There are several studies that suggest a single dose is as effective as more prolonged therapy for traveler's diarrhea.

- The combination of an antibiotic with an anti-motility drug may provide more rapid relief of diarrhea than either agent alone.

Definitive Therapy

- The choice of antibiotic, when indicated, should be based on in vitro sensitivity patterns (see Table 2 for specific pathogens and treatment choices).

Prevention

The following precautions apply to travelers who will be voyaging to less developed countries:

- Use a safe source of water for drinking and food preparation. If unsure, then bottled beverages, especially carbonated beverages or boiled water, should be used.

- Avoid ice cubes made from local tap water.

- Do not eat raw vegetables or salads.

- Eat only fruit that you wash or peel yourself.

- Avoid eating food from street vendors.

- Avoid eating open salsas (in Mexican restaurants).

Antimicrobial Prophylaxis

- Protection rates vary from 28%-100%; lower rates have been seen in studies that used less effective antimicrobial drugs or when a high level of resistance to the drug was present in local bacterial enteropathogens.

- Protection rates with norfloxacin or ciprofloxacin are 68%-94%.

- Rifaximin has recently been shown to provide 72% protection against traveler's diarrhea.

- Bismuth subsalicylate has also been used for prevention, based on its antimicrobial and antisecretory activities; however, it provides modest protection only when the traveler is conscientious about taking the higher dose needed for effective prevention.

- Since traveler's diarrhea is usually self-limited and highly responsive to antimicrobial therapy, prophylaxis is generally not recommended.

ID Board Pearls

- ETEC and EAggEC are the 2 most common etiologies of traveler's diarrhea, although half of cases or more do not have a specific pathogen identified.

- Travelers who are students or itinerant tourists, and are younger and fail to adhere to dietary precautions, are at increased risk for traveler's diarrhea.

- High risk fluids and foods include tap water, ice, undercooked or raw vegetables, meat, seafood, unpasteurized milk and dairy products, open salsas and unpeeled fruits.

- In addition to oral rehydration therapy, empiric therapy with a 3 day course of a fluoroquinolone or azithromycin is usually highly effective.

- Generally, antibiotics should not be used for prophylaxis of traveler's diarrhea.

6. Further Reading

DuPont HL. Travellers' diarrhoea: contemporary approaches to therapy and prevention. *Drugs*. 2006;66:303-314.

Guerrant RL, Van Gilder T, Steiner TS, et al. Practice guidelines for the management of infectious diarrhea. *Clin Infect Dis*. 2001;32:331-350.

Hamer DH, Gorbach SL. Intestinal infections, overview. In: Heggenhougen HK, Quah S, eds. *International Encyclopedia of Public Health*. San Diego, CA: Academic Press; 2008;683-695.

Hamer DH, Gorbach SL. Use of the quinolones for the treatment and prophylaxis of bacterial infections. In: Andriole VT, ed. *The Quinolones*. 3rd ed. San Diego, CA: Academic Press; 2000:303-323.

Kaper JB, Nataro JP, Mobley HL. Pathogenic Escherichia coli. *Nat Rev Microbiology*. 2004;2:123-140.

Niyogi SK. Shigellosis. *Microbiol*. 2005;43:133-143.

Sack DA, Sack RB, Nair GB, Siddique AK. Cholera. *Lancet*. 2004;363:223-233.

Thielman NM, Guerrant RL. Acute infectious diarrhea. *N Engl J Med*. 2004;350:38-47.

Chapter 21: Sexually Transmitted Diseases (STDs) for the ID Boards

Michael F. Rein, MD

Contents

1. Syphilis

Synonyms (street)

• Syph, bad blood.

Causative Organism

• *T pallidum* is a spirochete 5-15 μM long and less than 0.5 μM wide.

• Living organisms are visualized by reflected light using darkfield microscopy.

• The organism can also be identified by silver staining or by direct immunofluorescence.

Epidemiology

• Between 1991 and 2000, rates of syphilis declined in the United States, however, since 2004, overall rates have again increased, particularly among men who have sex with men and African American men.

• Possible reasons for the initial decline include the use of ceftriaxone for treatment of gonorrhea, HIV prevention education with personal protection measures being followed (eg, condom use), or HIV partner notification (which may allow for early therapy of new cases in contacts).

• Rates of infection remain highest:

　　* In the rural South

　　* Among lower socioeconomic, inner-city populations

　　* Among users of crack cocaine and sex-for-drugs prostitution

• Sexual transmission occurs by direct contact with a moist lesion.

• Transplacental transmission is the second major route of acquisition.

Key Clinical Features

• Syphilis is a chronic infection, but it is latent for most of its course.

• There are several clinically apparent stages.

• The incubation period usually lasts approximately 3 weeks but is said to range from 10-90 days. During this interval, infected patients have, by definition, neither clinical nor serologic evidence of disease.

• Because the incubation period can last for this prolonged interval, termed the *critical period*, it is the standard of care to treat people who have had sexual contact during the past 90 days with persons manifesting lesions of syphilis.

• This approach is termed *epidemiologic treatment*.

• Epidemiologic treatment is provided on the basis of risk rather than on the basis of diagnosis, and it is a cornerstone of the management of sexually transmitted diseases.

Primary Syphilis

• Primary syphilis manifests as one or more ulcerated lesions, called chancres.

• These develop at the site of initial infection and multiplication of the spirochetes.

• Although classically described as a single lesion, almost half of patients actually present with multiple chancres. Don't be misled by the presence of multiple lesions.

• The ulcers usually are only minimally painful or tender, in contrast to chancroid or herpes, in which lesions are usually painful.

• They are usually clean with distinctly indurated edges.

• Regional adenopathy develops within the first week, manifesting as several discrete nodes that are relatively nontender and rubbery.

• Inguinal adenopathy is usually bilateral, even if the chancre occurs on one side of the genital tract.

- The cervix, proximal third of the vagina and the glans penis are drained by deep iliac nodes, and chancres at these sites will not produce palpable adenopathy.

- Maintain a high index of suspicion for syphilis when confronting otherwise unexplained lesions around the mouth or anus.

- Untreated, the manifestations of primary syphilis usually resolve in 3-6 weeks in immunocompetent hosts.

- Nontreponemal serologic tests for syphilis are positive in only approximately 50% of patients at the time the chancre first appears.

    * A nonreactive test does not rule out syphilis in such patients.

Secondary Syphilis

- Secondary syphilis is a result of the early dissemination of *T pallidum* throughout the body.

- Dissemination may occur even before the chancre appears.

Generalized rash

- A rash appears, approximately 3-6 weeks and even after the resolution of the chancre.

    * It commonly involves the palms and soles

    * It almost always involves the oral mucous membranes and the genitalia

- The lesions are highly variable, making diagnosis challenging.

    * May resemble pityriasis rosea. Don't be fooled

    * Coppery or boiled ham color

    * Bilaterally symmetrical

    * Non- or minimally pruritic

- The dry lesions of secondary syphilis are not contagious.

- Distinctly unusual in secondary syphilis adults:

    * Bullae

    * Generalized rash sparing the mouth and genitalia

    * Marked pruritus

- Generally begins as a nonspecific, systemic illness:

    * Sore throat

    * Myalgias

    * Patchy alopecia is common

    * 75% of cases manifest generalized lymphadenopathy

- Condylomata lata may appear.

    * Hypertrophic lesions, resembling flat warts

    * Occur in moist areas, such as around the anus or under the breasts

    * Highly contagious

- Mucous patches may appear.

    * Painless shallow ulcers of the mucous membranes

    * Highly contagious, and in the past resulted in digital chancres among dentists ("dentist's finger")

- Asymptomatic involvement of the central nervous system is common.

    * Do not obtain examination of the cerebrospinal fluid in secondary syphilis

- Serologic tests are almost always reactive in secondary syphilis, usually in high titer.

- Rarely, patients have such high levels of antibody that antibody excess produces a falsely negative nontreponemal test

  * This prozone phenomenon can be avoided by performing quantitative nontreponemal tests, in which serial dilutions of serum are examined

  * Serial dilutions of serum will dilute out the excess antibody and high titers will then be observed

- The manifestations of secondary syphilis resolve without treatment.

- Nearly 25% of patients with untreated syphilis will again develop the manifestations of secondary syphilis during the first year of infection.

  * Such patients are said to have mucocutaneous relapse, and are again contagious to sexual partners

Latent Syphilis

- Latent syphilis is clinically silent and diagnosis can be made only on the basis of serologic tests.

Late (Tertiary) Syphilis
- Eventually develops in approximately one-third of untreated, infected patients.

- Antibiotics given for other reasons may prevent, delay or mask onset.

- Should be suspected in the following clinical settings:

  * Lymphocytic meningitis

  * May appear as meningovascular syphilis: A cerebrovascular accident in a young person without other cause should raise suspicion

  * Young people with HIV and syphilis may present with seizures or with diplopia or scotomata. Syphilis should be in the differential diagnosis of such patients

  * Stabbing (lightning) pains of the abdomen and extremities

- Destructive lesions of skin and bones may represent so-called late benign syphilis.

- The nontreponemal tests are insensitive in some forms of late syphilis.

- A patient being worked up for late syphilis should have a treponemal test performed, even if an initial, nontreponemal test is nonreactive.

- Approximately one-third of untreated syphilitic patients will remain seroreactive but will not develop late manifestations of syphilis.

- Nearly one-third of untreated syphilitic patients remain well and become nonreactive on nontreponemal testing.

Neurosyphilis

- Dementia may be due to paresis.

- Posterior column disease may result from tabes dorsalis. This may resemble the neurological sequellae of pernicious anemia. Don't be fooled.

- Small pupils responding to accommodation but not to light may be a Argyll-Robertson pupils, suggesting neurosyphilis.

- Latent syphilis with a nontreponemal test titre ≥1:32 is associated with a higher risk of having asymptomatic neurosyphilis.

Cardiovascular Syphilis

Aortitis

- Aneurysm of the proximal aorta vs. atheroscleotic disease, which more often affects the distal aorta.

- Syphilitic aneurysms dissect only rarely.

Aortic Regurgitation
- Aortic second sound with a drum-like quality (tambour sound).

- Aortic regurgitant murmur heard best at the right of the sternum.

Syphilis in HIV Infection
- The presence of active syphilis increases viral load and decreases CD4+ cell count.

  * Multiple or persistent chancres

  * Individual reports suggest that neurosyphilis may occur earlier

  * Cerebrospinal fluid examination should be performed on all HIV-infected patients with latent syphilis

  * There is a higher rate of failure of the serologic tests to respond to treatment

Key Laboratory Features

- Because *T pallidum* cannot be cultured *in vitro* and syphilis is subclinical for much of its course, laboratory diagnosis is critical.

- Syphilis can be diagnosed by identifying *T pallidum* in lesions.

Darkfield Examination

- Material from a lesion is examined using a microscope that sends light rays obliquely through the specimen, illuminating the organism by reflected light against a dark background.

- Obtaining the specimen and interpreting the test requires experience.

Other Evaluations

- Direct immunofluorescence has the same sensitivity, but specimens may be sent to a central laboratory.

- Silver staining is less sensitive and specific.

- Polymerase chain reaction (PCR) methods are far more sensitive and are available in a research setting.

Serodiagnosis
- Because syphilis is subclinical for much of its course, we have come to rely heavily on serologic diagnosis.

Nontreponemal Tests

- Often used as screening tests for syphilis

- Exploit the observation that patients with syphilis develop IgG antibodies reactive with a variety of poorly-defined lipids.

  * These antibodies are (unfortunately) classically called "reagin"

  * Not to be confused with IgE

- VDRL (Venereal Disease Research Laboratory).

- RPR (rapid plasma reagin).

- ART (automated reagin test).

- TRUST (toluidine red unheated serologic test).

- An ELISA for antiphospholipid antibody, the Spirotek Reagin II, is about 95% sensitive in early syphilis.

- Nontreponemal tests are nonspecific, and may be positive in:

  * Acute viral illnesses

  * Collagen vascular disease

  * Pregnancy

  * Intravenous drug use

  * Old age

  * Leprosy

- Considered diagnostic only in the presence of a highly suggestive clinical syndrome (eg, primary or secondary syphilis).

- Cannot be used to diagnose latent syphilis without confirmation by a treponemal test.

    * A reactive nontreponemal test and a nonreactive treponemal test is considered a false-positive nontreponemal test

- Usually quantitated.

    * Reported as the highest 2-fold dilution of serum yielding a positive reaction

    * Titers of 1:8 or higher are unusual among false positives

    * The highest titers ($\geq$1:128) may be seen in secondary syphilis

- Except for the ELISA, they are relatively insensitive in primary and late syphilis.

- When working up late syphilis, one should order a treponemal test even when the nontreponemal test is nonreactive.

Treponemal Tests

- Use *T pallidum*, or fractions thereof, as antigen.

- The treponemal tests are more specific and more sensitive than the nontreponemal tests, particularly in very early primary and late syphilis.

- They are not quantitated but are reported as reactive or nonreactive.

- The fluorescent treponemal antibody absorption test (FTA-abs) is the most sensitive test for antibody to T pallidum. It uses indirect immunofluorescence.

Agglutination Tests

- The microhemagglutination test for *T pallidum* (MHA-Tp) uses *T pallidum* attached to erythrocytes. Antibody to the organism causes the erythrocytes to agglutinate, a reaction which can be read grossly.

* It is subject to misleading results due to heterophile antibodies directed against the carrier red cells.

* It has been largely replaced by tests using particulate gelatin or latex, such as the Serodia TP-PA and the PK-TP, which are suitable as screening tests and are now used extensively by blood banks.

- These tests are about 97% specific.

Treponemal ELISA Tests

- The most commonly used is the Captia syphilis G test, which is 98% sensitive and about 100% specific.

- Several newer ELISA tests employ cloned *T pallidum* antigens and have high sensitivity and specificity.

- Western blot tests have very high specificity and may be used in problem cases.

- Treponemal tests are used to confirm a diagnosis of past or present treponemal infection in patients with reactive nontreponemal tests.

- The treponemal tests remain positive for prolonged periods, even after adequate treatment of syphilis.

    * A persistently reactive treponemal test does not indicate inadequate treatment, relapse or reinfection.

- The treponemal tests may be reactive in other diseases:

    * Nonvenereal treponematoses such as yaws, pinta or bejel

        • Be wary of interpreting reactive tests in persons from areas where these diseases are prevalent (eg, the Caribbean)

    * Some cases of Lyme disease, because of shared flagellar antigens

- The nontreponemal tests should be nonreactive in Lyme

Differential Diagnosis

- The differential diagnosis of early syphilis is difficult, and discussion is beyond the scope of this review. Sir William Osler said, "Know syphilis in all its manifestations and relations, and all things clinical will be added unto you." One should be suspicious of syphilis and consider serological diagnosis in any of the clinical settings listed above.

Empiric Therapy

- Empiric therapy is never appropriate.

Definitive Therapy

- Parenteral benzyl penicillin (penicillin G) is the treatment of choice for all stages of syphilis.

- Sexual partners of patients with syphilitic skin or mucous membrane lesions are infected about 25%-50% of the time.

- All patients presenting as contacts to syphilis within the past 90 days (the so-called critical period) are treated with a regimen effective for early syphilis.

- Patients whose exposure was more than 90 days previously may be evaluated serologically and if seronegative, need not be treated.

Early Syphilis (Primary, Secondary, and Latent Syphilis of <1 Year Duration)

- Benzathine penicillin G, 2.4 million units, IM, in 1 dose

- In penicillin allergy:

  * Doxycycline 100 mg PO BID for 2 weeks

  * Tetracycline 500 mg PO QID for 2 weeks

- There is likely to be poor compliance with this regimen because of the frequency of administration and the likelihood of gastrointestinal intolerance

  * There are recent reports of resistance to and treatment failure with macrolides/azalide antibiotics, and these drugs (azithromycin, erythromycin) should not be used to treat syphilis except in very rare circumstances

- Ceftriaxone 1 g QD, IM or IV for 10 days (data are limited, and the possibility of cross-hypersensitivity with the penicillins should be kept in mind).

  * This regimen should not be used in patients with a history of anaphylaxis to penicillin

- One should attempt to desensitize the pregnant woman with severe penicillin allergy so she can receive penicillin.

  * Tetracyclines are contraindicated in pregnancy

Latent Syphilis of Unknown Duration or of More Than 1 Year Duration, Late Benign Syphilis, Cardiovascular Syphilis

- Benzathine penicillin G, 7.2 million U total, administered as 3 doses of 2.4 million units IM, given 1 week apart for 3 consecutive weeks.

- Alternatively for penicillin-allergic, nonpregnant patients: doxycycline 100 mg PO BID for 4 weeks, or tetracycline 500 mg PO QID for 4 weeks.

- Management of the penicillin-allergic pregnant woman is uncertain and should probably involve desensitization to penicillin.

- One should examine cerebrospinal fluid in the following clinical settings:

  * Neurologic signs or symptoms

  * Treatment failure

  * Other evidence of active late syphilis (eg, aortitis, gumma, iritis)

* Non-penicillin therapy planned

* Concurrent HIV infection with syphilis of more than one year or unknown duration

Neurosyphilis

- Aqueous crystalline penicillin G, 12-24 million U/day IV for 10-14 days, administered 2-4 million units q4h or by continuous drip.

- In the HIV-positive patient, neurosyphilis may be particularly difficult to treat, and failures of therapy can occur, despite optimal therapy with high-dose IV aqueous penicillin.

- Procaine penicillin G 2.4 million U/d IM, and probenecid 500 mg PO QID, both for 10-14 days (perhaps a little barbaric).

- Ceftriaxone 1 g IM/day for 14 days.

  * This might be used in patients whose allergy to penicillin is not manifested by anaphylaxis

  * Data are limited

- Because the currently recommended regimen is shorter than that recommended for late syphilis in the absence of neurosyphilis, some experts administer one or more doses of benzathine penicillin, 2.4 million units IM, after completion of one of the above regimens.

The Jarisch-Herxheimer Reaction

- Onset 1-6 hours after beginning treatment for syphilis.

- Occurs in approximately 50% of patients with primary syphilis and in most patients with secondary syphilis.

- It presents as fever, increased rash, adenopathy and, sometimes, hypotension.

- It probably results from the release of treponemal antigens upon lysis of the organisms.

- It is self-limited and usually requires treatment only with antipyretics, but patients should be warned of its occurrence.

Serological Follow-up

- The titer of the nontreponemal test diminishes after adequate treatment of syphilis.

  * A 4-fold drop in titer documents adequate treatment

  * The drop should occur within 3 months of treatment of early syphilis

  * The drop should occur within 6 months of treatment of latent syphilis

- After treatment, one should follow nontreponemal serologic tests at 3 and 6 months, and then every 6 months thereafter until titers stabilize or disappear.

- The failure of the nontreponemal titer to drop 4-fold requires careful follow-up but is not associated with clinical relapse within 12 months.

- The RPR reverts to nonreactive within 2 years in:

  * Three-quarters of patients treated for primary syphilis

  * Half of patients treated for secondary syphilis

- A subsequent reappearance or 4-fold rise in titer of a nontreponemal test suggests relapse or reinfection.

- Follow-up with the same nontreponemal test that was used for the original testing, because the RPR can yield 2- to 8-fold higher titers on the same specimen than does the VDRL.

- There is a higher rate of failure of the serologic tests to respond to treatment in patients with syphilis and HIV infection.

- Syphilis in pregnancy should be managed according to the maternal stage of syphilis.

* Follow nontreponemal serologic tests monthly to rule out treatment failure or reinfection.

ID Board Pearls

• The treponemal tests remain positive even after adequate treatment, and persistence of reactivity is not an indication for retreatment.

• A reactive nontreponemal test is not diagnostic of syphilis except in a highly suggestive clinical scenario.

• The nontreponemal tests may be falsely negative in: very early primary syphilis, secondary syphilis with a prozone, and late syphilis.

• Almost 50% of patients with primary syphilis present with multiple chancres.

• Syphilis should not be treated with erythromycin or azithromycin.

2. Gonorrhea

Synonyms (street)

• Clap, dose, gleet.

Causative Organism

• *Neisseria gonorrhoeae*, a Gram-negative, kidney-shaped diplococcus with flattened adjacent edges.

• A negative culture in the face of a positive Gram stain does not rule out gonococcal urethritis (GCU).

• The organism has become resistant to many antibiotics formerly used as standard regimens.

   * Pencillins, tetracyclines and fluoroquinolones are no longer recommended for treatment of gonorrhea

Chromosomal Resistance

• Point mutations on the bacterial chromosome convey resistance to a variety of antimicrobial agents.

   * As organisms acquire more of these mutations, they become gradually more resistant to numerous antimicrobials

• Resistance to the fluoroquinolones is sufficiently common that these drugs should not be used to treat gonorrhea.

Plasmid-mediated Resistance

• Penicillinase production.

• Tetracycline resistance.

• Plasmids can be passed among gonococci and this form of resistance has rapidly become highly prevalent.

Epidemiology

• *N gonorrhoeae* can directly infect only certain epithelial surfaces *in the adult:*

   * Urethra

* Endocervix

* Conjunctiva

* Pharynx

* Rectum

Key Clinical Features

Urethritis
• Gonococcal urethritis (GCU) and nongonococcal urethritis (NGU) overlap clinically.

• Asymptomatic GCU must be considered in:

  * Partners of women whose infection is diagnosed through screening

  * Partners of women who present with complications

• 75% of symptomatic men with GCU develop symptoms within 4 days and 80%-90% within 2 weeks.

  * Incubation periods can be prolonged by subcurative doses of antibiotics

• Urethral discharge is described by 75% of patients.

  * Discharge present at the meatus without stripping suggests GCU

  * Women are usually unaware of urethral discharge

• Dysuria is common, and may resemble cystitis.

• Symptoms usually begin acutely.

• The clinical features of acute urethritis eventually will decrease or resolve without treatment.

  * Gleet is a thin discharge sometimes indicating chronic gonorrhea

• Gonococcal cervicitis often manifests as erythema around the cervical os and purulent or mucopurulent cervical discharge.

Pharyngeal Infection

• The major risk factor is fellatio.

• Most patients are asymptomatic.

• Erythema or exudate may occur.

• The identity of *N gonorrhoeae* on culture must be confirmed biochemically or immunologically because of the common presence of *N meningitidis*.

  * Nucleic acid amplification tests are not licensed for use in the pjharynx

Disseminated Gonococcal Infection

• Said to complicate 1%-3% of genital or pharyngeal infections.

• The organism resists killing by serum.

• A major risk factor is deficiency in the terminal components of complement, most frequently of C8.

  * Also predisposes to disseminated meningococcal infection

• Pustular or hemorrhagic lesions on distal extremities.

  * Most patients have few lesions.

• Arthritis or tenosynovitis.

  * Polyarthralgia and arthritis

  * Monarticular septic arthritis

• Meningitis or endocarditis rarely complicates this infection but must be treated longer.

Key Laboratory Features

• Urethral Gram stain in symptomatic men has a sensitivity of about 95%.

- Symptomatic men with Gram stain negative for gonococci may be treated for NGU.

- A cervical Gram stain negative for gonococci rules out the infection with a sensitivity of only 50%, and so such patients must still be treated for both gonococcal and nongonococcal cervicitis.

- Nucleic acid amplification techniques have supplanted the Gram stain and culture in many clinical settings.

  * Ligase chain reaction has a sensitivity of 99% and a specificity of 98%.

Differential Diagnosis

Urethritis
- GCU must be differentiated from NGU.

Cervicitis

- Consider chlamydial or herpetic infections.

- Disseminated infection: includes the differential diagnosis of fever, arthritis and rash.

  * Meningococcemia

  * Staphylococcal endocarditis

  * Rocky Mountain Spotted Fever

  * Dengue

  * Reiter's syndrome

Proctitis

- Consider gonococcal etiology in men with rectal symptoms who practice receptive anal intercourse.

Therapy

- Uncomplicated anogenital gonorrhea. Examples of currently acceptable regimens include:

  * Ceftriaxone 125 mg IM made up in 1% lidocaine as a single dose (the gold standard)

* Cefixime, 400 mg PO once

* Cefpodoxime, 400 mg PO once

* Azithromycin 2 g

  - Will cure coincident chlamydial infection

  - Very costly

  - Resistance is developing rapidly, and this regimen should be used with caution. A 1 gm regimen is no longer recommended

- Spectinomycin is not currently available in the United States.

- Because 10%-30% of heterosexual men and 40%-60% of women with gonorrhea (in STD clinics) are also infected with chlamydia, treatment for gonorrhea should include a second regimen effective against this organism unless the second infection has been ruled out by the now common combined probes.

- Disseminated gonococcal infection.

  * Ceftriaxone, 1 g IM or IV QD NGU

  * Ceftizoxime, 1 g IV TID

  * Cefotaxime, 1 g IV TID

  * Patients should also be treated for chlamydial infection

ID Board Pearls

- Fluoroquinolones should no longer be used to treat gonorrhea.

- Patients with uncomplicated gonorrhea should also be treated for chlamydial infection, unless this has been specifically excluded.

- Tenosynovitis accompanying arthritis suggests disseminated gonococcal infection.

- Remember gonococcal oculogenital syndrome: urethritis with autoinoculation of the eye.

- Consider asymptomatic gonococcal urethritis in the male sexual partners of women presenting with complications of gonorrhea (DGI or PID).

3. Nongonococcal Urethritis (NGU)

Causative Organisms

- Urethritis of all etiologies other than *N gonorrhoeae* is referred to as nongonococcal urethritis (NGU).

- The cause of perhaps 20% of cases has not been identified.

Chlamydia trachomatis

- Causes only about 25% of the cases of NGU in various studies.

    * Obligate intracellular parasite

    * DNA and RNA

    * Replicates by binary fission, like bacteria

    * Susceptible to a variety of antimicrobials:

        • Tetracyclines

        • Macrolides and azalides

        • Newer fluoroquinolones

        • Rifampin (few clinical data)

- Grown only in tissue culture.

- New diagnostic techniques are 95% sensitive on genital specimens and somewhat less sensitive on urine specimens from women:

    * Polymerase chain reaction (PCR)

    * Ligase chain reaction (LCR)

- The spectrum of diseases caused by *C trachomatis* closely parallels that caused by *N gonorrhoeae*. Coinfection with these 2 organisms is very common and affects management strategies.

Ureaplasma urealyticum

- May cause 15%-30% of cases, although this remains somewhat controversial.

* Free-living agent

* *Ureaplasma parvum* is a closely-related saprophyte which does not cause disease

* Cultures rarely performed except for research

* Some ureaplasma is resistant to the tetracyclines and must be treated with a macrolide/azalide or a fluoroquinolone

Mycoplasma genitalium

• Recently-characterized mycoplasma that is associated with up to 30% of NGU.

• Also associated with upper tract disease and infertility in women.

• Initially sensitive to the tetracyclines and macrolides.

* Recent data indicate that the organism may become resistant to azithromycin during therapy and may be a cause of treatment failure

* Such infections can be treated with moxifloxacin 400 mg orally per day for 10 days

Trichomonas vaginalis

• Usually is carried asymptomatically by men.

• Causes NGU that fails to respond to standard antibacterial treatment.

Herpes simplex virus

• Urethritis usually occurs in the setting of external lesions.

Rarer causes, usually not sexually transmitted:

• Enterobacteriaceae.

• Adenovirus.

• *Neisseria meningitidis*.

• *Streptococcus pneumoniae*.

• Microsporidia (in AIDS).

• *Staphylococcus saprophyticus*.

• *Haemophilus* spp.

• *Bacteroides*.

Epidemiology

• NGU is twice as common as GCU in the United States, especially among higher socioeconomic groups.

• GCU is relatively more common among homosexual than it is among heterosexual men with acute urethritis.

Key Clinical Features

• GCU and NGU cannot be differentiated reliably on clinical features alone.

• A significant proportion of men with NGU are asymptomatic.

Incubation Period

• 50% of symptomatic men with NGU develop symptoms within 4 days.

• The incubation period ranges from 2-35 days.

• Incubation periods can be prolonged by subcurative doses of antibiotics.

Urethral Discharge

• Discharge is described by 11%-33% of men with NGU.

• Mucopurulent discharge (purulent flecks in a mucoid matrix) is seen in 50% of cases of NGU, but also in 25% of cases of GCU.

• A completely clear urethral discharge suggests NGU.

• The discharge in NGU may be so slight as to be present only as a metal bead or a crust noted when the patient first arises.

Other Features

• Dysuria is common.

• Onset of NGU is often subacute.

• 30%-70% of men with NGU become asymptomatic over 1-3 months.

• Women usually are unaware of urethral discharge, and urethritis presents as dysuria with frequency.

• Infected women usually manifest pyuria.

• Some women have cystitis or urethritis caused by small numbers of *Enterobacteriaceae*

• NGU may respond initially to standard urinary tract treatments.

• Culture-negative urinary tract infection should suggest the possibility of sexually transmitted urethritis.

• Chlamydial infection should be considered in the differential diagnosis of acute epididymitis.

Key Laboratory Features

• Examination of the urethral specimen:

* The diagnostic criterion of 5 polymorphonuclear neutrophils (PMNs) per oil-immersion field is insensitive

* 16%-50% of men with NGU fail to show this number of PMNs in the densest portion of the slide

* The number of PMNs observed is reduced by recent micturition

* Even few PMNs on a urethral smear provide objective evidence of urethritis

* The complete absence of PMNs argues against urethritis

* If, in addition to PMNs, one sees characteristic Gram-negative, intracellular diplococci, the diagnosis of gonorrhea is established

* If such organisms are not observed, the patient is said to have NGU

• One cannot diagnose concurrent NGU by Gram staining in the presence of gonorrhea.

• Thus, one should assume that patients with gonorrhea are co-infected with nongonococcal pathogens, unless these have been excluded by laboratory testing.

Empiric Therapy

• Because it is impossible to differentiate among the common etiologies of NGU, the condition is treated syndromically.

Definitive Therapy

• Examples of regimens useful in the treatment of NGU include the following:

* Azithromycin 1 g orally provides the only single-dose regimen for chlamydial infections

* Doxycycline 100 mg PO BID for 7 days

• Tetracycline hydrochloride 500 mg PO QID for 7 days.

* Erythromycin 500 mg PO QID for 7 days or, if the larger dose is not tolerated, 250 mg PO QID for 7 days

* Ofloxacin 300 mg PO BID for 7 days. One may use equivalent (approximately half) doses of levofloxacin

* Minocycline 100 mg PO QHS for 7 days

• Additional regimens that may be used if the infection is known to be chlamydial:

* Clindamycin 450 mg PO TID for 10 days

  • Expensive

  • Safe in pregnancy

* Amoxicillin 500 mg PO TID for 7 days. Limited data, but looks good for treatment in pregnancy

* Sulfisoxazole 500 mg PO QID for 10 days. TMP-SMX has no greater efficacy

• Epidemiologic treatment of sexual partners of men with urethritis is essential.

  * Since only about 25% of NGU is chlamydial, a negative test for chlamydia in a partner does not obviate the need for treatment

  * Tests for other etiologies of NGU are currently available only in a research setting

• *C trachomatis* can be recovered from the endocervix of 60%-90% of the sexual partners of men with chlamydial urethritis.

• Subtle cervical abnormalities are observed in 80%-90% of infected women.

Management of Recurrent Disease

• Reinfection is the most common cause of recurrence.

• Initial response suggests infection with an antimicrobial-sensitive agent.

• Re-exposure followed by recurrence strongly suggests reinfection.

• Failure to respond to doxycycline (persistent PMNs on urethral smear) suggests infection with a tetracycline-resistant agent:

  * *U urealyticum*

  * *T vaginalis*

• Such patients should be empirically treated for both organisms with metronidazole, 2 g PO as a single dose, and erythromycin, azithromycin or an appropriate fluoroquinolone.

• Failure to respond to azithromycin suggests infection with *Trichomonas vaginalis* or azithromycin-resistant *Mycoplasma genitalium*.

  * Such patients should be treated with metronidazole 2 gm as a single dose and moxifloxacin 400 mg orally per day for 10 days

  * Sexual partners should be treated with the same regimen

ID Board Pearls

• *Chlamydia trachomatis* causes only about 25% of cases of NGU.

• Epidemiological treatment of sexual contacts to NGU is essential.

• *Mycoplasma genitalium* is a newly recognized cause of NGU.

• Failure of NGU to respond to treatment with azithromycin suggests infection with *T vaginalis* or *M genitalium*.

• Consider sexually transmitted urethritis in women with frequently recurring symptoms of UTI.

4. Chancroid

Synonyms

• Soft chancre; molle.

Causative Organism

• *Haemophilus ducreyi*, a Gram-negative rod.

Epidemiology

• The incidence of chancroid has increased in the United States.

• Small epidemics are often associated with prostitution.

• A major public health problem in the developing world.

• Significant association with HIV infection.

Key Clinical Features

• Incubation period is 4-7 days.

• Painful, ragged ulcers on the genitalia:

   * Dirty or necrotic-appearing

   * Not indurated

   * Vary in size

   * Sometimes superinfected with mixed anaerobic organisms

   * Kissing lesions of the thighs occur by autoinoculation

• Painful inguinal adenopathy occurs in more than 50% of patients.

   * Appears at about the same time as the lesions

   * Nodes often become fluctuant

   * Nodes may rupture

• The major differential diagnoses are herpes simplex genital infection and syphilis.

• Clinical differential diagnosis is unreliable.

Key Laboratory Features

• Darkfield examination can be used to rule out syphilis.

• Syphilis and chancroid may coexist.

   * The nontreponemal tests are insensitive early in primary syphilis

• Gram staining of the lesions is insensitive and non-specific, and it is not recommended.

• Culture of *Haemophilus ducreyi* is definitive.

   * Culture is difficult

   * Misses at least 20% of cases

• Newer tests are under development.

   * Polymerase chain reaction (PCR) is 90% sensitive

   * Antigen detection is 90% sensitive

   * Multiplex PCR can diagnose simultaneous infections

Definitive Treatment

• Complicated by resistance to traditional agents.

• Recommended in the United States:

   * Ciprofloxacin, 500 mg PO BID for 3 days

   * Ceftriaxone, 250 mg IM as a single dose

   * Erythromycin, 500 mg PO QID for 7 days

   * Azithromycin, 1 g PO as a single dose

• Patients co-infected with HIV may require longer courses of therapy.

• Epidemiologic treatment of sexual partners is important.

ID Board Pearls

- Resistance likely greater in other parts of the world.

- Ragged ulcers varying in size.

- About 10% of patients co-infected with syphilis or herpes.

- Asympomatic carriage of the organism appears to be relatively rare.

- Multiple infections of lesions are common.

5. Donovanosis

Synonyms

- Granuloma inguinale.

Causative Organism

- *Klebsiella (Calymmatobacterium) granulomatis.*

  * Obligate intracellular Gram-negative rod

  * Related to *Klebsiella*

Epidemiology

- Extremely rare in the United States.

- More common in India and Latin America.

Key Clinical Features

- Painless, destructive ulcers.

  * Exuberant granulation tissue formation

  * Serpiginous (healing in one area while progressing in another)

  * White border (helpful)

  * Often seen in inguinal areas

    - Not inguinal adenopathy, but overlying disease

  * Heal with scarring

- Osteomyelitis.

Key Laboratory Features

- Diagnosis is made by biopsy of involved tissue.

- Donovan bodies: intracellular rod-shaped chromatin condensations.

Definitive Therapy

- Azithromycin 1 g PO weekly for at least 3 weeks appears effective.

- Doxycycline, 100 mg PO BID for at least 3 weeks.

- TMP-SMX DS PO BID for at least 3 weeks.

- Ciprofloxacin 750 mg PO BID for at least 3 weeks.

- Sexual partners should probably be treated, although the value is not well defined.

ID Board Pearls

- Genital lesion with white border.

- Destructive of genitalia.

- Healing in one area while extending in another.

- Inguinal lesions are superficial, not adenopathy.

- Primarily in recent immigrants.

6. Genital Herpes Simplex Infection

Synonyms

- Herpes.

Causative Organisms

- Herpes simplex virus type 1 (HSV-1).

- Herpes simplex virus type 2 (HSV-2).

- These organisms are only relatively site specific.

    * Overall, about 30% of genital herpes is now caused by HSV-1

    * In some populations, (eg, younger college students) 70% of newly acquired genital infection is now caused by HSV-1

Epidemiology

- Type 1 genital infections may result from orogenital sexual contact.

- Serologic studies suggest that 20% of the population of the United States is infected with HSV type 2.

    * Most HSV-2 infection are genital

    * Genital HSV-1 infections recur less frequently than HSV-2

- Initial genital infections are classified as primary if the patient has no prior exposure to HSV (either type 1 or type 2).

    * Otherwise classified as nonprimary initial infection

- HSV-1 and HSV-2 share many antigens.

    * Prior infection with HSV-1 reduces but does not eliminate susceptibility to infection with HSV-2

    * Prior infection with HSV-1 reduces severity of infection with HSV-2

- Most genital HSV is acquired from persons who shed the virus asymptomatically.

    * Only about 20% of patients with genital herpes are aware of their infections

    * About 60% of patients with genital herpes have symptoms they do not recognize as HSV

    * About 20% of patients with genital herpes never have any clinical findings

- Asymptomatic shedding detected by culture occurs about 3% of the time in both people with symptomatic recurrences and people who are always asymptomatic.

    * Culture-independent techniques detect asymptomatic shedding up to 25% of the time

    * It is not clear which technique corresponds best with infectivity

- Among mutually monogamous couples having regular, unprotected sex when the partner with herpes is asymptomatic, the transmission rate is about 10% per year.

- It is essential that the clinician counsel patients regarding asymptomatic shedding and the need to inform partners of the diagnosis.

- A patient with few symptoms can transmit highly symptomatic infection to a partner.

- A patient having transmitted HSv to a partner will not be reinfected by that same partner.

Key Clinical Features

- Absolutely typical herpes can be diagnosed clinically with a positive predictive value of about 85%.

- Standard clinical evaluation can never rule out genital herpes.

- The rate of recurrence decreases over time.

Lesions

- Can appear 2-20 days after exposure.

- Mean incubation period is about 6 days.

- Lesions are initially vesicular, grouped, sometimes umbilicated and have an erythematous base.

- The vesicles quickly rupture to form clean, shallow, markedly painful ulcers.

    * Generally all about the same size

    * Not indurated

    * Ulcers may coalesce

    * Heal by crusting over

- Usually lesions are located on the penis or on the labia or vulva.

    * Adult vagina is involved in only about 5% of patients

    * Cervix is involved in 90% of primary infections

    * Urethral involvement is common

Other Features

- Inguinal lymphadenopathy, usually tender, generally develops toward the end of the first week of illness.

- Fever, malaise and anorexia are common in primary infection.

- Aseptic meningitis without encephalitis accompanies some primary infections with HSV type 2.

- Recurrent lymphocytic meningitis can be caused by HSV-2.

Recurrences

- Symptomatic recurrences are seen in approximately 90% of symptomatic patients with HSV-2 genital infections.

- Occur 4-8 times per year in most patients.

- Occur in only about 25%-50% of those genitally infected with HSV type 1, 10 times less frequently than with HSV-2.

- The rate of recurrence varies dramatically from patient to patient.

- May be triggered by stress.

- Sometimes preceded by a prodrome of itching, tingling or burning that begins 6-24 hours before lesions appear.

- Recurrences generally last 5-7 days and proceed through the same stages as primary disease.

- The diagnosis can usually be made clinically in symptomatic individuals.

Key Laboratory Features

Identification of Virus in Lesions
- Tzanck smear of a fresh vesicular lesion.

    * Stained with Wright or Giemsa stain

    * Multinucleated giant cells are seen in herpetic infection

    * Sensitivity of the test is only 40% when applied to ulcers

- Antigen detection by direct immunofluorescence and ELISA.

    * Sensitivity and specificity both about 70%-90%

- Viral DNA detected by PCR with 100% specificity and sensitivity, which is higher than any other direct technique.

- Culture sensitivity rapidly diminishes in recurrent disease.

- Serologic diagnosis has limited clinical utility.

    * Newer, commercially available tests reliably differentiate between type 1 and type 2 virus

    * An ELISA based on glycoprotein gG

    * A Western blot assay can differentiate between HSV-1 and HSV-2

    * Highly sensitive and specific

    * Some can be performed in the clinic

    * Become positive in 80% of infected patients after 2 weeks

- The type-specific tests are not useful for screening, because many patients are HSV-1 antibody-positive, and thus HSV-1 genital herpes cannot be ruled out.

Therapy

- Topical therapy has limited effectiveness and is not recommended.

- Effectiveness of regimens requires starting early in the relapse, preferably during the prodrome.

Oral Antiherpetic Agents

- Valacyclovir is a prodrug of acyclovir, and is therefore a more convenient but more expensive means of administration of acyclovir.

- Famciclovir is a prodrug of penciclovir.

Clinically equivalent oral regimens for initial infection
- 7-10 days of oral therapy with one of the following:

    * Acyclovir 400 mg TID

    * Acyclovir 200 mg 5 times a day

* Famciclovir 250 mg TID

* Valacyclovir 1 g BID

Recurrent episodes

• 5-day oral regimens:

    * Acyclovir 400 mg BID

    * Acyclovir 200 mg 5 times a day

    * Famciclovir 125 mg BID

    * Valacyclovir 500 mg BID or 1 g daily

Short course

• There are recent data supporting shorter courses of oral treatment for recurrent disease:

    * Valacyclovir 500 mg BID for 3 days

    * Acyclovir 800 mg TID for 2 days

    * Famciclovir 1000 mg BID for 1 day

Frequently recurring disease

• Long-term oral suppressive therapy:

    * Acyclovir 400 mg BID

    * Famciclovir 250 mg BID

    * Valacyclovir 500 mg BID, or 1000 mg QD

• Approximately 75% of patients will remain free of symptomatic recurrences.

    * Reduces, but does not eliminate, asymptomatic viral shedding

    * Patients should be warned that they might be contagious without knowing it

    * Reduces transmission to sexual partner by about half

• After 1 year of continuous daily therapy, consider discontinuing and reassessing.

ID Board Pearls

• Genital HSV-1 is now common and makes type-specific serology less useful.

• Only 20% of patients with genital herpes are aware of their diagnosis.

• Genital HSV is usually acquired from asymptomatic sources.

• Suppressive therapy reduces transmission by about 50%.

• Short course therapy is effective.

7. Molluscum Contagiosum

Causative Organism

• Poxvirus.

Epidemiology

• Seen frequently in children.

  * Nonvenereal

  * Trunk

• Sexually transmitted in adults.

  * Genital

Key Clinical Features

• Incubation period 2-8 weeks.

• 1- to 5-mm lesions.

  * Genitals, thighs, buttocks

  * Painless papules

  * Central umbilications

• Disseminated disease in HIV/AIDS.

  * Lesions resemble those of disseminated cryp-
    tococcosis.

Key Laboratory Features

• Crushing a lesion and staining with Wright's or
  Giemsa stain.

  * Molluscum bodies: intracytoplasmic inclu-
    sions

• Biopsy: histology.

• Fluorescent antibody.

• DNA hybridization.

Therapy

• Curettage.

• Cryotherapy.

• Cidofovir (limited data).

• Imiquimod (limited data; probably less effective).

ID Board Pearls

• Umbilicated papules look like lesions of disseminated cryptococosis in advanced HIV.

• Disseminated disease in advanced HIV.

• Not sexually transmitted when seen on the trunk in
  children, but genital lesions should raise question
  of sexual abuse.

8. Condylomata Acuminata

Synonyms

• Venereal warts.

• Genital warts.

• HPV.

Causative Organism

• Human papillomaviruses (HPV).

  * Double-stranded DNA viruses

  * Have not been cultured

  * Over 100 types have been identified

    • Less than 90% DNA homology with other types

• Types 6 and 11 cause most benign genital warts.

• Types 16, 18, 31, 33 and 35, among others, cause cervical cancer in the United States.

  * Other types relatively more prevalent in the developing world

• Oncogenic types cause smaller proportions of other cancers:

  * Anal (70%)

  * Vulvar (50%)

  * Vaginal (50%)

  * Oropharyngeal (20%)

• Cervical HPV infection is self-limited in women with normal immunity.

  * Median duration of about 8-10 months

  * Persistence associated with premalignant and malignant lesions

  * Premalignant lesions often develop within 1-2 years of infection

  * Invasive carcinoma of the cervix develops within about 10 years

Epidemiology

• Sexually transmitted.

• Warts found in about two-thirds of sexual partners.

• Reinfection between monogamous sexual partners does not seem to occur and does not cause relapse.

• Treatment of sexual partners is most important for preventing spread to other partners.

Key Clinical Features

• Incubation period appears to be 4-6 weeks.

• Soft papules with irregular, verrucous surfaces.

• Located around the external genitalia, inside the urethra or vagina, on the cervix or rarely in the mouth.

• Perianal warts.

  * In women, may reflect spread from a primary genital focus

  * In men, strongly suggest receptive anal intercourse, which is a significant HIV risk factor

    • Men with perianal warts should undergo anoscopy

• Daughter lesions appear near older lesions.

• Most patients have HPV DNA identified in normal epithelium near visible lesions.

  * The contagiousness of HPV DNA is undefined

• Diagnosis is made clinically.

  * Cervical and atypical lesions require biopsy

• Subclinical infections may be identified by swabbing the vagina, cervix or penis with 3-5% acetic acid, which turns infected areas white.

* Highly nonspecific and requires histologic confirmation

Key Laboratory Findings

Histology

• Characteristic koilocytosis, clear zones around pyknotic nuclei of infected cells.

• DNA hybridization kits now commercially available.

* Can supplement or replace standard cervical cytology in some circumstances

* Self-collected vaginal specimens can be tested for DNA

Differential Diagnosis

• Molluscum contagiosum.

• Squamous cell carcinoma.

• Bowen's disease.

Treatment

• Largely unsatisfactory.

• The benefit of treating subclinical infection has not been demonstrated.

• The goal of therapy is elimination of overt warts.

• The cervix should not be treated before cytologic studies have ruled out malignancy.

• The relapse rate with the treatments listed in this section approaches 75%.

Physician-applied

• Cryotherapy with liquid nitrogen or cryoprobe.

* Low toxicity

* Safe in pregnancy

* Destroys warts with a single treatment

• Podophyllin, 10%-25% in tincture of benzoin.

* Crude extract of *Podophyllum peltatum*

* Contains carcinogens

* Applied directly to the warts at weekly intervals

* Washed off after about 6 hours

* 50% of patients get complete resolution of warts with repeated treatment

* Absorption occurs; contraindicated in pregnancy

• Trichloroacetic acid, 80%-90%.

* Applied carefully to warts

* Neutralization by topical sodium bicarbonate

* Treatment can be repeated at weekly intervals

* Safe in pregnancy

* Relatively painful

• Laser therapy.

* May have a lower relapse rate because DNA-containing, normal-appearing skin is ablated

* Painful

* Expensive

• Intralesional interferon.

* Expensive and time-consuming

* Useful primarily with limited numbers of warts

Patient-applied

• Imiquimod 5% cream.

* Immunostimulator; induces interleukins and interferon

* Applied by the patient 3 times a week

* Response rate is the same as with podophyllin

* Expensive

• Podofilox 0.5% solution or gel.

* Active ingredient in podophyllin

* Nontoxic to normal skin

* Applied twice daily for 3 days followed by a 4-day rest

* May be repeated up to 4 times

* Expensive

• Green Tea Extract (Veregen®)

* Recently FDA-approved

*Very limited data

*No advantage over older regimens

*Very expensive

Complications

Carcinogenesis
• DNA from oncogenic types inserts into host DNA.

* Insertion permits increased synthesis of proteins that inactivate host oncogene suppressors

• Type 16 most commonly associated with cervical malignancy.

• Type 18 associated with most rapid development of premalignant lesions.

• Laryngeal papillomatosis in infants born vaginally to infected women.

Vaccine

• Quadrivalent (types 6, 11, 16, 18) is almost 100% effective in preventing sustained infection in women.

* 3 doses, cost $360

* Trials in men and older women are in progress.

• Preventive, not curative.

* Can still be given to women with warts to provide protection against subsequent infection with other types

* Does not increase rate of resolution of established warts

* Probably provides partial protection against some other cross-reacting types

• Has resulted in a decrease in incidence of premalignant cervical lesions.

• Bivalent (16, 18) not yet released in the United States because of concern over adjuvent.

• Debate surrounds making it mandatory for entering school.

ID Board Pearls

• Most therapies result in complete clearance of warts in about 50% of cases.

• Cervical (and possibly other) HPV infection is self-limited in most patients with normal immune systems.

• Most important cause of cervical cancer, but distribution of involved types vary internationally.

• LSIL pregresses to HSIL in only about 3% of cases.

• HPV is also associated with cancers other than cervical.

9. Pubic Lice

Synonyms

• Crabs, lice, pediculosis pubis.

Causative Organism

• *Pthirus pubis* (the crab louse).

Epidemiology

• Direct contact with infected persons, clothing, bed linens.

Key Clinical Features

• Incubation period about 4 weeks.

• Markedly pruritic.

• Lice: 1- to 2-mm long gray-brown organisms.

• Nits: 0.5 mm brown or white ovoids attached to the hair shafts.

   * Brown: Intact

   * White: Hatched

• Usually laid at the base of the pubic hair, which grows at about 1 mm/day.

   * Nits confined to the upper shafts: old infection

   * Height of nits suggests duration of infection

• Excreta: tiny red dots on the skin among the hair.

• Maculae caeruleae:

   * Blue-gray macules

   * Possibly an immunologic response

   * Rare

• Infestation of hairy areas may be widespread, including:

   * Pubic

   * Perianal

   * Abdominal

   * Chest

   * Axillary

   * Superciliary

   * Eyelashes

Differential Diagnosis

• Fungal infections.

Therapy

• Carefully examine the eyelids.

• Clothing or bed linen contaminated within the past 48 hours should be washed before reuse.

• Examine for other STIs.

• Sexual partners should be treated.

• Equally effective regimens:

   * Permethrin 1% cream rinse, applied to affected areas and washed off after 10 minutes

   * Pyrethrins and piperonyl butoxide applied to affected areas and washed off after 10 minutes

   * Malathione 0.5% lotion applied for 8-12 hours and washed off

   * Ivermectin 250 mcg/kg orally as a single dose, repeated in 2 weeks

   * Lindane (gamma-benzene hexachloride) 1% shampoo applied for 4 minutes and washed off in the shower. Reserve for those intolerant of other regimens

• Lice in eyebrows and eyelashes may be asphyxiated by coating with petroleum jelly or other occlusive ointment BID for 10 days.

• Spraying of living areas is not useful.

• Re-evaluate persistently symptomatic patients after 1 week.

• Indications for retreatment:

  * Lice

• Nits at the base of the hair shafts.

ID Board Pearls

• Persistence of nits high up on hair shaft do not indicate a need for retreatment.

• Examine underwear for nits and droppings.

• Examine axillae, eyebrows and eyelashes.

• Lindane may be more toxic than other regimens.

• Clothing or bed linens not used for more than 72 hours need not be decontaminated.

10. Scabies

Synonyms

• The itch, the 7-year itch.

Causative Organism *Therapy*

• *Sarcoptes scabiei* (the itch mite).

Epidemiology

• Direct contact with infected persons, clothing, bed linens.

Key Clinical Features

• Incubation period of about 4 weeks.

• Severe pruritus of the infected areas.

• Often worse at night or after bathing.

• Scattered moist-appearing papules and crusted lesions of:

  * Genital area, labia, penis, scrotum

  * Belt line

  * Wrists and ankles

  * Interdigital webs

• Pale linear burrows.

  * Burrow ink test: rub ink from fountain pen over affected areas; wash off; ink penetrates burrows, making them dark

• The diagnosis is usually made clinically.

Key Laboratory Features

• Scrapings from lesions.

  * Burrows are best sites

  * Unexcoriated papules

  * Superficial shave biopsy with a needle or a scalpel blade

* Suspend in immersion oil and cover with glass coverslip

* Can use 10% potassium hydroxide to dissolve skin cells

* Examine at 400x

* Female mite (rarely seen)

* Eggs

Therapy (Adults)

• Evaluate for other STIs.

• Clothing or bed linens contaminated within the previous 48 hours should be washed before reuse.

• Treat sexual partners and close household contacts.

Regimens

• Permethrin 5% cream applied to all areas of the body below the chin and washed off after 8-14 hours.

• Lindane (gamma-benzene hexachloride) 1% lotion or cream applied to all areas of the body below the chin, and washed off after 8 hours. This should be considered an alternative therapy, avoided in pregnancy and in patients with dermatitis, and used when other regimens are not tolerated.

• Application must be complete, including the interdigital spaces

• Patients should be cautioned not to wash their hands after applying the medication

• Ivermectin as a single oral dose of 200 mcg/kg, repeated in 2 weeks.

* Effective in crusted scabies

• Crotamiton 10%, applied to all areas of the body below the chin for 2 successive nights and washed off thoroughly 24 hours after the second application.

* Less effective than the agents listed above

• Pruritus may persist for several weeks after adequate treatment.

* Consider administering a single retreatment if pruritus is not improved after 1-2 weeks

Complications

• Superinfection.

• Crusted scabies.

* Formerly referred to as "Norwegian scabies"; avoid this term

* Severe disseminated disease

• Often resistant to topical therapies; consider ivermectin.

• A particular problem in advanced HIV infection.

ID Board Pearls

• Avoid lindane in setting of pregnancy, breast feeding or dermatitis.

• Itching may persist for 7-14 days after curative therapy.

• Advise patients not to wash hands after applying medication.

• Suspect crusted scabies in immunocompromised patients.

• Nosocomial transmission has been reported.

11. Trichomoniasis

Synonyms

• Trich.

Causative Organism

• *Trichomonas vaginalis*.

• Anaerobic, flagellated, motile protozoan.

• Approximately the size of a polymorphonuclear neutrophil.

Epidemiology

• The incidence has declined, possibly because of the widespread use of metronidazole for bacterial vaginosis.

• Prevalent in populations at risk for other STDs.

• Almost always sexually acquired.

    * Sexual partners should be treated

    * Evaluate for other STDs

Key Clinical Features

• Men usually asymptomatic.

    * Isolated from up to 20% of men in STD clinics

    * Infrequent cause of NGU (see above) that is resistant to standard antibacterial treatments

• 10%-50% of infected women asymptomatic.

• Incubation period of 5-28 days.

• Vaginal discharge.

• Vulvovaginal soreness or irritation.

• Dysuria.

• Dyspareunia.

• Odor (may actually be more suggestive of bacterial vaginosis).

• Symptoms often begin or exacerbate after the menstrual period.

• Occasional abdominal discomfort.

    * Evaluate for pelvic inflammatory disease

• Copious, rather loose discharge pooling in the posterior vaginal fornix.

    * Often yellow or green (indicating polymorphonuclear neutrophils)

    * Bubbles are observed in 10%-33%

    * pH elevated above 4.5 in 90%

    * May have a relatively thick discharge that may be confused with candidiasis

• Erythema and edema of the vaginal walls and the exocervix.

• Punctate hemorrhages (colpitis macularis).

    * Strawberry cervix

    * Detected colposcopically in 45% of infected women

    * Detected by physical examination in only 2%

Key Laboratory Features

• Demonstration of the organism.

• Wet mount:

    * Characteristic twitching motility

    * 60% sensitive

    * Large numbers of white blood cells

• Papanicolaou smear is specific but insensitive.

- Direct fluorescent antibody staining 80%-90% sensitive.

- Latex agglutination 80%-90% sensitive.

- ELISA 80%-90% sensitive but less sensitive than culture.

- DNA probes and PCR most sensitive.

Culture

- Commercially available kits have increased the ease with which the organism can be cultured.

Differential Diagnosis

- Candidiasis.

- Bacterial vaginosis.

- Purulent or desquamative vaginitis.

Therapy

- Sexual partners should be treated.

- Metronidazole, 2 g PO as a single dose.

- Metronidazole, 250 mg PO TID or 500 mg PO BID for 7 days.

- Tinidazole 2 g PO as a single dose.

- Metronidazole may be used in pregnancy.

- Metronidazole resistance is increasing in prevalence.

    * Retreat with metronidazole, 500 mg BID for 7 days

    * Single 2-g dose of metronidazole QD for 3-5 days

    * Combined oral and vaginal nitroimidazole

    * Consider consultation with a specialist

ID Board Pearls

- Resistance to metronidazole increasingly prevalent.

- Sexual partners must be treated.

- Diagnosis is difficult in men.

- Strawberry cervix rarely seen on physical examination.

- Elevated vaginal pH a clue.

12. Bacterial Vaginosis

Synonyms

• BV.

• Previously and incorrectly called nonspecific vaginitis.

Causative Organisms

• Complex polymicrobial infection.

   * Loss of hydrogen peroxide-producing lacto-bacilli key to pathogenesis

   * Many organisms cannot be cultured and have been identified only by nucleic acid studies

   * *Gardnerella vaginalis*: often present but not the cause

   * Anaerobic bacteria: eg, *Prevotella, Bacteroides*

   * Mycoplasmas

Epidemiology

• Most common vaginal infection in the United States.

• The precise contribution of sexual transmission to the overall epidemiology of the condition remains controversial.

   * Seen primarily in sexually active women

   * BV is common in populations with a high prevalence of STDs

   * Recurrence in the absence of sexual re-exposure is well described

   * It is not demonstrably necessary to treat male sexual partners initially

   * Recurrence more common in lesbians and heterosexual women with single sexual partners

Key Clinical Features

• Prominent vaginal odor.

• Mild to moderate discharge.

   * Often present at the introitus and visible on the labia minora

   * Grayish white, thin, homogeneous, adherent

   * Small bubbles

   * May be apparent only as increased light reflection off of vaginal walls

• The endocervix is unaffected by the process.

• pH is elevated above normal (4.5) in approximately 90% of cases.

• Inflammation and perivaginal irritation are mild, if present at all.

• Vaginal walls are not inflamed.

• Rare dysuria and dyspareunia.

• Abdominal discomfort, if present, is usually mild.

   * Adnexal tenderness should prompt concern for pelvic inflammatory disease

• Positive whiff test.

   * Adding 10 KOH to discharge elicits a pungent, amine-like odor

   * About 80% sensitive

   * Also seen in trichomoniasis, but not in candidiasis

Key Laboratory Features

• Wet mount:

   * Clue cells, vaginal epithelial cells studded with tiny coccobacilli 90% sensitive

* Rods supplanted by clumps of coccobacilli

* Few PMNs: Many PMN should suggest coincident trichomoniasis or cervicitis

- Gram stain: Normal Gram-positive rods replaced by Gram-variable coccobacilli.

- Culture for *G vaginalis* does not prove that the patient has BV or suggest a need for treatment.

Therapy

- Male sexual contacts do not require therapy for the initial episode.

Oral Regimens

- Metronidazole, 500 mg PO BID for 7 days.

- Metronidazole, 250 mg PO TID for 7 days.

- Clindamycin, 300 mg PO BID for 7 days.

- Cefadroxil, 500 mg PO BID for 7 days.

    * Very limited data

Topical Regimens

- Metronidazole 0.75% vaginal gel, 5 g (1 full applicator) vaginally BID or QHS for 5 days.

- Clindamycin 2% vaginal cream, 5 g (1 full applicator) vaginally QHS for 7 days.

    * Should not be used in pregnancy because it is less effective than metronidazole in preventing gestational complications

- Clindamycin ovules 100 g intravaginally QHS for 3 days.

    * Should probably not be used in pregnancy because it is less effective than metronidazole in preventing gestational complications

Complications

- Pregnancy:

* Preterm labor

* Preterm delivery

* Premature rupture of membranes

* Postpartum endometritis

- Nonpregnant women:

    * Increased risk of pelvic inflammatory disease

ID Board Pearls

- Not a benign disease: complications include PID and premature rupture of membranes.

- Not, strictly speaking, sexually transmitted.

- *Gardnerella vaginalis* not the cause; complex microbiology.

- No need to treat sexual partners initially.

- Recurrences common.

13. Further Reading

1. Barr E. Sings HL. Prophylactic HPV vaccines: new interventions for cancer control. *Vaccine*. 2008;26:6244-6257.

2. Centers for Disease Control and Prevention. Symptomatic early neurosyphilis among HIV-positive men who have sex with men--four cities, United States, January 2002-June 2004. MMWR. 2007;56:625-628.

3. Centers for Disease Control and Prevention. Update to CDC's sexually transmitted diseases treatment guidelines, 2006: fluoroquinolones no longer recommended for treatment of gonococcal infections. *MMWR*. 2007;56:332-336.

4. Centers for Disease Control and Prevention. Sexually Transmitted Disease Treatment Guidelines, 2006. *MMWR*. 2006; 55(RR-11):1-94. Note subsequent addenda and revisions, usually in MMWR.

5. Fethers KA, Fairley CK, Hocking JS, Gurrin LC. Bradshaw CS. Sexual risk factors and bacterial vaginosis: a systematic review and meta-analysis. *Clin Infect Dis*. 2008;47:1426-35

6. Gur I. The epidemiology of Molluscum contagiosum in HIV-seropositive patients: a unique entity or insignificant finding? *Internat J STD AIDs*. 2008; 19:503-506.

7. Jensen JS, Bradshaw CS, Tabrizi SN, Fairley CK, Hamasuna R. Azithromycin treatment failure in Mycoplasma genitalium-positive patients with nongonococcal urethritis is associated with induced macrolide resistance. *Clin Infect Dis*. 2008; 47:1546-1553.

8. Martinez V, Caumes E, Chosidow O. Treatment to prevent recurrent genital herpes. *Curr Opinion Infect Dis*. 2008;21:42-48.

9. O'Farrell N, Morison L, Moodley P, et al. Genital ulcers and concomitant complaints in men attending a sexually transmitted infections clinic: implications for sexually transmitted infections management. *Sex Transm Dis*. 2008;35:545-549.

10. Tjioe M, Vissers WH. Scabies outbreaks in nursing homes for the elderly: recognition, treatment options and control of reinfestation. *Drugs Aging*. 2008; 25:299-306.

Chapter 22: Antibiotics for the ID Boards

Burke A. Cunha, MD
Brian P. McDermott, DO
Francisco M. Pherez, MD

Contents

1. General Concepts

- Microbiologic susceptibility data are *not* ordinarily available prior to initial treatment with antibiotics.

- *Empiric* therapy is based on directing coverage against the *most likely pathogens*, and takes into consideration drug allergy history, hepatic and renal function, possible antibiotic side effects, resistance potential and cost.

- If a patient is moderately/severely ill, empiric therapy is usually initiated intravenously.

- Patients who are mildly/moderately ill, whether hospitalized or ambulatory, may be *started* on *oral* antibiotics with *high bioavailability* (>90%).

- Cultures of appropriate clinical specimens (eg, sputum, urine) should be obtained *prior* to starting empiric therapy to provide bacterial isolates for *in vitro* susceptibility testing.

Specific Therapy

- Refers to antibiotic therapy directed against a *known pathogen with antibiotic susceptibility*.

- There is no rationale for changing antibiotics from empiric to specific *if* empiric antibiotic is as effective against the pathogens with the specific antibiotic, especially if the empiric antibiotic is less expensive, given less often and has fewer side effects than the specific antibiotic.

- There is no benefit to changing from empiric therapy to specific therapy with a narrower spectrum to decreased antibiotic resistance *if* the empiric antibiotic chosen has a low resistance potential, eg, cefazolin (*S pneumoniae*, MSSA); meropenem (*P aeruginosa*, MSSA, VSE); respiratory quinolone (MSSA, VSE/VRE); daptomycin (MSSA, VSE, VRE); linezolid (MSSA, VSE/VRE, *S pneumoniae*, *H influenzae*).

Staph aureus' main mech of resistance is thru plasmid encoded β lactamases

2. Penicillins

(PCNs) bind PBP → ⊖ cell wall synth

Mechanism of Action:

- All beta lactam antibiotics utilize the same mechanism of action, the binding of penicillin-binding proteins (PBP), thereby inhibiting cell wall synthesis.

Resistance Mechanism:

- The most common Gram-positive resistance mechanism is through the alteration of PBPs, reducing binding affinity and thereby rendering the antibiotic ineffective. The classic example of this is methicillin resistant *S aureus* (MRSA). The *mecA* gene mutation substitutes a new PBP, termed PBP2a, which produces a protein with a conformational change that prohibits beta-lactam binding, rendering all beta-lactams ineffective.

- Gram-negative bacteria resistance through multiple mechanisms making it difficult to attribute resistance to any one mechanism. In addition to alterations in PBPs, bacteria utilize 3 other mechanisms of resistance: beta-lactamases, efflux pumps and decreased membrane permeability.

- Beta-lactamases are most commonly found on nearly all resistant Gram-negative bacteria. These are enzymes produced and released by the bacteria that bind and/or inactivate beta-lactam antibiotics prior to them reaching their intracellular penicillin binding sites. *main mech of resistance for GNRs to PCNs*

- Extended spectrum betalactamases (ESBL) are a subset of beta-lactamases that confer resistance, not only to penicillin-based beta-lactams, except perhaps piperacillin/tazobactam, but also to third generation cephalosporins and aztreonam. These are most common in *Klebsiella species* and *Proteus Species*, but have now been transferred to Enterobacteriaceae via plasmid. Carbapenems retain activity against these organisms and remain the preferred antibiotic for ESBLs. Carbapenemase producing *Klebsiella species* (KPC) are evolving, hydrolyze carbapenems via a metalloproteinase, rendering them ineffective.

- Efflux pumps contribute to antibiotic resistance to multiple drug classes including beta-lactams. Efflux pumps actively excrete intracellularly accumulated antibiotic so they do not reach a significant concentration to reach their binding site.

GN's

- Lastly, reduced membrane permeability to antibiotics confers resistance. Beta-lactam antibiotics must penetrate the outer membrane of Gram-negative organisms through channels or porins to reach their penicillin binding site. Alteration or loss of specific porins reduces or eliminates the ability of beta-lactams to reach their target binding site. *Pseudomonas aeruginosa* displays a notable resistance to imipenem through the loss of the OprD porin specific for imipenem, but not meropenem which retains its activity.

Natural Penicillins

Parenteral

Penicillin G
- Usual dose: 1-2 mU (IV) q4h QID

- Meningeal dose: 4 mU (IV) q4h

Oral

Penicillin V
- Usual dose: 500 mg (PO) QID

Hits
(usual clinical spectrum due to susceptible strains)

- Meningococci

- Group A, B, C, G streptococci

- Viridans streptococci

- *Streptococcus bovis*

- *S pneumoniae*

- *Listeria*

- *Bacillus anthracis*

- *Erysipelothrix rhusiopathiae*

- *Streptobacillus moniliformis*

- *Spirillum minus (rat-bite fever)*

- *Pasteurella multocida*

- *Actinomyces*

- *Clostridium*

- *Treponema*

- *Leptospira*

- *Borrelia*

Misses
- *Haemophilus influenzae* GNR

- *Enterococcus faecalis* (VSE) — *Enterococcus*

- *E faecium* (VRE) — *Staph*

- *Staphylococcus aureus* (MSSA/MRSA)

- *Klebsiella-Enterobacter-Serratia* GNR.

- *Pseudomonas aeruginosa*

- *Acinetobacter*

- *Bacillus fragilis* anaerobes

Major Clinical Uses
- Streptococcal infections

- Syphilis

- Oral anaerobes (dental infections)

- Meningococcal infections

- Actinomycosis

- Rat-bite fever

ID Board Pearls

- Not active against *H influenzae* or *E faecalis* (VSE), even when appearing susceptible *in vitro*.

- *P multocida* one of the very few aerobic GNBs susceptible to penicillin.

Antistaphylococcal Penicillins (ASPs)

Parenteral

Oxacillin/Nafcillin
- Usual dose: 1-2 g (IV) q4h QID

- Meningeal dose: 2 g (IV) q4h

Oral

Cloxacillin/Dicloxacillin
- Usual dose: 500 mg (PO) QID

Hits
(usual clinical spectrum due to susceptible strains)

- *S aureus (MSSA)*

- Group A streptococci

Misses
- *S aureus* (MRSA)

- *E faecalis* (VSE)

- *E faecium* (VRE)

- *Legionella*/atypicals

- Common coliforms

- *P aeruginosa*

- *B fragilis*

Major Clinical Uses
- MSSA infections

ID Board Pearls

- Nafcillin has the greatest anti-group A *streptococcal* activity among the ASPs.

- Nafcillin is the only ASP *hepatically* eliminated (*no dose change* in renal insufficiency).

- Nafcillin side effects are rare, but if present are renal, *not hepatic*.

[handwritten: Nafcillin/Methicillin are not cleared by S. aureus β lactamase so that makes it more effective than regular PCNs staph strep]

- Oxacillin is eliminated renally. Side effects are rare, but if present are hepatic, *not renal*.

Aminopenicillins

Parenteral

Ampicillin
- Usual dose: 2 g (IV) q4h

- Meningeal dose: 2 g (IV) q4h

Oral

Amoxicillin
- Usual dose: 1 g (PO) q8h

Drug Interactions

- Probenecid (↑ levels)

Hits
(usual clinical spectrum due to susceptible strains)

- Spectrum *same as penicillin plus anti-E faecalis (VSE) activity*

- *H influenzae* (ß-lactamase negative)

- Common aerobic GNBs

- *Listeria*

Misses
- *E faecium* (VRE)   *[handwritten: not for most GN Rs]*

- *S aureus* (MSSA/MRSA)

- *Legionella*/atypicals

- *Klebsiella-Enterobacter-Serratia*

- *P aeruginosa*

- *B fragilis*

Major Clinical Uses
- *E faecalis* (VSE)

- *Listeria*

- Upper respiratory tracts (acute sinusitis, otitis, bronchitis)

- Endocarditis prophylaxis (amoxicillin)

- Coliform UTIs/*E faecalis* (VSE)

ID Board Pearls

- Avoid ampicillin due to high incidence of resistance among Gram-negative bacilli.

- Ampicillin should be used primarily for *E faecalis* (VSE) SBE.

- Amoxicillin should be used instead of ampicillin IV → PO switch.

- Amoxicillin 1 g (IV) TID ~ serum levels as ampicillin (IM).

- Amoxicillin (vs. ampicillin) is well absorbed without GI side effects.

Antipseudomonal Penicillins (ASPs)

Parenteral

Ticarcillin (Ticar)
- Usual dose: 3 g (IV) QID

Mezlocillin (Mezlin)
- Usual dose: 3 g (IV) QID

Piperacillin
- Usual dose: 4 g (IV) TID

- Meningeal dose: 2 mU (IV) q4h

Oral

Carbenicillin (Geopen®) (UTIs only)
- Usual dose: 382 mg (PO) QID

Hits
(usual clinical spectrum due to susceptible strains)

- Most aerobic/anaerobic GNBs

- *B fragilis*

- *P aeruginosa*

- *Klebsiella-Enterobacter-Serratia*

- *E faecalis* (VSE)

- *S aureus* (MSSA)

Misses
- *Klebsiella-Enterobacter-Serratia*

- *E faecium* (VRE)

- *S aureus* (MRSA)

- *Legionella/atypicals*

Major Clinical Uses

- Aerobic Gram-negative bacillary infections

- Pseudomonas infections

- Nosocomial pneumonias

- Intraabdominal/pelvic infections

ID Board Pearls

- Among the ASPs, piperacillin has the *highest degree of anti-P aeruginosa and E faecalis (VSE) activity.*

- ASPs have *little activity* against *Klebsiella-Enterobacter-Serratia.*

- *Anti-S aureus (MSSA) of ASPs is modest.*

- *P aeruginosa* resistance *not* a problem with ASPs.

3. Cephalosporins

Mechanism of Action:
- All beta lactam antibiotics utilize the same mechanism of action, the binding of penicillin-binding proteins (PBP), thereby inhibiting cell wall synthesis.

Resistance Mechanism:
- The most common Gram-positive resistance mechanism is through the alteration of PBPs, reducing binding affinity, and thereby rendering the antibiotic ineffective. The classic example of this is methicillin resistant *S aureus* (MRSA). The *mecA* gene mutation substitutes a new PBP, termed PBP2a, which produces a protein with a conformational change that prohibits beta-lactam binding, rendering all beta-lactams ineffective.

GNR (R) to β lactams

- Gram-negative bacteria produce resistance through multiple mechanisms, making it difficult to attribute resistance to any one mechanism. In addition to alterations in PBPs, bacteria utilize 3 other mechanisms of resistance: beta-lactamases, efflux pumps and decreased membrane permeability.

- Beta-lactamases are most commonly found on nearly all resistant Gram-negative bacteria. These are enzymes produced and released by the bacteria that bind and/or inactivate beta-lactam antibiotics prior to them reaching their intracellular penicillin binding sites.

- Extended spectrum betalactamases (ESBL) are a subset of beta-lactamases that confer resistance not only to penicillin-based beta-lactams, except perhaps piperacillin/tazobactam, but also to third generation cephalosporins and aztreonam. These are most common in *Klebsiella species* and *Proteus Species*, but have now been transferred to Enterobacteriaceae via plasmid. Carbapenems retain activity against these organisms and remain the preferred antibiotic for ESBLs. Carbapenemase producing *Klebsiella species* (KPC) are evolving, hydrolyze carbapenems via a metalloproteinase, rendering them ineffective.

- Efflux pumps contribute to antibiotic resistance to multiple drug classes including beta-lactams.

Efflux pumps actively excrete intracellularly accumulated antibiotic so they do not reach a significant concentration to reach their binding site.

- Lastly, reduced membrane permeability to antibiotics confers resistance. Beta-lactam antibiotics must penetrate the outer membrane of Gram-negative organisms through channels or porins to reach their penicillin binding site. Alteration or loss of specific porins reduces or eliminates the ability of beta-lactams to reach their target binding site. *Pseudomonas aeruginosa* displays a notable resistance to imipenem through the loss of the OprD porin specific for imipenem, but not meropenem which retains its activity.

First-Generation Cephalosporins

Parenteral

Cefazolin (Ancef®, Kefzol)
- Usual dose: 1 g (IV) TID

Cephalothin (Keflin®)
- Usual dose: 1 g (IV) QID

Cephapirin (Cefadyl)
- Usual dose: 1 g (IV) QID

Oral

Cephalexin (Keflex)
- Usual dose: 0.5-1 g (PO) QID

Cefadroxil (Duricef)
- Usual dose: 0.5 g (PO) BID

Cephradine (Anspor, Velosef)
- Usual dose: 0.5 g (PO) BID

Hits *(usual clinical spectrum due to susceptible strains)*
- *S aureus (MSSA)*

- *Streptococci (group A, B, C, G, viridans)*

- *S pneumoniae*

- *E coli*

- *Klebsiella pneumoniae*

- *Proteus mirabilis*

- *Oral anaerobes*

Misses
- *Listeria*

- *E faecalis* (VSE)

- *E faecium* (VRE)

- *S aureus* (MRSA)

- *Legionella*/atypicals

- *H influenzae*

- *Providencia*

- *Morganella*

- *Enterobacter* spp.

- *Serratia marcescens*

- *P aeruginosa*

Major Clinical Uses
- Skin/soft tissue infections

- *S aureus* (MSSA)

- Antibiotic prophylaxis for implant related procedures

- *K pneumoniae*

- Group A streptococci

ID Board Pearls

- A fast way to differentiate *Klebsiella* from *Enterobacter*/*Serratia* is susceptibility to first generation cephalosporins (*Klebsiella* = S; *Enterobacter*/*Serratia* = R.)

- Cefazolin has *minimal* anti-*H influenzae* activity.

Second-Generation Cephalosporins

Parenteral

Cefamandole (Mandol)
- Usual dose: 2 g (IV) QID

Cefuroxime (Zinacef)
- Usual dose: 1.5 g (IV) TID

Cefoxitin (Mefoxin®)
- Usual dose: 2 g (IV) QID

Cefotetan (Cefotan®)
- Usual dose: 2 g (IV) BID

Oral

Cefaclor (Ceclor®)
- Usual dose: 500 mg (PO) QID

Cefuroxime axetil (Ceftin®)
- Usual dose: 500 mg (PO) BID

Cefprozil (Cefzil)
- Usual dose: 500 mg (PO) BID

Loracarbef (Lorabid)
- Usual dose: 400 mg (PO) BID

Hits
(usual clinical spectrum due to susceptible strains)

- Same spectrum as first-generation cephalosporins plus *H influenzae*

- Cefoxitin and cefotetan cover *B fragilis*

- All cover oral anaerobes

Misses
- *Listeria*

- *E faecalis* (VSE)

- *E faecium* (VRE)

- *S aureus* (MRSA)

- *B fragilis* (except cefoxitin and cefotetan)

- *Legionella*/atypical

- *Enterobacter*

- *Serratia*

- *P aeruginosa*

Major Clinical Uses
- Community-acquired pneumonia

- MSSA infections

- Cefoxitin or cefotetan (monotherapy for *mild to moderate* intraabdominal/pelvic infections)

- Skin and soft tissue infections

ID Board Pearls

- Cefamandole associated resistance to *H influenzae* and *Enterobacter* spp.

- Cefotetan has an MTT side chain (disulfiram) reaction.

- Only cefotetan has anti-B *fragilis* activity, but misses *B fragilis* "D.O.T." species; *B distasonis*; *Bovatus, B thetaiotaomicron*.

Third-Generation Cephalosporins

Parenteral

Cefotaxime (Claforan®)
- Usual dose: 2 g (IV) QID

Ceftizoxime (Cefizox®)
- Usual dose: 2 g (IV) TID

Cefoperazone (Cefobid)
- Usual dose: 2 g (IV) BID

Ceftazidime (Fortaz®, Tazidime®, Tazicef)
- Usual dose: 2 g (IV) TID

Ceftriaxone (Rocephin®)
- Usual dose: 1-2 g (IV) QD

- Meningeal dose: 2 g (IV) q4h (all 3rd GC cephalosporins except ceftriaxone)

- Ceftriaxone: 2 g (IV) BID

Oral

Cefixime (Suprax®)
- Usual dose: 400 mg (PO) BID

Cefpodoxime (Vantin®)
- Usual dose: 200 mg (PO) BID

Cefdinir (Omnicef)
- Usual dose: 600 mg (PO) QD

Cefditoren (Spectracef)
- Usual dose: 400 mg (PO) BID

Hits
(usual clinical spectrum due to susceptible strains)

- All cover oral anaerobes

- All cover *E coli*, *Klebsiella*, *Enterobacter*, *Serratia*, *Proteus*, *Providencia*

- All cover MSSA (*except* ceftazidime)

Misses
- *E faecium* (VRE)

- *E frecalis* (VSE)

- *Listeria*

- *S aureus* (MRSA)

- *Legionella*/atypicals

Major Clinical Uses
- Typical CAP pathogens

- Bacterial meningitis (*excluding Listeria*)

- Lyme disease

- Viridans streptococcal SBE

- Intraabdominal/pelvic infections (ceftriaxone *plus* either metronidazole or clindamycin)

- Hospital-acquired pneumonia (*only* ceftazidime or cefoperazone)

- Ceftriaxone or cefixime for anogenital gonorrhea

ID Board Pearls

- All have anti-*S aureus* (MSSA) activity: all *except* ceftazidime.

- Oral 3rd-generation cephalosporins have anti-MSSA activity *except* cefpodoxime.

- Anti-*P aeruginosa* activity: *only* cefoperazone, ceftazidime.

- Anti-*B fragilis* activity all *except* cefotaxime, ceftazidime.

- Anti-*E faecalis* activity (VSE): *only* cefoperazone.

- Only ceftriaxone and cefoperazone do *not* require dose adjustments in patients with renal insufficiency.

Fourth-Generation Cephalosporins

Parenteral

Cefepime (Maxipime)
- Usual dose: 2 g (IV) BID

- Meningeal dose: 2 g (IV) TID

Hits
(*usual clinical spectrum due to susceptible strains*)

- Same as third-generation cephalosporins, plus *P aeruginosa* (including ceftazidime-resistant *P aeruginosa*)

Misses
- MRSA

- *Stenotrophomonas (Xanthomonas) maltophilia*

- *E faecalis* (VSE)

- *E faecium* (VRE)

- *Legionella*/atypical

- *B fragilis*

Major Clinical Uses
- Nosocomial pneumonia

- Febrile neutropenia

- *P aeruginosa* infections

ID Board Pearls

- Increasing resistance secondary to ESBLS.

- For GNBs, use 2g (IV) BID, but for *P aeruginosa* or febrile neutropenia, use 2g (IV) TID.

Ceftobiprole

Usual dose:

Skin and soft tissue infections
500 mg (IV) BID

Nosocomial pneumonias[a]
500 mg (IV) TID

Mixed aerobic/anaerobic infections[b]
500 mg (IV) TID

[a]With an anti-*P aeruginosa* antibiotic

[b]If *B fragilis* suspected, add an anti-*B fragilis* antibiotic

Hits:
- MSSA

- VISA

- *E faecalis* (ampicillin susceptible)

- MRSA

- CoNS

- Most aerobic GNBs (*except* see below)

- Most anerobes (*except B fragilis*)

Misses
- *Proteus vulgaris*

- *E faecium* (ampicillin resistant)

- *Acinetobacter baumannii*

- *B (Pseudomonas) cepacia*

- *S (Xanthomonas) maltophilia*

- *B fragilis*

Major Clinical Uses
- MSSA/MRSA infections

- cSSSIs

- Nosocomial pneumonias

ID Board Pearls

- Misses ESBL producing strains of *E coli*, *Klebsiella pneumoniae* and *Enterobacter* spp.

- Cross resistance to ceftazidime and cefepime with *P aeruginosa*

4. Beta-Lactam/Beta-Lactamase Inhibitor Combinations

Mechanism of Action:
- All beta lactam antibiotics utilize the same mechanism of action, the binding of penicillin-binding proteins (PBP), thereby inhibiting cell wall synthesis.

Resistance Mechanism:
- The most common Gram-positive resistance mechanism is through the alteration of PBPs, reducing binding affinity, and thereby rendering the antibiotic ineffective. The classic example of this is methicillin resistant *S aureus*, (MRSA). The *mecA* gene mutation substitutes a new PBP, termed PBP2a, which produces a protein with a conformational change that prohibits beta-lactam binding, rendering all beta-lactams ineffective.

- Gram-negative bacteria resistance through multiple mechanisms, making it difficult to attribute resistance to any one mechanism. In addition to alterations in PBPs, bacteria utilize 3 other mechanisms of resistance: beta-lactamases, efflux pumps and decreased membrane permeability.

- Beta-lactamases are most commonly found on nearly all resistant Gram-negative bacteria. These are enzymes produced and released by the bacteria that bind and/or inactivate beta-lactam antibiotics prior to them reaching their intracellular penicillin binding sites.

- Extended spectrum betalactamases (ESBL) are a subset of beta-lactamases that confer resistance not only to penicillin-based beta-lactams, except perhaps piperacillin/tazobactam, but also to third generation cephalosporins and aztreonam. These are most common in *Klebsiella* species and *Proteus Species*, but have now been transferred to Enterobacteriaceae via plasmid. Carbapenems retain activity against these organisms and remain the preferred antibiotic for ESBLs. Carbapenemase-producing *Klebsiella* species (KPC) are evolving, hydrolyze carbapenems via a metalloproteinase, rendering them ineffective.

- Efflux pumps contribute to antibiotic resistance to multiple drug classes including beta-lactams. Efflux pumps actively excrete intracellularly accumulated antibiotic so they do not reach a significant concentration to reach their binding site.

- Lastly, reduced membrane permeability to antibiotics confers resistance. Beta-lactam antibiotics must penetrate the outer membrane of Gram-negative organisms through channels or porins to reach their penicillin binding site. Alteration or loss of specific porins reduces or eliminates the ability of beta-lactams to reach their target binding site. *Pseudomonas aeruginosa* displays a notable resistance to imipenem through the loss of the OprD porin specific for imipenem, but not meropenem which retains its activity.

B lactam/B lactamose Inhibitor Combinations

Parenteral

Ampicillin sulbactam (Unasyn®)
- Usual dose: 1.5-3 g (IV) QID

Ticarcillin clavulanic acid (Timentin®)
- Usual dose: 3.1 g (IV) QID

Piperacillin/tazobactam (Zosyn®)
- Usual dose: 4.5 g (IV) TID

Oral

Amoxicillin/clavulanic acid (Augmentin®)
- Usual dose: 875/125 mg (PO) BID

Hits
(usual clinical spectrum due to susceptible strains)

- Ampicillin/sulbactam: *same as ampicillin plus* MSSA, *Klebsiella, H influenzae, Moraxella catarrhalis* and *B fragilis*

- Ticarcillin/clavulanic acid: *same as ticarcillin* plus MSSA, *H influenzae, Klebsiella*

- Piperacillin/tazobactam: *same as piperacillin plus enhanced activity against* MSSA, *Klebsiella, Enterobacter, Serratia*

Misses
- *E faecium* (VRE)

- *S aureus* (MRSA)

- *Legionella*/atypical

Major Clinical Uses
- **Amoxicillin-clavulanic acid**

- Skin and soft tissue infections

- *Human or animal bites*

- **Ampicillin/sulbactam (Unasyn®) and ticarcillin/clavulanic acid (Timentin®)**

- Skin and soft tissue infections

- Intraabdominal/pelvic infections

- Diabetic foot infections

- Human or animal bites

- **Piperacillin/tazobactam (Zosyn®)**

- Skin and soft tissue infections

- Nosocomial pneumonias

- Intraabdominal/pelvic infections

- Diabetic foot infections

- Human or animal bites

ID Board Pearls

- Piperacillin/tazobactam *doesn't* predispose to MRSA/VRE or *C difficile*.

- Ampicillin/sulbactam is particularly useful for carbapenem resistant *Acinetobacter*.

- Tazobactam does *not* enhance the anti-*P aeruginosa* activity of piperacillin.

5. Macrolides

Mechanism of Action:
- Bind to the 50S subunit of the 70S ribosome, inhibiting RNA-dependent protein synthesis.

Resistance Mechanism:
- Efflux pumps.

- Decreased ribosomal binding. Most notable is the *erm* gene mutation which alters the 23S rRNA subunit leaving the ribosome resistant to the antibiotic. The *erm* mutation also produces cross resistance to lincosamide antibiotics (clindamycin and lincomycin) and streptogramins. This resistance can be inducible and not readily apparent on initial sensitivity testing. For strains that initially show erythromycin resistance but clindamycin sensitivity, additional testing with the D-test will clarify true underlying clindamycin resistant strains.

- Reduced cell permeability.

Macrolides

Parenteral

Erythromycin
- Usual dose: 1 g (IV/PO) QID 500 mg (PO) QID

Azithromycin (Zithromax)
- Usual dose: 500 mg (IV/PO) QD

Clarithromycin (Biaxin XL®)
- Usual dose: 1 g (IV) QD

Hits
(usual clinical spectrum due to susceptible strains)

- *S pneumoniae (misses ~20%)*

- Group A streptococci (most)

- Most *S aureus* (MSSA) (most)

- Mycobacterium-avium-intracellulare (MAI)

- *H influenzae only (azithromycin)*

- Oral anaerobes

- Legionella/atypical

Misses
- GNBs

- *B fragilis*

- Some *S aureus* (MSSA)

- Some group A streptococci

- *E faecium* (VRE)

Major Clinical Uses
- Non-zoonotic atypical CAPs

- Skin/soft tissue infection in penicillin-allergic patients

- Sinusitis, otitis, pharyngitis

- Bacillary angiomatosis

- MAI treatment and prophylaxis in HIV (clarithromycin or azithromycin)

ID Board Pearls

- Macrolides miss ~20% of *S pneumoniae* due to *intrinsic/natural resistance*, *plus* 15%-25% *S pneumoniae*, more strains become resistant due to *acquired* resistance (2° to use).

- Macrolides *unreliable* against *MSSA, Group A streptococci*, and *S pneumonia*.

- Macrolides *frequently ineffective* in Lyme disease.

- Erythromycin and clarithromycin have *little/no* anti-*H influenzae* activity.

- Macrolides are *the only* antibiotics *ineffective* against *P multocida*.

6. Tetracyclines

Mechanism of Action:
- Inhibit ribosomal protein synthesis by binding the 50S ribosomal subunit.

Resistance Mechanism:
- Several gene mutations alter the ribosomal binding site, protecting the bacteria protein synthesis inhibition.

- Efflux pumps

Tetracyclines

Parenteral/Oral

Minocycline (Minocin®)
Doxycycline (Vibramycin®)
- Usual dose: 100 mg (IV/PO) BID

- Meningeal dose: 100 mg (IV/PO) BID

Tetracycline
- Usual dose: 500 mg (PO) QID

- Usual dose: 100 mg (IV/PO) BID

- Meningeal dose: 100 mg (IV/PO)

Hits
(usual clinical spectrum due to susceptible strains)

- Oral anaerobes

- *Mycoplasma*

- *Legionella*

- *Rickettsia*

- *S aureus* (MSSA) (minocycline > doxycycline)

- *S aureus* (MRSA) (minocycline > doxycycline)

- *E faecium* (VRE) (doxycycline > minocycline)

- *B fragilis* (minocycline > doxycycline > tetracycline)

- *Vibrio*

- *Anthrax*

- *Borrelia*

- *Chlamydia*

- Spirochetes

- *E histolytica*

- *P falciparum* malaria *(doxycycline)*

Misses
- Group A streptococci

- *E faecalis* (VSE)

- *S aureus* (MRSA) (tetracycline, doxycycline)

- Campylobacter

- *P aeruginosa*

- *Klebsiella-Enterobacter-Serratia*

Major Clinical Uses
- CAP (typicals/atypicals)

- RMSF

- Ehrlichiosis/anaplasmosis

- Syphilis

- Lyme disease

- Chlamydia

- Zoonoses

- *E faecium* (VRE) (*only* doxycycline)

- *S aureus* (MRSA) (*only* minocycline)

ID Board Pearls

- *Oral* doxycycline useful for *neuroborreliosis* and *neurosyphilis*.

- *Doxycycline* has *good* anti-*CA-MRSA* activity; not good *CO/HA-MRSA* activity.

- *Minocycline has good anti-CO-MRSA, HA-MRSA and CA-MRSA activity.*

- *Campylobacter* is the commonest bacterial cause of traveler's diarrhea, *not covered by doxycycline*.

Mechanism of Action:
- Bind to the 50S subunit of the 70S ribosome, inhibiting RNA-dependent protein synthesis.

Resistance Mechanism:
- Efflux pumps

- Decreased ribosomal binding. Most notable is the erm gene mutation which alters the 23S rRNA subunit leaving the ribosome resistant to the antibiotic. The erm mutation also produces cross resistance to lincosamide antibiotics (clindamycin and lincomycin) and streptogramins. This resistance can be inducible and not readily apparent on initial sensitivity testing. For strains that initially show erythromycin resistance but clindamycin sensitivity, additional testing with the D-test will clarify true underlying clindamycin resistant strains.

- Reduced cell permeability.

Lincosamides

Parenteral/Oral

Clindamycin (Cleocin®)
- Usual dose: 600 mg (IV) TID 300 mg (PO) TID

Hits
(usual clinical spectrum due to susceptible strains)

- Group A streptococci

- *S aureus* (MSSA)

- *S pneumoniae* (some penicillin-resistant strains)

- CA-MRSA

- *B fragilis*

- *Toxoplasma gondii*

- PCP

- Babesia

- Malaria

Misses
- Most CoNS

- VSE/VRE

- Some *Fusobacterium* spp.

- Some *Clostridium* spp.

- All aerobic Gram-negative bacilli

- S aureus (CO/HA-MRSA)

Major Clinical Uses
- Skin and soft tissue infections

- Polymicrobial intraabdominal/pelvic infection (with an anti-GNB antibiotic)

- Combined with pyrimethamine for CNS *toxoplasmosis*

- Combined with primaquine for PCP

- Combined with quinine for *babesiosis*

ID Board Pearls

- Clindamycin useful for toxoplasmosis.

- Clindamycin useful for PCP.

- Clindamycin useful for babesiosis.

- ↑ risk of neuromuscular blockade with intraperitoneal lavage.

8. Chloramphenicol

Mechanism of Action:
- Binds the 50S ribosomal subunit preventing protein synthesis.

Resistance Mechanism:
- There are uncommon reports of decreased protein binding.

- Reduced permeability.

- Chloramphenicol acetyltransferase causing drug inactivation.

- Efflux pump.

Chloramphenicol

Parenteral/Oral

Chloramphenicol
- Usual dose: 500 mg – 1 g(IV/PO) QID

- Meningeal dose: 500 mg – 1 g (IV/PO) QID

Hits
(usual clinical spectrum due to susceptible strains)

- *Rickettsia*

- *E faecalis* (VSE)

- Nearly all Gram-positive and Gram-negative aerobes and anaerobes

- *B fragilis*

- *E faecium* (VRE)

Misses
- P aeruginosa

Major Clinical Uses
- Bacterial meningitis

- *Listeria* meningitis

- *E faecium* (VRE) infections

ID Board Pearls

- Chloramphenicol-induced *aplastic* anemia is idiosyncratic (not dose dependent) and irreversible.

- Chloramphenicol-induced anemia *is dose dependent and reversible*.

- Only antibiotic with *higher* serum levels PO than IV.

- Excellent *CNS penetration*, but *penetrates poorly/inactivated into bile/urine*.

Mechanism of Action:
- The antibiotic enters cells by passive diffusion, then, in anaerobic cells, the antibiotic is reduced by pyruvate ferredoxin oxidoreductase to form free radicals that then destabilize the cell, leading to cell death.

Resistance Mechanism:
- Alterations in the reductase are thought to convey resistance.

Metronidazole

Parenteral

Metronidazole (Flagyl®) IV/PO
- Usual dose: 1 g (IV) QD 250-500 mg (PO) TID-BID

- Meningeal dose: 1 g (IV) QD

Hits
(usual clinical spectrum due to susceptible strains)

- *B fragilis*

- *C difficile*

- *Gardnerella*

- *Trichomonas*

- *Giardia*

- *Entamoeba histolytica*

Misses
- *All* streptococci

- *All* aerobic Gram-negative and Gram-positive bacilli

- *S aureus* (MSSA/MRSA)

Major Clinical Uses
- C difficile (diarrhea/colitis)

- Bacterial vaginosis

- Amebic liver abscess

- *Mixed* aerobic/anaerobic infections (*in combination with an aerobic GNB agent*)

- Giardiasis

- *Trichomonas*

ID Board Pearls

- Metronidazole serum levels IV = PO.

- *Excellent CNS penetration* for amebic brain abscesses.

- Seizures and encephalopathy *common* side effects.

- Metronidazole therapy for *C difficile* diarrhea frequently fails.

- Metronidazole used for *C difficile* predisposes to ↑ VRE prevalence.

- Metronidzole preferred therapy for *C difficile* colitis (*not diarrhea*).

10. Aminoglycosides

Mechanism of Action:
- Inhibit ribosomal protein synthesis by binding the 30S ribosomal subunit.

Mechanism of Resistance:
- Efflux pumps.

- Acetylating, adenalating, and phosphorylating enzymes which alter the antibiotic, decreasing its affinity for the ribosomal binding.

- Ribosomal alteration that prevents or protects binding site.

- Decreased membrane permeability.

Aminoglycosides

Parenteral

Gentamicin (Garamycin®)
- Usual dose: 240 mg (IV) QD

Tobramycin (Nebcin®)
- Usual dose: 240 mg (IV) QD

Amikacin (Amikin®)
- Usual dose: 1 g (IV) QD

Streptomycin
- Usual dose: 1 g (IM) QD

Hits
(usual clinical spectrum due to susceptible strains)

- *S aureus* (MSSA)

- *Enterobacter*

- *Providencia*

- *Morganella*

- *Proteus*

- *Klebsiella*

- *Enterobacter*

- *Serratia*

- P aeruginosa

- Acinetobacter

Misses

- All streptococci

- All anaerobes (including *B fragilis*)

- *S aureus* (MRSA)

- *E faecium* (VRE)

- *Salmonella*

- *Shigella*

Major Clinical Uses
- P aeruginosa infections

- Aerobic GNB infections

- Combined with vancomycin/rifampin for treatment of *E faecalis* SBE

ID Board Pearls

- Gentamicin: *highest* degree of anti-*Serratia marcescens* and *S aureus* (MSSA) activity among aminoglycosides.

- Streptomycin has the highest degree of activity *against TB, tularemia, plague, brucellosis.*

- *Inhaled* tobramycin *predisposes* to *P aeruginosa resistance.*

- Amikacin has the *greatest degree of P aeruginosa activity and lowest resistance potential.*

11. Trimethoprim-Sulfamethoxazole (TMP-SMX)

Mechanism of Action:
- Each component inhibits a different step in folate synthesis.

Resistance Mechanism:
- Efflux pumps.

- Reduced permeability.

- Reduced target site binding.

TMP-SMX

Parenteral/Oral

TMP-SMX (Bactrim®, Septra®)
- Usual dose: 2.5mg/kg (IV/PO) QID

- PCP/Meningeal dose: 2.5mg/kg (IV/PO) QID

Hits
(usual clinical spectrum due to susceptible strains)

- *Most* aerobic GNBs

- *Some E faecalis* (VSE)

- *S aureus* (MSSA)

- Most CA-MRSA

- *Listeria*

- PCP

- *Nocardia*

- *Legionella*/atypical

Misses
- *S aureus* (CO/HA-MRSA)

- *E faecium* (VRE)

- *P aeruginosa*

- *B fragilis*

- *Klebsiella pneumoniae*

Major Clinical Uses

- *Most* aerobic gram-negative bacillary infections

- UTIs (pyelonephritis, prostatitis, etc.)

- PCP (prophylaxis and treatment)

- *Isospora belli*

- *Listeria* meningitis

- Nocardiosis

ID Board Pearls

- TMP-SMX same spectrum as ceftriaxone (*except* TPM-SMX is active against *Listeria*).

- TMP-SMX active against *all aerobic GNBs except P aeruginosa*.

12. Quinolones

Mechanisms of Action:
- Inhibit DNA Gyrase and topoisomerase IV resulting in DNA breakage and cell death.

Resistance Mechanism:
- Alteration in target site binding.

- Efflux pumps.

- Reduced permeability.

Quinolones

Parenteral/Oral

Ofloxacin (Floxin®)
- Usual dose: 400 mg (IV/PO) BID

Gatifloxacin (Tequin®)
- Usual dose: 400 mg (IV/PO) QD

Ciprofloxacin (Cipro®)
- Usual dose: 400 mg (IV) BID or 500-750 mg (PO) BID

Moxifloxacin (Avelox®)
- Usual dose: 400 mg (IV/PO) QD

Levofloxacin (Levaquin®)
- Usual dose: 500 mg (IV/PO) QD

Hits
(usual clinical spectrum due to susceptible strains)

- Enterobacteriaceae

- *P aeruginosa*

- *Neisseria gonorrhoeae* (PPNG)

- *Legionella*/atypicals

- *Campylobacter, Salmonella, Shigella*

- Anthrax

- *Brucella*

- *S aureus* (MSSA)

• *E faecalis* (VSE)

Misses
• *Bacteroides fragilis* (*except* moxifloxacin)

• *S aureus* (MRSA)

• Some *E faecium* (VRE)

Major Clinical Uses
• Oral anaerobes

• CAP (except ciprofloxacin

• Sinusitis, AECB, otitis media

• Osteomyelitis (due to susceptible organisms)

• Respiratory quinolones (levofloxacin, moxifloxacin) highly active against *S pneumoniae*/ MDR *S pneumoniae*

• Bacterial diarrheas

• Anthrax

• Skin/soft tissue infections

• UTIs (except moxifloxacin)

ID Board Pearls

• *Only quinolones* highly active against *P aeruginosa* are *levofloxacin* and ciprofloxacin.

• Quinolones have *some* activity against *E faecalis* (VSE) but *none* are active against *E faecium* (VRE).

• Moxifloxacin *doesn't* concentrate well in urine (avoid for UTIs).

• Moxifloxacin is *the only* quinolone with good anti-*B fragilis* activity.

13. Colistin

Mechanism of Action:
• Acts similar to a membrane detergent, binding to the phospholipid content of the cell wall leading to increased permeability and cell death.

Resistance Mechanism:
• Resistance is likely due to decreased permeability.

Colistin

Parenteral

Colistin
• Usual dose: 1.7 mg/kg (IV) TID (1 mg = 12,500)

• Meningeal dose: usual systemic dose + 10 mg (IT) QD

Hits
(usual clinical spectrum due to susceptible strains)

• *P aeruginosa*

• *Acinetobacter*

• *K pneumoniae*

Misses
• *Proteus*

• *Serratia*

• Gram-positive cocci

• VSE/VRE

• *B fragilis*

Major Clinical Uses
• MDR *P aeruginosa*

• MDR *Acinetobacter*

• MDR *Klebsiella*

14. Polymyxin B

Mechanism of Action:
• Acts similar to a membrane detergent, binding to the phospholipid content of the cell wall leading to increased permeability and cell death.

Resistance Mechanism:
• Resistance is likely due to decreased permeability.

Polymyxin B

Parenteral

Polymyxin B
• Usual dose: 1.25 mg/kg (IV) BID (mg = 10,000 μ)

• Meningeal dose: usual dose + 50 mg (IT) QD for 3 days then once every other day

Hits
(usual clinical spectrum due to susceptible strains)

• *P aeruginosa*

• *Acinetobacter*

• *K pneumoniae*

Misses
• *Proteus*

• *Serratia*

• Gram-positive cocci

• VSE/VRE

• *B fragilis*

Major Clinical Uses
• MDR *P aeruginosa*

• MDR *Acinetobacter baumannii*

• MDR *Klebsiella pneumoniae*

ID Board Pearls

- Polymyxin B *not* nephrotoxic *if* dosed according to CrCl.

- Avoid aerosolized Polymyxin B, which ↑ resistance *P aeruginosa* potential.

- If being used for meningitis, use IT dose with IV dose.

- Polymyxin B *highly active against all aerobic GNBs, except Proteus and Serratia.*

Mechanism of Action:
- All beta lactam antibiotics utilize the same mechanism of action, the binding of penicillin-binding proteins (PBP), thereby inhibiting cell wall synthesis.

Resistance Mechanism:
- The most common Gram-positive resistance mechanism is through the alteration of PBPs, reducing binding affinity, and thereby rendering the antibiotic ineffective.

- In addition to alterations in PBPs, bacteria utilize 3 other mechanisms of resistance, beta-lactamases, efflux pumps and decreased membrane permeability.

- Beta-lactamases are most commonly found on nearly all resistant Gram-negative bacteria. These are enzymes produced and released by the bacteria that bind and/or inactivate beta-lactam antibiotics prior to them reaching their intracellular penicillin binding sites. Extended spectrum betalactamases (ESBL) are a subset of beta-lactamases that confer resistance not only to penicillin-based beta-lactams, but also to third generation cephalosporins and aztreonam. These are most common in *Klebsiella* species and Proteus Species, but have now been transferred to most Enterobacteriaceae via plasmids. Carbapenems retain activity against these organisms and remain the preferred antibiotic and ESBL-producing bacteria. However, carbapenemase-producing *Klebsiella* (KPC) are evolving through a metalloproteinase, hydrolyze carbapenem antibiotic, rendering them ineffective as well.

- Efflux pumps contribute to antibiotic resistance to multiple drug classes, including beta-lactams. Efflux pumps actively excrete intracellularly accumulated antibiotic so they do not reach a significant concentration to reach their binding site.

- Lastly, reduced membrane permeability to antibiotics confers resistance. Beta-lactam antibiotics must penetrate the outer membrane of Gram-negative organisms through channels or porins to reach their penicillin binding site. Alteration or loss of specific porins reduces or eliminates the ability of beta-lactams to reach their target binding site.

• *Pseudomonas aeruginosa* displays a notable resistance to imipenem through the loss of the OprD porin, which is specific for imipenem, but not meropenem which retains activity.

Carbapenems

Parenteral

Imipenem (Primaxin®)
• Administered with cilastatin (dehydropeptidase inhibitor)

• Usual dose: 0.5-1 g (IV) QID

Meropenem (Merrem®)
• Usual dose: 500 mg-1 g (IV) TID

• Meningeal dose: 2 g (IV) TID

Doripenem (Doribax®)
• Usual dose: 500 mg-1 g (IV) TID

Ertapenem (Invanz)
• Usual dose: 1 g (IV) QD

Hits
(usual clinical spectrum due to susceptible strains)

• All streptococci

• *E faecalis* (VSE) (*except* ertapenem)

• *S aureus* (MSSA)

• Most GNBs

• *P aeruginosa* (*except* ertapenem)

• *B fragilis*

• Acinetobacter (*except* ertapenem)

• Listeria

Misses
• S aureus (MRSA)

• Stenotrophomonas (Xanthomonas) maltophilia

• Burkholderia (Pseudomonas) cepacia

• Enterococcus faecium (VRE)

• Legionella/atypicals

Major Clinical Uses
• CIAIs

• CSSSIs

• Nosocomial pneumonias,(meropem or doripenem)

• Meropenem (ABM secondary susceptible to Gram-positive/Gram-negative meningeal pathogens at meningeal doses).

• *E faecalis* (VSE) (except ertapenem)

• Empiric therapy for infections in penicillin-allergic patients.

ID Board Pearls

• Ertapenem (*not active* against *enterococci*, *Acinetobacter or P aeruginosa*).

• Meropenem (meningeal doses) is *the only* carbapenem useful in meningitis, due to susceptible organisms (GNB, Listeria).

• Imipenem, (*not* meropenem or ertapenem), associated with seizures (incidence ↑ with renal insufficiency/CNS disorders).

• Except ertapenem Carbapenems have good anti-*E faecalis* (VSE) activity; *none* have activity against *E faecium* (VRE).

• Meropenem *safe* in penicillin-allergic patients.

• Meropenem and dovipenem imipenem are highly active against *P aeruginosa* (*not* ertapenem).

• Doripenem is particularly active against MDR Acinetobacter and MDR *P aeruginosa*.

16. Monobactams

Mechanism of Action:
- All beta lactam antibiotics utilize the same mechanism of action, the binding of penicillin-binding proteins (PBP), thereby inhibiting cell wall synthesis.

Resistance Mechanism:
- The most common Gram-positive resistance mechanism is through the alteration of PBPs, reducing binding affinity, and thereby rendering the antibiotic ineffective. The classic example of this is *Methicillin Resistant S aureus* (MRSA). The *mecA* gene mutation substitutes a new PBP, termed PBP2a, which produces a protein with a conformational change that prohibits beta-lactam binding, rendering all beta-lactams ineffective.

- Gram-negative bacteria resistance through multiple mechanisms, making it difficult to attribute resistance to any one mechanism. In addition to alterations in PBPs, bacteria utilize 3 other mechanisms of resistance: beta-lactamases, efflux pumps and decreased membrane permeability.

- Beta-lactamases are most commonly found on nearly all resistant Gram-negative bacteria. These are enzymes produced and released by the bacteria that bind and/or inactivate beta-lactam antibiotics prior to them reaching their intracellular penicillin binding sites.

- Extended spectrum betalactamases (ESBL) are a subset of beta-lactamases that confer resistance not only to penicillin-based beta-lactams, except perhaps piperacillin/tazobactam, but also to third generation cephalosporins and aztreonam. These are most common in *Klebsiella* species and *Proteus Species*, but have now been transferred to Enterobacteriaceae via plasmid. Carbapenems retain activity against these organisms and remain the preferred antibiotic for ESBLs. Carbapenemase-producing Klebsiella species (KPC) are evolving through hydrolyze carbapenems via a metalloproteinase, rendering them ineffective.

- Efflux pumps contribute to antibiotic resistance to multiple drug classes, including beta-lactams. Efflux pumps actively excrete intracellularly accumulated antibiotic, so they do not reach a significant concentration to reach their binding site.

- Lastly, reduced membrane permeability to antibiotics confers resistance. Beta-lactam antibiotics must penetrate the outer membrane of Gram-negative organisms through channels or porins to reach their penicillin binding site. Alteration or loss of specific porins reduces or eliminates the ability of beta-lactams to reach their target binding site. *Pseudomonas aeruginosa* displays a notable resistance to imipenem through the loss of the OprD porin specific for imipenem, but not meropenem which retains its activity.

Monobactam

Parenteral

Aztreonam (Azactam®)
- Usual dose: 2 g (IV) TID

- Meningeal dose: 2 g (IV) QID

Hits
(usual clinical spectrum due to aerobic strains)

- GNBs

- *P aeruginosa*

Misses
- All Gram-positive cocci

- *B fragilis*

- *Legionella/atypicals*

Major Clinical Uses
- Aerobic GNBs

- Aerobic GNBs infections in penicillin-allergic patients

ID Board Pearls

- Aztreonam has *no activity* against Gram-positive cocci.

- No cross reactivity in penicillin-allergic patients.

17. Vancomycin

Mechanism of Action:
- During cell wall synthesis, vancomycin binds the crosslinking D-alanyl-D-alanine terminal chain, thereby inhibiting cell wall synthesis.

Resistance Mechanism:
- Resistance to Vancomycin is most prevalent in *enterococci faecium*. Resistance genes termed *VanA* through *VanG* have been described, with *VanA* and *VanB* being the most noteworthy. All the mutations are expressed by an alternate, terminal amino acid substitution in the D-alanyl-D-alanine crosslink, which vancomycin does not then bind.

- *VanA* confers high grade resistance to vancomycin, and *VanB* conveys a more variable level of resistance. *Van* gene mutations are plasmid-mediated, and therefore easily transferred between bacteria, facilitating spread.

- Resistance to vancomycin by *S aureus* is of growing concern. Heterogeneous resistance typically manifests as hVISA, heterogeneous, vancomycin intermediate-sensitivity *S aureus*(VISA) stains.

- Reduced susceptibility to vancomycin is achieved through an increased cell wall thickness, which limits vancomycin access to intercellular binding sites.

- *Vancomycin* resistant *S aureus* (VRSA) is still extremely rare, with only a handful of documented cases. In all documented cases though, the mechanism of (VRSA) resistance is through transfer of the enterococcus *VanA* plasmid to *S aureus*.

Vancomycin

Parenteral

Vancomycin
- Usual dose: 1 g (IV) BID

- Meningeal dose: Usual IV dose plus 20 mg (intrathecal) QD

Oral
- 125-250 mg (PO) QID (not systemically absorbed)

Hits
(usual clinical spectrum due to susceptible strains)

- Oral anaerobes

- *S aureus* (MSSA)

- *S aureus* (MRSA)

- Enterococci (except VRE)

- *S pneumoniae* (+ PRSP)

- *Clostridium difficile*

- All streptococci

- *S epidermidis*

- Corynebacterium JK

Misses
- *All aerobic* GNBs

- *Legionella*/atypicals

- B fragilis

- Erysipelothrix rhusiopathiae

- E faecium (VRE)

Major Clinical Uses

- Staphylococcal infections (including MRSA)

- Endocarditis prophylaxis for *penicillin-allergic* patients

- *Prosthetic valve* endocarditis (combined with rifampin and gentamicin)

- VSE endocarditis in penicillin-allergic patients

- Vancomycin PO for *C difficile* diarrhea (*not colitis*)

ID Board Pearls

• *S aureus* bacteremias often respond slowly/not at all to vancomycin.

• Vancomycin use increases cell wall thickness in staphylococci, resulting in *penetration-mediated resistance*.

• Vancomycin (*IV not PO*) use increases *VRE prevalence*.

• Properly dosed vancomycin is not, in itself, *nephrotoxic* (as part of combination therapy, with a known *nephrotoxic* drug, if nephrotoxicity occurs it is *not due* to *vancomycin*).

18. Quinupristin/Dalfopristin

Mechanism of Action:
• Streptogramin antibiotics bind the 50S ribosomal subunit inhibiting protein synthesis.

Resistance Mechanism:
• Streptogramins are related to the macrolides and lincosamides and are susceptible to the same inducible erm gene mutation described earlier.

• Efflux pumps account for the difference in susceptibility between Enterococcus faecium and *Enterococcus faecalis* (USE).

• Enzymatic degradation and inactivation.

Quinupristin/dalfopristin

Parenteral

Quinupristin/dalfopristin (Synercid®)
• Usual dose: 7.5 mg/kg (IV) TID

Hits
(usual clinical spectrum due to susceptible strains)

• Group A streptococci

• *S pneumoniae*

• *S aureus* (MSSA/MRSA)

• *E faecium* (VRE)

Misses
• *E faecalis* (VSE)

• All aerobic GNBs

• All anaerobes (including *B fragilis*)

Major Clinical Uses
• Serious infections due to MSSA/MRSA

• Serious VRE infections

• Often used for MRSA in vancomycin intolerant patients

ID Board Pearls

• Quinupristin/dalfopristin induced *myalgias* are rare but *severe/prolonged*; often continuing for days after quinupristin/dalfopristin has been discontinued.

• Quinupristin/dalfopristin highly active against *E faecium* (VRE) but not *E faecalis* (VSE).

• Quinupristin/dalfopristin useful in MRSA ABE unresponsive to daptomycin.

19. Linezolid

Mechanism of Action:
• Binds the 30S ribosomal subunit inhibiting protein synthesis.

Resistance Mechanism:
• A single point mutation leads to decreased ribosomal binding, conferring resistance.

• Certain bacteria such as E coli have an intrinsic efflux pump.

Oxazolidinones

Parenteral/Oral

Linezolid (Zyvox)
• Usual dose: 600 mg (IV/PO) BID

• Meningeal dose: same

Hits
(usual clinical spectrum due to susceptible strains)

• *S aureus* (MSSA/MRSA)

• MDR *S pneumoniae*

• Group A, B, C, G streptococci

• *E faecalis* (VSE)

• *E faecium* (VRE)

Misses
• All aerobic and anaerobic GNBs

• Legionella/atypicals

• *B fragilis*

Major Clinical Uses *(due to susceptible strains)*
• MRSA/MSSA infections

• *E faecalis* (VSE) infections

• *E faecium* (VRE) infections

- Linezolid *serum levels IV same as PO* (100% bioavailability).

- Linezolid is one of the few antibiotics with *activity against Listeria*.

- Excellent CSF penetration; *useful in CNS infections due to gram-positive cocci*.

- Only 1 of 2 *oral* anti-MRSA antibiotics.

Linezolid = Listeria

20. Daptomycin

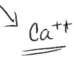

Ca^{++}

Mechanism of Action:
- Disrupts calcium-dependent cell membrane function by an unknown mechanism.

Resistance Mechanism:
- Cell wall thickening is thought to limit daptomycin access to the cell membrane.

- Alterations in the cytoplasmic membrane voltage potential decrease susceptibility in resistant strains.

Daptomycin

Parenteral

Daptomycin (Cubicin®)
- Usual dose: 4 mg/kg (IV) QD (skin/soft tissue infection)

- 6 mg/kg (IV) QD (bacteremia ABE)

Hits
(usual clinical spectrum due to susceptible strains)

- *S aureus* (MSSA/MRSA)

- *E faecalis* (VSE)

- *E faecium* (VRE)

Misses
- All aerobic GNBs

- All anaerobic GNBs (including *B fragilis*)

Major Clinical Uses
- Serious MSSA/MRSA infection (including ABE)

- MDR *S pneumoniae* CAP

ID Board Pearls

- *If CrCl <30 mL/min*, give indicated dose *once every other day*.

- Daptomycin *doesn't penetrate CNS (don't use for CNS infections)*.

• Most rapidly bactericidal anti-*S aureus* antibiotic.

• *Don't* use for *pneumonias* (lung surfactant containing Ca+ antagonizes daptomycin).

• No allergic cross reactions with other antibiotics.

• Useful in treating *S aureus* bacteremias/ABE *unresponsive to vanconycin*.

Dapto — cidal against enterococcus [handwritten]

21. Tigecycline

other tetra's are SO [handwritten]

Mechanism of Action:
• Binds the 30S ribosomal subunit inhibiting protein synthesis.

Resistance Mechanisms:
• Alterations in the 30S ribosomal binding site, but most alteration resulting in tetracycline resistance remain tigecycline-susceptible.

• Efflux pumps, most notable for pseudomonas and proteus species.

Glycylcyclines

Parenteral

Tigecycline (Tygacil)
• Usual dose: 100 mg (IV) for 1 dose (loading dose); then 50 mg (IV) BID

Hits
(usual clinical spectrum due to susceptible strains)

• VSE/VRE

• *S aureus* (MSSA/MRSA)

• Aerobic GNBs (*except P aeruginosa and some Proteus*)

• *B fragilis*

Misses
• *P aeruginosa*

Major Clinical Uses
• Mixed aerobic/anaerobic (cIAIs infection)

• Mixed aerobic/anaerobic (cSSSIs infections)

• MDR GNBs

• MSSA/MRSA infection

ID Board Pearls

• Tigecycline *highly effective against ESBL -producing strains of E coli, Klebsiella sp, Enterobacter sp., but potential for Acinetobacter resistance*

- Tigecycline can be used safely in *penicillin/sulfa-allergic* patients.

- Tigecycline has *no cross reactivity* with other antibiotics.

- *No dosing adjustments in mild or moderate renal/hepatic insufficiency* with tigecycline.

- Tigecycline is highly effective against MDR and Klebsiella.

- Tigecycline often the *only antibiotic effective against carbapenemase-producing* GNBs (KPC).

- No P450 interactions

22. Spectrum Summaries

Anti-Enterococcal VSE/VRE Antibiotics

Antibiotics with *little/no* anti-*E faecalis* (VSE) activity
- Penicillin *(alone)*

- Metronidazole

- Cephalosporin *(except cefoperazone)*

- Aztreonam

- Clindamycin

- Ertapenem

- Quinupristin/dalfopristin

- Colistin

- Polymyxin B

Antibiotics with *some* anti-*E faecalis* (VSE) activity
- TMP-SMX

- Macrolides

- Quinolones

- Ceftobiprole

Antibiotics with *good* anti-*E faecalis* (VSE) activity
- Ampicillin

- Cefoperazone

- Amoxicillin

- Nitrofurantoin

- Penicillin + aminoglycoside (*only* in combination)

- Linezolid

- Ampicillin/sulbactam

- Daptomycin

- Amoxicillin/clavulanate

- Imipenem

- Piperacillin/tazobactam

- Meropenem

- Ticarcillin/clavulanate

- Doripenem

- Chloramphenicol

- Tigecycline

- Vancomycin

Antibiotics with *little/no* anti-*E faecium* (VRE) activity
- β-Lactams

- Colistin

- Quinolones

- Polymyxin B

- Aminoglycosides

- TMP-SMX

- Vancomycin

- Macrolides

- Clindamycin

- Carbapenems

- Aztreonam

Antibiotics with *good* anti-*E faecium* (VRE) activity
- Nitrofurantoin

- Linezolid

- Chloramphenicol

- Daptomycin

- Doxycycline

- Tigecycline

- Quinupristin/dalfopristin

- Ceftobiprole (*except* ampicillin resistant *E faecium*

Anti-staphylococcal MSSA/MRSA antibiotics

Antibiotics with *little/no* anti-MSSA activity
- Penicillin

- Metronidazole

- Ampicillin

- Oral 3rd generation cephalosporins (cefpodoxime, cefixime)

- Aztreonam

Antibiotics with *some* anti-MSSA activity
- Amoxacillin/clavulanic acid

- Macrolides• Ampicillin/sulbactam

- Doxycycline

- Ceftazidime

- Tobramycin

- Ciprofloxacin

- Amikacin

Antibiotics with *good* anti-MSSA activity
- 1st generation cephalosporins

- Clindamycin

- 2nd generation cephalosporins

- Gentamicin

- 3rd generation cephalosporins (except ceftazidime)

- Vancomycin

- Televancin

- Carbapenems

- Piperacillin/tazobactam

- Quinupristin/dalfopristin

- Chloramphenicol

- Linezolid

- TMP-SMX

- Daptomycin

- Rifampin

- Minocycline

Antibiotics with *good* anti-MRSA activity (HA-MRSA, CO-MRSA and CA-MRSA)
- Minocycline

- Quinupristin/dalfopristin

- Linezolid

- Tigecycline

- Daptomycin

- Vancomycin

Antibiotics with anti-CA-MRSA activity (*ineffective* against CO-MRSA and HR-MRSA)
- Doxycycline

- TMP-SMX

- Clindamycin

Anti-Klebsiella pneumoniae antibiotics

Antibiotics with *little/no* anti-*Klebsiella pneumo-*

niae **activity**
- Penicillin

- Macrolides

- Ampicillin

- Vancomycin

- Clindamycin

Antibiotics with some anti-*Klebsiella pneumoniae* activity
- Ampicillin/sulbactam

- TMP-SMX

- Anti-pseudomonal penicillin (APPs)

- Chloramphenicol

Antibiotics with *good* anti-*Klebsiella pneumoniae* activity
- 1st, 2nd, 3rd generation cephalosporins

- Colistin, Polymyxin B

- Ceftobiprole (except ESBL + strains)

- Quinolones

- Aminoglycosides

- Carbapenems

- Aztreonam

- Tigecycline

Antibiotics with *good* anti-MDR *Klebsiella pneumoniae* activity
- Gentamicin

- Carbapenems

- Colistin

- Tigecycline

- Polymyxin B

Anti-*Pseudomonas aeruginosa* antibiotics

Antibiotics with *little/no* anti-*P aeruginosa* activity
- Penicillin

- Linezolid

- Ampicillin/sulbactam

- Daptomycin

- Nitrofurantoin

- Vancomycin

- TMP-SMX

- Tigecycline

- Moxifloxacin

- Ertapenem

- 1st, 2nd and 3rd generation cephalosporins (except ceftazidime and cefoperazone)

Antibiotics with *Good* anti-*P aeruginosa* activity
- Aminoglycosides (amikacin, tobramycin, gentamicin)

- Anti-pseudomonal penicillins (APPs)

- Ciprofloxacin

- Ticarcillin/clavulanate

- Levofloxacin

Antibiotics with *Good* anti-MDR *P aeruginosa* activity
- Amikacin

- Colistin

- Meropenem

- Polymyxin B

- Doripenem

Anti-Acinetobacter baumannii antibiotics

Antibiotics with *little/no* anti-*Acinetobacter baumannii* activity
- Penicillins

- 1st generation cephalosporins

- 2nd generation cephalosporins

- Anti-pseudomonal penicillins (APPs)

Antibiotics with *some* anti-Acinetobacter baumannii activity
- TMP-SMX

- Moxifloxacin

- Aztreonam

- Levofloxacin

- Ceftobiprole

- Cefepime

Antibiotics with *good* anti-*Acinetobacter* activity[a]
- Aminoglycosides

- Colistin

- Tigecycline

- Polymyxin B

- 3rd generation cephalosporins

- Meropenem

- Cefepime

- Doripenem

• Ampicillin/sulbactam

[a]In general, *A baumannii* are more susceptible than *A lwoffii*.

Anti-S maltophilia antibiotics

Antibiotics with *little/no Stenotrophomonas (Xanthomonas) maltophilia* activity
• β-lactams

• Carbapenems

• Aminoglycosides

• Ceftobiprole

Antibiotics with *some Stenotrophomonas (Xanthomonas) maltophilia* activity
• Respiratory quinolones

• Cefepime

• TMP-SMX

Antibiotics with good *Stenotrophomonas (Xanthomonas) maltophilia* activity
• Sulbactam/ampicillin

• Minocycline

• TMP-SMX

• Polymyxin B

• Colistin

Anti-Listeria monocytogenes antibiotics

Antibiotics with *little/no* anti-*Listeria monocytogenes* activity
• β-lactams

• 1st, 2nd, 3rd, 4th generation cephalosporins

• Clindamycin

• Vancomycin

Antibiotics with some anti-*Listeria monocytogenes*
activity
• Quinolones

• Aminoglycosides

Antibiotics with good anti-*Listeria monocytogenes* activity
• Ampicillin

• Linezolid

• Chloramphenicol

• Meropenem

• TMP-SMX

Anti-Burkholderia (Pseudomonas) cepacia antibiotics

Antibiotics with *little/no* anti-*Burkholderia (Pseudomonas) cepacia* activity
• Aminoglycosides

• Polymyxin B

• Colistin

• Ceftobiprole

Antibiotics with good anti-*Burkholderia (Pseudomonas) cepacia* activity
• TMP-SMX

• Respiratory quinolones

• Minocycline

Anti-B fragilis antibiotics

Antibiotics with *little/no* anti-*B fragilis* activity
• Penicillin

• 1st generation cephalosporins

• Ampicillin

• 2nd generation cephalosporins (except cefoxitin, cefotan)

- Aztreonam

- 3rd/4th generation cephalosporins ceftazidime, ceftriaxone, cefepime (except ceftizoxime, cefoperazone)

- Ciprofloxacin

- Ceftobiprole

- Levofloxacin

Antibiotics with *some* anti-*B fragilis* activity
- Macrolides

- Cefotaxime

Antibiotics with good anti-*B fragilis* activity
- Ampicillin/sulbactam

- Moxifloxacin

- Amoxicillin/clavulanate

- Cefotetan

- Ticarcillin/clavulanate

- Cefoxitin

- Piperacillin/tazobactam

- Cefoperazone

- Clindamycin

- Ceftizoxime

- Metronidazole

- Carbapenems

- Doxycycline

- Tigecycline

- Minocycline

- Chloramphenicol

23. Tissue Penetration

Antibiotic CSF Penetration

General Concepts

- Except for cholramphenicol, linezolid, minocycline, TMP-SMX, anti-TB drugs, antibiotics *don't* penetrate the CSF in adequate concentration when administered in the *usual* doses.

ID Board Pearls

- Third- and fourth-generation cephalosporins penetrate the CSF in "meningeal doses"

- Meropenem penetrates the CSF in "*meningeal doses*"

- Only ceftriaxone penetrates the CSF in therapeutically useful concentrations with usual dose

Antibiotic Lung Penetration

General Concepts

- Penetration not a problem. Lung parenchymal levels approximate serum levels.

- Lungs are *well-vascularized and perfused*.

- With usual dosing, most antimicrobials penetrate lung well.

ID Board Pearls

- Aminoglycosides: ↓activity, not ↓levels

- Surfactant (Ca++)↓ activity of daptomycin.

- Low vancomycin lung levels with under dosing.

Antibiotic Bone Penetration

General Concepts

- β-Lactam levels about ¼ of simultaneous serum levels.

ID Board Pearls

- Limited data available on other agents, ↓ *but nearly all penetrate bone well*.

Antibiotic Synovial Fluid Penetration

General Concepts

- Penetration not a problem with most antibiotics. Synovial fluid levels ~ serum levels.

ID Board Pearls

- Aminoglycosides: activity, not levels

- Vancomycin and erythromycin do not penetrate synovial fluid well

Antibiotic Biliary Tract Penetration

General Concepts

- Bile levels differ from gallbladder wall levels.

- The only antibiotics that achieve therapeutic concentrations in an obstructed biliary tract are cefoperazone and clindamycin.

ID Board Pearls

- Most hepatically-eliminated drugs concentrate in bile if no obstruction is present.

- Chloramphenicol not good for biliary tract infections.

- Most chloramphenicol in bile is in the form of inactive metabolites.

Antibiotic Urinary Penetration

General Concepts

- Most *renally* eliminated drugs achieve *supra* serum levels in urine.

- With *renally* eliminated antibiotics, urinary spectrum >serum spectrum, because susceptibility is in part concentration-dependent.

- For *P aeruginosa* catheter-associated bacteriuria (CAB) in urine (*not* systemic infection), doxycycline is effective.

- Ciprofloxacin equally active as levofloxacin for *P aeruginosa* UTIs.

- *Hepatically*-inactivated or eliminated drugs may not achieve high urine concentration (eg, moxifloxacin).

ID Board Pearls

- *Alkaline* urine increases activity of *erythromycin* against aerobic Gram-negative bacilli.

- *Alkaline* urine *neutralizes* the effects of *methenamine* salts; acidified urine necessary for antibacterial effects.

Antibiotic Prostate and Kidney Penetration

General Concepts

- *Acute* infection with increased vascular permeability (secondary to inflammatory mediators) permits good penetration of nearly all antibiotics.

- Chronic prostatitis or chronic pyelonephritis has *little* or no inflammatory component, use: quinolones, doxycycline, TMP-SMX, linezolid.

ID Board Pearls

- Suboptimal antibiotic penetration into chronically infected prostate and kidney with macrolides and β-Lactams.

24. Duration of Therapy

- *Most* bacterial infections in normal hosts are treated with antibiotics for 1-2 weeks.

- The duration of therapy may need to be extended in patients with impaired immunity (eg, diabetes, SLE, alcoholic liver disease, neutropenia, diminished splenic function, etc.), *chronic* bacterial infections (eg, endocarditis, osteomyelitis), chronic viral and fungal infections, or *certain* bacterial *intracellular pathogens*.

- Infections such as HIV and CMV in compromised hosts *may require lifelong suppressive therapy*. Antibiotic therapy should ordinarily not be for more than 2 weeks, even if low-grade fever persists.

- Prolonged antibiotic therapy offers no benefit, and increases the risk of adverse side effects, drug interactions and superinfections.

Table 1

Bioavailability of Oral Antimicrobials

Bioavailability

Excellent (>90%)[1]	Amoxicillin[c]	TMP[a,e]	Linezolid[c,d,e,f]
	Cephalexine	TMP-SMX[a,e]	Fluconazole
	Cefproxile	Doxycycline[d,e,f]	Voriconazole
	Cefadroxil[e]	Minocycline[d,e]	Rifampine[e]
	Clindamycin[e]	Chloramphenicol[e]	
	Quinolonese	Metronidazole	
Good (60%-90%)[2]	Most β-lactams[e]	Valacyclovir	5-Fluctosine
	Cefixime[e]	Famciclovir	Posaconazole
	Cefpodoxime[e]	Valganciclovir	Itraconazole (solution)
	Cefuroxime[e]	Acyclovir	Macrolides[b]
		Cefaclor[e]	
Poor (<60%)[3]	Vancomycin[c,e]	Cefdinir[e]	Cefditroren[e]

Adapted from Cunha, ed. Antibiotic Essentials. 8th ed. Sudbury, MA: Jones & Bartlett; 2009.

1. Oral administration results in equivalent blood/tissue levels as the same dose given IV (PO = IV)
2. Oral administration results in lower but therapeutically effective blood/tissue levels than the same dose given IV (PO < IV)
3. Oral administration results in inadequate blood/tissue levels.

[a] Variable anti-MRSA activity
[b] Variable anti-MSSA activity
[c] Anti-VSE activity
[d] Anti-VRE activity
[e] Anti-MSSA activity
[f] Anti-MRSA activity

25. Oral or IV PO Therapy

- For IV → PO switch therapy, select a PO antibiotic (with the *same spectrum* as its IV formulation equivalent) with *high bioavailability.*

- Oral therapy is *equally* efficacious (≥90%) as IV therapy using antibiotics with the *same spectrum* and *high bioavailability.*

26. Further Reading

Bryskier A, ed. *Antimicrobial Agents.* Washington, DC: ASM Press; 2005.

Cohen J, Powderly WG. *Infectious Diseases,* 2nd ed. New York, NY: Mosby; 2004.

Cunha BA, ed. *Antibiotic Essentials.* 8th ed. Sudbury, MA: Jones & Bartlett; 2009.

Finch RG, Greenwood D, Norrby SR, Whitley RJ. *Antibiotic and Chemotherapy.* 8th ed. London, England: Churchill Livingstone; 2003.

Gorbach SL, Bartlett JG, Blacklow NR. *Infectious Diseases.* 3rd ed. New York, NY: Lippincott Williams & Wilkins; 2004.

Kucers A, Crowe S, Grayson ML, Hoy J, eds. *The Use of Antibiotics: A Clinical Review of Antibacterial, Antifungal, and Antiviral Drugs.* 5th ed. Oxford, England: Butterworth-Heinemann; 1997.

Mandell GL. *Principles and Practice of Infectious Diseases.* 6th ed. Philadelphia, PA: Churchill Livingstone; 2005.

Ristuccia AM, Cunha BA, eds. *Antimicrobial Therapy.* New York, NY: Raven Press; 1984.

Schlossberg D, ed. *Current Therapy of Infectious Disease.* 3rd ed. St. Louis, MO: Mosby-Yearbook; 2007.

Yu VL, Merigan Jr. TC, Barriere SL, eds. *Antimicrobial Therapy and Vaccines.* Baltimore, MD: Williams & Wilkins; 1999.

Chapter 23: Antibiotic Adverse Effects for the ID Boards

Burke A. Cunha, MD

Contents

1. Leukopenia and Thrombocytopenia

General Concepts

- Leukopenia and thrombocytopenia are *the most common hematologic side effects* related to antimicrobial therapy.

ID Board Pearls

- β-Lactam antibiotics and the sulfamethoxazole (SMX) component of trimethoprim- sulfamethoxazole (TMP-SMX) are *the most common cause of isolated leucopenia or thrombocytopenia.*

2. Anemia

- β-Lactams may cause *autoimmune* hemolytic anemia.

- TMP-SMX may be associated with folate deficiency/megaloblastic anemia.

- Chloramphenicol *rarely* causes irreversible aplastic anemia.

    * Aplastic anemia is from an *idiosyncratic reaction* and is *not* dose related.

    * Serial hemograms are of *no value in predicting or preventing chloramphenicol-induced aplastic anemia.*

    * Chloramphenicol *dose-related anemia is reversible.*

    * Chloramphenicol-related aplastic anemia may occur with PO, PR, ocular *or administration,* but *not* if given IV.

3. Platelet Dysfunction

General Concepts

- Impaired platelet aggregation occurs *most commonly with antipseudomonal penicillins* (APPs) and *is dose-related* (≥30 g/d).

- The APPs (eg, azlocillin, mezlocillin, piperacillin), since the usual dosage is 18 g/d, have *less potential for decreased platelet aggregation.*

ID Board Pearls

- The antipseudomonal penicillins have *little potential for clinical bleeding (unless given to patients with a bleeding problem).*

4. Clinical Bleeding

General Concepts

- Many antibiotics, *particularly* the *β-lactams,* may increase the INR/prothrombin time (PT) *by interfering with the synthesis of vitamin K dependent clotting factors.*

- Beta-lactams with the methyl tetrathiazole (MTT) side chain (cefamandole, cefoperazone, cefotetan) may increase PT/INR but do *not* cause *clinical bleeding.*

ID Board Pearls

- Elevations of the INR or PT *rapidly normalize* after discontinuation of the antibiotic and *intramuscular vitamin K.*

- *Clinical bleeding relates to the severity of the clinical illness,* (not to the MTT side chain).

5. Drug Fever

General Concepts

- Drug fever is the *most common* antibiotic mediated *hypersensitivity* side effect.

- Drug fevers account for 10%-15% of unexplained fevers in hospitalized patients.

- *Drug fevers are hypersensitivity reactions to medications whose primary clinical manifestation is fever* (without rash).

ID Board Pearls

- Drug fevers may occur with any antibiotic but are most *common with lactams and sulfonamides*.

- *Most* drug fevers are caused by *non*-antibiotics:

    * Sulfa-containing diuretics (eg, thiazides, Lasi)

    * Sulfa-containing stool softeners (eg, Colace)

    * Anti-seizure medications

    * Anti-arrhythmics

    * Sedatives

    * Antihypertensives

    * Pain medications

6. Drug Rash

General Concepts

- Drug *rash* may be caused by any of the medications causing drug fever, but is particularly common with *β-lactams* or the sulfamethoxazole (SMX) *component of TMP-SMX*.

ID Board Pearls

- "Red Neck" or "Red Man" syndrome is a *histamine-mediated* reaction to the *rapid infusion* of vancomycin, and is *not an allergic reaction to* vancomycin.

7. Serum Sickness

General Concepts

- Serum sickness (*not* just from serum derivatives) reactions may occur with *any* medication, but are continually usually due to β-lactams and symptoms usually occur 2 *weeks after the exposure* to the causative medication.

- Serum sickness is usually accompanied by non-specific systemic findings that include *arthralgias/myalgias with no/low-grade fevers*.

ID Board Pearls

- Serum sickness should be *suspected* in patients with *low-grade fevers and arthralgias occurring ~2 weeks after antimicrobial administration in patients with decreased serum complement*.

8. Drug-induced SLE

General Concepts

• Many medications may induce a systemic lupus erythematosus (SLE)-like syndrome.

• Antibiotics are a *rare* cause of *drug*-related SLE.

ID Board Pearls

• Antibiotic causes of *drug-induced SLE include*:

    * Minocycline

    * INH

    * Nitrofurantoin

    * Griseofulvin

9. Neurologic Side Effects

General Concepts

• Antibiotic-induced *seizures* may be due to ciprofloxacin (but *not* other quinolones), imipenem (but *not* other carbapenems).

• Quinolones (*except* ciprofloxacin) and carbapenems (except imipenem) are safe to use in seizure patients.

• Neuromuscular blockade may occur following *aminoglycoside* therapy, *if* large amounts of the aminoglycoside are absorbed (eg, via *aerosolization into the lung or peritoneal lavage*).

• *Chronic* high-dose nitrofurantoin use in *renal insufficiency* may result in *peripheral neuropathy*.

ID Board Pearls

• Encephalopathy is not uncommon and may occur with metronidazole.

• *Clindamycin*, when used in *peritoneal lavage*, may cause *neuromuscular blockade or respiratory arrest*.

• Peripheral neuropathy *is most* commonly associated with INH, griseofulvin, metronidazole or cycloserine.

• Muscular tremors and spasticity have been associated with amantadine.

10. Ototoxicity

- Ototoxicity may be *cochlear or vestibular* and is most commonly associated with aminoglycosides or *parenteral* erythromycin.

- (Deafness) cochlear toxicity may be *irreversible* and is associated with *prolonged and very highly-elevated* aminoglycoside peak serum levels.

- Deafness may follow *rapid infusions of intravenous erythromycin.*

- *Dizziness and vestibular toxicity is commonly associated with minocycline.*

11. Ocular Toxicity

General Concepts

- EMB (>15 mg/kg) may lead to color blindness.

ID Board Pearls

- Ethambutol's ocular toxicity may (decreased visual acuity), occur in patients receiving ≥25 mg/kg *not* if ≤15 mg/kg.

12. Pulmonary Side Effects

General Concepts

- *Nitrofurantoin* pulmonary reactions may be *acute or chronic*:

- *Acute* nitrofurantoin pulmonary reactions usually present with fever *accompanied by pulmonary infiltrates, pleural effusions* and peripheral eosinophilia and are *transient and readily reversible* when nitrofurantoin is discontinued.

- Patients should not be getting nitrofurantoin if the (CrCl <30 mL/min).

ID Board Pearls

- The most common pulmonary side effect causing a flu-like illness with rifampin.

- *Chronic* nitrofurantoin pulmonary reactions may result in *irreversible pulmonary fibrosis* are *not* characterized by fever, peripheral eosinophilia or pleural effusions.

- *Chronic nitrofurantoin pulmonary toxicity* is most common in patients with *renal insufficiency receiving prolonged/ high dose* nitrofurantoin.

13. Cardiac Side Effects

General Concepts

- Prolonged QTc interval may result in ventricular arrhythmias (eg, torsades de pointes).

- Antimicrobials *most* commonly associated with prolongation of the QTc interval include IV erythromycin, clarithromycin, terbinafine and quinolones.

- Quinolones that increase the QTc interval *within the normal range* ≤500 ms should be *avoided* in patients with bradycardia, hypokalemia, heart block or *in patients receiving other drugs that increase QTc interval, eg, amiodarone*.

- *Torsades de pointes* or ventricular arrhythmias may occur due to the *additive* effects *of multiple agents* that may increase the QTc interval (eg, quinolone plus amiodarone).

ID Board Pearls

- Myocarditis is a *rare* complication of nevirapine therapy.

- Antimicrobial-induced *hypotension* may occur with *pentamidine*.

- Amphotericin B also may induce *hypotension*.

14. Gastrointestinal Side Effects

General Concepts

- Many *orally* administered antimicrobials and anti-retrovirals are associated with nausea/vomiting.

- Among antibiotics, PO *macrolides* are most often associated with *GI side effects*.

- *Doxycycline* and minocycline may cause gastrointestinal upset on an *empty* stomach and *should always be administered with food*.

- Tetracycline should be administered *without* food (ie, 1 hour before or 2 hours after a meal).

- Antibiotic-induced (*not* secondary to *C difficile*) diarrhea may be due to *antibiotic-induced changes in colonic flora, high osmotic load* or due to *poor absorption* (irritative to the colon in high concentrations).

- Many antibiotics may cause *C difficile* diarrhea, but this is most commonly associated with the β-lactams, *except piperacillin/tazobactam and cetriaxone*.

- *C difficile* diarrhea is *rare* with *doxycycline, minocycline, monobactams, carbapenems, aminoglycosides, TMP-SMX, macrolides, linezolid, piperacillin/tazobactam, tigecycline and ceftriaxone*.

ID Board Pearls

- Clarithromycin may cause *gastric discomfort and taste perversion*.

- *Non-C difficile* diarrhea is common with ampicillin, amoxicillin-clavulanic acid, ceftriaxone, macrolides or clindamycin.

- Metronidazole may *cause* and is *therapy* for *C difficile* diarrhea. Metronidazole may increase VRE prevalence.

- Acute chemical or clinical pancreatitis may be caused by pentamidine, TMP-SMX.

15. Hepatic Side Effects

General Concepts

• Mild/transient elevations of serum transaminases are *common* (eg, associated with antibiotic therapy).

• Erythromycin, nitrofurantoin and thiabendazole are the *most* common causes of antimicrobial-induced *cholestasis*.

• *Acute hepatic necrosis* or liver failure may occur with PAS, ketoconazole and telithromycin.

ID Board Pearls

• Tetracycline has *dose-related* hepatotoxicity and may occur with doses of ≥2 g/d, and for this reason *doxycycline or minocycline are not hepatotoxic*.

• Oxacillin (renally eliminated) is associated with hepatitis (not interstitial nephritis).

16. Renal Side Effects

General Concepts

• *Nitrofurantoin* is unique among the antimicrobials causing *chronic active hepatitis*.

• Nephrotoxicity may be manifested as *glomerular or tubular* toxicity.

• Aminoglycoside-induced *tubular dysfunction* is best assessed by *urinary cast excretion counts*.

• Serum *creatinine is increased for a variety of reasons in hospitalized patients* and is *not* a good indicator of *tubular* dysfunction.

• *Tubular* toxicity is *more common* and is associated with *prolonged* aminoglycoside therapy.

• *Nephrotoxic potential* is similar among aminoglycosides and may occur with *prolonged/very high* **trough** *levels*.

• *Once-daily* intravenous aminoglycoside regimens have *virtually eliminated* the *nephrotoxic potential of aminoglycosides*.

• Vancomycin alone has *little or no* nephrotoxic potential. *Other medications* being *given concurrently with the vancomycin are usually the cause*.

• *Interstitial nephritis* may occur with a wide variety of antimicrobials, but is *most* commonly associated with *β-lactam therapy*.

• *Eosinophiluria* is a cardinal finding *acute allergic interstitial nephritis*.

ID Board Pearls

• Aminoglycoside *tubular* dysfunction may occur *after 2 weeks of multiple daily dosed aminoglycoside therapy*.

• Nafcillin (hepatically eliminated) is associated with interstitial nephritis (not hepatitis).

• Crystaluria is commonly associated with *acyclovir or indinavir*.

17. Miscellaneous Side Effects

General Concepts

- *Short* course quinolone therapy (ie, ≤2 weeks) does *not* cause cartilage damage/arthropathy.

- Acute onset of fever/sweats, mental confusion, hallucinations, muscle rigidity and hyperreflexia in patients on linezolid suggests serotonin syndrome.

ID Board Pearls

- Skin discoloration may occur after *prolonged* minocycline use, and *may not be reversible* after discontinuation of treatment.

18. Further Reading

Cunha BA. *Antibiotic Essentials*. 8th ed. Jones & Bartlett, Sudbury, MA; 2009.

Kucers A, Crowe SM, Grayson ML, et al, eds. *The Use of Antibiotics*. 5th ed. Oxford, England: Butterworth-Heinemann; 1997.

Root RK, ed. *Clinical Infectious Diseases*. New York, NY: Oxford University Press; 1999.

O'Grady F, Finch RG, Lambert HP, et al, eds. *Antibiotic and Chemotherapy*. 7th ed. New York, NY: Churchill Livingstone; 1997.

Chapter 24:
Anti-infective Drug-Drug Interactions for the ID Boards

Keith A. Rodvold, PharmD

Contents

- Drug-drug interactions are an increasingly complex challenge for the infectious disease clinician

- In addition to anti-infective agents to treat infections, patients are often receiving therapy for comorbid conditions and/or prophylaxis of opportunistic infections (eg, patient with HIV infection)

- The benefit vs. risk must be carefully evaluated when significant or life-threatening drug-drug interactions are involved.

ID Board Pearls

- The most important strategy in successful prevention of drug-drug interactions is to conduct a thorough medication history at every visit, including questions about prescription, over-the-counter, herbal and recreational drugs, and prescriptions received from other health care providers

1. Classification of Drug-Drug Interactions

- A drug-drug interaction is defined as concomitantly administered drugs that interfere with one another's efficacy or safety profile. Generally, the object drug is the medication that is affected by the interaction, whereas the precipitant drug is the medication that causes the interaction

- Drug-drug interactions can be classified into 2 broad categories: 1.) interactions affecting pharmacodynamics; and 2.) interactions altering pharmacokinetics

- Pharmacodynamic interactions occur when 1 agent causes an alteration in the efficacy or safety (eg, pharmacological effects) of a second agent, without a resultant change in drug concentrations or pharmacokinetic parameters

- The effects of pharmacodynamic interactions can be: 1.) additive (2 agents leads to enhanced pharmacological effect [eg, increased bone marrow suppression with concurrent use of zidovudine and ganciclovir]); 2.) synergistic (use of 2 or more agents results in drug effect greater than [e.g., exponential vs. additive] the addition of all of the drugs together [eg, combined effect with concurrent use of indinavir, lamivudine and zidovudine vs. the sum of their individual effects]); or 3.) antagonistic (the pharmacological effect of 1 agent is reduced due to concurrent therapy with another agent [eg, concurrent use of zidovudine and stavudine reduces antiviral effect])

- Pharmacokinetic drug-drug interactions are associated with changes in the concentration of a drug in body fluids and tissues. Pharmacokinetic interactions can be classified according to whether they affect the absorption, distribution, metabolism or elimination of other drugs. The most common drug-drug interactions of anti-infective agents involve those that affect absorption or metabolism

- Absorption interactions generally occur in the gut. Absorption drug-drug interactions occur when 1 agent changes the amount or rate of absorption or reduces the bioavailability of a second agent. Common mechanisms associated with reduced absorption include: 1.) alterations in gastric pH caused by antacids, H_2-antagonists or proton pump inhibitors (eg, occurs with some oral cephalosporins); 2.) chelation of drug (eg, tetracyclines or fluoruquinolones) caused by bivalent or trivalent cations such as calcium, magnesium or iron; 3.) antibiotic alteration of the normal gastrointestinal flora (eg, cephalosporins or tetracyclines and warfarin); and 4.) inhibition of a transport pump, such as P-glycoprotein (eg, effect of rifampin on plasma digoxin concentrations).

• Distribution type of drug-drug interactions most often involves alterations in protein-binding (sulfamethoxazole/trimethoprim can displace warfarin from its protein-binding sites and increased INR). Drug interactions involving protein binding and drug displacement have become less important clinically, because steady-state unbound drug concentrations often redistribute and remain unaltered.

• Drug metabolism is a site where many pharmacokinetic interactions evolve and is difficult to predict. Metabolism of drugs is divided into 2 reaction phases (Phase I and II) and drug-drug interactions can occur in both reactions.

• Phase I reactions increase the polarity of medications through oxidative transformation and generally go through the cytochrome P-450 (CYP) enzyme system. CYP-450 enzymes are expressed both in the liver and in the enterocytes of the small intestine.

• The isoenzyme responsible for the majority of drug metabolism is CYP3A4, although CYP2D6, CYP2C9, CYP2C19 and CYP1A2 are commonly involved (see Figure 1).

• Phase II reactions further increase the polarity of medications by conjugating them with endogenous groups, such as glucuronides or sulfates. Phase II reactions are most commonly mediated by uridine diphosphate (UDP)-glucuronosyltransferase, sulfotransferase, N-acetyltransferase and glutathione-S-transferase.

• Drugs can interact with cytochrome p-450 enzymes as substrates, inhibitors or inducers. Some agents may have 2 or more of these properties and may interact with different CYP enzymes (Table 1).

Figure 1

The relative proportions of clinically used drugs metabolized by various cytochrome P450 enzymes.

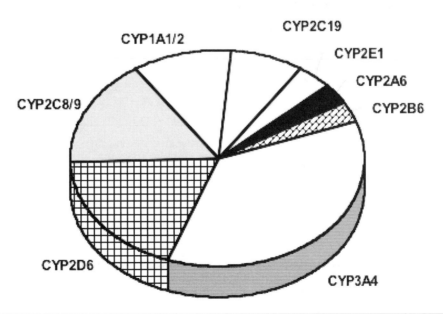

Table 1

Examples of Anti-infective Agents as Substrates, Inhibitors and Inducers of Cytochrome P450 Enzymes and P-glycoprotein

Enzymes or Transporter	Substrates	Inhibitors	Inducers
CYP1A2	Ritonavir	Erythromycin, clarithromycin, ciprofloxacin, norfloxacin, ritonavir	Ritonavir, rifampin
CYP2C9	Nelfinavir, ritonavir, fluconazole, voriconazole, dapsone	Erythromycin, metronidazole, sulfamethoxazole, SMX-TMP, fluconazole, miconazole, voriconazole, isoniazid,	Rifampin, rifapentine
CYP2C19	Chloramphenicol, nelfinavir, ritonavir, fluconazole, voriconazole	Chloramphenicol, ritonavir, fluconazole, ketoconazole, voriconazole	Rifampin
CYP2D6	Ritonavir	Primaquine, ritonavir	Rifampin
CYP2E1	Ritonavir, isoniazid, dapsone	Ritonavir, isoniazid	Isoniazid
CYP3A4	Erythromycin, clarithromycin, telithromycin, clindamycin, protease inhibitors, delavirdine, nevirapine, NNRTIs, maravoric, miconazole, ketoconazole, intraconazole, fluconazole, voriconazole, posoconazole, dapsone, quinine	Chloramphenicol, erythromycin, clarithromycin, telithromycin, norfloxacin, ciprofloxacin, amprenaivr, nelfinavir, lopinavir/ritonavir, ritonavir, saquinavir, indinavir, delaviridine, efavirenz, quinupristin/dalfopristin, clotrimazole, miconazole, intraconazole, ketoconazole, fluconazole, voriconazole, posaconazole	Efavirenz, nevirapine, rifampin, rifabutin, rifapentine, ritonavir
UGT	Posoconazole	Fluconazole	
P-GP	Clarithromycin, erythromycin, indinavir, nelfinavir, ritonavir, saquinavir, maravoric, ketoconazole, intraconazole, fluconazole, posaconazole,	Clarithromycin, erythromycin, ketoconazole, itraconazole, indinavir, nelfinavir, ritonavir, saquinavir	Rifampin, ritonavir

Abbreviations: CYP = cytochrome P450; UGT = uridine diphosphate glucoronosyltransferase; P-GP = P-glycoprotein

- Substrates are drugs metabolized by a cytochrome P-450 isoenzyme, and can be influenced by other drugs that inhibit or induce the specific CYP isoenzyme that metabolizes the substrate.

- Drugs that inhibit cytochromes cause decreased drug clearance and increased plasma concentrations of substrate drugs (and metabolites) metabolized by the inhibited pathway. The onset and dissipation of inhibition reactions are quick (based on substrate half-life), with maximal effect occurring when highest concentrations of the inhibitor are reached.

- Transporter-based drug-drug interactions have been increasingly documented. These transport proteins play a role in the tissue distribution, as well as absorption and excretion of medications. Various reported drug-drug interactions attributed earlier to other mechanisms of interaction may be due in part to the inhibition or induction of transport proteins, such as P-glycoprotein (P-gp), organic anion transporter (OAT), organic anion transporting polypeptide (OATP), organic cation transporter (OCT), multidrug resistance-associated proteins (MDR) or breast cancer-resistant protein (BCRP). Examples of transporter-based interactions include: penicillin with probenecid, fexofenadine with ketoconazole or erythromycin.

- Drug-drug interactions involving renal excretion are usually competitive interactions that occur rapidly and often involve the active secretion of drugs. The organic anion transport proteins (OAT1 and OAT3) are primarily located in the kidney and facilitate excretion of weakly acidic drugs (eg, penicillins, cidofivir). Probenecid is an inhibitor of OAT1 and thus leads to decreased renal clearance of OAT1 substrates (eg, probenecid increases plasma penicillin concentrations by being an inhibitor of renal tubular secretion).

ID Board Pearls

- Selective substrates of CYP3A4 can be associated with major or life-threatening interactions when co-administered with a CYP3A inhibitor (see Table 2).

- Drugs that induce cytochromes cause increased drug clearance and decreased plasma concentrations of substrate drugs. The effect of enzyme induction occurs more gradually than inhibition, and maximal effect may not be apparent until 7-14 days later. Rifampin is a classic potent enzyme inducer and has effects on both Phase I and II metabolism (see Table 3).

Table 2

Substrates of CYP3A4 with Major or Life-Threatening Interactions When Co-administered with a CYP3A Inhibitor[a]

CYP3A4 Substrate	Pharmacologic effect	Management recommendation
Astemizole[b], terfenadine[b], cisapride[b], bepridil[b], pimozide	QTc interval prolongation, arrhythmias, sudden death, torsade de pointes	Contraindicated
Cyclosporine, sirolimus, tacrolimus	Increased serum concentration and immunosuppression	Monitor immunosuppressive agent serum concentration; adjust dose as needed
Ergot alkaloids	Ergotism, peripheral ischemia	Contraindicated
Lovastatin, simvastatin	Risk of rhabdomyolysis	Use other HMG-Co-A reductase inhibitors, such as pravastatin or fluvastatin
Midazolam, triazolam	Excessive sedation	Use other benzodiazepines, such as lorazepam, oxazepam or temazepam
Rifabutin	Uveitis, neutropenia, flu-like syndrome	Reduce dose of rifabutin
Sidenafil, tadalafil, vardenafil	Hypotension, priapism	Reduce dose or avoid use entirely
Vincristine, vinblastine	Neurotoxicity	Reduce dose and monitor for vinca toxicity

[a] *Examples of anti-infective agents that are potent CYP3A4 inhibitors include clarithromycin, erythromycin, telithromycin, protease inhibitors, delavudine, ketoconazole, itraconazole, and voriconazole*

[b] *Drug is not or no longer commercially available in the United States*

Abbreviations: HMG Co-A reductase inhibitors = 3 hydroxy-3 methylglutaryl coenzyme A

Table 3

Drug-drug Interactions of Rifampin

Interacting Drug	Comments and Management Strategy
Anti-infective Agents	
Atovaquone	Monitor clinical response; increase dose if needed; consider alternative agent
Casofungin	Monitor clinical response; increase dose to 70 mg daily
Chloramphenicol	Monitor chloramphenicol serum concentrations; increase dose if needed
Clarithromycin	Monitor clinical and microbiologic response; increase dose if needed
Dapsone	Monitor clinical response and hematologic toxic effects
Delaviridine	Avoid rifampin; use rifabutin or alternative agent and monitor viral response
Doxycycline	Monitor clinical and microbiologic response; increase dose if needed
Efavirenz	Monitor viral response; increase dose if needed (eg, 800 mg if >60 kg)
Etravirine	Avoid rifampin; use rifabutin or alternative agent and monitor viral response
Fluconazole	Monitor clinical and microbiologic response; increase dose if needed
Itraconazole/Voriconazole	Avoid rifampin; if used, increase dose of azole and monitor response
Maraviroc	Monitor viral response; increase dose to 600 mg BID if used without a strong CYP3A inhibitor; lower dose to 150 mg BID with a strong CYP3A inhibitor
Mefloquinine	Consider avoiding combination; larger study needed
Metronidazole	Monitor clinical and microbiologic response; increase dose if needed
Nevirapine	Avoid rifampin; use rifabutin or alternative agent and monitor viral response
Praziquantel	Consider alternative agent if possible; monitor clinical response
Protease Inhibitors	Avoid rifampin; use rifabutin or alternative agent and monitor viral response
Quinine	Monitor clinical response; consider alternative agent if possible
Raltegavir	Consider using rifabutin; if rifampin is used, monitor viral response
Trimethoprim/Sulfamethoxazole	Monitor clinical and microbiologic response; increase dose if needed

Table 3 (continued)

Drug-drug Interactions of Rifampin

Interacting Drug	Comments and Management Strategy
Analgesics	
Codeine	Monitor pain control and clinical response
COX 2 Inhibitors[a]	Monitor clinical response; increase dose if needed
Fentanyl	Monitor pain control; increase dose if needed
Methadone	Increase methadone dose; monitor and control withdrawal symptoms
Morphine	Monitor pain control and clinical response
Anticonvulsants	
Phenytoin	Monitor phenytoin serum concentrations and seizure activity; increase dose if needed
Antidiabetic Agents	
Sulfonylureas[b]	Monitor blood glucose levels; dose adjust based blood glucose control
Meglitidinides[c]	Monitor blood glucose levels; dose adjust based blood glucose control
Thiazolidinediones[d]	Monitor blood glucose levels; dose adjust based blood glucose control
Anticoagulants (oral)	Monitor INR; increase anticoagulant dose as needed
Cardiovascular Drugs	
Beta-blocking Agents	Monitor clinical response; increase propranolol or metoprolol dose if needed
Digitoxin	Monitor clinical response and/or arrhythmia control, and digitoxin serum concentration
Digoxin (oral)	Monitor clinical response and/or arrhythmia control, and digoxin serum concentration
Diltiazem	Use alternative agent; monitor patient for clinical response
Disopyramide	Monitor arrhythmia control; increase dose if needed
Losartan	Monitor clinical response; increase dose if needed

Table 3 (continued)

Drug-drug Interactions of Rifampin

Interacting Drug	Comments and Management Strategy
Nifedipine	Alternative class of agents should be considered; if use, monitor clinical response; increase dose if needed
Nilvadipine	Monitor clinical response; increase dose if needed
Propafenone	Monitor clinical response; increase dose if needed; consider alternative agent
Quinidine	Monitor quinidine serum concentration and arrhythmia control; increase dose if needed
Tocainide	Monitor arrhythmia control; increase dose if needed
Verapamil	Use alternative agent; monitor patient for clinical response
Contraceptives (oral)	Use alternative form(s) of birth control; counsel patient and document
Glucocorticoids	Increase dose of glucocorticoid 2- to 3-fold
HMG-CoA Reductase Inhibitors[e]	Monitor lipid panel; increase dose if needed (likely for simvastatin)
Immunosuppressants	
Cyclosporine	Monitor cyclosporine serum concentration; increased dose if needed
Tacrolimus	Monitor tacrolimus serum concentration; increase dose if needed
Everolimus	Monitor everolimus serum concentration; increase dose if needed
Psychotropic Agents	
Buspirone	Monitor clinical response; increase dose likely needed; use alternative agent if possible
Clozapine	Monitor clinical response; increase dose if needed or use alternative agent if possible
Haloperidol	Monitor clinical response; increase dose if needed
Nortriptyline	Monitor clinical response and nortriptyline serum concentration
Sertraline	Monitor clinical response; increase dose if needed

Table 3 (continued)

Drug-drug Interactions of Rifampin

Interacting Drug	Comments and Management Strategy
Others	
5 HT$_3$ Antiemetics[f]	Monitor clinical response; increase dose if needed; use alternative agent if needed
Diazepam	Monitor clinical response; increase dose if needed
Gefitinib	Avoid combination; if must use, increase dose
Imatinib	Avoid combination; if must use, increase dose
Levothyroxine	Monitor TSH; increased dose likely needed
Lorazepam	Monitor clinical response; increase dose if needed
Midazolam	Avoid combination; use alternative agent if possible
Tamoxifen/toremifene	Monitor clinical response; increased dose likely needed
Theophylline	Monitor theophylline serum concentration; increase dose if needed
Triazolam	Avoid combination; use alternative agent if possible
Zolpidem	Monitor clinical response; increase dose if needed or use alternative agent if possible

Adapted from Baciewicz AM, Chrisman CR, Finch CK, Self TH. Update on rifampin and rifampin drug interactions. Am J Med Sci. *2008;335:126-136.*

[a] *Examples include celecoxib and rofecoxib (no longer available)*
[b] *Examples include tolbutamide, chlorpropamide, gliclazide, and glimepiride*
[c] *Examples include repaglinide and nateglinide*
[d] *Examples include rosiglitazone and pioglitazone*
[e] *Examples include simvastatin, atorvastatin, and pravastatin*
[f] *Examples include ondansetron and dolasetron*

2. Antituberculosis Agents

- The majority of drug-drug interactions of this class are associated with rifampin, rifabuten and isoniazid (Table 4)

- Rifampin is a potent inducer of CYP enzymes (hepatic and intestinal) and the P-glycoprotein transport system, mediated by activation of the nuclear pregnane X receptor.

- Rifampin has also been shown to induce glucuronidation, which is mediated by uridine 5'-diphosphate-glucuronosyltransfereases (UGTs)

- Rifabutin is also an important inducer of CYP enzyme and P-glycoprotein transport system however is less potent than rifampin (eg, rifampin>rifapentine>>rifabutin) and the magnitude of decreasing drug concentrations is significantly less (eg, 30%-50% of rifampin's effect)

- Since rifabutin is a less potent inducer than rifampin, it is often recommended as the alternative to rifampin for the treatment of tuberculosis in HIV-infected patients being treated with protease inhibitors or nucleoside and nucleotide reverse transcriptase inhibitors.

- Isoniazid inhibits CYP2C9, CYP2C19 and CYP3A4. The potential for drug-drug interactions is greater in slow acetylators, who compose 30%-50% of Caucasians and African Americans

ID Board Pearls

- Whenever rifampin, rifapentine or rifabutin are prescribed, the possibility of drug-drug interactions must be proactively considered and monitored.

Table 4

Drug-drug Interactions of Antituberculosis Agents

Antituberculosis Agent	Interacting Drug	Interaction and Management Strategy
Aminosalicyclic acid	Probenecid	Increased aminosalicyclic acid serum concentrations (transiently); monitor for toxicity
	Diphendyramine	Decreased absorption of aminosalicyclic acid; avoid concomitant use
	Digoxin	Increased digoxin serum concentration and toxicity; monitor digoxin serum concentration and adjust dose appropriately
	Warfarin	Enhanced anticoagulation; monitor prothrombin time/international normalized ratio (PT/INR) and adjust warfarin dose appropriately
	Ammonium chloride	Increased probability of crystalluria; avoid concomitant use
Capreomycin	Nephrotoxic agents[a]	Direct or additive injury to the renal tubule; concomitant therapy should be avoided or used with caution and includes monitoring of renal function and dosage adjustment based body weight and creatinine clearance estimation

Table 4 (continued)

Drug-drug Interactions of Antituberculosis Agents

Antituberculosis Agent	Interacting Drug	Interaction and Management Strategy
Capreomycin	Ototoxic agents[b]	Increase risk of ototoxicity; concomitant therapy should be avoided or used with caution at the lowest possible dose; consider alternative agent if possible
	Neuromuscular-blocking Agents[c]	Increase respiratory suppression produced by neuromuscular agent; concomitant therapy should be avoided or used with caution and monitoring for respiratory depression
Cycloserine	Isoniazid	Increased CNS adverse effects (eg, dizziness, drowsiness) when both drugs are used concurrently; monitor toxicity
	Ethionamide	Increased CNS adverse effects (eg, seizures) when both drugs are used concurrently; monitor toxicity
	Phenytoin/ fosphenytoin	Increased phenytoin serum concentration; monitor toxicity and phenytoin serum concentration and adjust dose as needed
Ethambutol	Antacids	Decreased ethambutol serum concentrations with aluminum-containing antacids; space administration by at least 4 hours
	Ethionamide	Increased adverse effects (eg, GI distress, headache, confusion, neuritis, hepatotoxicity) when both drugs are used concurrently; monitor toxicity and avoid concomitant use when possible
Ethionamide	Aminosalicyclic acid, ethambutol, isoniazid, pyrazinamide, rifampin	Potentiate the adverse effects of other antituberculosis agents (hepatotoxicity, peripheral neuritis, GI distress, headache, confusion, neuritis, seizures, encephalopathy); monitor toxicity
	Excessive alcohol	Increased psychotic reactions; avoid concomitant use
	Isoniazid	Increased isoniazid serum concentrations (temporarily); monitor for toxicity

Table 4 (continued)

Drug-drug Interactions of Antituberculosis Agents

Antituberculosis Agent	Interacting Drug	Interaction and Management Strategy
Isoniazid	Cycloserine, ethionamide	Increased CNS adverse effects; monitor toxicity
	Carbamazepine	Increased carbamazepine serum concentration and toxicity (eg, ataxia, headache, blurred vision, drowsiness, confusion); monitor toxicity, carbamazepine serum concentration, and decrease dose if needed
	Phenytoin/fosphenytoin	Increased phenytoin serum concentration and toxicity; monitor toxicity, phenytoin serum concentration, and decrease dose if needed
	Primidone	Increased primidone serum concentration; monitor toxicity, primidone serum concentration, and adjust dose if needed
	Meperidine	Increase toxicity (eg, serotonin syndrome); monitor toxicity and adjust dose if needed
	Itraconazole	Decreased itraconazole serum concentration and loss of antimycotic efficacy; alternative antifungal agent or interacting drug should be considerate
	Warfarin	Enhanced anticoagulation; monitor prothrombin time/international normalized ratio (PT/INR) and adjust warfarin dose appropriately
	Disulfiram	Increased CNS changes (eg, coordination difficulties, mood or behavioral changes); monitor toxicity and consider dose reduction or discontinuation of disulfiram
	Acetaminophen	Increased risk for hepatotoxicity; avoid concomitant use or limit use of acetaminophen
	Diazepam	Increased diazepam serum concentration; monitor toxicity and adjust dose if needed
	Levadopa	Decreased toxicity (e.g., flushing, palpitations, hypertension); monitor toxicity and adjust dose if needed
	Aluminum hydroxide	Decreased isoniazid serum concentrations; space administration by at least 1 hour

Table 4 (continued)

Drug-drug Interactions of Antituberculosis Agents

Antituberculosis Agent	Interacting Drug	Interaction and Management Strategy
Pyrazinamide	Ethionamide or rifampin	Increased heptotoxicity; monitor liver enzymes and toxicity
	Cyclosporine	Decreased cyclosporine serum concentrations; monitor clinical response and cyclosporine serum concentrations; adjust dose as needed
	Zidovudine	Decreased pyrazinamide serum concentrations and efficacy; consider alternative antituberculosis agent if possible
	Probenecid	Decreased efficacy of probenecid (eg, increased serum uric acid levels; worsening symptoms of gout); monitor serum uric acid levels and adjust probenecid dose as needed
Rifabutin	Ritonavir-boosted protease inhibitors (ATV±r, FPV/r, DRV/r, IDV/r, LPV/r, SQV/r, TPV/r)	Increased rifabutin serum concentration; rifabutin dosing to 150 mg QOD or 3 times weekly; monitor viral response and CBC
	Fosamprenavir	Increased rifabutin serum concentratios; rifabutin dosing to 150 mg QD or 300 mg 3 times weekly; monitor viral response and CBC
	Indinavir	Increased rifabutin serum concentratios and decrease indinavir serum concentration; rifabutin dosing to 150 mg QD or 300 mg 3 times weekly; indinavir 1000 mg TID or consider ritonavir boosing; monitor viral response and CBC
	Nelfinavir	Increased rifabutin serum concentration and decreased nelfinavir serum concentration; rifabutin dosing to 150 mg QD or 300 mg 3 times weekly; monitor viral response and CBC
	Delaviridine	Increased rifabutin serum concentration and decreased delaviridine serum concentrations; coadministration is not recommended
	Efavirenz	Decreased rifabutin serum concentration; dose rifabutin 450-600 mg QD or 600 mg 3 times weekly if efavirenz is not coadministered with a protease inhibitor; monitor viral response and CBC

Table 4 (continued)

Drug-drug Interactions of Antituberculosis Agents

Antituberculosis Agent	Interacting Drug	Interaction and Management Strategy
	Etravirine	Decreased rifabutin and metabolite serum concentration and decreased etravinine serum concentration; dose rifabutin 300 mg QD if not coadministered with a ritonavir-boosted protease inhibitor; if coadministered with lopinavir plus ritonavir, dose rifabutin 150 mg QOD or 3 times weekly
	Nevirapine	Increased rifabutin serum concentration and decreased nevirapine serum concentrations; no dosage adjustment is not recommended; monitor viral response and CBC
	Maraviroc	Maraviroc dose of 300 mg BID if used without a strong CYP3A inducer or inhibitor; maraviroc dose of 150 mg BID if used with a strong CYP3A inhibitor; monitor viral response
	Fluconazole	Increased rifabutin serum concentration and potential rifabutin toxicity (uveitis, ocular pain, photophobia, visual disturbances); monitor toxicity and CBC
	Itraconazole, voriconazole, posaconazole	Increased rifabutin serum concentration and potential rifabutin toxicity (uveitis, ocular pain, photophobia, visual disturbances); decreased azole serum concentration and/or loss of antimycotic efficacy; alternative antifungal agent should be considered
	Clarithromycin	Decreased clarithromycin serum concentrations and increased risk of rifabutin toxicity (rash, GI disturbances, hematologic abnormalities). Monitor efficacy, toxicity and CBC
	Cyclosporine	Decreased cyclosporine serum concentrations; monitor clinical response and cyclosporine serum concentrations; adjust dose as needed
	Warfarin	Decreased anticoagulation; monitor prothrombi time/international normalized ratio (PT/INR) and adjust warfarin dose appropriately
	Oral contraceptives	Use alternative form(s) of birth control; counsel patient and document
Rifampin	See Table 3	

3. Antibacterial Agents

- Absorption drug-drug interactions with antibacterial agents include: 1.) alterations in gastric pH caused by antacids, H_2-antagonists or proton pump inhibitors (eg, oral cephalosporins); 2.) chelation of drug (eg, tetracyclines or fluoruquinolones) caused by bivalent or trivalent cations, such as calcium, magnesium or iron; and 3.) inhibition of a transport pump, such as P-glycoprotein (eg, effect of clarithromycin on plasma digoxin concentrations) (Table 5)

- Drug-drug interactions that involve CYP enzyme transport system include macrolides or ketolides (eg, erythromycin, clarithromycin or telithromycin), older fluoroquinolones (eg, ciprofloxacin or norfloxacin), and quinupristin-dalfopristin.

- Newer agents, such as daptomycin, linezolid and tigecycline do not have activity to inhibit common human CYP isoforms (1A2, 2C9, 2C19, 2D6 and 3A4).

Table 5

Drug-drug Interactions of Antibacterial Agents

Antibacterial Agent	Interacting Drug	Interaction and Management Strategy
Oral cephalosporins prodrugs[a]	H_2-antagonists or antacids	Decreased absorption of cephalosporin; space administration by at least 2 hours
Penicillins, cephalosporins, and carbapenems[b]	Probenecid	Increased serum concentrations of beta-lactam agent; avoid concomitant use when higher concentrations are not desirable or increase risk in toxicity (eg, CNS) may occur
Ampicillin or amoxicillin	Allopurinol	Increased risk (3-fold higher) for rash; monitor for rash; consider alternative agent if possible
Carbapenems[c]	Valproic acid	Decreased serum concentrations of valproic acid; monitor serum valproic acid concentrations and seizure activity; increase dose of valproic acid if needed or avoid concomitant use
Imipenem	Ganciclovir or cyclosporine	Increased risk for CNS toxicity; concomitant use of these agents is not recommended
Erythromycin, clarithromycin or telithromycin	Substrates of CYP3A4	See Table 3
	Calcium channel blockers[d]	Increased serum concentrations of calcium channel blocker; monitored for hypotension, tachycardia, edema, flushing and dizziness; increased risk of sudden cardiac death (diltiazim, verapamil); consider alternative agent if possible
	Anti-arrhythmic agents[e]	Increased serum concentrations of antiarrhythmic agents leading to the risk of QTc prolongation, torsades de pointes and death; alternative agents should be considered

Table 5 (continued)

Drug-drug Interactions of Antibacterial Agents

Antibacterial Agent	Interacting Drug	Interaction and Management Strategy
	Tricyclic antidepressants and antipsychotic agents[f]	Increased serum concentration of antidepressant or antipsychotic agent; risk of QTc prolongation and torsades de pointes; alternative agents should be considered
	Warfarin	Enhanced anticoagulation; monitor prothrombin time/international normalized ration (PT/INR) and adjust warfarin dose appropriately
	Theophylline	Increased theophylline serum concentrations and risk of toxicity; monitor serum theophylline concentrations and toxicity; decrease dose of theophylline as needed
	Digoxin	Increased digoxin serum concentrations and risk of toxicity; monitor serum digoxin concentrations and toxicity; decrease dose of digoxin as needed
Fluoroquinolones[g]	Multivalent cations[h]	Decreased absorption of fluoroquinolone; space administration by at least 2-4 hours
	Class Ia and IIIa anti-arrhythmic agents	Increased serum concentration of antiarrhythmic agents; risk of QTc prolongation and torsades de pointes; alternative agents should be considered in patients who at risk (e.g., history QTc prolongation or uncorrected electrolyte abnormalities)
Ciprofloxacin, norfloxacin	Theophylline	Increased theophylline serum concentrations and risk of toxicity; monitor serum theophylline concentrations and toxicity; decrease dose of theophylline as needed
Aminoglycosides[i], polymyxin, colistin	Nephrotoxic agents[j]	Direct or additive injury to the renal tubule; concomitant therapy should be avoided or used with caution and includes monitoring of renal function and dosage adjustment based body weight, creatinine clearance estimation and/or serum aminoglycoside concentration
	Ototoxic agents[k]	Increased risk of ototoxicity; concomitant therapy should be avoided or used with caution at the lowest possible dose; consider alternative agent if possible
	Neuromuscular blocking agents[l]	Increased respiratory suppression produced by neuromuscular agent; concomitant therapy should be avoided or used with caution and monitoring for respiratory depression

Table 5 (continued)

Drug-drug Interactions of Antibacterial Agents

Antibacterial Agent	Interacting Drug	Interaction and Management Strategy
Vancomycin	Aminoglycosides	Direct or additive injury to the renal tubule; concomitant therapy should be used with caution and includes monitoring of renal function and dosage adjustment based body weight, creatinine clearance estimation, and/or serum aminoglycoside and vancomycin concentrations
Daptomycin	HMG-CoA reductase inhibitors[m]	May increase creatinine phosphokinase concentrations or cause rhabdomylosis; monitor for signs and symptoms and consider temporarily discontinuation of HMG-Co-A reductase inhibitor during daptomycin therapy
Linezolid	Selective serotinin reuptake inhibitors (SSRIs)[n]	Increase in serotonin concentrations and development of serotonin syndrome (hyperpyrexia, cognitive dysfunction); concomitant therapy should be avoided or used with caution and monitoring for serotonin syndrome
	Sympathomimetic agents[o]	Enhance pharmacological (eg, enhanced vasopressor effect); concomitant therapy should be avoided or used with caution; counsel patients regarding choice of over-the-counter (OTC) products
Quinupristin-Dalfopristin	Substrates of CYP3A4	See Table 2
Tigecycline	Warfarin	Potential decreased clearance of warfarin; monitor PT/INR and adjust warfarin dose appropriately
Tetracyclines	Multivalent cations[h], colestipol, kaolin-pectin, activated charcoal and sodium biocarbonate	Decreased absorption of tetracyclines; space administration by at least 2 hours
	Atovaquone	Decreased atovaquone concentration; parasitemia should be closely monitored and consider alternative agent if possible
	Digoxin	Increased digoxin serum concentration and toxicity; monitor digoxin serum concentration and adjust dose appropriately
	Ergotamine tartate	Increased ergotism; monitor for ergotism and use alternative therapy when possible

Table 5 (continued)

Drug-drug Interactions of Antibacterial Agents

Antibacterial Agent	Interacting Drug	Interaction and Management Strategy
Tetracyclines		Isotretinoin, acitretin Additive effects of pseudotumor cerebri (benign intracranial hypertension); avoid concurrent use
	Lithium	Increased lithium serum concentrations and toxicity; monitor lithium serum concentration and adjust dose appropriately
	Methotrexate	Increased methotrexate serum concentrations and toxicity; monitor methotrexate serum concentration and use leucovorin rescue as needed
	Quinine	Increased quinine serum concentration; monitor for quinine toxicity
	Theophylline	Increased theophylline serum concentration; monitor toxicity and theophylline serum concentration; adjust dose appropriately
	Warfarin	Enhanced anticoagulation; monitor PT/INR and adjust warfarin dose appropriately
Doxycycline	Barbiturates, chronic ethanol ingestion, carbamazepine, phenytoin/fosphenytoin, rifampin/rifabutin	Decrease doxycycline serum concentrations; use other tetracycline product or alternative agent if possible
Metronidazole	Ethanol, OTC and prescription products containing ethanol or propylene glycol[p]	Produces a disulfiram-like reaction (eg, flushing, palpitation, tachycardia, nausea, vomiting); avoid concomitant therapy within 2 or 3 days of taking metronidazole; counsel patients about these potential side effects
	Warfarin	Enhanced anticoagulation; monitor PT/INR and adjust warfarin dose appropriately
	Lithium, busulfan, cyclosporine, tacrolimus, phenytoin, carbazepine	Increase serum concentrations of interacting drugs; monitor toxicity and serum drug concentration; adjust dose appropriately
	5-fluorouracil	Increased toxicity; avoid concomitant use

Table 5 (continued)

Drug-drug interactions of antibacterial agents

Antibacterial Agent	Interacting Drug	Interaction and Management Strategy
Metronidazole	Phenobarbital, phenytoin, rifampin, prednisone	Decreased metronidazole serum concentrations; monitor efficacy; doses of metronidazole may need to be increased
Chloramphenicol	Acetaminophen	Equivocal changes to chloramphenicol serum concentration; monitor chloramphenicol serum concentration and adjust dose appropriately; use other analgesic or antipyretic agents
	Cyclosporine, tacrolimus, phenobarbital, phenytoin	Increased serum drug concentrations of the interacting drug; monitor toxicity, serum drug concentration and adjust dose appropriately
	Phenobarbital, phenytoin, rifampin	Decreased chloramphenicol serum concentrations; monitor efficacy, chloramphenicol serum concentrations and adjust dose appropriately
	Sulfonylurea hypoglycemic^q	Enhanced hypoglycemia; monitor efficacy and blood glucose concentration
	Warfarin	Enhanced anticoagulation; monitor PT/INR and adjust warfarin dose appropriately
	Cyclophosphamide	Decreased effectiveness of cyclophosphamide; avoid concomitant use
	Cimetidine	Bone marrow suppression and increased risk for aplastic anemia; avoid concomitant use and consider use of other anti-ulcer medications
	Folic acid, iron, cyanocobalamin	Delay response of anemias; avoid concomitant use
Trimethoprim-sulfamethoxazole	Amantadine, dapsone, digoxin, defetilide, lamuvidine, methotrexate, phenytoin/fosphenytoin, procainamide, zidovudine	Increased serum drug concentration of the interacting drug; monitor for toxicity, drug concentrations (eg, digoxin, procainamide and its metabolite, NAPA) or appropriate laboratory test (dapsone:methemoglobin level; zidovudine: complete blood count), and adjust dose appropriately; avoid concomitant use (eg, dofeetilide, methotrexate) if possible
	Azathiprine	Increased leukopenia; monitor complete blood count

Table 5 (continued)

Drug-drug Interactions of Antibacterial Agents

Antibacterial Agent	Interacting Drug	Interaction and Management Strategy
Trimethoprim -sulfamethoxazole	Cyclosporine	Decreased cyclosporine serum concentration and azotemia; monitor cyclosporine serum concentration and renal function; adjust dose appropriately
	Enalapril (ACE inhibitors), potassium, potassium-sparing diuretics	Hyperkalemia; monitor serum potassium level
	Methenamine	Crystallation of sulfonamides in urine; avoid concomitant use
	Metronidazole	Disulfiram reaction (ethanol in intravenous TMP-SMX product); use alternative therapy when possible
	Procaine, tetracaine	Decreased effect of sulfonamides; use alterantive therapy when possible
	Pryimethamine	Megaloblastic anemia and pancytopenia; monitor complete blood count and consider adding leucovorin rescue; avoid concomitant use
	Repaglinide, rosiglitazone, sulfonylurea hypoglycemic[q]	Increased serum concentrations of interacting drug and increased hypoglycemic effect;monitoir serum glucose concentration and adverse effects
	Rifabutin	Increased sulfamethoxazole hydroxylamine concentration; monitor for SMX toxicity
	Rifampin	Increased rifampin concentration and decreased TMP-SMX concentrations; monitor TMP-SMX efficacy

Table 5 (continued)

Drug-drug Interactions of Antibacterial Agents

Antibacterial Agent	Interacting Drug	Interaction and Management Strategy
Trimeothoprim- -sulfamethoxazole	Thiazide diuretics	Hyponatremia; monitor serum sodium level
	Warfarin	Enhanced anticoagulation; monitor PT/INR and adjust warfarin dose appropriately

a Oral cephalosporins prodrugs, such as cefpodoxime proxetil, cefuroxime axetil, cefditoren pivoxil

b Inhibition of tubular secretion of most renally eliminated beta-lactam agents

c Imipenem, meropenem, ertapenem and doripenem

d Examples include nifedipine, felodipine, diltiazem, and verapamil

e Examples include quinidine, ibulitide, sotalol, dofetilide, amiodarone and bretylium

f Examples include amitryptilline, haloperidol, respiridone, and quetapine

g Norfloxacin, ciprofloxacin, levolfoxacin, moxifloxacin and gatifloxacin

h Examples include antacids (containing aluminum or magnesium or calcium), iron, zinc, bismuth subsalicylate, multivitamin products, laxatives, sucralfate, didanosine, sevelamer and quinapril

i Gentamicin, tobramycin, amikacin

j Examples include amphotericin B, cisplatin, cyclosporine, vancomycin, foscarnet, intravenous pentamidine, cidofivir, polymyxin B, colistin, radio contrast and aminoglycosides

k Examples include ethacrynic acid , furosemide, urea, mannitol and cisplatin11

l Examples include succinylcholine, d-tubocurarine, vecuronium, pancuronium and atracurium

m HMG-CoA = hydroxymethyglytaryl-coenzyme A reductase inhibitors (or the "statins"), such as simvastatin, lovastatin, pravastatin and fluvastatin

n Examples include sertraline, paroxetine, citalopram and fluoxetine

o Examples include dopamine, epinephrine, and over-the-counter (OTC) cough and cold preparations that contain pseudoephedrine or phenylpropanolamine

p Examples include oral (cough and cold OTC preparations, ritonavir solution) and intravenous products (diazepam, nitroglycerin, phenytoin, trimethoprim-sulfamethoxazole). Amprenavir oral solution contains high content of propylene glycol.

q Examples include tolbutamide, chlorpropamide, glipizide, glyburide

4. Antifungal Agents

- Drug-drug interactions of amphotericin B and flucytosine involve pharmacodynamic effect (eg, increase risk of toxicities) (Table 6)

- Fluconazole is a substrate and inhibitor of CYP3A4, CYP2C9 and CYP2C19. It is also a substrate of P-glycoprotein and inhibitor of uridine diphosphate glucuonosyltransferease (UGT). It is a much less potent inhibitor of CYP3A4 than itraconazole and stronger inhibitor of CYP2C9 than voriconazole.

- Itraconazole is a substrate and potent inhibitor of CYP3A4 (hepatic and intestinal) and P-glycoprotein.

- Voriconazole is metabolized by a inhibitor of CYP2C19, CYP3A4 and CYP2C9

- Posaconazole is metabolized by phase II biotransformation using uridine diphosphate glucuonosyltransferease (UGT) and is an inhibitor of CYP3A4.

- Triazoles are involved in clinically significant pharmacokinetic interactions that include: induction (eg, reduce serum concentration by rifamycins), inhibition of CYP2C9 (e.g., warfarin by voriconazole), inhibition of CYP and breast cancer resistance protein (eg, lovastatin and itraconazole), inhibition of CYP and P-glycoprotein (eg, quinidine and itraconazole), inhibition P-glycoprotein (eg, digoxin and itraconazole), inhibition of UGT (eg, zidovudine and fluconazole) and 2-way interactions (eg, induction of CYP or UGT by phenytoin and inhibition of CYP3A4 by triazole).

- Anidulafungin and micafungin are not clinically important substrates, inducers or inhibitors of CYP isoenzymes

ID Board Pearls

- Whenever triazoles (itraconazole, voriconazole and to a lesser extent, fluconazole and posaconazole) are prescribed, the possibility of drug-drug interactions must be proactively considered and monitored.

Table 6

Drug-drug Interactions of Antibacterial Agents

Antifungal Agent	Interacting Drug	Interaction and Management Strategy
Amphotericin B	Nephrotoxic agents[a]	Direct or additive injury to the renal tubule; concomitant therapy should be avoided or used with caution and includes monitoring of renal function and dosage adjustment based on toxicity, body weight and creatinine clearance estimation
	Flucytosine	May increase flucytosine toxicity; monitor complete blood cell count and flucytosine serum concentrations; initiate flucytosine at a low dosage (eg, 75-100 mg/kg) and adjust dose as needed
Flucytosine	Amphotericin B	May increase flucytosine toxicity; monitor complete blood cell count and flucytosine serum concentrations; initiate flucytosine at a low dosage (eg, 75-100 mg/kg) and adjust dose as needed
	Cytarabine	Antagonizes the antifungal activity of flucytosine; avoid concomitant use

Table 6

Drug-drug Interactions of Antibacterial Agents

Antifungal Agent	Interacting Drug	Interaction and Management Strategy
Fluconazole	Substrates of CYP3A4	See Table 2; fluconazole is contraindicated for concomitant use with ergot alkaloids and drugs (eg, astemizole, terfenadine, cisapride, quinidine, pimozide, mesoridazine, bepridil, thioridazine, levomethadyl, ziprasaidone) that are CYP3A4 substrates and prolong the QTc interval
	Phenytoin/ fosphenytoin	Increased phenytoin serum concentration and phenytoin toxicity; monitor toxicity and phenytoin serum concentration and adjust dose as needed
	Cyclosporine, tacrolimus, sirolimus, everolimus	Increased cyclosporine, tacrolimus, sirolimus or everolimus serum concentrations; monitor toxicity and serum drug concentrations, adjust dose as needed
	Warfarin	Enhanced anticoagulation; monitor prothrombin time/international normalized ratio (PT/INR) and adjust warfarin dose appropriately
	Rifampin, rifapentine	Decreased fluconazole serum concentration; monitor efficacy and increase dose as needed
	Zidovudine	Increased zidovudine serum concentration; monitor for toxicity and adjust dose as needed
	Sulfonylurea hypoglycemic[b]	Enhanced hypoglycemia; monitor efficacy and blood glucose concentration
	Theophylline	Increased theophylline serum concentrations and risk of toxicity; monitor serum theophylline concentrations and toxicity; decrease dose of theophylline as needed
Itraconazole	Substrates of CYP3A4	See Table 2; itraconazole is contraindicated for concomitant use with ergot alkaloids, HMG-CoA reductase inhibitors metabolize by CYP3A4 (lovastatin, simvastatin), oral midazolam, triazolam, alprazolam, astemizole, terfenadine, cisapride, quinidine, pimozide, defetilide, levomethadyl, silodosin, eplerenone, nisoldipine, ranolazine, alfuzosin or conivaptan

Table 6 (continued)

Drug-drug Interactions of Antibacterial Agents

Antifungal Agent	Interacting Drug	Interaction and Management Strategy
	Rifampin, rifabutin, isoniazid, carbamazepine, phenobarbital, efavirenz, nevirapine, St. John's wart	Decreased itraconazole serum concentration and loss of antimycotic efficacy; alternative antifungal agent or interacting drug should be considerate
	Antacids, H2-antagonist (eg, famotidine), proton pump inhibitor (eg, omeprazole), didanosine (buffered formulation)	Decreased itraconazole absorption and serum concentration; loss of antimycotic efficacy; alternative antifungal agent or interacting drug should be considerate; space antacid administration by at least 2 hours; administer itraconazole with a cola beverage if receiving H^2-antagonist; use new didanosine formulation with buffer
	Cyclosporine, tacrolimus, sirolimus, everolimus	Increased cyclosporine, tacrolimus, sirolimus or everolimus serum concentrations; monitor toxicity and serum drug concentrations, adjust dose as needed
	Buspirone, haloperidol, risperidone, diazepam	Increased serum concentrations of interacting agents; monitor toxicity and adjust dose as needed
	Warfarin	Enhanced anticoagulation; monitor prothrombin time/international normalized ratio (PT/INR) and adjust warfarin dose appropriately
	Calcium channel blockers[c]	Increased serum concentrations of calcium channel blocking agents; monitor toxicity and adjust dose as needed
	Busulfan, docetaxel	Increase serum concentrations of interacting drugs and toxicity; monitor toxicity and complete blood count; adjust dose appropriately
	Digoxin	Increased digoxin serum concentration and toxicity; monitor digoxin serum concentration and adjust dose appropriately
	Loperamide	Increase loperamide serum concentration; monitor for increased loperamide toxicity (eg, nausea, vomiting, dry mouth, dizziness or drowsiness)
	Protease inhibitors (indinavir, ritonavir, saquinavir)	Increased serum concentrations of protease inhibitors and/or itraconazole; monitor toxicity and adjust dose as needed

Table 6 (continued)

Drug-drug Interactions of Antibacterial Agents

Antifungal Agent	Interacting Drug	Interaction and Management Strategy
Voriconazole	Substrates of CYP3A4	See Table 2; voriconazole is contraindicated for concomitant use with ergot alkaloids, ritonavir (400 mg BID), sirolimus, and drugs (eg, astemizole, terfenadine, cisapride, quinidine, pimozide, ranolazine) that are CYP3A4 substrates and prolong the QTc interval
	Rifampin, rifabutin, carbamazepine, phenobarbital, mephobarbital, efavirenz, St. John's wart	Decreased voriconazole serum concentrations; voriconazole is contraindicated for concomitant use with these interacting drugs
	Phenytoin/ fosphenytoin	Decreased voriconazole serum concentration and increased phenytoin serum concentration; increase voriconazole dose to 400 mg BID (oral) or 5 mg/kg BID (intravenous), monitor efficacy, toxicity and phenytoin serum concentration and adjust dose as needed
	Warfarin	Enhanced anticoagulation; monitor prothrombin time/international normalized ratio (PT/INR) and adjust warfarin dose appropriately
	Omeprazole	Increased omeprazole serum concentrations; reduce omeprazole dose in half
	Methadone	Increased R-methadone concentrations and risk of toxicity (eg, QTc prolongation, respiratory depression); monitor for toxicity and adjust dose as needed
	Cyclosporine, tacrolimus	Increased cyclosporine or tacrolimus serum concentrations; reduce dose of cyclosporine or tacrolimus by 33%-50%, monitor toxicity and cyclosporine or tacrolimus serum concentrations, and adjust dose as needed
Posaconazole	Substrates of CYP3A4	See Table 2; posaconazole is contraindicated for concomitant use with ergot alkaloids, sirolimus, and drugs (eg, astemizole, terfenadine, cisapride, quinidine, pimozide, halofantrine) that are CYP3A4 substrates and prolong the QTc interval
	Cimetidine	Decreased posaconazole serum concentration; avoid concomitant use and consider use of other antiulcer medications

Table 6 (continued)

Drug-drug Interactions of Antibacterial Agents

Antifungal Agent	Interacting Drug	Interaction and Management Strategy
	Phenytoin/ fosphenytoin	Decreased posaconazole serum concentration and increased phenytoin serum concentration; avoid concomitant use; if concomitant use required, monitor efficacy, toxicity and phenytoin serum concentration and adjust dose as needed
	Cyclosporine, tacrolimus	Increased cyclosporine or tacrolimus serum concentrations; reduce dose of cyclosporine (by 25%) or tacrolimus (by 66%), monitor toxicity and cyclosporine or tacrolimus serum concentrations, and adjust dose as needed
Caspofungin	Rifampin (and potentially other potent inducers)	Decreased serum concentration of caspofungin; monitor clinical response and increase caspofungin maintenance dose to 70 mg daily if needed
	Tacrolimus	Increased tacrolimus blood concentrations; monitor tacrolimus blood concentrations and adjust as needed
	Cyclosporine	Increased caspofungin serum concentrations and transient elevations in liver enzymes (e.g., ALT and AST); monitor for toxicity and liver enzymes
Anidulafungin	Cyclosporine	Slight increase in anidulafungin serum concentration; no dose adjustment required
Micafungin	Cyclosporine	Decreased oral clearance and increased half-life of cyclosporine; monitor cyclosporine serum concentration and adjust dose as needed
	Nifedipine	Increase nifedipine serum concentrations; monitor for nifedipine toxicity and reduce dose if needed

[a] *Examples include amphotericin B, cisplatin, cyclosporine, vancomycin, foscarnet, intravenous pentamidine, cidofivir, polymyxin B, colistin, radio contrast, and aminoglycosides*
[b] *Examples include tolbutamide, chlorpropamide, glipizide or glyburide*
[c] *Examples include nifedipine, felodipine, diltiazem, and verapamil*

5. Nucleoside and Nucleotide Reverse Transcriptase Inhibitors NRTIs

• Nucleoside and nucleotide reverse transcriptase inhibitors do not undergo metabolism or inhibit common human CYP isoforms (1A2, 2C9, 2C19, 2D6, and 3A4) (Table 7)

• Majority of interactions involve drug absorption (eg, didanosine), antagonism of intracellular phosphorylation (eg, zidovudine and stavudine) or increased toxicity.

• Mechanisms of many of the drug-drug interactions of NRTIs remain unclear.

Table 7

Drug-drug Interactions of (NNRTIs)

Antiviral Agent	Interacting Drug	Interaction and Management Strategy
Abacavir	Methadone	Decreased methadone serum concentration; monitor for methadone withdrawal and titrate methadone dosed as needed
	Tripranaivir/ritonavir	Decreased abacavir serum concentration; monitor for abacavir efficacy; appropriate dose for this combination is not established
Didanosine	Ganciclovir/ valganciclovir (oral)	Increased didanosine serum concentration and decreased ganciclovir serum concentration after oral administration; monitor ganciclovir efficacy and didansine toxicity
	Ribavirin	Increased didanosine intraceullular concentration; concomitant administration is not recommended because of serious didanosine toxicities
	Hydroxyurea	Peripheral neuropathy, lactic acidosis, and pancreatitis has been seen with this combination (with or without stavudine); avoid co-administration if possible
	Stavudine	Peripheral neuropathy, lactic acidosis, and pancreatitis has been seen with this combination (with or without hydroxyurea); avoid co-administration if possible
	Allopurinol	Increased didanosine serum concentrations and increased risk for toxicity (pancreatitis, neuropathy); reduce didanosine dose by 50% and monitor toxicity

Table 7 (continued)

Drug-drug interactions of (NNRTIs)

Antiviral Agent	Interacting Drug	Interaction and Management Strategy
Didanosine	Atazanavir	Decreased didanosine serum concentration with simultaneous co-administration; space administration by 2 hours before or 1 hour after didanosine
	Tipranavir/ritonavir	Decreased didanosine and tipranavir serum concentrations; space administration by at least 2 hours
	Indinavir	Decreased indinavir serum concentration after pediatric solution; space administration by at least 1 hour
	Delavirdine	Decreased delavirdine serum concentration after didanosine pediatric solution; space administration by at least 1 hour
	Tenofovir	Increased didanosine serum concentration; decrease didanosine dose (e.g., delayed-release capsules: if CL_{CR}>60 mL/min: 250 mg/day if patient weighs >60 kg; 200 mg if patient weighs <60 kg)
	Methadone	Decreased didanosine serum concentration with didanosine pediatric solution; monitor didanosine efficacy
	Fluoroquinolones	Decreased fluoroquinolone serum concentration with simultaneous co-administration of dadinosine pediatric solution but not delayed-release capsules; space administration by at least 2-6 hours
	Tetracyclines	Decreased tetracycline serum concentration with simultaneous co-administration of didanosine pediatric solution; space administration by at least 1-2 hours
	Itraconazole	Decreased itraconazole serum concentration with concurrent administration of didanosine pediatric
Emtricitabine	No major interactions	
Lamivudine	Trimethoprim/ Sulfamethoxazole	Increased lamivudine serum concentrations; ; monitor lamivudine toxicities

Table 7 (continued)

Drug-drug interactions of nucleoside and nucleotide reverse transcriptase inhibitors (NNRTIs)

Antiviral Agent	Interacting Drug	Interaction and Management Strategy
Stavudine	Zidovudine	Antagonism may occur ; competitive inhibition of intracellular phosphorylation of stavudine by zidovudine; avoid concomitant administration
	Methadone	Decreased stavudine serum concentration; monitor stavudine efficacy
	Didanosine	Peripheral neuropathy, lactic acidosis, and pancreatitis has been seen with this combination (with or without hydroxyurea); avoid co-administration if possible
Tenofovir	Didanosine	Increased didanosine serum concentration; decrease didanosine dose (e.g., delayed-release capsules: if CL_{CR}>60 mL/min: 250 mg/day if patient weighs >60 kg; 200 mg if patient weighs <60 kg)
	Atazanavir/Ritonavir	Decreased atazanavir serum concentration and increased tenofovir serum concentration; recommended dosage regimen: atazanavir 300 mg, ritonavir 100 mg, tenofovir 300 mg given once daily with food; monitor for tenofovir toxicities; avoid concomitant administration without ritonavir
	Darunavir/Ritonavir	Increased tenofovir serum concentration; monitor tenofovir toxicities
	Lopinanvir/Ritonavir	Increased tenofovir serum concentration; monitor tenofovir toxicities
	Tipranavir/Ritonavir	Decreased tenofovir serum concentration; monitor tenofovir efficacy
Zidovudine	Stavudine	Antagonism may occur ; competitive inhibition of intracellular phosphorylation of stavudine by zidovudine; avoid concomitant administration
	Ganciclovir/ Valganciclovir	Increase risk of hematologic toxicity (e.g., anemia, neutropenia, pancytopenia) and GI toxicity; concomitant therapy should be avoided or used with caution with careful monitoring of hematologic function and at the lowest possible dose; consider alternative antiretroviral agent

Table 7 (continued)

Drug-drug interactions of nucleoside and nucleotide reverse transcriptase inhibitors (NNRTIs)

Antiviral Agent	Interacting Drug	Interaction and Management Strategy
	Acyclovir	Increase risk of neurotoxicity (e.g., drowsiness, lethargy); monitor for adverse events
	Ribavirin	Rabivirin inhibits intracellular phosphorylation of zidovudine; avoid concomitant administration; if administered together, monitor virologic efficacy and hematologic toxicities
	Methadone	Increased zidovudine serum concentration; monitor zidovudine toxicities
	Atazanavir	Decreased zidovudine serum concentration; monitor zidovudine efficacy
	Tipranaivir/Ritonavir	Decreased zidovudine and tipranavir serum concentrations; monitor virologic efficacy
	Atovaquone	Increased zidovudine serum concentration; monitor zidovudine toxicities
	Probenecid	Increased zidovudine serum concentration; monitor zidovudine toxicities
	Cidofovir	Manufacturer recommends that on days of cidofovir plus probenecid (see interaction above) co-administration, zidovudine should be temporarily discontinued or given at a 50% reduced dose
	Fluconazole	Increased zidovudine serum concentration; monitor zidovudine toxicities
	Valproic acid	Decreased zidovudine serum concentration; monitor virologic efficacy

---

6. Non-nucleoside Reverse Transcriptase Inhibitors (NNRTIs] (Table 8)

- Delavirdine, nevirapine and efavirenz are substrates of CYP3A4 (Table 8)

- Etravirine is a substrate of CYP3A4, CYP2C9 and CYP2C19.

- Delavirdine is a potent inhibitor of CYP3A4, nevirapine is an inducer of CYP3A4, efavirenz is a mixed inducer and inhibitor of CYP3A4, and etravirine is an inducer of CYP3A4 and an inhibitor of CYP2C9 and CYP2C19

- The reader should refer to the most recent report by the Panel on Antiretroviral Guidelines for Adults and Adolescents: A Working Group of the Office of AIDS Research Advisory Council for up-to-date guidelines on prescribing and important drug-drug interactions of NNRTIs.

ID Board Pearls

- All NNRTIs are metabolized by the liver by the cytochrome P450 system, particularly by CYP3A4. Whenever NNRTIs are prescribed, the possibility of drug-drug interactions must be proactively considered and monitored. The list of potential drug-drug interactions is extensive and continues to increase.

Table 8

Drug-drug Interactions of NNRTIs[a]

NNRTI	Interacting Drug	Interaction and Management Strategy
Delavirdine	Substrates of CYP3A4	See Table 2; delaviridine is contraindicated for concomitant use with ergot alkaloids, drugs (e.g., astemizole, terfenadine, cisapride, pimozide, bepridil) that are CYP3A4 substrates and prolong the QTc interval, simvastatin, lovastatin, rifampin, rifapentine, rifabutin, alprazolam, oral midazolam, triazolam, St. John's wort, fosamprenavir, carbamazepine, phenobarbital and phenytoin
	Antacids/didanosine	Decreased delavirdine concentrations; space administration by at 1 hour
	Clarithromycin	Increased clarithromycin and delaviridine concentrations; reduce clarithromycin dose by 50% if CLCR 30-60 ml/min and by 75% if CLCR <30 ml/min
	Benzodiazepines: Alprazolam Diazepam	Avoid concomitant use; consider alternative agent Consider alternative agent (eg, lorazepam)
	Hormonal contraceptives	Consider using additional methods
	Atorvastatin	Use lowest possible dose; use alternative lipid lowering agent

Table 8 (continued)

Drug-drug Interactions of NNRTIs[a]

NNRTI	Interacting Drug	Interaction and Management Strategy
Delavirdine	Protease inhibitors	See Table 9
	Maraviroc	Increase maraviroc serum concentration; use lower maraviroc dose (eg, 150 mg BID)
	Methadone	Monitor for methadone toxicity; adjust dose as needed
	Warfarin	Monitor PT/INR; adjust dose as needed
Efavirenz	Itraconazole, posaconazole	Decrease itraconzole, OH-itraconazole, and posaconazole serum concentration; adjust dose as needed
	Voriconazole	Contraindicated at standard dose; use voriconazole 400 mg BID and efavirenz 300 mg daily
	Carbamazepine, phenobarbital, phenytoin	Decreased carbamazepine concentration; monitor anticonvulsant serum concentrations; adjust dose as needed or use alternative anticonvulsant
	Clarithromycin	Decrease clarithromycin serum concentration; monitor efficacy or use alternative agent
	Rifabutin	Decrease rifabutin serum concentration; increase dose
	Rifampin	Decrease rifampin serum concentration; increase dose
	Oral midazolam	Do not administered with oral midazolam
	St. John's wort	Avoid combination
	Hormonal contraceptives	Use alternative or additional methods
	Atorvastatin	Adjust atorvstatin dose according to lipid response
	Lovastatin, simvastatin	Adjust statin dose according to lipid response
	Pravastatin, rosuvastatin	Adjust statin dose according to lipid response
	Protease inhibitors	See Table 9
	Methadone	Decreased methadone serum concentration; adjust dose as needed; monitor for withdrawal

Table 8 (continued)

Drug-drug Interactions of NNRTIs[a]

NNRTI	Interacting Drug	Interaction and Management Strategy
	Warfarin	Monitor PT/INR; adjust dose as needed
Efavirenz	Anti-arrhythmic	Decreased anti-arrhythmic serum concentrations; use with caution, monitor antiarrhythmic serum concentrations, and adjust dose as needed
	Dexamethasone	Decreased etravirine serum concentration; use with caution or consider alternative corticosteroid for long-term use
	Itraconazole	Decreased itraconazole and increase etravirine serum concentration; adjust dose as needed
	Voriconazole	Decreased itraconazole and etravirine serum concentration; adjust voriconazole dose as needed
	Carbamazepine, phenobarbital, phenytoin	Do not coadminister; consider alternative anticonvulsant
	Clarithromycin	Decreased clarithromycin and increased 0H-clarithomycin serum concentration; increased etravrine serum concentration; consider alternative agen
	Rifabutin	Use alternative agent or adjust dose appropriately
	Rifampin	Do not coadminister
	Diazepam	Increased diazepam serum concentrations; decrease dose
	St. John's wort	Avoid combination
	Hormonal contraceptives	Increased ethinyl estadiol serum concentration; No dosage adjustment needed
	Atorvastatin, fluvastatin	Increased atorvastatin serum concentration; standard dose; adjust dose according to response
	Lovastatin, simvastatin	Decreased statin serum concentration; adjust dose according to response

Table 8 (continue)

Drug-drug Interactions of NNRTIs[a]

NNRTI	Interacting Drug	Interaction and Management Strategy
Etravirine	Sildenafil	Decrease sildenafil serum concentration; may need to increase sildenafil dose based on clinical effect
	Protease Inhibitors	See Table 9
	Warfarin	Monitor PT/INR; adjust dose as needed
Nevirapine	Fluconazole	Increased nevirapine serum concentration and hepatotoxicity; monitor hepatotoxicity
	Carbamazepine, phenytoin, phenobarbital	Decreased nevirapine serum concentration; contraindicated; do not coadminister
	Clarithromycin	Increased nevirapine and decreased clarithromycin serum concentration; monitor efficacy or use alternative agent
	Rifampin	Decreased nevirapine concentration; do not coadminister
	St. John's wort	Avoid combination
	Protease inhibitors	See Table 9
	Methadone	Decreased methadone serum concentrations; monitor for opiate withdrawal and increased methadone dose as needed
	Warfarin	Monitor PT/INR; adjust dose as needed

[a] Adapted from: Panel on Antiretroviral Guidelines for Adults and Adolescents: A Working Group of the Office of AIDS Research Advisory Council (OARAC), Department of Health and Human Services. Guidelines for the use of antiretroviral agents in HIV-1-infected adults and adolescents. November 3, 2008. Please refer to the product package insert and literature for complete details and a potential list of both studied and theoretical drug-drug interactions

7. Protease Inhibitors

- All protease inhibitors are substrates of CYP3A4 and are subject to drug-drug interactions involving inhibition or induction of CYP3A4 (Table 9)

- Most protease inhibitors are inhibitors of CYP3A4 and some are inducers of other CYP isoenzymes, P-glycoprotein or other transporters.

- Ritonavir is commonly used in low doses (eg, 100 or 200 mg) for its inhibitory effect on the CYP3A4 metabolism of other protease inhibitors. This beneficial drug-drug interaction is used to increase drug concentrations of other protease inhibitors (booster effect) and prolong the elimination of the other protease inhibitor.

- Benefits from booster ritonavir dosing with other protease inhibitors include: higher minimum (trough) serum concentration, reduction in the development of drug resistance by increasing drug exposure, less frequent dosing and enhanced adherence to the drug regimen.

- The reader should refer to the most recent report by the Panel on Antiretroviral Guidelines for Adults and Adolescents: A Working Group of the Office of AIDS Research Advisory Council for up-to-date guidelines on prescribing and important drug-drug interactions of protease inhibitors.

ID Board Pearls

- All protease inhibitors are metabolized by the liver by the cytochrome P450 system, particularly by CYP3A4. Whenever protease inhibitors are prescribed, the possibility of drug-drug interactions must be proactively considered and monitored. The list of potential drug-drug interactions is extensive and continues to increase.

Table 9

Drug-drug Interactions of Protease Inhibitors[a]

Protease Inhibitor	Interacting Drug	Interaction and Management Strategy
Atazanavir	Substrates of CYP3A4	See Table 2; atazanavir is contraindicated for concomitant use with ergot alkaloids, drugs (eg, astemizole, terfenadine, cisapride, pimozide, bepridil) that are CYP3A4 substrates and prolong the QTc interval, simvastatin, lovastatin, rifampin, rifapentine, oral midazolam, triazolam, St. John's wort and fluticasone
	Antacids	Decreased atazanavir concentrations; space administration by 2 hours before or 1 hour after antacid
	Didanosine	Decreased didanosine serum concentration with simultaneous coadministration; space administration by 2 hours before or 1 hour after didanosine

Table 9 (continued)

Drug-drug Interactions of Protease Inhibitors[a]

Protease Inhibitor	Interacting Drug	Interaction and Management Strategy
Atazanavir	H2-Receptor Antagonist	Decreased atazanavir concentrations; three dosing recommendations:
		H2-receptor antagonist dose should not exceed a dose equivalent to famotidine 40 mg BID in treatment-naïve patients or 20 mg BID in treatment-experience patients;
		Atazanavir 300 mg plus ritonavir 100 mg should be administered simultaneously with and/or >10 hours after the H_2-receptor antagonist;
		In treatment-experience patients, if tenofoovir is used with H_2-receptor antagonists, atazanavir 400 mg plus ritonavir 100 mg should be used
	Proton Pump Inhibitors	Decreased atazanavir concentrations; proton pump inhibitors are not recommended in patients receiving unboosted atazanavir or in treatment-experienced patients
		For atazanivir plus ritonavir, proton pump inhibitors should not exceed a dose equivalent to omeprazole 20 mg daily in treatment-naïve patients; proton pump should be administered >12 hours prior to atazanavir plus ritonavir
	Itraconazole	Potential bi-directional inhibition between itraconazole and atazanavir plus ritonavir; high-dose itraconazole (>200 mg /day) are not recommended; monitor itraconazole serum concentration if possible
	Voriconazole	Atazanavir plus ritonavir 100-200 mg: decreased voriconazole serum concentrations; concomitant administration is not recommended; atazanavir plus ritonavir 400mg BID or higher is contraindicated
	Carbamazepine, phenytoin, phenobarbital	Monitor anticonvulsant and tipranavir serum concentration and virologic response; consider alternative anticonvulsant and ritonavir boosting regimen
	Clarithromycin	Increased clarithromycin serum concentration and may prolong QTc; reduce clarithromycin dose by 50%; consider alternative therapy

Table 9 (continued)

Drug-drug Interactions of Protease Inhibitors[a]

Protease Inhibitor	Interacting Drug	Interaction and Management Strategy
Atazanavir	Rifabutin	Increased rifabutin serum concentrations; dose rifabutin 150 mg QOD or 3 times per week
	Benzodiazepines: Alprazolam Diazepam	Avoid concomitant use; consider alternative agent (eg, lorazepam, oxazepam or temazepam)
	Calciium channel blockers: Dihydropyridine Diltiazem	Caution; dose titration with ECG monitoring Increase diltiazem serum concentrations with atazanavir plus ritonavir; decrease diltiazem dose by 50%; ECG monitoring recommended
	Hormonal contraceptives	Boosted regimen: decreased ethinyl estradiol and increase progestin serum concentrations; oral contraceptive should contain at least 35 mcg of ethinyl estradiol; consider using alternative or additional methods
		Unboosted regimen: increase ethinyl estadiol serum concentration; oral contraceptive should contain at least 30 mcg of ethinyl estradiol; consider using alternative or additional methods
	Atorvastatin, rosuvastatin	Use lowest possible dose with careful monitoring; use alternative lipid-lowering agent
	Indinavir	Coadministration is not recommended because of potential additive hyperbilirubinema
	Efavirenz	Decreased atazanavir serum concentration; in treatment-naïve patients: atazanavir 400 mg plus ritonavir 100 mg plus standard dose of efavirenz; Do not coadminister in treatment-experienced patients
	Etravirine	Decreased atazanavir and increased etravirine serum concentration; do not coadminister with boosted or unboosted atazanavir regimens
	Maraviroc	Increase maraviroc serum concentration; use lower maraviroc dose (eg, 150 mg BID)

Table 9 (continued)

Drug-drug Interactions of Protease Inhibitors[a]

Protease Inhibitor	Interacting Drug	Interaction and Management Strategy
Atazanavir	Methadone	Boosted regimen: decrease methadone serum concentration; monitor for methadone withdrawal; adjust dose as needed
	Warfarin	Monitor PT/INR; adjust dose as needed
Darunavir	Substrates of CYP3A4	See Table 2; atazanavir is contraindicated for concomitant use with ergot alkaloids, drugs (eg, astemizole, terfenadine, cisapride, pimozide) that are CYP3A4 substrates and prolong the QTc interval, simvastatin, lovastatin, rifampin, rifapentine, oral midazolam, triazolam, St. John's wort, fluticasone, carbamazepine, phenytoin and phenobarbital
	Itraconazole	Potential bidirectional inhibition between itraconazole and darunavir plus ritonavir; high-dose itraconazole (>200 mg /day) are not recommended; monitor itraconazole serum concentration if possible
	Voriconazole	Daruanvir plus ritonavir 100-200 mg: decreased voriconazole serum concentrations; concomitant administration is not recommended; atazanavir plus ritonavir 400mg BID or higher is contraindicated
	Clarithromycin	Increased clarithromycin serum concentration; reduce clarithromycin dose by 50% if CLCR 30-60 mL/min; reduce clarithromycin dose by 75% if CLCR <30 mL/min; consider alternative therapy
	Rifabutin	Increased rifabutin serum concentrations; dose rifabutin 150 mg QOD or 3 times per week
	Benzodiazepines: Alprazolam Diazepam	Avoid concomitant use; consider alternative agent (eg, lorazepam, oxazepam or temazepam)
	Hormonal contraceptives	Consider using alternative or additional methods

Table 9 (continued)

Drug-drug Interactions of Protease Inhibitors[a]

Protease Inhibitor	Interacting Drug	Interaction and Management Strategy
Darunavir	Atorvastatin, pravastatin, rosuvastatin	Use lowest possible dose with careful monitoirng; use alternative lipid lowering agent
	Paroxetine, sertaline	Decrease paroxetine and sertraline serum concentrations; minitor efficacy and titrate dose as needed
	Lopinavir/ritonavir; saquinavir	Decreased darunavir; increased lopinavir. Coadministration is not recommended because dosing is not established
	Efavirenz	Decreased darunavir and increased efavirenz serum concentrations; use standard doses and monitor virologic response
	Etravirine	Decreased etravirine serum concentrations; use standard doses and monitor virologic response
	Nevirapine	Increased nevirapine serum concentration; use standard doses and monitor virologic response
	Maraviroc	Increase maraviroc serum concentration; use lower maraviroc dose (eg, 150 mg BID)
	Methadone	Boosted regimen: decrease methadone serum concentration; monitor for methadone withdrawal; adjust dose as needed
	Warfarin	Monitor PT/INR; adjust dose as needed
Fosamprenavir	Substrates of CYP3A4	See Table 2; atazanavir is contraindicated for concomitant use with ergot alkaloids, drugs (eg, astemizole, terfenadine, cisapride, pimozide, bepridil) that are CYP3A4 substrates and prolong the QTc interval, simvastatin, lovastatin, rifampin, rifapentine, oral midazolam, triazolam, St. John's wort, fluticasone, delavirdine and oral contraceptives
	Antacids	Decreased amprenavir concentrations; space administration by 2 hours before or 1 hour after antacid

Table 9 (continued)

Drug-drug Interactions of Protease Inhibitors[a]

Protease Inhibitor	Interacting Drug	Interaction and Management Strategy
Fosamprenavir	Didanosine	Decreased didanosine serum concentration with simultaneous co-administration; space administration by 2 hours before or 1 hour after didanosine
	H$_2$-receptor antagonist	Decreased amprenavir serum concentrations in unboosted regimen; separate administration if coadministration is necessary; consider boosting with ritonavir
	Itraconazole	Potential bi-directional inhibition between itraconazole and fosamprenavir plus ritonavir; high-dose itraconazole (>200 mg /day) are not recommended; monitor itraconazole serum concentration if possible
	Voriconazole	Fosamprenavir plus ritonavir 100-200 mg: decreased voriconazole serum concentrations; concomitant administration is not recommended; Fosamprenavir plus ritonavir 400 mg BID or higher is contraindicated
	Carbamazepine, phenytoin, phenobarbital	Boosted regimen: decreased phenytoin and increased amprenavir serum concentration; monitor anticonvulsant and dose adjust as needed. Unboosted regimen: increased aprenavir serum concentration; no dosage adjustment
	Rifabutin	Boosted regimen: Increased rifabutin serum concentrations; dose rifabutin 150 mg QOD or 3 times per week Unboosted regimen: increased rifabutin serum concentration; dose rifabutin 150 mg daily or 300 mg 3 times per week
	Benzodiazepines: Alprazolam Diazepam	Avoid concomitant use; consider alternative agent (eg, lorazepam, oxazepam or temazepam)

Table 9 (continued)

Drug-drug Interactions of Protease Inhibitors[a]

Protease Inhibitor	Interacting Drug	Interaction and Management Strategy
Fosamprenavir	Hormonal contraceptives	Boosted regimen: decreased ethinyl estradiol and norethindrone serum concentrations; usr alternative or additional methods
		Unboosted regimen: increase ethinyl estadiol, norethindrone and amprenavir serum concentration; use alternative or additional methods
	Atorvastatin, rosuvastatin	Use lowest possible dose with careful monitoring; use alternative lipid lowering agent
	Delaviridine	Increase amprenavir and delavirdine serum concentration; avoid concomitant administration
	Efavirenz	Decreased amprenavir serum concentrations; dose: fosamprenavir 1400 mg plus ritonavir 300 mg QD or fosamprenavir 700 mg plus ritonavir 100 mg BID plus standard dose of efavirenz
	Etravirine	Increased amprenavir serum concentrations; do not coadminister with boosted or un boosted atazanavir regimens
	Maraviroc	Use lower maraviroc dose (eg, 150 mg BID)
	Methadone	Decrease methadone serum concentration; monitor for methadone withdrawal; adjust dose as needed
	Warfarin	Monitor PT/INR; adjust dose as needed
Indinavir	Substrates of CYP3A4	See Table 2; indivair is contraindicated for concomitant use with ergot alkaloids, drugs (e.g., astemizole, terfenadine, cisapride, pimozide, amiodarone) that are CYP3A4 substrates and prolong the QTc interval, simvastatin, lovastatin, rifampin, rifapentine, oral midazolam, triazolam, St. John's wort, and atazanavir
	Itraconazole	Potential bi-directional inhibition between itraconazole and indinavir plus ritonavir; high-dose itraconazole (>200 mg /day) are not recommended; monitor itraconazole serum concentration if possible

Table 9 (continued)

Drug-drug Interactions of Protease Inhibitors[a]

Protease Inhibitor	Interacting Drug	Interaction and Management Strategy
Indinavir	Voriconazole	Indinavir plus ritonavir 100-200 mg: decreased voriconazole serum concentrations; concomitant administration is not recommended; indinavir plus ritonavir 400 mg BID or higher is contraindicated
	Carbamazepine, phenytoin, phenobarbital	Monitor anticonvulsant and indinavir serum concentration and virologic response; consider alternative anticonvulsant and ritonavir-boosting regimen
	Clarithromycin	Increased clarithromycin serum concentration; reduce clarithromycin dose by 50% if CLCR 30-60 mL/min; reduce clarithromycin dose by 75% if CLCR <30 mL/min; consider alternative therapy
	Rifabutin	Boosted regimen: increased rifabutin serum concentrations; dose rifabutin 150 mg QOD or 3 times per week
		Unboosted regimen: increased rifabutin and decreased indinavir serum concentration; rifabutin 150 mg daily or 300 mg 3 times weekly plus indinavir 1000 mg TID or consider ritonavir boosting
	Benzodiazepines: Alprazolam Diazepam	Avoid concomitant use; consider alternative agent (eg, lorazepam, oxazepam or temazepam)
	Calciium channel blockers: Dihydropyridine	Caution; dose titration with ECG monitoring Increase amlodipine serum concentrations with indinavir plus ritonavir
	Hormonal Contraceptives	For ritonavir boosted regimen: consider using alternative or additional methods
		For unboosted regimen: increase ethinyl estadiol and indinavir serum concentration; no dose adjustments needed
	Atorvastatin, Rosuvastatin	Use lowest possible dose with careful monitoring; use alternative lipid lowering agent

Table 9 (continued)

Drug-drug Interactions of Protease Inhibitors[a]

Protease Inhibitor	Interacting Drug	Interaction and Management Strategy
Ritonavir[a]	Atazanavir	Coadministration is not recommended because of potential additive hyperbilirubinema
	Delavirdine	Increased indinavir serum concentration; dose: indinavir 600 mg q8h; standard dose for delvirdine
	Efavirenz	Decreased indinavir serum concentration; dose: indinavir 1000 mg q8h; consider boosting regimen; standard efavirenz dose
	Nevirapine	Decreased indinavir serum concentration; dose: indinavir 1000 mg q8h; consider boosting regimen; standard nevirapine dose
	Maraviroc	Possibly increased maraviroc serum concentration; araviroc dose (eg, 150 mg BID)
	Methadone	For ritonavir boosted regimen: decrease methadone serum concentration; monitor for methadone withdrawal; adjust dose as needed
	Warfarin	Monitor PT/INR; adjust dose as needed
Lopinavir/Ritonavir	Substrates of CYP3A4	See Table 2; lopinavir/ritonavir is contraindicated for concomitant use with ergot alkaloids, drugs (eg, astemizole, terfenadine, cisapride, pimozide, flecainide, propafenone) that are CYP3A4 substrates and prolong the QTc interval, simvastatin, lovastatin, rifampin, rifapentine, oral midazolam, triazolam, St. John's wort and fluticasone
	Itraconazole	Increased itraconazole serum concentration; do not exceed 200 mg/day; monitor itraconazole serum concentration if possible
	Voriconazole	Atazanavir plus ritonavir 100-200 mg: decreased voriconazole serum concentrations; concomitant administration is not recommended; atazanavir plus ritonavir 400mg BID or higher is contraindicated

Table 9 (continued)

Drug-drug Interactions of Protease Inhibitors[a]

Protease Inhibitor	Interacting Drug	Interaction and Management Strategy
Lopinavir/ ritonavir	Carbamazepine, phenytoin, phenobarbital	Increased carbamazepine, decreased phenytoin, Phenobarbital, and lopinavir serum concentration; monitor anticonvulsant and lopinavir serum concentration and virologic response; consider alternative anticonvulsant
	Clarithromycin	Increased clarithromycin serum concentration; reduce clarithromycin dose by 50% if CLCR 30-60 mL/min; reduce clarithromycin dose by 75% if CLCR <30 mL/min; consider alternative therapy
	Rifabutin	Increased rifabutin serum concentrations; dose rifabutin 150 mg QOD or 3 times per week
	Benzodiazepines: Alprazolam Diazepam	Avoid concomitant use; consider alternative agent (eg, lorazepam, oxazepam or temazepam)
	Calciium channel blockers: Dihydropyridine	Increase amlodipine serum concentration; caution is warranted and clinical monitoring is required
	Hormonal Contraceptives	Decreased ethinyl estradiol ; use alternative or additional methods
	Atorvastatin, rosuvastatin	Use lowest possible dose with careful monitoring; use alternative lipid-lowering agent
	Ritonavir	Additional ritonavir is not recommended
	Tipranavir	Decreased lopinavir serum concentration; avoid concomitant administration
	Maraviroc	Increase maraviroc serum concentration; use lower maraviroc dose (eg, 150 mg BID)
	Methadone	For ritonavir boosted regimen: decrease methadone erum concentration; monitor for methadone withdrawal; adjust dose as needed
	Warfarin	Monitor PT/INR; adjust dose as needed

Table 9 (continued)

Drug-drug Interactions of Protease Inhibitors[a]

Protease Inhibitor	Interacting Drug	Interaction and Management Strategy
Nelfinavir	Substrates of CYP3A4	See Table 2; nelfinavir is contraindicated for concomitant use with ergot alkaloids, drugs (eg, astemizole, terfenadine, cisapride, pimozide) that are CYP3A4 substrates and prolong the QTc interval, simvastatin, lovastatin, rifampin, rifapentine, oral midazolam, triazolam and St. John's wort
	Proton pump inhibitors	Decreased nelfinavir and metabolite (M8) concentrations; avoid concomitant administration of proton pump inhibitors and nelfinavir
	Itraconazole	Potential bi-directional inhibition between itraconazole and nelfinavir plus ritonavir; high-dose itraconazole (>200 mg day) are not recommended; monitor itraconazole serum concentration if possible
	Voriconazole	Nelfinavir plus ritonavir 100-200 mg: decreased voriconazole serum concentrations; concomitant administration is not recommended; nelfinavir plus ritonavir 400 mg BID or higher is contraindicated
	Carbamazepine, phenytoin, phenobarbital	Monitor anticonvulsant and nelfinavir serum concentration and virologic response; consider alternative anticonvulsant and ritonavir boosting regimen
	Rifabutin	Increased rifabutin serum concentration and decreased nelfinavir concentration; dose rifabutin 150 mg QD or 300 mg 3 times per week
	Benzodiazepines: Alprazolam Diazepam	Avoid concomitant use; consider alternative agent (eg, lorazepam, oxazepam or temazepam)
	Hormonal contraceptives	Boosted regimen: decreased ethinyl estradiol and progestin serum concentration; use alternative or additional methods Unboosted regimen: decreased ethinyl estadiol and norethindrone serum concentration; use alternative or additional methods

Table 9 (continued)

Drug-drug Interactions of Protease Inhibitors[a]

Protease Inhibitor	Interacting Drug	Interaction and Management Strategy
Nelfinavir	Atorvastatin, rosuvastatin	Use lowest possible dose with careful monitoring; use alternative lipid-lowering agent
	Delavirdine	Decreased delavirdine and increased nelfinavir serum concentrations; monitor delvirdine virologic efficacy and nelfinavir toxicities
	Efavirenz	Increased nelfinavir serum concentration; use standard doses of each agent
	Nevirapine	Increased nelfinavir serum concentration; use standard doses of each agent
	Maraviroc	Use lower maraviroc dose (eg, 150 mg BID)
	Methadone	Decreased methadone serum concentration; monitor for methadone withdrawal; adjust dose as needed
	Warfarin	Monitor PT/INR; adjust dose as needed
Ritonavir[a]	Substrates of CYP3A4	See Table 2; atazanavir is contraindicated for concomitant use with ergot alkaloids, drugs (eg, astemizole, terfenadine, cisapride, pimozide, bepridil, amiodarone, flecainide, propafenone, quinidine) that are CYP3A4 substrates and prolong the QTc interval, simvastatin, lovastatin,rifampin, rifapentine, oral midazolam, triazolam, St. John's wort, fluticasone, alfuzosin and voriconazole (with ritonavir >400 mg BID)
	Desipramine	Increased desipramine serum concentrations; reduce desipramine dose and monitor toxicities
	Trazodone	Increased trazodone serum concentrations; use lowest dose of trazodone and monitor CNS and cardiovascular toxicities
	Theophylline	Decreased theophylline serum concentrations; monitor theophylline serum concentrations and adjust dose as needed
	Hormonal contraceptives	Use alternative or additional methods

Table 9 (continued)

![separator bar]

Drug-drug Interactions of Protease Inhibitors[a]

Protease Inhibitor	Interacting Drug	Interaction and Management Strategy
	Delavirdine	Increased ritonavir serum concentration; no data on dosing recommendations
	Efavirenz	Increased ritonavir and efavirenz serum concentration; use standard doses
	Nevirapine	Decreased ritonavir serum concentration; use standard doses
	Maraviroc	Increase maraviroc serum concentration; use lower maraviroc dose (e.g., 150 mg BID)
Saquinavir	Substrates of CYP3A4	See Table 2; saquinavir/ritonavir is contraindicated for concomitant use with ergot alkaloids, drugs (e.g., astemizole, terfenadine, cisapride, pimozide) that are CYP3A4 substrates and prolong the QTc interval, simvastatin, lovastatin, rifampin, rifapentine, oral midazolam, triazolam, St. John's wort, and fluticasone
	Proton Pump Inhibitors	Boosted regimen: Increased saquinavir serum concentrations; monitor for toxicities
	Itraconazole	Potential bi-directional inhibition between itraconazole and saquinavir plus ritonavir; use lower doses of itraconazole; monitor itraconazole serum concentration if possible
	Voriconazole	Saquinavir plus ritonavir 100-200 mg: decreased voriconazole serum concentrations; concomitant administration is not recommended; atazanavir plus ritonavir 400 mg BID or higher is contraindicated
	Carbamazepine, phenytoin, phenobarbital	Monitor anticonvulsant and saquinavir serum concentration and virologic response; consider alternative anticonvulsant and ritonavir boosting regimen
	Clarithromycin	Increased clarithromycin serum concentration; reduce clarithromycin dose by 50% if CLCR 30-60 mL/min; reduce clarithromycin dose by 75% if CLCR <30 mL/min; consider alternative therapy
	Rifabutin	Increased rifabutin serum concentrations; dose rifabutin 150 mg QOD or 3 times per week

Table 9 (continued)

Drug-drug Interactions of Protease Inhibitors[a]

Protease Inhibitor	Interacting Drug	Interaction and Management Strategy
Saquinavir	Benzodiazepines: Alprazolam Diazepam	Avoid concomitant use; consider alternative agent (eg, lorazepam, oxazepam or temazepam)
	Calciium channel blockers: Dihydropyridine Diltiazem	Caution; dose titration with ECG monitoring Increase diltiazem serum concentrations with atazanavir plus ritonavir; decrease diltiazem dose by 50%; ECG monitoring recommended
	Hormonal contraceptives	Boosted regimen: decreased ethinyl estradiol serum concentrations; use alternative or additional methods
	Atorvastatin, rosuvastatin	Use lowest possible dose with careful monitoring; use alternative lipid-lowering agent
	Delavirdine	Increased saquinavir serum concentration; recommended dose: saquinavir/ritonavir 1000 mg/100 mg BID
	Efavirenz	Decreased saquinavir and efavirenz serum concentration; recommended dose: saquinavir/ritonavir 1000 mg/100 mg BID
	Etravirine	Decreased saquinavir and etravirine serum concentration; recommended dose: saquinavir/ritonavir 1000 mg/100 mg BID
	Maraviroc	Increase maraviroc serum concentration; use lower maraviroc dose (eg, 150 mg BID)
	Methadone	For ritonavir-boosted regimen: decrease methadone serum concentration; monitor for methadone withdrawal; adjust dose as needed
	Warfarin	Monitor PT/INR; adjust dose as needed
Tipranavir/ritonavir	Substrates of CYP3A4	See Table 2; atazanavir is contraindicated for concomitant use with ergot alkaloids, drugs (eg, astemizole, terfenadine, cisapride, pimozide, bepridil, amiodarone, flecainide, propafenone, quindine) that are CYP3A4 substrates and prolong the QTc interval, simvastatin, lovastatin, rifampin, rifapentine, oral midazolam, triazolam, St. John's wort and fluticasone

Table 9 (continued)

Drug-drug Interactions of Protease Inhibitors[a]

Protease Inhibitor	Interacting Drug	Interaction and Management Strategy
	Antacids	Decreased tipranavir concentrations; space administration by 2 hours before or 1 hour after antacid
	Proton pump inhibitors	Decreased omeprazole serum concentration; may need to increase the dose of omeprazole
	Itraconazole	Potential bi-directional inhibition between itraconazole and tipranavir plus ritonavir; high-dose itraconazole (>200 mg /day) are not recommended; monitor itraconazole serum concentration if possible
	Voriconazole	Tipranavir plus ritonavir 100-200 mg: decreased voriconazole serum concentrations; concomitant administration is not recommended; atazanavir plus ritonavir 400 mg BID or higher is contraindicated
	Carbamazepine, phenytoin, phenobarbital	Monitor anticonvulsant and tipranavir serum concentration and virologic response; consider alternative anticonvulsant and ritonavir boosting regimen
	Clarithromycin	Increased clarithromycin serum concentration; reduce clarithromycin dose by 50% if CLCR 30-60 mL/min; reduce clarithromycin dose by 75% if CLCR <30 mL/min; consider alternative therapy
	Rifabutin	Increased rifabutin serum concentrations; dose rifabutin 150 mg QOD or 3 times per week
	Benzodiazepines: Alprazolam Diazepam	Avoid concomitant use; consider alternative agent (eg, lorazepam, oxazepam or temazepam)
	Hormonal contraceptives	Boosted regimen: decreased ethinyl estradiol serum concentrations; use alternative or additional methods
	Atorvastatin, Rosuvastatin	Use lowest possible dose with careful monitoring; use alternative lipid-lowering agent
	Efavirenz	Decreased or no change in tipranavir serum concentration; use standard doses
	Etravirine	Decreased etravirine and increased tipranavir serum concentration; avoid coadministration

Table 9 (continued)

Drug-drug Interactions of Protease Inhibitors[a]

Protease Inhibitor	Interacting Drug	Interaction and Management Strategy
Tipranavir/ritonavir	Maraviroc	Use standard doses of maraviroc dose (eg, 300 mg BID)
	Methadone	For ritonavir-boosted regimen: decrease methadone erum concentration; monitor for methadone withdrawal; adjust dose as needed
	Warfarin	Monitor PT/INR; adjust dose as needed

[a] *Adapted from: Panel on Antiretroviral Guidelines for Adults and Adolescents: A Working Group of the Office of AIDS Research Advisory Council (OARAC), Department of Health and Human Services. Guidelines for the use of antiretroviral agents in HIV-1-infected adults and adolescents. November 3, 2008. Please refer to the product package insert and literature for complete details and a potential list of both studied and theoretical drug-drug interactions*

[b] *Ritonavir is used at low doses (eg, 100 to 200 mg) to increase serum concentration of most protease inhibitors so review other protease inhibitor recommendations; over 200 drugs used in HIV-infected patients have been identify for potential drug-drug interactions; please review the product package insert and literature for complete details and potential list of studied and theoretical interactions*

8. CCR5 Antagonist

- Maraviroc is a substrate of CYP3A enzymes and the P-glycoprotein transport system (Table 10)

- Maraviroc is neither an inhibitor or inducer of CYP3A enzymes.

- Maraviroc serum concentrations are significantly decreased by potent CYP3A inducers and significantly increased by potent CYP3A inhibitors.

9. Fusion and Integrase Inhibitors

- Enfuvirtide is currently the only available fusion inhibitor.

- Enfuvirtide undergoes catabolism of its amino acid constituent and is not associated with drug-drug interactions.

- Raltegravir is the only HIV integrase strand transfer inhibitor, and is primarily eliminated by glucuronidation (UGT1A1).

- Inducers of UGT1A1 (eg, rifampin, rifabutin, efavirenz or tipranavir/ritonavir) can reduce raltegravir serum concentrations, and these combinations should be carefully monitored and used cautiously.

Table 10

Dosing Recommendations for Maraviroc Associated with Drug-drug Interactions

Maraviroc Dosage	Dosing Recommendation for Interacting Drugs
300 mg BID	Standard dose of maraviroc with no concomitant administration of CYP3A inhibitors or inducers; recommended dosage of maraviroc with concomitant administration of tipranavir-ritonavir or nevirapine
150 mg BID	Reduced dose of maraviroc with concomitant administration of CYP3A4 inhibitors (with or without a CYP3A inducer) including protease inhibitors (exception: tipranavir-ritonavir [see above dosage recommendation]), delaviridine, ketoconazole, itraconazole, clarithromycin (including with etravirine plus ritonavir-boosted protease inhibitors or with efavirenz plus either lopinavir-ritonavir or saquinavir-ritonavir), and other strong CYP3A inhibitors (eg, nefazadone, telithromycin)
600 mg BID	Increased dose of maraviroc with CYP3A inducers (without a CYP3A inhibitor) including rifampin, carbamazepine, phenytoin, phenobarbital, efavirenz and etravirine

10. Antiherpesvirus Agents

- Most drug-drug interactions for antiherpesvirus agents involved inhibition of renal elimination (eg, probenecid or cimetidine) or increased pharmacodynamic effect (eg, increase risk of toxicities) (Table 11)

11. Anti-Influenza Agents

- Very few interactions are associated with anti-influenza agents (Table 12)

- Oseltamivir and zanamivir do not undergo metabolism or inhibit common human CYP isoforms (1A2, 2C9, 2C19, 2D6, and 3A4) and have a wide margin of safety.

Table 11

Drug-drug Interactions of Antiherpesvirus Agents

Antiviral Agent	Interacting Drug	Interaction and Management Strategy
Acyclovir, valacyclovir, famciclovir	Probenecid	Increased antiviral agent serum concentration; avoid concomitant use when high-dose acyclovir or patients who require a dose adjustment because of renal impairment or current adverse effects; monitor for adverse events
	Cimetidine	Increased antiviral agents serum concentration; avoid concomitant use when high-dose acyclovir or patients who require a dose adjustment because of renal impairment or current adverse effects; monitor for adverse events
	Mycophenolate	Increased serum concentration of antiviral agent and glucuronide metabolite of mycophenolate; monitor for adverse events and CBC
Acyclovir	Phenytoin, fosphenytoin, valproic acid	Increase risk of seizures; monitor seizure acitivity and serum concentration of the anticonvulsant agents; adjust dose as needed
	Theophylline	Increased theophylline serum concentration and risk of toxicity; monitor theophylline serum concentration and toxicity; decrease dose of theophylline as needed
	Zidovudine	Increase risk of neurotoxicity (eg, drowsiness, lethargy); monitor for adverse events
	Tizanidine	Increase tizanidine serum concentrations and risk of toxicity (eg, hypotension, sedation); concomitant therapy should be avoided; consider alternative agent for managing spasticity
Ganciclovir, valganciclovir	Zidovudine	Increase risk of hematologic toxicity (eg, anemia, neutropenia, pancytopenia) and GI toxicity; concomitant therapy should be avoided or used with caution with careful monitoring of hematologic function and at the lowest possible dose; consider alternative antiretroviral agent
	Nephrotoxic agents[a]	Additive injury to the renal tubule; concomitant therapy should be avoided or used with caution and includes monitoring of renal function and dosage adjustment creatinine clearance estimation

Table 11 (continued)

Drug-drug interactions of antiherpesvirus agents

Antiviral Agent	Interacting Drug	Interaction and Management Strategy
	Myelosuppressive agents[2]	Increase risk of blood dyscrasias; concomitant therapy should be avoided or used with caution at the lowest possible dose; consider alternative agent if possible
	Didanosine	Increase didanosine and slight decrease ganciclovir serum concentration; monitor for didanosine toxicity
	Probenecid	Increased ganciclovir serum concentration; monitor for ganciclovir toxicity
	Imipenem/cliastin	Increased risk of seizures; monitor adverse events and consider alternative antibacterial agent
Foscarnet	Nephrotoxic agents[1]	Direct or additive injury to the renal tubule; concomitant therapy should be avoided or used with caution and includes monitoring of renal function and dosage adjustment creatinine clearance estimation
	Intravenous pentamidine	Increased risk for severe symptomatic hypocalcemia; monitor electrolytes, calcium, and magnesium to minimize adverse events
	Saquinavir and/or ritonavir	Increased risk of abnormal renal function; monitor renal function and consider alternative antiretroviral agents
Cidofovir	Nephrotoxic agents[1]	Concomitant administration of cidofovir with potentially nephrotoxic drugs is contraindicated, and the manufacturer recommends waiting at least 7 days between exposure to these agents and administration of cidofovir
	Probenecid	Concomitant probenecid is used to decrease the risk of renal toxicity of cidofovir by decreasing its concentration within proximal tubular cells; careful monitoring for other drug-drug interactions of probenecid and dose adjust as needed

[1] *Examples include amphotericin B, cisplatin, cyclosporine, vancomycin, foscarnet, intravenous pentamidine, cidofivir, polymyxin B, colistin, radio contrast, and aminoglycosides*
[11] *Examples include antineoplastics, amphotericin B, flucytosine, dapsone, trimethoprim-sulfamethoxazole, intravenous pentamidine, primaquine, and pyrimethamine*

Table 12

Drug-drug Interactions of Aanti-Influenza Agents

Antiviral Agent	Interacting Drug	Interaction and Management Strategy
Amantadine	Anticholinergic agents[a] or antihistamines[b]	Increased CNS adverse effects (eg, additive anticholinergic effects); avoid combination or use lowest possible dose or alternative agent
	Buproprion	Increased risk of neurotoxicity (eg, restlessness, agitation, gait disturbances, dizziness); avoid combination or use alternative agent
	Triamterene-hydrochlorothiazine, quinidine, quinine or trimethroprim (alone or in combination with sulfamethoxazole)	Increased amantadine serum concentration and CNS toxicities; avoid combination or use lowest possible dose or alternative agent
Rimantadine	No major interactions	
Oseltamivir	Probenecid	Increased oseltamivir carboxylate metabolite serum concentration; no dose adjustment or monitoring is recommended because of wide margin of safety
Zanamivir	No major interactions	

[a] *Examples include benztropine, biperiden, and trihexyphenidyl*
[b] *Examples include chlorpheniramine and phenylpropanolamine*

12. Further Reading

Baciewicz AM, Chrisman CR, Finch CK, Self TH. Update on rifampin and rifabutin drug interactins. *Am J Med Sci*. 2008;335(2):126-136.

HIV InSite. University of California, San Francisco available at http://hivinsite.ucsf.edu. Accessed January 23, 2009.

Indiana University Department of Medicine. Cytochrome P450 drug interactions. Accessed January 23, 2009.

Nivoix Y, Leveque D, Herbrecht R, Koffel J-C, Beretz L, Ubeaud-Sequier G. The enzymatic basis of drug-drug intactions with systemic triazole antifungals. *Clin Pharmacokinet*. 2008;47(12):779-792.

Pai MP, Momary KM, Rodvold KA. Antibiotic drug interactions. *Med Clin N Am*. 2006;90:1223-1255.

Panel on Antiretroviral Guidelines for Adults and Adolescents: A Working Group of the Office of AIDS Research Advisory Council (OARAC), Department of Health and Human Services. Guidelines for the use of antiretroviral agents in HIV-1-infected adults and adolescents. November 3, 2008;1-146. Available at http://aidsinfo.nih.gov/contentfiles/AdultandAdolescentGL.pdf. Accessed on May 13, 2009.

Piscitelli SC, Gallicano KD. Interactions among drugs for HIV and opportunistic infections. *N Engl J Med* 2001;344(13):984-996.

Piscitelli SC, Rodvold, eds. Drug Interaction in Infectious Diseases, 2nd Totowa, New Jersey. : Humana Press Inc.; 2005.

Sousa M, Pozniak A, Boffito M. Pharmacokinetics and pharmacodynamics of drug interactions involving rifampin, rifabutin and antimalarial drugs. *J Antimicrob Chemother*. 2008;62:872-878.

Chapter 25: Immunizations for the ID Boards

Maria D. Mileno, MD

Contents

1. Introduction and General Concepts

- Immunizations are one of the most cost-effective health interventions available. There are 17 FDA-licensed vaccines in routine use in 2009. Additional vaccines for travelers include yellow fever vaccine, which requires a separate license for administration, and others. This chapter reviews, in outline form, all routine immunizations and those that may be helpful based upon individual itineraries and length of stay in endemic countries.

- It has become a specialist's task to advise travelers, and this is beyond the scope of this chapter. Individuals with altered immune status require special consideration, and the pertinent vaccine issues are noted in the individual vaccine sections here. **Live vaccines generally should be deferred until immune function has improved.** Certain vaccines, such as inactivated influenza and pneumococcal vaccines, are specifically recommended for persons with altered immunocompetence. All inactivated vaccines can be administered safely to such individuals, although they might be less effective during the period of altered immunocompetence.

- Immunizations reduce disease rates beyond the individual, for example:

    * Pneumococcal vaccine in adults aged 55 and over decreases rates of invasive pneumococcal disease

    * Children given pneumococcal conjugate and had associated 55% decrease of invasive pneumococcal disease **in adults** aged 50 and older.

- Ongoing vaccination efforts are important: recent outbreaks of measles in Indiana, polio in Minnesota, mumps on US college campuses occurred in undervaccinated communities.

2. Vaccine Update and Review

Influenza Virus Vaccines

Expansion of indications:

- Recommended for **all children** ages 6 months-18 years
    * Live or inactivated products are equally effective and may be used if immunocompetent

    * Age <9 years receiving vaccine for the first time require 2 doses separated by 4-6 weeks

- 1 dose annually is recommended for **all adults** over age 50 and those under age 50 with other risk factors:

    * Chronic medical conditions

    * Pregnant women (give inactivated product only)

    * Occupational risk: all health care workers

    * Lifestyle: nursing home residents, household contacts and caregivers of children

    * **Travelers taking long flights during flu season**

- **Inactivated: trivalent influenza virus** vaccine is composed of inactivated disrupted "split" influenza viruses or purified surface antigens. The antigenic content of the vaccine is changed annually to reflect the influenza A and B strains in circulation. Efficacy is directly related to the degree of concordance between the virus strains included in the vaccine and the strains circulating in the community. When major changes in structure occur in nature, vaccine made from other antigens can have decreased effectiveness; however, some cross protection may still result. AEs are infrequent and can include local injection site tenderness and low grade fever in 3%-5 % of recipients.

- **Live Attenuated Influenza** vaccine is administered intranasally and consists of 6 internal genes from a cold-adapted, temperature-sensitive attenuated mutant virus. The hemagglutinin and neuraminidase are derived from recently circulating wild strains. Cold adaptation supports growth of the vaccine viruses in the upper airways; temperature sensitivity decreases their growth in the lower airways.

- **AEs result from live product only can include coryza, nasal congestion, headache and sore throat. Children aged 12-59 months reported increased reactive airways disease over placebo, which has not been seen in older age groups.**

Diphtheria Tetanus Pertussis

- **Pertussis** is the only vaccine preventable childhood illness with increasing rates in the U.S.

- Vaccine available since the 1940s.

- Acellular product made from purified components of *Bordetella pertussis* and detoxified pertussis toxin.

- Whole cell products (killed whole *B pertussis* suspensions) no longer used in U.S., but are still used internationally.

- Children: DTaP 3 doses IM age 2, 4 and 6 months of age, and fourth dose at age 15-18 months; fifth dose at age 4-6 years,

    * "big" D = larger dose of diphtheria for primary vaccination

    * age >10: use Tdap

        • Boostrix age 10-18 approved

        • Adacel age 11-64

* Tdap is replacing Td, which is indicated every 10 years (unless traveling, consider boosting within 5 years of travel). Can safely administer Tdap to all who have not had vaccine in 2 years, and we should target adults in contact with infants, **postpartum women** and health care workers with direct patient contact.

- **Pregnant women** who received the last Td vaccination 10 or more years previously can receive **Td during the second or third trimester, or Tdap in the immediate postpartum period**.

Tetanus and Diphtheria Toxoid (Td)

- One of the most effective immunizing agents known, this aluminum precipitated preparation is recommended for use in all US residents without contraindication in the primary course of 2 doses administered 4-8 weeks apart and a third dose given 6-12 months apart. **Tdap** (see above) should replace a **single dose** of Td for adults ages 19-64 years who have not received a dose of Tdap previously. Adults with uncertain or incomplete history of primary vaccination can have the first 2 doses at least 4 weeks apart and the third dose at 6-12 months after the second: Tdap can substitute for any **one** of the 3 doses. Can use either Td or Tdap for booster doses after 10 years.

- Td or Tdap can be used as prophylaxis in wound management (see ACIP statement), which generally is given for soiled injuries if 5 years have passed since the last tetanus dose.

- **Travelers who have received Td or Tdap within 5 years can avoid needles in foreign countries if cut or injured**
- Common **AE's**: local reactions and fever

- Sometimes after multiple doses: Arthus-like reaction

- Rare: brachial plexus neuropathy

- GBS

- **Contraindications:** severe hypersensitivity reactions

Hepatitis A and B combination vaccine (Twinrix) is commonly recommended for travelers. Frequent short term travel poses risk, not only for food- and water-borne illness from ubiquitous environmental hepatitis A in endemic countries, but also inadvertent medical interventions, unplanned and intentional sexual contact and cultural activities that may lead to hepatitis B exposure. **The accelerated 4-**

dose schedule is now included in the routine guidelines and can be useful for travelers who are leaving in 1 month. Administer on Day 0, 7, 21 to 30 and at month 12, or, if time permits, routine schedule is Day 0, 1 month and 6 months.

Hepatitis A Vaccine

- Hepatitis A is the most common vaccine preventable illness worldwide.

- 2 inactivated hepatitis A vaccines are available in the U.S. and are equivalent in safety and efficacy. More than 97% of individuals age 2 and over acquire protective titres after a single dose. A second dose given 6-12 months later (Havris) or 6-18 months later (Vaqta) confers long-term protection.

- Recommended for:

  * **All children age 1 and over and adults**, especially those traveling to endemic regions; communities in the southwestern U.S. have higher rates of hepatitis A, and the vaccine is recommended to those schoolchildren

  * Indiviudals with **chronic liver disease**

  * **Men who have sex with men**

  * **Illegal drug users**

  * Individuals who work with hepatitis A-infected primates or do laboratory research with the virus

Hepatitis B Vaccine

- Purified inactivated HBsAg particles.

  * In the U.S., all yeast derived through recombinant DNA technology

  * Abroad, some plasma derived products are still used

- Recommended for all newborns in the U.S.

- Must also continue to target high-risk individuals:

  * Health care workers

  * **Hemodialysis patients**

  * Parenteral drug users

  * Household and sexual contacts of chronic Hep B carriers

  * Travelers: both frequent short term travelers as well as those who plan prolonged stays

- Infants born to HBsAg positive mothers: give Hep B vaccine **as well as Hep B IG within 12 hours.**

- 3-dose schedule: dose at time, 0 (or at birth in newborn), 1 month, 6 months confers protective antibody: greater than 10 m IU/ml at following rates:

  * >95% of infants and children

  * >90% of adults <40 years old

  * 75%-90% of adults >40

- No booster doses recommended.

- **Adults receiving hemodialysis or with other immunocompromising conditions: 1 dose of 40 ug/ml (Recombivax) or 2 doses of 20 ug/ml (Energix B) administered simultaneously on a 4-dose schedule can be given at Day 0, 1, 2 and 6 months.**

- Few AES, primarily local reactions and low grade fever, **rare** anaphylaxis; alopecia

- Contraindication: hypersensitivity to yeast

Human Papilloma Virus (HPV)

- High risk genotypes include types 16, 18, 31, 33, 45 and other associated with oncogenic changes of the cervix.

- HPV is identified 99.7% of cervical cancers, 70% of cervical cancer associated with types 16 and 18, quadrivalent HPV vaccine – targets types 6, 11, 16, 18

* Use in females aged 9-26.

* Contain NO viral DNA, only antigens/virus-like particles

* Ideal immunization: prior to potential HPV in sexual encounters may be extended to older ages for partial benefit; not licensed indication

* Females with evidence of HPV (+ PAP, genital warts) **should also** receive vaccination: unlikely to have all 4 genotypes

* 3-dose series: 0, 2 months and 6 months

* **Not** recommended during pregnancy

* Contraindicated if history of life-threatening allergic reaction to yeast or prior dose

Herpes Zoster Vaccine (varicella-zoster or shingles)

• Approved for adults over age 60

• Boosts waning cell-mediated immunity to VZV

• Lyophilized prep of live attenuated VZV: has considerably more plaque-forming units of virus than the varicella (chicken pox vaccine) although made from the same strain (Oka/Merck strain)

• Incidence of shingles was reduced by 51% in vaccine recipients; highest efficacy in subjects 60-69 years old.

• **Contraindications:**

   * **Immunocompromise**

   * Severe allergy

   * Tuberculosis

   * **Pregnancy**

• **AEs:** local reactions; no vaccine virus detected in recipients who went on to develop zoster, no evidence of vaccine spread to others

Measles Vaccine

This live attenuated virus vaccine offers greater than 95% efficacy when administered to a child aged 12-15 months or older. Yet, 2%-5 % of vaccinated persons fail to seroconvert after an initial dose, and there is evidence that measles transmission can be sustained in communities due to this issue. Beginning in 1989, a 2-dose schedule was recommended in the U.S. Mortality rates from measles declined from 2000 to 2007 by 74%, most significantly in heavily stricken areas including southeast Asia and sub-Saharan Africa, yet industrialized European countries including Switzerland, the United Kingdom, Italy and Germany have had large outbreaks and deaths, often because parents chose not to vaccinate their children against measles.

• Administer 2 doses at 12-15 months and at 4-6 years.

• Can be administered additionally as early as 6 months of age if traveling to measles endemic regions, and would require re-dosing at above ages upon return.

Indications

• Adults born before 1957 are considered immune.

• **Adults born during or after 1957 should receive 1 MMR dose unless:**
   * **Medically contraindicated (immunocompromised or pregnant)**

   * Have 2 documented doses of MMR

   * Have a history of measles based on health care provider diagnosis

   * Have laboratory evidence of immunity

• **2 MMR doses are indicated for the following individuals:**
   *Adults who have been recently exposed to measles

*Adults who have been vaccinated with killed measles vaccine or unknown type of vaccine (1963-1967 product)

* College or postgraduate students

* Health care workers

* International travelers

• **AEs:** high fever (to 39.4° C or greater) and transient rashes occur in 5% of vaccine recipients beginning 7-12 days after vaccination and lasting 1-2 days.

* Rare: anaphylaxis and thrombocytopenic purpura

* 1 in 2 million reported encephalopathy with onset 10 days after vaccination (no causal role for measles vaccine established.)

* **NO evidence for causal role in autism.**

* Anaphylaxis to eggs is not a contraindication: can give vaccine with added observation.

Mumps

• Live attenuated virus age 12 months or over, as MMR.

• 2 dose schedule; second dose at age 4-6 years.

• Travelers as young as 6 months (see travel) can receive vaccine, but dose doesn't count and must be repeated on schedule or after travel.

• Adults born during or after 1957: 1 dose unless history of mumps or contraindication.

• Consider revaccination during outbreak or + titre.

• **Contraindications:**
    * Pregnancy

    * Immunocompromise

• **AEs:**
    * Rare parotitis and orchitis

*TTP and anaphylaxis, exceedingly rare

Rubella Vaccine

• Live attenuated, part of MMR, administer at age 12 months.

* Confers 95% immunity, long-lasting after single dose

* Persons born before 1957 considered immune, **however**, still must check titers in females with childbearing potential

* Avoid vaccine during pregnancy but inadvertent administration should not be a reason to consider termination of pregnancy

• **AEs:**
    * Low-grade fever and rash 5%-10%.

    * Joint pains 25%

    * Acute arthritis 10%; risk of arthritis after *vaccine* substantially lower than risk after natural rubella

Pneumococcal Vaccine

Current guidelines expand use of pneumococcal polysaccharide vaccination to all persons with asthma and history of cigarette smoking. Alaskan Natives and American Indians no longer require routine use of PPSV under age 65, unless there are warranting medical conditions or public health authorities identify and announce areas in which the risk of invasive disease is increased.

• **Polysaccharide Vaccine**
    * Contains 23 serotypes of pneumococcal capsular polysaccharide

    * Responsible for 85-90% of bacteremic disease from pneumococcus in the U.S.

    * 80%-95% of healthy recipients demonstrate protective antibodies

    * Indications:

- Adults and children >2 years old at high risk due to underlying medical conditions as well as immunocompromise

- HIV-infected persons, as close to time of diagnosis as possible

- Healthy elderly >65

- Revaccination:

  * For persons over age 65, one time revaccination if they were under age 65 at time of primary vaccination

  * For persons with underlying medical conditions and immunocompromise, one time revaccination after 5 years

  - AEs: mild erythema and pain at injection site is 50%

    * Rare: anaphylaxis

- **Conjugate:** pneumococcal capsular polysaccharide is covalently linked to protein carriers

  *7 polysaccharide types account for 80% of invasive infection in children <6 years

  * 4-dose series age 2, 4, 6 and 12-15 years

  * Also continue to use in older children with high risk of pneumococcal disease

- **AEs:** if administered with other childhood vaccines, can be associated with fever >100.4° F within 48 hours.

Polio

- **One dose during adulthood is indicated for travel**

- Only inactivated product (enhanced potency IPV) is used in U.S.

- OPV can rarely cause paralytic polio

  * Greatest risk after 1st dose

* Overall risk 1:750,000 first doses

- **Adults can contract vaccine associated polio from babies/others given OPV, commonly given outside of the U.S.**

Varicella Vaccine (Chicken Pox)

- Recent guidelines advise adults who had only one dose in the past to receive a **second dose** unless medically contraindicated.

  * Highly effective against *severe* varicella 95%-100% and less so against mild disease (70%-90%).

  * Minimum age: 12 months

  * 2-dose schedule 12-15 months and 4-6 years

  * Second dose can be given sooner but at least 3 months after first

  ***Adults without evidence of immunity who are not pregnant or immunocompromised should receive 2 doses.**

  * Evidence of immunity:

    - 2 documented vaccine doses 4 to 8 weeks apart

    - Born in U.S. before 1980 (exception: check titers for healthcare workers and pregnant women)

    - History of varicella or herpes zoster diagnosed by a physician

Haemophilus influenzae Type b Vaccine

- Conjugated vaccines have replaced earlier polysaccharide vaccines.

  * Elicit higher antibody titers

  * Effective in young infants

  * Polysaccharide is covalently linked to protein carriers and are T cell-dependent antigens

* 3-dose series: age 2, 4 and 6 months

* **IF** the following combination products are used at 2 and 4 months:

* PedvaxHIB

* Com Vax

* Then, the 6 month dose can be omitted.

- * Use triHiBit only for booster doses not primary inoculation

• **Consider adult vaccination prior to splenectomy along with pneumococcal and meningococcal immunization.**

Rotavirus

• New, live oral pentavalent is now available

• 3-dose series beginning at age 6 weeks targets strains responsible for >90% rotavirus gastroenteritis in the U.S.

• **Earlier monovalent and tetravalent produces were withdrawn due to increased risk of intussusception.**

•**AEs:** diarrhea, vomiting, otitis media, nasopharyngitis, bronchospasm.

• **Contraindications:** serious allergic reaction.

• Full protection lasts 1 year to decrease hospital and ER care by 95% for this disease; 88% protection during the second year post-vaccination.

Meningococcal

• Newest Guidelines: revaccinate every 5 years if indicated for travel

• Both vaccines protect against serogroups **A, C, Y, W-135**

• **Tetravalent polysaccharide MPSV4 is recommended for ages 2-10 and over age 55 and is an acceptable alternative for ages 11-55.**

• Indications: persons with terminal complement deficiencies, asplenia or planning splenectomy, and travelers to countries where N meningitidis is hyperendemic or epidemic, and especially if contact with local population will be prolonged.

• **Conjugate MCV4** available since 2005 for ages 11-55 A, C, Y, W-135 induces greater duration of immunity

*Indicated for all 11-12 year olds or upon high school entry if previously unvaccinated; for college freshmen living in dormitories and military recruits

* Expensive

* Contains large amounts of diphtheria toxoid however we can give Tdap simultaneously if indicated.

• **AEs:** case reports of Guillain-Barré Syndrome (GBS) after MCV4

* From 2005: do not give this conjugate product if patient has a h/o GBS.

3. Vaccines in Immunocompromised Hosts

• **Severe compromise:** The following individuals:[a]

    * Must avoid live viral or live bacterial vaccines

    * May require additional vaccines when healthy

    * May receive decreased protection from vaccines

[a] Persons with **active** leukemia, lymphoma, generalized malignancy, aplastic anemia, graft vs. host disease, congenital immunodeficiency or persons who have received current or recent radiation therapy, solid organ transplant (SOT) or bone marrow transplant within 2 years of transplantation, or persons whose transplants are of longer duration but who are still taking immunosuppressive drugs.

• SOT: much higher risk of infection occurs within the first year of transplant so high risk travel might be postponed until after that time.

Persons on Compromising Medications:

High dose steroids: given for more than 2 weeks: wait at least 1 month after discontinuation before administration of any live virus vaccination; greater than physiologic doses can blunt immune response to vaccines. The immunosuppressive effects of steroid treatment vary, but the majority of clinicians consider a dose equivalent to either >2 mg/kg of body weight or 20 mg/day of prednisone or equivalent for persons who weigh >10 kg when administered for >2 weeks as sufficiently immunosuppressive to raise concern about the safety of vaccination with live-virus vaccines.

TNF-blocking Agents[b] and IL-1 Receptor Antagonists:

• Safety of live vaccine is unknown: most practicing clinicians reluctant to use live vaccines

[b] Agents such as etanercept, adalimumab and infliximab are known to activate latent mycobacterial infection as well as to increase overall susceptibility to fungal and other serious infections.

• Other agents causing severe immunosuppression, which result in increased rates of infection and blunting of response to killed vaccines:

    *Alkylating agents (eg, cyclophosphamide)

    *Antimetabolites (eg, azathioprine, 6-mercaptopurine)

    * Transplant-related immunosuppressive drugs (eg, cyclosporine, tacrolimus, sirolimus and mycophenolate mofetil)

    * Mitoxantrone (used in multiple sclerosis), and most cancer chemotherapeutic agents (excluding tamoxifen).

    * Methotrexate, including low-dose weekly regimens, is classified as severely immunosuppressive, as evidenced by increased rates of opportunistic infections and blunting of responses to killed vaccines.

• **AIDS**: persons with CD4+ cell counts less than 200 or who have had history of an AIDS-defining illness or symptomatic HIV are severely compromised: newly diagnosed individuals can delay travel pending reconstitution of their CD4+ cell counts with antiretroviral therapy to minimize risk of infection and avoid immune reconstitution illness during travel.

• **Moderately compromised:** chronic diseases with limited immune deficits: asplenia, chronic renal disease, chronic hepatic disease from cirrhosis and alcoholism, diabetes and nutritional deficiencies; persons taking ribavirin and interferon for hepatitis C infection risk **neutropenia**. Theoretical risk but no information on decreased vaccine efficacy or increased adverse events with live viral antigens is available.

• **Not compromised**: for the purpose of vaccination, persons with the following conditions are not considered to be immunocompromised:

    * Corticosteroid therapy under the following circumstances:

- Short- or long-term daily or alternate day therapy with 20 mg or less of prednisone or equivalent

- Long-term, alternate day treatment with short-acting preparations

- Maintenance physiologic doses (replacement therapy)

- Steroid inhalers

- Topical steroids (skin, ears or eyes)

- Intraarticular, bursal or tendon injection of steroids; or if longer than 1 month has passed since high-dose steroids (greater than 20 mg per day of prednisone or equivalent for longer than 2 weeks) have been used

* Some experts will wait 2 weeks prior to the administration of measles vaccine following short-term (less than 2 weeks) of therapy with daily or alternate day dosing of greater than 20 mg of prednisone or equivalent

* HIV patients with >500 CD4+ cell count lymphocytes

* Longer than 3 months since chemotherapy for leukemia/lymphoma or cancer, and the malignancy is in remission. Although some clinicians suggest waiting only 1 month since a last dose of immunosuppressive medications (including TNF-blockers) that are not being used for the chemotherapy of cancer, data are inconclusive. This recommendation may primarily refer to corticosteroids, but it remains unknown exactly how long is safest.

* Bone marrow transplant, if longer than 2 years post-transplant, not on immunosuppressive drugs and without graft vs. host disease.

* Definitive data do not exist with respect to autoimmune diseases in the absence of any overlay of immunosuppressive drugs (eg, systemic lupus erythematosus, inflammatory bowel disease, rheumatoid arthritis or multiple sclerosis). The ACIP's advice for the normal use of all live-virus as well as killed vaccines in multiple sclerosis (MS) patients who are not undergoing a current exacerbation of disease is reinforced by the National MS Society (www.nationalmssociety.org/Sourcebook-vaccinations.asp), a source well respected by MS patients and their physicians. In the past, many practicing neurologists have strongly advised their MS patients against the use of live-virus vaccines at any time. If possible, MS patients should not receive any vaccine for 6 weeks after the onset of a disease exacerbation. Immunomodulatory agents commonly used in MS patients, such as interferons and glatiramer acetate, are not thought to affect vaccine response or safety, but definitive data are lacking. In these special circumstances, travel health advisors should confer with the traveler's other physicians in developing an appropriate plan.

- **Recommend:** Hib, Meningococcal, Pneumococcal, influenza

    * Consideration and warning about yellow fever.

4. Vaccines in Pregnancy

• **Contraindicated vaccines: MMR, varicella**

• Vaccines for which **data are not available**

  * **Tdap:** offer Td, however, if pertussis risk is great in some situations recommend during second or third trimester

  * **Hepatitis A:** weigh benefit or give immune globulin

  * **Japanese encephalitis:** weigh benefit

  * **Meningococcal conjugate** weigh benefit; polysaccharide indicated especially in outbreak

  * **Typhoid (Ty21a) oral** product no data however injectable polysaccharide (ViCPS) is indicated for travel

• **Postponement of travel preferable** to vaccination but indicated if exposure can't be avoided: **Yellow fever**

• **Safe and indicated** for pregnant individuals:

  * Immune globulin

  * Td (prefer administration during second or third trimester)

  * Influenza

  * Meningococcal typhoid and pneumococcal *polysaccharide* products

5. Additional Commonly Used Travel Vaccines

• **Yellow fever**

• **Typhoid**

• **Japanese Encephalitis**

Yellow Fever Vaccine

• Because of recent reports of deaths due to YF vaccination travelers to high risk areas should be encouraged and targeted accurately.

• YF is a viral disease with illness ranging from influenza-like syndrome to severe hepatitis, liver failure and hemorrhagic fever (case fatality rate approximately 20%), occurs only in sub-Saharan Africa and tropical South America where it is endemic and intermittently epidemic.

• Vaccine fully prevents yellow fever with single 0.5 ml subcutaneous injection of reconstituted products.

• International health regulation allows countries to require proof of vaccination for entry and/or from travelers arriving from certain countries. Travelers without an approved, completed international certificate of vaccination (ICV) for yellow fever may be quarantined or refused entry unless they submit to onsite vaccination. Must be administered at an approved (licensed) yellow fever vaccination center, certificate is valid 10 days after vaccination and for subsequent 10 years. Certificate may be required even for travelers only transiting endemic region.

• **AEs:** mostly mild reactions

  * Headache, myalgia, low grade fever, can last 5-10 days

  * 1% must curtail regular activities

  * Rash, urticaria, asthma uncommon <0.8/100,000

• Vaccine-associated neurologic disease

• Encephalitis-historically only in infants too young to have vaccine.

* Since 1992: 6 cases reported in adult recipients

* 10 cases of autoimmune neurologic disease including GBS and acute disseminated encephalitis

* All began 4-27 days after vaccination and all were first-time recipients

* 0.5/100,000 doses

* Vaccine associated viscerotropic disease

* Multisystem organ failure reported in 12 cases since 1996

* Disease similar to naturally acquired YF

* 24 suspected cases identified worldwide since 2006

* Higher in persons older than 60 (1.8 cases/100,000 in this age group)

• **Contraindications**:
  * Age younger than 6 months: absolutely contraindicated

  * Should delay immunization until infant is 9 months and if considering vaccination any younger should seek advice at CDC

  * **Increased age poses increased risk** of AE but benefits and risks should be weighed

  * **Immunosuppression:** avoid YF vaccine – **see section on immunosuppression**

  * **History of Thymus Disease, recently identified as a contraindication**

  * **Pregnancy** – avoid, waive if only required for country protection requirements; if she must travel to areas where risk of infection is high, vaccinate and follow infant closely with guidance from CDC

  * **Breastfeeding** – avoid vaccine

* **HIV with less than 200 CD4+ cells** – avoid and CD4 >200 and cannot avoid exposure – offer vaccine and monitor closely for AE. If country requirements only – waive. Seroconversion rate may be reduced

* **Hypersensitivity** – egg allergy or chicken hypersensitivity.

* Administration with other Vaccines, MMR, varicella

  • Ideally administer YF with other live vaccines **concurrently** or 4 weeks apart or may risk impaired immune response

  • All commonly used vaccines can safely and effectively be given simultaneously and is encouraged at separate sites preferably

Typhoid

Persons traveling to endemic regions for 2 or more weeks or who may be adventurous eaters/unable to comply with strict food and water precautions may benefit from typhoid vaccination. Two available vaccines confer only 60%-70% protection which waves over time.

• Typhoid polysaccharide injectable (Typhim Vi) is given as 1 dose prior to travel and lasts 2 years.

  * **AEs:** local injection site soreness, mild fever, chills

• Oral typhoid vaccine (Ty21a/Vivotif) is a live attenuated vaccine consisting of 4 doses given every other day over the course of 1 week to confer local intestinal immunity. Protection lasts 5 years. Dose must be taken on an empty stomach (fasting >3 hours) or dose will be digested and thus ineffective)

  * AEs: nausea and vomiting occasionally occur

• Whole cell injectable product is no longer available and had the most significant AE's including hypotension, rash, fever and systemic symptoms.

Japanese Encephalitis

- Vaccine is currently indicated for travelers to Asia and India who will spend 3 or more weeks in agricultural regions during season of transmission.

- Vaccine is given on Day 0, 7, 21 and persons must have 10 additional days before travel out of U.S. to exclude late onset of adverse events.

- AE's anaphylaxis approximately 1%, delayed type hypersensitivity reactions have occurred.

- Of note, a presentation of ASTMH in December 2008 revealed that recommendations may require updating: a retrospective review of cases of Japanese encephalitis showed that half of the cases in Western travelers may have acquired Japanese encephalitis during journeys that did not fulfill the above criteria for indications for Japanese encephalitis vaccination. 3 recovered, 4 died and 11 were left with severe neurologic sequelae.

6. Further Reading

All of the latest immunization schedules can be found on this CDC website http://www.cdc.gov/vaccines/recs/schedules/child-schedule.htm.

CDC. Prevention and control of influenza: recommendations of the Advisory Committee on Immunization Practices (ACIP), 2008. *MMWR*. 2008;57(No. RR-7):8.

CDC. Recommended Adult Immunization Schedule-United States, 2009. *MMWR*. Jan 9, 2009; 57(53):Q1-Q4.

CDC. Recommended Immunization Schedules for Persons Aged 0-18 Years – United States 2009. *MMWR*. Jan 2, 2009:57(51):Q1-Q4.

CDC. Health Information for International Travel 2008. Atlanta, GA: US Department of Health and Human Services, Public Health Service, 2007.

Cortese MM, Jordan HT, Curns AT, et al. Mumps vaccine performance among university students during a mumps outbreak. *Clin Infect Dis*. 2008;46(8):1172-1180.

Dayan GH, Rubin S. Mumps Outbreaks in Vaccinated Populations: are available mumps vaccines effective enough to prevent outbreaks? *Clin Infect Dis*. 2008;1(47):1458-1467.

Hicks L, Mileno MD. Preparing the immunocompromised traveler. In: Keystone JS, Kozarsky, PE, Freedman DO, Nothdurft HD, Connor BA, eds. *Travel Medicine*. 2nd ed. New York, NY: Elsevier; 2009.

Middleman AB. Immunization update: pertussis, meningococcus and human papillomavirus. *Adolesc Med Clin*. 2006;17(3):547-563.

Mileno MD, Bia FJ. The compromised traveler. *Infect Dis Clin North Am*. 1998;12:369-412.

Chapter 26:
Questions for the ID Boards

Stephen M. Smith, MD

Chapter numbers refer to "Principles and Practices of Infectious Diseases", sixth edition, edited by Mandell, Bennett, and Dolin, Elsevier/Churchill Livingstone, Philadelphia, PA, 2005.

1. Penicillin kills bacteria by:
   a. Blocking protein synthesis.
   b. Creating holes in bacterial cell membrane.
   c. Blocking peptidoglycan cross-linking.
   d. Causing autolysis.
   e. Unknown mechanisms.

2. Bacteria are resistant to β-lactams through all of the following ways, except:
   a. Destruction of β-lactam ring by β-lactamase.
   b. Inability of antibiotic to penetrate cell wall.
   c. Mutation of ribosomal proteins.
   d. Low affinity penicillin-binding proteins.

3. *S. aureus'* main mechanism of resistance to penicillin is through:
   a. Alterations of PBPs.
   b. Chromosomally encoded β-lactamase.
   c. Plasmid encoded β-lactamase.
   d. Increased cell wall thickness, which inhibits penetration of penicillin.

4. The β-lactamases of Gram-positive bacteria:
   a. Are located in the periplasmic space between the outer and inner lipid membranes.
   b. Are not common.
   c. Freely diffuse in the surrounding environment.
   d. Play little role in antibiotic resistance.

5. Mechanisms by which Gram-negative bacteria mediate resistance to β-lactam antibiotics include all of the following, except:
   a. Destruction of antibiotic by β-lactamase.
   b. Exclusion of antibiotic by porin mutation.
   c. Increased cell thickness.
   d. Transport of drug out of periplasmic space.
   e. Mutations in bacterial gyrases.

6. Semi-synthetic penicillins, such as nafcillin and methicillin, are active against most strains of penicillin resistant *S. aureus*, because they:
   a. Have increased affinity for the *S. aureus* PBPs.
   b. Are not cleaved by the *S. aureus* β-lactamase.
   c. Penetrate the outer membrane more efficiently.
   d. Have increased plasma and tissue concentrations.

7. Untoward reactions to penicillins include all of the following, except:
   a. Induction of seizures.
   b. Interstitial nephritis.
   c. Skin rash.
   d. Neutropenia.
   e. Interstitial pneumonitis.

8. Cefoxitin covers most isolates of the following bacteria, except:
   a. *B. fragilis*.
   b. *E. coli*.
   c. *S. aureus*.
   d. *Enterococcus* spp.

9. Which of the following does not have allergic cross reactivity with other β-lactam antibiotics?
   a. Meropenem.
   b. Ertapenem.
   c. Imipenem.
   d. Aztreonam.
   e. Cefotetan.

10. In patients with a history of a morbilliform rash to penicillin, one should:
    a. Avoid cephalosporins completely.
    b. Perform a skin test with penicillin major and minor determinants, and use a cephalosporin if the skin test is negative.
    c. Use a cephalosporin without testing.
    d. Desensitize with an oral penicillin protocol.

Chapter numbers refer to "Principles and Practices of Infectious Diseases", sixth edition, edited by Mandell, Bennett, and Dolin, Elsevier/Churchill Livingstone, Philadelphia, PA, 2005.

Questions 11-14: True or False

Answers:

1.	E
2.	C
3.	C
4.	C
5.	C
6.	B
7.	E
8.	D
9.	D
10.	C
11.	B
12.	B
13.	A
14.	B
15.	E

11. Most patients with a history of penicillin allergy are skin test positive.
    a. True
    b. False

12. 1-3% of skin test negative patients develop anaphylaxis after receiving penicillin.
    a. True
    b. False

13. In patients with history of penicillin allergy and positive skin test, the rate of acute immediate or accelerated allergic reaction is over 50%.
    a. True
    b. False

14. In skin test positive patients, carbapenems can be used.
    a. True
    b. False

15. A morbilliform rash secondary to penicillin is an example of which of the following types of immune or allergic reaction?
    a. Type I.
    b. Type II.
    c. Type III.
    d. Type IV.
    e. None of the above.

Chapter numbers refer to "Principles and Practices of Infectious Diseases", sixth edition, edited by Mandell, Bennett, and Dolin, Elsevier/Churchill Livingstone, Philadelphia, PA, 2005.

1. Tetracyclines inhibit bacteria by:
   a. Blocking DNA gyrase and topoisomerase activity.
   b. Binding to the 50s ribosomal subunit.
   c. Binding to the 30s ribosomal subunit.
   d. Blocking cell wall synthesis.

2. The most common side-effects of tetracyclines include all of the following, except:
   a. Photoxicity.
   b. Discoloration of growing teeth.
   c. Induction of seizures.
   d. Hepatitis.
   e. Nausea and vomiting.

3. Chloramphenicol inhibits bacteria by all of the following, except:
   a. Reversibly binding to the 50s ribosomal subunit.
   b. Preventing attachment of the aminoacyl-transfer RNA.
   c. Causing autolysis of bacterial cells.
   d. Blocking protein synthesis.

4. Chloramphenicol bone marrow toxicity:
   a. Is never dose related.
   b. Is always irreversible.
   c. Is less common in newborns.
   d. Can be idiosyncratic.

5. Rifamycins inhibit bacteria by:
   a. Reversibly binding to the 50s ribosomal subunit.
   b. Preventing attachment of the aminoacyl-transfer RNA.
   c. Causing autolysis of bacterial cells.
   d. Blocking RNA transcription.
   e. Blocking DNA gyrase and topoisomerase IV.

6. Rifampin has clearly been shown to:
   a. Improve response rates in osteomyelitis, when used with other agents.
   b. Hasten clearance of bacteremia in *S. aureus* endocarditis when used with vancomycin or nafcillin.
   c. Effectively eradicate meningococcal carriage.
   d. Be the drug of choice for chancroid.

7. Metronidazole kills bacteria by:
   a. Reversibly binding to the 50s ribosomal subunit.
   b. Preventing attachment of the aminoacyl-transfer RNA.
   c. Damaging bacterial DNA through production of free radicals.
   d. Blocking RNA transcription.
   e. Blocking DNA gyrase and topoisomerase IV.

8. Macrolides inhibit bacteria by:
   a. Reversibly binding to the 50s ribosomal subunit.
   b. Preventing attachment of the aminoacyl-transfer RNA.
   c. Damaging bacterial DNA through production of free radicals.
   d. Blocking RNA transcription.
   e. Blocking DNA gyrase.

9. Azithromycin covers all of the following bacteria, except:
   a. *H. influenzae*.
   b. Erythromycin resistant *S. pneumoniae*.
   c. *S. pyogenes*.
   d. *M. catarrhalis*.
   e. *L. pneumophila*.

10. Properties of linezolid include all of the following, except:
    a. Bactericidal activity against susceptible *S. aureus* strains.
    b. Inhibition of protein synthesis.
    c. Being an oxazolidinone.
    d. Causing bone marrow suppression.

Chapter numbers refer to "Principles and Practices of Infectious Diseases", sixth edition, edited by Mandell, Bennett, and Dolin, Elsevier/Churchill Livingstone, Philadelphia, PA, 2005.

11. Trimethroprim-sulfamethoxazole inhibits bacteria by:
    a. Sequential blockage of cell wall synthesis.
    b. Inhibition of protein synthesis.
    c. Sequential blockage of folic acid synthesis.
    d. Inhibition of DNA gyrase and topoisomerase IV.

12. Which quinolone has the most potency against Gram-negative bacteria?
    a. Moxifloxacin.
    b. Gatifloxacin.
    c. Levofloxacin.
    d. Ciprofloxacin.
    e. Trovafloxacin.

Answers:

1.	C
2.	C
3.	C
4.	D
5.	D
6.	C
7.	C
8.	A
9.	B
10.	A
11.	C
12.	D

Chapter numbers refer to "Principles and Practices of Infectious Diseases", sixth edition, edited by Mandell, Bennett, and Dolin, Elsevier/Churchill Livingstone, Philadelphia, PA, 2005.

1. Isoniazid kills *M. tuberculosis* through inhibition of:
    a. Folic acid synthesis.
    b. Mycolic acid synthesis.
    c. DNA synthesis.
    d. Arabinosyl transferase.
    e. Cell wall synthesis.
    f. Unknown pathways.

2. Pyrazinamide kills *M. tuberculosis* through inhibition of:
    a. Folic acid synthesis.
    b. Mycolic acid synthesis.
    c. DNA synthesis.
    d. Arabinosyl transferase.
    e. Cell wall synthesis.
    f. Unknown pathways.

3. Ethambutol inhibits *M. tuberculosis* through inhibition of:
    a. Folic acid synthesis.
    b. Mycolic acid synthesis.
    c. DNA synthesis.
    d. Arabinosyl transferase.
    e. Cell wall synthesis.
    f. Unknown pathways.

4. Amphotericin B kills fungi by:
    a. Disrupting the cell membrane.
    b. Inhibiting C-14α demethylase.
    c. Interfering with DNA synthesis.
    d. Inhibiting the synthesis of β (1, 3)-D-glucan.
    e. Inhibiting squalene epoxidase.

5. Azoles inhibit fungi by:
    a. Disrupting the cell membrane.
    b. Inhibiting C-14α demethylase.
    c. Interfering with DNA synthesis.
    d. Inhibiting the synthesis of β (1, 3)-D-glucan.
    e. Inhibiting squalene epoxidase.

6. Caspofungin inhibits fungi by:
    a. Disrupting the cell membrane.
    b. Inhibiting C-14α demethylase.
    c. Interfering with DNA synthesis.
    d. Inhibiting the synthesis of β (1, 3)-D-glucan.
    e. Inhibiting squalene epoxidase.

Questions 7-8: True or False

7. "Slow acetylators" have higher levels of isoniazid and better outcomes as a result.
    a. True
    b. False

8. Rifampin increases the level of many drugs through its effects on the cytochrome P-450 complex.
    a. True
    b. False

9. Pyrazinamide causes which of the following abnormalities in up to 50% of patients?
    a. Anemia.
    b. Thrombocytopenia.
    c. Peripheral neuropathy.
    d. Hepatitis.
    e. Increased uric acid levels.

Questions 10-11: True or False

10. Streptomycin has less renal toxicity than other aminoglycosides but more vestibular toxicity.
    a. True
    b. False

11. Ofloxacin is the most active quinolone against *M. tuberculosis*.
    a. True
    b. False

12. Caspofungin has reduced activity against which *Candida* species?
    a. *C. albicans*.
    b. *C. parapsilosis*.
    c. *C. krusei*.
    d. *C. tropicalis*.
    e. *C. glabrata*.

13. Acyclovir is a nucleoside analogue of:
    a. Cytosine.
    b. Guanosine.
    c. Thymidine.
    d. Adenosine.

Quiz 3
Topic: Antiviral/Antifungal/Antimycobacterial Agents (Chapters 36-38)

Chapter numbers refer to "Principles and Practices of Infectious Diseases", sixth edition, edited by Mandell, Bennett, and Dolin, Elsevier/Churchill Livingstone, Philadelphia, PA, 2005.

14. Which of the following drugs is an improved oral form of acyclovir?
    a. Cidofovir.
    b. Ganciclovir.
    c. Famciclovir.
    d. Valacyclovir.

15. Cidofovir is a nucleoside analogue of:
    a. Cytosine.
    b. Guanosine.
    c. Thymidine.
    d. Adenosine.

16. Thymidine kinase minus HSV strains are resistant to all of the following drugs, except:
    a. Ganciclovir.
    b. Valacyclovir.
    c. Penciclovir.
    d. Cidofovir.

17. Foscarnet inhibits which herpes virus enzyme?
    a. Reverse transcriptase.
    b. Thymidine kinase.
    c. DNA polymerase.
    d. Protease.

18. Interferon-γ inhibits hepatitis C virus *in vivo* by:
    a. Inhibiting reverse transcription.
    b. Blocking viral entry.
    c. Disrupting ribosomal function.
    d. Stimulating host cell genes.
    e. Causing autolysis.

Questions 19-20: True or False

19. Amantadine inhibits only influenza A viruses.
    a. True
    b. False

20. Imiquimod is a topical immune response modifier.
    a. True
    b. False

Answers:

1.	B
2.	F
3.	D
4.	A
5.	B
6.	D
7.	B
8.	B
9.	E
10.	A
11.	B
12.	B
13.	B
14.	D
15.	A
16.	D
17.	C
18.	D
19.	A
20.	A

Quiz 4
Topic: Antiretroviral Agents (Chapter 124)

Chapter numbers refer to "Principles and Practices of Infectious Diseases", sixth edition, edited by Mandell, Bennett, and Dolin, Elsevier/Churchill Livingstone, Philadelphia, PA, 2005.

1. All of the following are true about nucleoside reverse transcriptase inhibitors (NRTIs), except:
   a. They are active against a broad range of retroviruses, including HIV-1, HIV-2 & HTLV-1.
   b. Some may be associated with lactic acidosis.
   c. They block necessary cleavage of viral proteins.
   d. They lead to premature chain termination of HIV DNA.

2. Which of the following is true concerning non-nucleoside RT inhibitors (NNRTIs)?
   a. They are non-competitive inhibitors of RT.
   b. They have activity against HIV-2.
   c. They require phosphorylation to become active.
   d. None of the above.

3. Which of the following is true concerning protease inhibitors (PIs)?
   a. They are active against HIV-1 and HIV-2.
   b. They may be associated with hyperlipidemia.
   c. They block necessary cleavage of viral proteins.
   d. They are usually not metabolized by cytochrome p450.
   e. a, b & c.

4. All of the following are true about zidovudine, except:
   a. It causes macrocytosis and anemia.
   b. It decreases the odds of transmission in occupational exposure.
   c. It decreases the rate of transmission to newborns.
   d. It causes fetal malformation.

Questions 5-8: True or False

5. The most problematic side effect of efavirenz is rash.
   a. True
   b. False

6. Nevirapine is teratogenic in animals.
   a. True
   b. False

7. Nelfinavir has been associated with nephrolithiasis.
   a. True
   b. False

8. Zidovudine and stavudine may be used together.
   a. True
   b. False

9. All of the following are features of abacavir hypersensitivity, except:
   a. Fever.
   b. Malaise.
   c. Acidosis.
   d. Myalgias.
   e. Rash.

10. Lamivudine commonly causes:
    a. Neutropenia.
    b. Nephrolithiasis.
    c. CNS disturbances.
    d. Neuropathy.
    e. None of the above.

11. Predictors of failure of anti-retroviral therapy (ART) include all of the following, except:
    a. Prior therapy with NRTIs.
    b. Advanced HIV disease.
    c. Non-adherence to ART regimen.
    d. Older age.

12. Which of the following is true concerning (PIs)?
    a. They decrease plasma levels of some antihistamines.
    b. They may be associated with hypoglycemia.
    c. They are not active against HIV-2.
    d. They are associated with lipodystrophy.
    e. All of the above.

Chapter numbers refer to "Principles and Practices of Infectious Diseases", sixth edition, edited by Mandell, Bennett, and Dolin, Elsevier/Churchill Livingstone, Philadelphia, PA, 2005.

13. Peripheral neuropathy may be associated with which of the following agents?
    a. Stavudine.
    b. Zalcitabine.
    c. Didanosine.
    d. Abacavir.
    e. a, b & c.

Answers:

1.	C
2.	A
3.	E
4.	D
5.	B
6.	B
7.	B
8.	B
9.	C
10.	E
11.	D
12.	D
13.	E

Chapter numbers refer to "Principles and Practices of Infectious Diseases", sixth edition, edited by Mandell, Bennett, and Dolin, Elsevier/Churchill Livingstone, Philadelphia, PA, 2005.

1. Rhinoviruses account for which percentage of the common cold?
   a. 20%.
   b. 40%.
   c. 60%.
   d. 80%.

2. Which of the following viruses is not thought to be a causative agent of the common cold?
   a. Respiratory syncitial virus.
   b. Coronavirus.
   c. Parainfluenza virus.
   d. Alphavirus.
   e. Adenovirus.

3. A CT scan of the sinuses is a useful way to distinguish bacterial from viral upper respiratory infections (URIs).
   a. True
   b. False

4. The most significant barrier to a rhinoviral vaccine is:
   a. Polysaccharide capsule.
   b. Viral mutation rate.
   c. Existence of over 100 serotypes.
   d. Lack of an animal model.

5. Which of the following streptococcal groups is not associated with pharyngitis?
   a. Group A.
   b. Group B.
   c. Group C.
   d. Group G.

6. Pharyngitis with conjunctivitis is most commonly caused by which of the following agents?
   a. *N. gonorrhoeae*.
   b. RSV.
   c. Rhinovirus.
   d. Parainfluenza virus.
   e. Adenovirus.

7. Treatment of *S. pyogenes* pharyngitis after 5 days of symptoms has no effect on preventing rheumatic fever.
   a. True
   b. False

8. Which of the following does not typically cause acute pharyngitis?
   a. Epstein-Barr virus.
   b. *Arcanobacterium haemolyticum*.
   c. *C. pneumoniae*.
   d. *M. pneumoniae*.
   e. *S. pneumoniae*.

9. The most common etiology of acute laryngotracheobronchitis (croup) is:
   a. Influenza A virus.
   b. RSV.
   c. Parainfluenza virus.
   d. Adenovirus.
   e. *M. pneumoniae*.

10. The age group most commonly affected by croup is which of the following?
   a. 0- 6 months.
   b. 6 months-1 year old.
   c. 1-2 years old.
   d. 2-3 years old.
   e. 3-4 years old.

Answers:

1.	B
2.	D
3.	B
4.	C
5.	B
6.	E
7.	B
8.	E
9.	C
10.	C

Quiz 6
Topic: Upper Respiratory Infections II (Chapters 54-57)

Chapter numbers refer to "Principles and Practices of Infectious Diseases", sixth edition, edited by Mandell, Bennett, and Dolin, Elsevier/Churchill Livingstone, Philadelphia, PA, 2005.

1. The microbial flora of the external canal:
   a. Is similar to skin flora elsewhere.
   b. Is predominantly staphylococci, corynebacterium, and anaerobic bacteria.
   c. Does not commonly include *H. influenzae*, *M. catarrhalis*, and *S. pneumoniae*.
   d. All of the above.
   e. None of the above.

2. All of the following are true regarding "malignant" otitis externa, except:
   a. It is usually caused by *Pseudomonas aeruginosa*.
   b. Systemic therapy with pseudomonal coverage should be used for 4 to 6 weeks.
   c. Elderly, diabetic, debilitated, and immunocompromised patients are at greater risk for the disease.
   d. It usually presents with few clinical signs and symptoms.

3. Which of the following is true about otitis media?
   a. It has peak incidence in the first 3 years of life.
   b. The vast majority of children with recurrent and severe bouts have obvious immunological defects.
   c. It is more common in females than males.
   d. No association exists between passive exposure to smoke as well as attendance of large daycare groups and increased risk of otitis media.

4. All of the following are true about treatment of acute otitis media, except:
   a. Gram-negative enteric bacilli must be considered in newborn patients, patients with depressed immune response and in patients with suppurative complications of otitis media.
   b. The antibiotics must be active against *S. pneumoniae*, *H. influenzae*, and *M. catarrhalis*.
   c. The antibiotics should achieve concentrations in middle ear fluid above expected minimal inhibitory concentrations of likely pathogens.
   d. Amoxicillin is the initial drug of choice.
   e. There is no need to re-evaluate children who do not improve in 48-72 hours.

Questions 5-9: True or False: Acute Sinusitis
5. It is most often caused by viruses or bacteria.
   a. True
   b. False

6. It is challenging to diagnose and manage secondary to difficulty in making an etiologic diagnosis with accuracy and evaluating effectiveness of treatment with precision.
   a. True
   b. False

7. It can be caused by viruses, including rhinovirus, parainfluenza virus, and influenza virus.
   a. True
   b. False

8. It is never caused by fungi.
   a. True
   b. False

9. In the nosocomial setting, acute sinusitis is typically caused by pathogens, including *S. aureus*, *P. aeruginosa*, *Serratia marcescens*, and *Klebsiella pneumoniae*.
   a. True
   b. False

10. Which of the following is true about sinusitis?
    a. In nosocomial sinusitis, cultures of sinus aspirate are not recommended.
    b. Acute fungal sinusitis frequently occurs in otherwise healthy patients.
    c. Non-infectious causes of sinusitis include chemical irritation, nasal and sinus tumors, foreign bodies, and Wegner's granulomatosis.

Chapter numbers refer to "Principles and Practices of Infectious Diseases", sixth edition, edited by Mandell, Bennett, and Dolin, Elsevier/Churchill Livingstone, Philadelphia, PA, 2005.

d. Acute community acquired bacterial sinusitis cannot lead to intracranial, orbital, and respiratory complications.

11. All of the following are true about epiglottitis, except:
    a. Acute epiglottitis is a cellulitis of the epiglottis and adjacent structures.
    b. It has potential for causing abrupt airway obstruction.
    c. The diagnosis is established by visualizing an edematous cherry-red epiglottis.
    d. *H. influenzae* type b is the most frequently isolated bacterial pathogen.
    e. *H. influenzae* bacteremia occurs very infrequently in children with epiglottitis.

12. Which of the following is true about odontogenic infections?
    a. Complications can occur either by hematogenous spread or by direct extension.
    b. Prophylactic antibiotic therapy is the standard of care for all patients, including those without valvular disease.
    c. Acute mediastinitis and intracranial suppuration secondary to odontogenic infections are very common currently.
    d. Transient bacteremia is uncommon during various dental procedures.

13. Which of the following is true about suppurative jugular thrombophlebitis?
    a. It usually arises from the lateral pharyngeal space.
    b. It occurs with acute onset, with shaking chills, fevers, and prostration.
    c. Localizing signs of pain are usually present but may be subtle.
    d. Fusobacterium necrophilum has been the organism most frequently isolated from blood cultures.
    e. All of the above.

14. All of the following are true about parotitis, except:
    a. Staphylococci have been the predominant pathogen isolated in acute bacterial parotitis.
    b. Viral causes for parotitis include mumps, influenza and enterovirus.
    c. Chronic parotitis may be confused with Sjögren's syndrome.
    d. Early surgical drainage and decompression of the gland are not generally required in acute bacterial parotitis.

Answers:

1.	E
2.	D
3.	A
4.	E
5.	A
6.	A
7.	A
8.	B
9.	A
10.	C
11.	E
12.	A
13.	E
14.	D

Quiz 7
Topic: Pleuropulmonary Infections I (Chapters 58-60)

Chapter numbers refer to "Principles and Practices of Infectious Diseases", sixth edition, edited by Mandell, Bennett, and Dolin, Elsevier/Churchill Livingstone, Philadelphia, PA, 2005.

Questions 1-4: Match the syndrome with the clinical feature: Acute Infectious Bronchitis (AIB) vs. Common Cold (CC)

1. Cough is severe and becomes the predominant complaint.
    a. AIB
    b. CC

2. Cough persists for up to a month or longer.
    a. AIB
    b. CC

3. It may progress into adult asthma.
    a. AIB
    b. CC

4. Cough is one of several symptoms.
    a. AIB
    b. CC

5. Which of the following pathogens may cause acute bronchitis?
    a. *Bordetella pertussis*, *Mycoplasma pneumoniae*, *Chlamydia pneumoniae*, adenovirus.
    b. Rhinovirus.
    c. Corona virus.
    d. All of the above.

6. All of the following may be associated with recurrent respiratory infections and persistent chronic bronchitis, except:
    a. Immunoglobulin deficiency.
    b. Cigarette smoking.
    c. Cilia or epithelial cell defect.
    d. Abnormal PMN production.
    e. Interferon gamma deficiency.

Questions 7-10: True or False

7. It is difficult to document the microbial cause of many respiratory infections.
    a. True
    b. False

8. *Haemophilus influenzae* and *Streptococcus pneumoniae* chronically colonize at least ½ of patients with chronic bronchitis.
    a. True
    b. False

9. There is no need to include coverage for *Moraxella catarrhalis* and *Bordetella pertussis* in treatment of acute exacerbation of chronic bronchitis (AECB).
    a. True
    b. False

10. *S. aureus* and streptococci are frequent causes of acute infection in chronic bronchitis.
    a. True
    b. False

11. Which of the following is true regarding antibiotic therapy in AECB?
    a. It does not hasten recovery.
    b. It does not improve clinical outcome.
    c. It is usually used for approximately 7 days.
    d. It should always be given intravenously.

12. Which of the following is/are considerations in starting appropriate antibiotics in AECB?
    a. Spectrum of activity.
    b. Frequency of administration and cost.
    c. Mode of action.
    d. Tissue penetration.
    e. All of the above.

13. Bronchiolitis:
    a. Is an inflammatory condition of the tracheobronchial tree that usually is associated with an acute respiratory infection.
    b. Features cough and excessive secretion of mucus from the tracheobronchial airways that is not associated to other specific diseases.
    c. Is an active viral lower respiratory tract illness occurring during the 1st two years of life.
    d. None of the above.

Chapter numbers refer to "Principles and Practices of Infectious Diseases", sixth edition, edited by Mandell, Bennett, and Dolin, Elsevier/Churchill Livingstone, Philadelphia, PA, 2005.

14. The most common pathogen of bronchiolitis is:
    a. *Streptococcus pneumoniae*.
    b. *Bordetella pertussis*.
    c. Mumps virus.
    d. Respiratory syncytial virus (RSV).
    e. Corona virus.

15. Increased risk factors for hospitalization in young infants with bronchiolitis include all of the following, except:
    a. Lack of breastfeeding.
    b. Illness caused by RSV.
    c. Living in crowded and polluted surround-ings.
    d. Post-dates delivery.
    e. Young age (first several months of life).

16. All of the following are true about bronchiolitis, except:
    a. It has a prodromal period of one to seven days marked by mild fever.
    b. It is usually associated with coryza and cough.
    c. Tachypnea and tachycardia may be present with progression of disease.
    d. Wheezing may be auscultated.
    e. Cyanosis is commonly seen.
    f. Aerosolized ribavirin may be used for treat-ment if illness is due to RSV.

Answers:

1.	A
2.	A
3.	A
4.	B
5.	D
6.	E
7.	A
8.	A
9.	B
10.	B
11.	C
12.	E
13.	C
14.	D
15.	D
16.	E

Quiz 8
Topic: Pleuropulmonary Infections II (Chapters 61-64)

Chapter numbers refer to "Principles and Practices of Infectious Diseases", sixth edition, edited by Mandell, Bennett, and Dolin, Elsevier/Churchill Livingstone, Philadelphia, PA, 2005.

1. All of the following are part of the pulmonary host defense mechanisms, except:
   a. Mucociliary apparatus.
   b. Epiglottic reflexes.
   c. Immunoglobulin production.
   d. Mast cells.
   e. Alveolar macrophages.

2. All of the following are true about Gram stains of expectorated sputum samples in patients with suspected pneumonia, except:
   a. They should have >25 PMNs and < 10 epithelial cells per low power field.
   b. They detect approximately 60% of pneumococcal pneumonias.
   c. They have a higher sensitivity for *H. influenzae* pneumonia than pneumococcal pneumonia.
   d. They show only PMNs in Legionella pneumonia.
   e. They show mixed morphology in anaerobic pneumonias.

3. Which of following percentages is incorrect regarding the etiologies of typical, community-acquired pneumonia?
   a. 16-60% *S. pneumoniae*.
   b. 3-15% *H. influenzae*.
   c. 2-8% *Legionella* spp.
   d. 25% *S. aureus*.
   e. 7-18% Gram-negative rods.

4. Pneumococcal resistance to penicillin:
   a. Is associated with resistance to other antibiotics in 5% of strains.
   b. Is caused by plasmid encoded β-lactamase.
   c. Is not clearly associated with a worse clinical outcome.
   d. Is associated with quinolone resistance.

5. In adults, parapneumonic effusion is seen commonly with each of the following agents, except:
   a. *S. aureus*.
   b. *S. pyogenes*.
   c. *S. pneumoniae*.
   d. *H. influenzae*.

6. Drainage of parapneumonic effusion is recommended for any of the following observations, except when:
   a. Pleural fluid is gross pus.
   b. Gram stain of pleural fluid is positive.
   c. Culture of pleural fluid is positive.
   d. Pleural fluid WBC > 10,000 cells/mm^3.
   e. Pleural fluid pH is < 7.2.

7. The most common etiology of lung abscesses is:
   a. *S. aureus*.
   b. *S. pneumoniae*.
   c. *H. influenzae*.
   d. Oral flora.
   e. *Bacteroides fragilis*.

8. Lung abscesses should be treated with:
   a. Open drainage and IV antibiotics.
   b. 2 weeks of po amoxicillin.
   c. 2-4 months of clindamycin and penicillin.
   d. Needle aspiration.

9. Each of the following has been shown to cause chronic pneumonia, except:
   a. *Mycobacterium marinum*.
   b. *Mycobacterium avium* complex.
   c. *Blastomyces dermatitidis*.
   d. *Cryptococcus neoformans*.
   e. *Histoplasma capsulatum*.

10. A 53-year old man comes in with 4-month history of malaise, low-grade fever, cough, and progressive left chest wall pain. He has severe dental caries, and has abused both alcohol and tobacco. On exam, he has crackles at the left lung base and drainage from a left chest wall mass. The most likely etiology is:
    a. *Sporotrichrix shenckii*.
    b. *Nocardia* spp.
    c. *Actinomyces* spp.
    d. *Rhodococcus equi*.
    e. *M. tuberculosis*.

Chapter numbers refer to "Principles and Practices of Infectious Diseases", sixth edition, edited by Mandell, Bennett, and Dolin, Elsevier/Churchill Livingstone, Philadelphia, PA, 2005.

Answers:

1.   D
2.   C
3.   D
4.   C
5.   D
6.   D
7.   D
8.   C
9.   A
10. C

Quiz 9
Topic: UTI/Sepsis/Abdominal Infections (Chapters 66-68)

Chapter numbers refer to "Principles and Practices of Infectious Diseases", sixth edition, edited by Mandell, Bennett, and Dolin, Elsevier/Churchill Livingstone, Philadelphia, PA, 2005.

Questions 1-4: True or False

1. Urine of uninfected women is always sterile.
   a. True
   b. False

2. Nonoxynol-9 increases the rate of UTI by decreasing vaginal pH.
   a. True
   b. False

3. Women with dysuria, frequency, and urgency, and whose urine has fewer than 105 bacteria per ml of urine have a 33% chance of having a bacterial infection.
   a. True
   b. False

4. The 105 CFU per ml of urine cut-off applies to all forms of bacteria and to *Candida*.
   a. True
   b. False

5. If there are more than 105 bacteria per ml in a clean catch urine specimen of an asymptomatic woman, the probability that this woman has true bacteriuria is:
   a. 40%.
   b. 60%.
   c. 80%.
   d. 95%.

6. Asymptomatic elderly patients with bacteriuria should be:
   a. Observed closely with repeat urinalysis and culture.
   b. Treated once with antibiotics, and no more if the bacteriuria recurs.
   c. Not treated at all.
   d. Put on cranberry juice chronically.

7. Each of the following is a recommended first-line choice to treat lower UTIs, except:
   a. Amoxicillin.
   b. TMP/SMX.
   c. Ciprofloxacin.
   d. Norfloxacin.
   e. Trimethoprim.

8. Ecthyma gangrenosum has which of the following appearances?
   a. Dark eschar.
   b. Bull's eye.
   c. Erythema with serpiginous border.
   d. Necrosis with large bullae.

9. Primary peritonitis occurs in approximately what percentage of alcoholic cirrhotics?
   a. 10%.
   b. 25%.
   c. 50%.
   d. 85%.

10. Which of the following pathogens is a common cause of peritonitis?
    a. *S. aureus*.
    b. *S. pneumoniae*.
    c. *C. perfringens*.
    d. *B. fragilis*.
    e. *C. fetus*.

11. A peritoneal fluid WBC > 500 cells/mm³ is indicative of primary peritonitis.
    a. True
    b. False

12. Aminoglycosides are typically NOT used to treat abdominal abscesses, because of which of the following?
    a. They are highly toxic.
    b. They lack activity against strict anaerobes.
    c. They have poor activity against *Enterococcus*.
    d. They are inactive in acidic environments.

Chapter numbers refer to "Principles and Practices of Infectious Diseases", sixth edition, edited by Mandell, Bennett, and Dolin, Elsevier/Churchill Livingstone, Philadelphia, PA, 2005.

13. Patients on peritoneal dialysis who develop peritonitis:
    a. Should have their catheter removed in order to achieve a cure.
    b. Should be treated with systemic and intraperitoneal antibiotics.
    c. May have peritoneal fluid WBC < 500.
    d. Should be placed on enterococcal coverage.

Questions 14-16: True or False

14. Amebic liver abscess occurs more often in men than women.
    a. True
    b. False

15. In patients with acute cholecystitis, the AST is usually elevated.
    a. True
    b. False

16. In uncomplicated acute cholecystitis, recent series suggest that a delay in surgery improves outcome.
    a. True
    b. False

Answers:

1.	B
2.	B
3.	A
4.	B
5.	C
6.	C
7.	A
8.	B
9.	A
10.	B
11.	A
12.	D
13.	C
14.	A
15.	B
16.	B

Chapter numbers refer to "Principles and Practices of Infectious Diseases", sixth edition, edited by Mandell, Bennett, and Dolin, Elsevier/Churchill Livingstone, Philadelphia, PA, 2005.

1. In patients with native valve infective endocarditis, audible heart murmurs are heard in:
   a. 15%.
   b. 25%.
   c. 55%.
   d. 65%.
   e. 85%.

2. *Viridans streptococci* are the etiologic agent in which of the following percentages of cases of native valve infective endocarditis?
   a. 10-20%.
   b. 20-30%.
   c. 30-40%.
   d. 40-50%.
   e. 50-60%.
   f. 60-70%.

3. Each of the following is true about transesophageal echocardiography (TEE) in the diagnosis of infective endocarditis, except:
   a. TEE has higher sensitivity than transthoracic echocardiography.
   b. TEE has lower specificity than transthoracic echocardiography.
   c. TEE has better spatial resolution than transthoracic echocardiography.
   d. TEE is well tolerated.

4. In a patient with suspected endocarditis, when Gram-positive cocci grow on initial blood culture but fail to grow on subculture, which of the following is probably true?
   a. The initial isolate is a contaminant.
   b. The isolate is an enterococcal species.
   c. Empiric therapy should include vancomycin.
   d. Subculture should be repeated on chocolate agar and held for 3 weeks.
   e. Subculture should be repeated on media with L-cysteine or pyridoxine.

5. For native valve endocarditis caused by one of the HACEK, the regimen of choice is which of the following?
   a. Ceftriaxone for 3-4 weeks.
   b. Ampicillin plus streptomycin or gentamicin for 4-6 weeks.
   c. Vancomycin for 4 weeks.
   d. Ceftazidime for 4-6 weeks.

6. The risk of prosthetic valve endocarditis (PVE) is:
   a. 5-10% in the first 12 months after surgery.
   b. Higher in patients with mechanical valves than in those with bioprosthetics between years 1-5 after surgery.
   c. Relatively constant after the first 12 months post-surgery.
   d. 4-5% per year after the first 12 months post-surgery.

7. All of the following are true about the etiologies of PVE, except:
   a. *S. epidermidis* is the most common etiology in the first 2 months post-surgery.
   b. At >12 months post-surgery, *S. aureus* is the most common pathogen.
   c. Corynebacterium cause "late" PVE in 10-11% of cases.
   d. Fungal etiologies are difficult to culture.

Questions 8-11: True or False

8. Mycotic aneurysms are secondary to fungal pathogens.
   a. True
   b. False

9. The majority of intracranial hemorrhages associated with endocarditis are secondary to ruptured mycotic aneurysms.
   a. True
   b. False

10. Mycotic aneurysms should be treated with prompt surgery.
    a. True
    b. False

Quiz 10
Topic: Cardiovascular Infections 1 (Chapters 74-76)

Chapter numbers refer to "Principles and Practices of Infectious Diseases", sixth edition, edited by Mandell, Bennett, and Dolin, Elsevier/Churchill Livingstone, Philadelphia, PA, 2005.

11. Pelvic suppurative thrombophlebitis should be treated with a combination of broad-spectrum antibiotics and heparin.
    a. True
    b. False

Choose the risk category of infective endocarditis (High, Intermediate or Low) for each cardiac disorder:

12. Prosthetic heart valve.
    a. High
    b. Intermediate
    c. Low

13. MV prolapse without regurgitation.
    a. High
    b. Intermediate
    c. Low

14. Surgically repaired intracardiac lesions, with minimal or no hemodynamic abnormality > 6 months post-operative.
    a. High
    b. Intermediate
    c. Low

15. Cardiac pacemaker.
    a. High
    b. Intermediate
    c. Low

16. Bicuspid aortic valve.
    a. High
    b. Intermediate
    c. Low

17. Ventricular septal defect.
    a. High
    b. Intermediate
    c. Low

Answers:

#	Answer
1.	E
2.	C
3.	B
4.	E
5.	A
6.	C
7.	B
8.	B
9.	B
10.	B
11.	B
12.	A
13.	C
14.	C
15.	C
16.	B
17.	A

Quiz 11
Topic: Cardiovascular Infections II (Chapters 77-78)

Chapter numbers refer to "Principles and Practices of Infectious Diseases", sixth edition, edited by Mandell, Bennett, and Dolin, Elsevier/Churchill Livingstone, Philadelphia, PA, 2005.

1. All of the following have been firmly established as etiologic agents of myocarditis, except:
   a. *Trichinella spiralis*.
   b. Mumps virus.
   c. Coxsackie A virus.
   d. Coxsackie B virus.
   e. HIV.
   f. *Toxoplasma gondii*.

2. Which of the following is true regarding myocarditis?
   a. It usually presents with fever, chest pain, SOB, and PVCs.
   b. Endomyocardial biopsy is routinely done and helpful in diagnosis.
   c. Dilated cardiomyopathy can develop at the end stage of viral myocarditis.
   d. It usually does not cause ECG changes.

3. Non-infectious causes of myocarditis include all of the following, except:
   a. Systemic lupus erythematosus.
   b. Rheumatoid arthritis.
   c. Cocaine.
   d. Alcohol.
   e. Wegener's granulomatosis.

4. Infectious causes of pericarditis include all of the following, except:
   a. *Histoplasma capsulatum*.
   b. HIV.
   c. *S. pneumoniae*.
   d. *Listeria monocytogenes*.
   e. *Toxoplasma gondii*.
   f. Coxsackie A virus.

5. Acute pericarditis is associated with all of the following, except:
   a. Three-component pericardial friction rub.
   b. Chest pain, often retrosternal.
   c. Elevated CK-MB isoenzymes.
   d. Dyspnea.
   e. Dysphagia.

6. ECG changes found in acute pericarditis include all of the following, except:
   a. ST segment elevation.
   b. Q waves.
   c. PR segment depression.
   d. T-wave flattening.
   e. Electrical alternans.
   f. Low voltage QRS.

7. Which of the following is TRUE regarding tuberculous pericarditis?
   a. Prednisone has no effect on outcome.
   b. In the third pathologic stage, mycobacteria are easily seen in biopsy specimens.
   c. Constrictive pericarditis rarely occurs in those who receive an anti-TB regimen.
   d. Early surgical intervention is advocated in patients with hemodynamic compromise from progressive pericardial thickening.

8. Which is the major route for descending infections which cause mediastinitis?
   a. The retropharyngeal space.
   b. The lateral pharyngeal space.
   c. The pretracheal space.

Questions 9-12: True or False:

Post-sternotomy mediastinitis:

9. Usually presents within the first 2 weeks.
   a. True
   b. False

10. Is commonly caused by *Candida albicans*.
    a. True
    b. False

11. May present even a year after surgery.
    a. True
    b. False

12. Can usually be treated with antibiotics alone.
    a. True
    b. False

Chapter numbers refer to "Principles and Practices of Infectious Diseases", sixth edition, edited by Mandell, Bennett, and Dolin, Elsevier/Churchill Livingstone, Philadelphia, PA, 2005.

Questions 13-16: True or False:	**Answers:**	

Sclerosing mediastinitis:

	1.	E
	2.	C
13. Is cured with prolonged courses of antifungal agents.	3.	E
	4.	B
a. True	5.	C
b. False	6.	B
	7.	D
14. Is caused by chronic, active *H. capsulatum* infection.	8.	A
	9.	A
a. True	10.	B
b. False	11.	A
	12.	B
15. Often presents with superior vena cava syndrome.	13.	B
	14.	B
a. True	15.	A
b. False	16.	B

16. Is successfully treated with prolonged courses of prednisone.
   a. True
   b. False

Quiz 12
Topic: CNS Infections I (Chapters 79, 80, 82 & 83)

Chapter numbers refer to "Principles and Practices of Infectious Diseases", sixth edition, edited by Mandell, Bennett, and Dolin, Elsevier/Churchill Livingstone, Philadelphia, PA, 2005.

Questions 1-4: True or False:

1. Most CSF is produced by the choroid plexus.
   a. True
   b. False

2. Most CSF is produced by the arachnoid villi.
   a. True
   b. False

3. Parameningeal infections may cause a pleocytosis and increased CSF protein.
   a. True
   b. False

4. Corticosteroids have a proven beneficial effect as adjunctive therapy in treating bacterial meningitis.
   a. True
   b. False

5. Meningismus occurs in which percentage of adult patients with bacterial meningitis?
   a. 55%.
   b. 65%.
   c. 75%.
   d. 85%.
   e. 95%.

6. In a patient with fever, headache, and facial nerve palsy, which of the following pathogens should be considered as the most probable agent?
   a. *S. pneumoniae*.
   b. *B. burgdorferi*.
   c. *N. meningitidis*.
   d. *L. monocytogenes*.
   e. *H. influenzae*.

7. In a patient with suspected meningitis who has a normal neurological exam and no papilledema, what is the next step in evaluation following the exam?
   a. Obtain blood cultures and perform lumbar puncture.
   b. Obtain blood cultures and start empirical antibiotics.

c. Start empirical antibiotics and obtain a CT scan of the head, and if the CT scan is negative, perform a lumbar puncture.

8. Above which age should ampicillin be added as part of the empirical regimen for meningitis?
   a. 20 years.
   b. 30 years.
   c. 40 years.
   d. 50 years.
   e. 65 years.

9. Which of the following is the drug of choice for Listeria meningitis in penicillin allergic patients?
   a. Vancomycin.
   b. Chloramphenicol.
   c. Linezolid.
   d. Clindamycin.
   e. Trimethoprim-sulfamethoxazole.

10. In chronic meningitis, all of the following are associated with an eosinophilic pleocytosis, except:
   a. *Cryptococcus neoformans*.
   b. *Coccidioides immitis*.
   c. Lymphoma.
   d. Schistosoma.
   e. *Angiostrongylus cantonensis*.

11. All of the following are true regarding Mollaret's meningitis, except:
   a. Symptoms include fever, headache, & nuchal rigidity.
   b. CSF findings include a mixed lymphocytic and neutrophilic pleocytosis.
   c. Attacks persist for a few days and resolve without sequelae and then rarely recur.
   d. CSF protein levels are usually less than 100 mg/ml.

Chapter numbers refer to "Principles and Practices of Infectious Diseases", sixth edition, edited by Mandell, Bennett, and Dolin, Elsevier/Churchill Livingstone, Philadelphia, PA, 2005..

Questions 12-14: True or False:

Answers:

12. Tuberculous meningitis has unique, characteristic CSF findings.
    a. True
    b. False

13. Coccidioidal meningitis is typically diagnosed by culture.
    a. True
    b. False

14. Neurocysticercosis is diagnosed by CSF antibodies to *T. saginata*.
    a. True
    b. False

15. In which season is enterovirus encephalitis most common?
    a. Winter.
    b. Spring.
    c. Summer.
    d. Fall.

1.	A
2.	B
3.	A
4.	B
5.	D
6.	B
7.	A
8.	D
9.	E
10.	A
11.	C
12.	B
13.	B
14.	B
15.	C

Quiz 13
Topic: CNS Infections II (Chapters 84-85)

Chapter numbers refer to "Principles and Practices of Infectious Diseases", sixth edition, edited by Mandell, Bennett, and Dolin, Elsevier/Churchill Livingstone, Philadelphia, PA, 2005.

Questions 1-6: True or False

1. Streptococci are the bacteria most commonly cultured from brain abscesses.
    a. True
    b. False

2. Coagulase-negative staphylococci account for 10-15% of brain abscesses.
    a. True
    b. False

3. Anaerobes are frequently isolated from brain abscesses.
    a. True
    b. False

4. Enteric Gram-negative bacteria are isolated from brain abscesses in approximately 23-33% of cases.
    a. True
    b. False

5. Brain abscesses are not caused by *Nocardia* species.
    a. True
    b. False

6. Most patients (>50%) with brain abscesses present with fever, headache, and focal neurologic deficit.
    a. True
    b. False

7. Risk factors for brain abscess include all of the following, except:
    a. Diabetes mellitus.
    b. Hematologic neoplasms.
    c. Renal transplantation.
    d. Use of deferoxamine.
    e. Cystic fibrosis.

8. Which of the following statements is/are correct?
    a. Subdural empyema is often caused by spread of infection through the paranasal sinuses.
    b. Subdural empyema never coexists with meningitis in adults.
    c. Subdural empyema may develop after intracranial procedures.
    d. Subdural empyema is more common in women.
    e. All of the above.
    f. a & c.

Questions 9-14: True or False:

9. An epidural abscess represents localized infection between the outermost two layers of the meninges.
    a. True
    b. False

10. An epidural abscess is almost always accompanied by focal osteomyelitis.
    a. True
    b. False

11. An epidural abscess may be secondary to sinusitis.
    a. True
    b. False

12. Current opinion recommends against the use of anticoagulants in the treatment of cavernous vein thrombosis.
    a. True
    b. False

13. The thoracic spine is the most common site for spinal epidural abscess.
    a. True
    b. False

14. Plain x-rays are the diagnostic procedure of choice for epidural abscess.
    a. True
    b. False

Chapter numbers refer to "Principles and Practices of Infectious Diseases", sixth edition, edited by Mandell, Bennett, and Dolin, Elsevier/Churchill Livingstone, Philadelphia, PA, 2005.

15. Initial therapy for suspected cavernous venous thrombophlebitis should cover which of the following agents?
    a. *S. aureus*.
    b. Aerobic streptococci.
    c. Anaerobes.
    d. Fungi.
    e. All of the above.
    f. a, b & c.

Questions 16-19: Choose the anatomic location corresponding to the infection.

16. Epidural abscess
    a. Between arachnoid & pia mater.
    b. Between dura mater & arachnoid.
    c. Between dura mater & skull/spine.
    d. Below the pia mater.

17. Subdural abscess
    a. Between arachnoid & pia mater.
    b. Between dura mater & arachnoid.
    c. Between dura mater & skull/spine.
    d. Below the pia mater.

18. Brain abscess
    a. Between arachnoid & pia mater.
    b. Between dura mater & arachnoid.
    c. Between dura mater & skull/spine.
    d. Below pia mater.

Answers:

1.	A
2.	B
3.	A
4.	A
5.	B
6.	B
7.	E
8.	F
9.	B
10.	A
11.	A
12.	B
13.	A
14.	B
15.	F
16.	C
17.	B
18.	D

Quiz 14
Topic: Skin & Soft Tissue Infections (Chapters 86-88)

Chapter numbers refer to "Principles and Practices of Infectious Diseases", sixth edition, edited by Mandell, Bennett, and Dolin, Elsevier/Churchill Livingstone, Philadelphia, PA, 2005.

1. Crepitus is associated with which of the following infections?
   a. Streptococcal gangrene.
   b. Clostridial myonecrosis.
   c. Cutaneous mucormycosis.
   d. Pseudomonas cellulitis with bacteremia.
   e. Progressive bacterial synergistic gangrene.

Questions 2-13: True or False

2. Erysipelas is deeper than cellulitis.
   a. True
   b. False

3. Erysipelas is usually caused by *S. aureus*.
   a. True
   b. False

4. Erysipelas is usually confined to the lymphatics and dermis.
   a. True
   b. False

5. Necrotizing fasciitis is seen in most patients with streptococcal toxic shock cases.
   a. True
   b. False

6. Streptococcal toxic shock is usually seen in patients with underlying illness.
   a. True
   b. False

7. A primary site of infection is found in >95% of patients with streptococcal toxic shock.
   a. True
   b. False

8. Pyomyositis is seen more often in tropical climates.
   a. True
   b. False

9. *S. aureus* is the etiology in 95% of cases of tropical pyomyositis.
   a. True
   b. False

10. Penetrating trauma precedes most cases of pyomyositis.
    a. True
    b. False

11. *S. pyogenes* is most common cause of pyogenic lymphadenitis.
    a. True
    b. False

12. Fever is rare in patients with pyogenic lymphadenitis.
    a. True
    b. False

13. In the USA, *M. tuberculosis* is the most common cause of scrofula.
    a. True
    b. False

Answers:

1.	B
2.	B
3.	B
4.	A
5.	B
6.	B
7.	B
8.	A
9.	A
10.	B
11.	B
12.	B
13.	B

Chapter numbers refer to "Principles and Practices of Infectious Diseases", sixth edition, edited by Mandell, Bennett, and Dolin, Elsevier/Churchill Livingstone, Philadelphia, PA, 2005.

Questions 1-3: True or False

1. The infectious dose for *Shigella* is much higher than that of *Salmonella*.
   a. True
   b. False

2. Enterotoxigenic *E. coli* (ETEC) may produce one of three strains of toxin.
   a. True
   b. False

3. ETEC LT toxin activates adenylate cyclase, which is similar to cholera toxin.
   a. True
   b. False

4. All of the following cause non-inflammatory diarrhea, except:
   a. *Giardia lamblia*.
   b. Rotavirus.
   c. ETEC.
   d. *Salmonella* spp.
   e. Norwalk-like viruses.

5. Fecal polymorphonuclear cells are found in all of the following infections, except:
   a. *Shigella flexneri*.
   b. *Salmonella typhi*.
   c. *Yersinia enterocolitica*.
   d. *Vibrio cholerae*.
   e. *Campylobacter jejuni*.

Questions 6-8: True or False

6. In AIDS patients with esophagitis, *Candida* esophagitis can be diagnosed by visualization alone.
   a. True
   b. False

7. The presence of fever rules out traveler's diarrhea caused by ETEC.
   a. True
   b. False

8. In non-inflammatory diarrhea, the organism typically adheres to the colonic epithelium.
   a. True
   b. False

9. *Giardia lamblia* infection is best diagnosed by:
   a. Culture of the organism from stool specimen.
   b. Wet mount examination of stool specimen.
   c. Wet mount examination of small bowel aspirate.
   d. Serology.

10. The drug of choice for *Giardia* infection is which of the following?
    a. Albendazole.
    b. Metronidazole.
    c. Paromomycin.
    d. Doxycycline.

11. A positive fecal lactoferrin assay indicates which of the following?
    a. *C. difficile* colitis.
    b. Amebic colitis.
    c. Toxigenic *E. coli* infection.
    d. Strongyloides infection.
    e. Inflammatory diarrhea.

Answers:

1.	B
2.	A
3.	A
4.	D
5.	D
6.	B
7.	B
8.	A
9.	C
10.	B
11.	E

Quiz 16
Topic: Gastrointestinal Infections II (Chapters 94-96)

Chapter numbers refer to "Principles and Practices of Infectious Diseases", sixth edition, edited by Mandell, Bennett, and Dolin, Elsevier/Churchill Livingstone, Philadelphia, PA, 2005.

1. *S. aureus* is a frequent cause of antibiotic-associated diarrhea not caused by *C. difficile*.
   a. True
   b. False

2. In patients with antibiotic-associated diarrhea, in which percentage of cases is *C. difficile* implicated?
   a. 10-20%.
   b. 20-30%.
   c. 50-60%.
   d. >90%.

3. Fever is seen in which percentage of patients with *C. difficile*-associated diarrhea?
   a. 10-30%.
   b. 30-50%.
   c. 50-70%.
   d. 70-90%.

4. Abdominal pain is very rarely seen in patients with *C. difficile* colitis.
   a. True
   b. False

5. Which of the following is the most sensitive and specific test for *C. difficile*-associated diarrhea?
   a. EIA toxin test.
   b. Cell culture cytotoxin test.
   c. Latex test for *C. difficile* antigen.
   d. Endoscopy.
   e. PCR of the toxin gene.

6. All of the following are causes of acute dysentery, except:
   a. *Campylobacter jejuni*.
   b. *Balantidium coli*.
   c. *Entamoeba histolytica*.
   d. *Shigella flexneri*.
   e. *Entamoeba dispar*.

7. Classic enteric fever presents with all of the following symptoms, except:
   a. Fever.
   b. Diarrhea.
   c. Relative bradycardia.
   d. Leukopenia.
   e. Splenomegaly.

Questions 8-11: True or False

8. Rose spots are pathognomonic for *Salmonella* enteric fever.
   a. True
   b. False

9. *Salmonella* enteric fever is typically diagnosed by stool cultures.
   a. True
   b. False

10. *Y. enterocolicita* is a more frequent human pathogen than *Y. pseudotuberculosis*.
    a. True
    b. False

11. *S. stercoralis* infection is usually diagnosed by the demonstration of larvae in the host's stool.
    a. True
    b. False

12. First line agents for the treatment of typhoid fever include all of the following, except:
    a. TMP-SMX.
    b. Ceftriaxone.
    c. Aztreonam.
    d. Ciprofloxacin.

Chapter numbers refer to "Principles and Practices of Infectious Diseases", sixth edition, edited by Mandell, Bennett, and Dolin, Elsevier/Churchill Livingstone, Philadelphia, PA, 2005.

Answers:

1.	B
2.	B
3.	B
4.	B
5.	B
6.	E
7.	B
8.	B
9.	B
10.	A
11.	A
12.	A

Quiz 17
Topic: Gastrointestinal Infections III (Chapters 95-97)

Chapter numbers refer to "Principles and Practices of Infectious Diseases", sixth edition, edited by Mandell, Bennett, and Dolin, Elsevier/Churchill Livingstone, Philadelphia, PA, 2005.

1. All of the following can cause food poisoning by the formation of a preformed toxin, except:
   a. *B. cereus.*
   b. *S. epidermidis.*
   c. *C. jejuni.*
   d. *S. aureus.*
   e. *C. botulinum.*

2. *B. cereus* can cause gastrointestinal disease via preformed toxin production or by *in vivo* toxin production.
   a. True
   b. False

3. Which of the following is most likely to cause nausea, vomiting, diarrhea and paralysis within 18-36 hours?
   a. Ciguatera.
   b. Histamine fish poisoning.
   c. *C. jejuni.*
   d. Shiga-toxin producing *E. coli.*
   e. *C. botulinum.*

4. Which of the following is the most commonly recognized pathogen in waterborne outbreaks?
   a. *G. lamblia.*
   b. *Shigella* spp.
   c. Hepatitis A virus.
   d. Norwalk-like agents.
   e. *C. jejuni.*

5. In persons with underlying liver disease, especially iron overload states, who have ingested oysters, which of the following agents causes fulminant myonecrosis or primary bacteremia?
   a. *V. cholerae.*
   b. *Y. enterocolitica.*
   c. Hepatitis A virus.
   d. *C. jejuni.*
   e. *V. vulnificus.*

Questions 6-7: True or False

6. *S. aureus* food poisoning is classically associated with fried rice.
   a. True
   b. False

7. In tropical sprue, folate deficiency leads to bacterial overgrowth, which causes the malabsorption syndrome.
   a. True
   b. False

8. In Whipple's disease, the characteristic histologic finding is:
   a. Flattened duodenal villi.
   b. Partial villous atrophy.
   c. Edematous small bowel.
   d. PAS-positive macrophages.

9. The drug of choice for Whipple's disease is:
   a. Penicillin po for six months.
   b. Ceftriaxone IV for 2 weeks, followed by oral TMP/SMX for one year.
   c. Penicillin/Streptomycin IV/IM followed by oral tetracycline for one year.
   d. Oral metronidazole for one year.

10. Whipple's disease diagnosis is confirmed by which one (or more) of the following tests?
    a. PCR for *T. whipplei* DNA from biopsy lesions.
    b. Serology for *T. whipplei.*
    c. Electron microscopy of biopsy lesions, which shows characteristic rod-shaped bacillus within macrophages.
    d. Culture of *T. whipplei* from biopsy lesions.

Answers:

1.	C
2.	A
3.	E
4.	A
5.	E
6.	B
7.	B
8.	D
9.	B
10.	A, C

Chapter numbers refer to "Principles and Practices of Infectious Diseases", sixth edition, edited by Mandell, Bennett, and Dolin, Elsevier/Churchill Livingstone, Philadelphia, PA, 2005.

1. Synovial fluid cultures are usually positive in patients with disseminated gonococcal infection.
   a. True
   b. False

2. Sternoclavicular septic arthritis is associated with which of the following risk factors?
   a. Age.
   b. Diabetes mellitus.
   c. Corticosteroid therapy.
   d. Intravenous drug use.
   e. Sexually transmitted diseases.

3. Symmetric arthritis in women is a usual manifestation of which of the following infections?
   a. Adenovirus.
   b. Influenza.
   c. Rubeola.
   d. Parvovirus B19.

4. Sinus tract cultures of which of the following organisms are reliable for predicting the cause of osteomyelitis?
   a. *P. aeruginosa*.
   b. *C. albicans*.
   c. *S. aureus*.
   d. *P. mirabilis*.
   e. *B. fragilis*.

Questions 5-10: True or False

5. In patients with vertebral osteomyelitis, fever and elevated peripheral WBC are often absent.
   a. True
   b. False

6. Adults who had hematogenous osteomyelitis as children can have recurrences decades later at the same site, by the same organism.
   a. True
   b. False

7. Most prosthetic joint infections can be cured with 4-6 weeks of antibiotic therapy.
   a. True
   b. False

8. Patients with prosthetic joint infections usually present with fever.
   a. True
   b. False

9. The higher the ratio of bone to serum concentrations, the better the outcome in treating osteomyelitis.
   a. True
   b. False

10. In adults with vertebral osteomyelitis, the blood cultures are usually negative.
    a. True
    b. False

Answers:

1.	B
2.	D
3.	D
4.	C
5.	A
6.	A
7.	B
8.	B
9.	B
10.	A

Chapter numbers refer to "Principles and Practices of Infectious Diseases", sixth edition, edited by Mandell, Bennett, and Dolin, Elsevier/Churchill Livingstone, Philadelphia, PA, 2005.

1. Which of the following is NOT a cause of genital ulcer?
   a. Chancroid.
   b. HSV-2.
   c. Syphilis.
   d. *C. trachomatis* serovars A-C.

Questions 2-3: True or False

2. Gram stain of urethral discharge is a sensitive and specific test for diagnosing gonococcal urethritis.
   a. True
   b. False

3. In men with urethritis, the incubation period is a reliable factor in differentiating between GU and NGU.
   a. True
   b. False

4. *N. gonorrhoeae* isolation by culture is reduced because some gonococci are inhibited by which of the following antibiotics in the culture media?
   a. Metronidazole.
   b. Tetracycline.
   c. Chloramphenicol.
   d. Cephalothin.
   e. Vancomycin.

Questions 5-7: True or False

5. It is well established that *U. urealyticum* is the main cause of Chlamydia-negative NGU.
   a. True
   b. False

6. 95% of men with gonococcal urethritis who do not receive treatment will be symptom free within 6 months.
   a. True
   b. False

7. Most women with primary herpes simplex genital infection will have symptoms of dysuria.
   a. True
   b. False

8. The CDC recommends which of the following treatment for men with GU?
   a. Single dose of IM ceftriaxone or oral ciprofloxacin.
   b. Seven days of doxycycline.
   c. Single dose of IM ceftriaxone or oral ciprofloxacin plus single dose of oral azithromycin.
   d. Five days of levofloxacin.

Questions 9-11: True or False
9. Bacterial vaginosis (BV) is characterized by vaginal discharge, "fishy" odor, and decreased vaginal pH.
   a. True
   b. False

10. BV is caused by *G. vaginalis*.
    a. True
    b. False

11. BV is a sexually-transmitted disease.
    a. True
    b. False

12. Causes of acute cervicitis include all of the following, except:
    a. HSV-2.
    b. Chlamydia.
    c. *N. gonorrhoeae*.
    d. HPV.
    e. Molluscum contagiosum.

Answers:

1.	D	8.	C
2.	A	9.	B
3.	B	10.	B
4.	E	11.	B
5.	B	12.	E
6.	A		
7.	A		

Chapter numbers refer to "Principles and Practices of Infectious Diseases", sixth edition, edited by Mandell, Bennett, and Dolin, Elsevier/Churchill Livingstone, Philadelphia, PA, 2005.

1. Risk factors for intra-amniotic infection syndrome (IAIS) include all of the following, except:
   a. Pre-existing bacterial vaginosis.
   b. Prolonged rupture of membranes.
   c. Old age.
   d. Low socioeconomic class.

Questions 2-4: True or False

2. IAIS, caused by *E. coli* and Group B *streptococcus*, can often be cured with ampicillin and gentamicin.
   a. True
   b. False

3. Ovarian vein thrombophlebitis responds well to antibiotics alone.
   a. True
   b. False

4. Postabortal infection responds well to antibiotics alone.
   a. True
   b. False

5. Antibiotic therapy for pelvic inflammatory disease should cover the following organisms, except:
   a. *C. trachomatis*.
   b. *N. gonorrhoeae*.
   c. Anaerobes.
   d. *Actinomyces* spp.

6. All patients with PID and who are treated as outpatients should be reevaluated at:
   a. 24 hours.
   b. 48 hours.
   c. 72 hours.
   d. 96 hours.
   e. 7 days.

7. Most cases of mycotic prostatitis have been associated with each of the following mycoses, except:
   a. Aspergillosis.
   b. Blastomycosis.
   c. Cryptococcosis.
   d. Coccidioidomycosis.

Questions 8-10: True or False

8. Mumps orchitis usually results in sterility.
   a. True
   b. False

9. Acute bacterial prostatitis is often subtle and difficult to diagnose.
   a. True
   b. False

10. *C. trachomatis* is an important pathogen of epididymitis in men older than 35 years as well as those under 35 years.
    a. True
    b. False

Answers:

1.	C
2.	B
3.	B
4.	B
5.	D
6.	C
7.	A
8.	B
9.	B
10.	B

Quiz 21
Topic: Eye Infections (Chapters 106-110)

Chapter numbers refer to "Principles and Practices of Infectious Diseases", sixth edition, edited by Mandell, Bennett, and Dolin, Elsevier/Churchill Livingstone, Philadelphia, PA, 2005.

1. The principle causes of acute bacterial conjunctivitis include all of the following, except:
   a. *M. catarrhalis.*
   b. *S. pneumoniae.*
   c. *S. aureus.*
   d. *N. gonorrhoeae.*
   e. *H. influenzae.*

2. All of the following cause epidemic hemorrhagic conjunctivitis, except:
   a. Enterovirus 70.
   b. Coxsackie A24.
   c. Adenovirus 11.
   d. Measles virus.

Questions 3-4: True or False
3. *C. trachomatis* typically causes blindness after one episode of acute conjunctivitis.
   a. True
   b. False

4. Most cases of herpes virus keratitis are caused by HSV-2.
   a. True
   b. False

5. Parinaud's oculoglandular syndrome consists of the following symptoms and signs, except:
   a. Pharyngitis.
   b. Conjunctivitis.
   c. Fever.
   d. Preauricular lymphadenopathy.

6. The leading cause of bacterial endophthalmitis is:
   a. Surgery.
   b. Trauma.
   c. Contact lens use.
   d. Foreign body penetration.

Questions 7-11: True or False

7. Preseptal cellulitis is a surgical emergency.
   a. True
   b. False

8. A chalazion is usually sterile.
   a. True
   b. False

9. An external hordeolum (stye) is usually treated with oral antibiotics.
   a. True
   b. False

10. Patients with *Candida* chorioretinitis usually respond to medical therapy alone.
    a. True
    b. False

11. Patients with orbital cellulitis should receive broad spectrum antibiotics and have emergent surgery.
    a. True
    b. False

Answers:

1.	A
2.	D
3.	B
4.	B
5.	A
6.	A
7.	B
8.	A
9.	A
10.	A
11.	B

Chapter numbers refer to "Principles and Practices of Infectious Diseases", sixth edition, edited by Mandell, Bennett, and Dolin, Elsevier/Churchill Livingstone, Philadelphia, PA, 2005.

1. Hepatitis A virus (HAV) can be transmitted by all of the following routes, except:
   a. Blood transfusion.
   b. Sexual contact.
   c. Close contact with young children in day care centers.
   d. Skin-to-skin contact.
   e. Ingestion of contaminated water or food.

Questions 2-4: True or False

2. The diagnosis of acute hepatitis A infection is made by finding positive IgM against HAV in the serum.
   a. True
   b. False

3. Jaundice in acute HAV infection is rare in patients older than 4 years old.
   a. True
   b. False

4. Most patients with acute delta virus infection become chronic carriers.
   a. True
   b. False

5. Polyarteritis nodosa is associated with which of the following infections?
   a. Hepatitis A virus.
   b. Hepatitis B virus.
   c. Hepatitis C virus.
   d. Hepatitis D virus.
   e. Hepatitis E virus.

6. Hepatitis B virus infection occurs via all of the following routes, except:
   a. Needle sharing.
   b. Vaginal or rectal sex.
   c. Fecal-oral route.
   d. Blood transfusion.

7. Hepatitis D virus infection is seen in all of the following areas, except:
   a. China.
   b. Southern Italy.
   c. South America.
   d. Middle East countries.
   e. Central Africa.

8. Chronic delta virus infection is diagnosed by which of the following?
   a. Serology.
   b. RT-PCR of the viral genome in plasma.
   c. Viral antigen testing of the serum.
   d. RT-PCR of the viral genome in feces.

9. Which of the following is associated with an increased risk of mortality in acute hepatitis E virus infection?
   a. Iron-overload states.
   b. Alcoholism.
   c. Co-infection with hepatitis B.
   d. Pregnancy.
   e. Chronic hepatitis C infection.

Questions 10-13: True or False

10. Lamivudine therapy for chronic hepatitis B infection reduces viral DNA, but does not result in an increased rate of HbeAg seroconversion.
    a. True
    b. False

11. Mutations in the YMDD locus of the hepatitis B virus RT gene confer resistance to lamivudine and adefovir.
    a. True
    b. False

12. Maternal HIV co-infection increases the rate of hepatitis C virus (HCV) vertical transmission considerably.
    a. True
    b. False

Chapter numbers refer to "Principles and Practices of Infectious Diseases", sixth edition, edited by Mandell, Bennett, and Dolin, Elsevier/Churchill Livingstone, Philadelphia, PA, 2005.

13. Acute HCV infection is cleared in less than 5%
    of cases.
    a. True
    b. False

Answers:

1.	D
2.	A
3.	B
4.	B
5.	B
6.	C
7.	A
8.	A
9.	D
10.	B
11.	B
12.	A
13.	B

Quiz 23
Topic: Introduction to Viruses and Pox Viruses (Chapters 128-130)

Chapter numbers refer to "Principles and Practices of Infectious Diseases", sixth edition, edited by Mandell, Bennett, and Dolin, Elsevier/Churchill Livingstone, Philadelphia, PA, 2005.

Questions 1-5: True or False

1. Poxviridae are among the smallest human viruses.
   a. True
   b. False

2. Viral RNA (+) sense genomes can be directly translated by ribosomes.
   a. True
   b. False

3. Tropism of viruses is often determined by expression of a cellular protein, which serves as a receptor for the virus.
   a. True
   b. False

4. Most human cancers are caused by viruses.
   a. True
   b. False

5. Encephalitis secondary to vaccinia responds well to VIG therapy.
   a. True
   b. False

6. Poxviridae have which of the following genomes?
   a. Linear DS DNA.
   b. SS (+) RNA.
   c. SS (-) RNA.
   d. Circular DS DNA.

7. Monkeypox is found in squirrels and monkeys in which of the following areas?
   a. Central and West Africa.
   b. Southeast Asia.
   c. South America.
   d. Australia.
   e. Montclair.

8. The capacity of a virus to infect a distinct group of cells in the host is referred to as:
   a. Tropism.
   b. Replication capacity.
   c. Virulence.
   d. Attachment.

9. Which of the following viruses can cause chronic, active infection and latent infection?
   a. Hepatitis C virus.
   b. Herpes simplex type 1.
   c. CMV.
   d. HIV.
   e. Hepatitis B virus.

10. In which of the following countries did the last case of smallpox in the wild occur?
    a. Bangladesh.
    b. England.
    c. Yugoslavia.
    d. Somalia.
    e. Texas.

11. In what year was this case diagnosed?
    a. 1977.
    b. 1942.
    c. 1989.
    d. 1968.

Extra Credit: In what month of the year did the case occur? _____

Extra, extra credit: In which city did the case occur? _____

Extra, extra, extra credit: Did the patient survive? _____

Extra, extra, extra, extra credit: What was the patient's occupation? _____

Answers:

1.	B	Extra credit: October
2.	A	Extra, extra credit: Merca
3.	A	Extra, extra, extra credit: Yes
4.	B	Extra, extra, extra, extra credit: Cook
5.	B	
6.	A	
7.	A	
8.	A	
9.	D	
10.	D	
11.	A	

Quiz 24
Topic: Herpesviridae I (Chapters 131-133)

Chapter numbers refer to "Principles and Practices of Infectious Diseases", sixth edition, edited by Mandell, Bennett, and Dolin, Elsevier/Churchill Livingstone, Philadelphia, PA, 2005.

1. Which of the following does NOT cause life-long latent infection in humans?
   a. CMV.
   b. HSV-1.
   c. EBV.
   d. HHV-8.
   e. None of the above.

2. Which of the following is a cause of roseola infantum?
   a. CMV.
   b. EBV.
   c. VZV.
   d. HHV-6.
   e. HHV-8.

3. The genome structure for all herpes viruses is which of the following?
   a. ssRNA(+).
   b. ssRNA(-).
   c. ssDNA.
   d. dsDNA.

Questions 4-7: True or False

4. HSV-1 is commonly spread by fomites.
   a. True
   b. False

5. Transmission of HSV-2 can occur in the absence of visible skin lesions.
   a. True
   b. False

6. Pregnant women with HSV-2 should be screened weekly for cytologic and virologic studies near term.
   a. True
   b. False

7. Aseptic meningitis secondary to HSV-2 has a benign prognosis, even in the absence of therapy with intravenous acyclovir.
   a. True
   b. False

8. Acyclovir resistance in HSV usually occurs via mutations in which of the following genes?
   a. Cellular DNA polymerase.
   b. Viral DNA polymerase.
   c. Viral thymidine kinase.
   d. Cellular thymidine kinase.

9. VZV is typically transmitted by which route?
   a. Fecal-oral.
   b. Respiratory via aerosol.
   c. Skin-skin.
   d. Skin-mucous membranes via fomites.

10. When should VZIG be administered to an infant whose mother develops varicella?
    a. 5 days before and up to 48 hours after birth.
    b. In the third trimester.
    c. 7 days before and up to 72 hours after birth.
    d. If the newborn has lesions at the time of birth.

Questions 11-13: True or False

11. Patients with varicella are infectious only when the rash is present and the lesions have not yet crusted over.
    a. True
    b. False

12. A pregnant woman with no history of chicken-pox and recent exposure should be offered prophylaxis with VZIG, but should not receive the vaccine.
    a. True
    b. False

13. Epidemiologically, Reye's syndrome is associated with zoster and aspirin therapy.
    a. True
    b. False

Quiz 24
Topic: Herpesviridae I (Chapters 131-133)

Chapter numbers refer to "Principles and Practices of Infectious Diseases", sixth edition, edited by Mandell, Bennett, and Dolin, Elsevier/Churchill Livingstone, Philadelphia, PA, 2005.

Answers:

1.	E
2.	D
3.	D
4.	B
5.	A
6.	B
7.	A
8.	C
9.	B
10.	A
11.	B
12.	A
13.	B

Quiz 25
Topic: Herpesviridae II (Chapters 134-138)

Chapter numbers refer to "Principles and Practices of Infectious Diseases", sixth edition, edited by Mandell, Bennett, and Dolin, Elsevier/Churchill Livingstone, Philadelphia, PA, 2005.

1. EBV primarily infects which of the following cell types?
   a. T-cell.
   b. Basophil.
   c. Mast cell.
   d. B-cell.

Questions 2-4: True or False:

2. Unlike CMV, EBV is rarely shed from healthy, sero-positive adults.
   a. True
   b. False

3. EBV is the leading cause of "post-pump perfusion" mononucleosis.
   a. True
   b. False

4. HHV-6 typically is transmitted in early adulthood, similar to EBV.
   a. True
   b. False

5. Antibodies to EBV are found in which percentage of healthy USA adults?
   a. 20-40%.
   b. 40-60%.
   c. 60-80%.
   d. >90%.

6. Which complication of EBV infection is associated with X-linked immunodeficiency (Duncan) syndrome?
   a. African Burkitt's lymphoma.
   b. Nasopharyngeal carcinoma.
   c. Hodgkin's lymphoma.
   d. Uncontrolled lymphoproliferative syndrome.
   e. Autoimmune hemolytic anemia.

7. Which virus is associated with Castleman's disease?
   a. HHV-8.
   b. HHV-7.
   c. HHV-6.
   d. EBV.
   e. CMV.

8. Which animal is the natural host for herpes B virus?
   a. Squirrel monkeys.
   b. Chimpanzees.
   c. Macaques.
   d. Gorillas.

Questions 9-12: True or False

9. CMV retinitis is characterized by cotton wool spots.
   a. True
   b. False

10. A mutation in UL97 is the most common mechanism of ganciclovir resistance in CMV.
    a. True
    b. False

11. Culture of CMV from urine is proof of active CMV infection.
    a. True
    b. False

12. CMV resistant to ganciclovir is typically sensitive to cidofovir.
    a. True
    b. False

Answers:

1.	D
2.	B
3.	B
4.	B
5.	D
6.	D
7.	A
8.	C
9.	B
10.	A
11.	B
12.	A

CHAPTER 26: QUESTIONS FOR THE ID BOARDS **839**

Chapter numbers refer to "Principles and Practices of Infectious Diseases", sixth edition, edited by Mandell, Bennett, and Dolin, Elsevier/Churchill Livingstone, Philadelphia, PA, 2005.

Questions 1-2: True or False

1. The genome of adenoviruses is circular, ssDNA.
   a. True
   b. False

2. Adenoviral pneumonia responds well to ribavirin therapy.
   a. True
   b. False

3. Which immunocompromised state is associated with adenoviral chronic meningoencephalitis?
   a. Hypogammaglobulinemia.
   b. Severe combined immunodeficiency disease.
   c. Chronic granulomatous disease.
   d. Job's syndrome.
   e. AIDS.

Questions 4-6: True or False

4. Adeno-associated virus is associated with hydrops fetalis.
   a. True
   b. False

5. The genome of adeno-associated virus has significant homology to that of adenovirus.
   a. True
   b. False

6. Papillomavirus DNA is found in >70% of cervical intraepithelial neoplasias.
   a. True
   b. False

7. In renal transplant patients, BK virus is associated with:
   a. Chronic rejection.
   b. Acute rejection.
   c. Hemorrhagic cystitis.
   d. Ureteral stenosis.

Questions 8-10: True or False

8. PML responds well to Ara-C therapy.
   a. True
   b. False

9. JCV viruria in pregnancy is associated with gestational diabetes.
   a. True
   b. False

10. Anal cancer is closely associated with anogenital warts.
    a. True
    b. False

Answers:

1.   B
2.   B
3.   A
4.   B
5.   B
6.   A
7.   D
8.   B
9.   B
10. A

Chapter numbers refer to "Principles and Practices of Infectious Diseases", sixth edition, edited by Mandell, Bennett, and Dolin, Elsevier/Churchill Livingstone, Philadelphia, PA, 2005.

1. Most of the hepatitis B virus (HBV) surface antigen is found in subviral particles.
   a. True
   b. False

2. Replication of the HBV genome is achieved by which of the following enzymes and templates?
   a. Viral DNA polymerase from a viral DNA genome.
   b. Viral RNA polymerase from a viral RNA genome.
   c. Viral reverse transcriptase from a viral RNA pregenome.
   d. Viral reverse transcriptase from a viral RNA genome.
   e. None of the above.

3. Replication of the hepatitis D virus (HDV) genome is achieved by which of the following enzymes and templates?
   a. Viral DNA polymerase from a viral DNA genome.
   b. Viral RNA polymerase from a viral RNA genome.
   c. Viral reverse transcriptase from a viral RNA pregenome.
   d. Viral reverse transcriptase from a viral RNA genome.
   e. None of the above.

4. Regions of high prevalence of HDV include each of the following, except:
   a. South America.
   b. Asia.
   c. Mediterranean basin.
   d. North Africa.

Questions 5-7: True or False

5. The prevalence of HBV infection in an area is inversely correlated with average age at the time of infection.
   a. True
   b. False

6. The rate of chronic HBV infection is correlated with age at the time of infection, the higher the age, the greater the chance of chronic infection.
   a. True
   b. False

7. A person whose has isolated IgG anti-HBc without other serologic markers of HBV is not infectious.
   a. True
   b. False

8. The most common measure of success for chronic HBV treatments is which of the following?
   a. Elimination of HBeAg.
   b. Elimination of HBsAg.
   c. Elimination of HBV viral DNA.
   d. Normalization of serum aminotransferases.
   e. Improvement in liver histology.

Questions 9-11: True or False

9. Vaccinated individuals have protection against HBV infection even when the antibody level has fallen to below 10 IU/L.
   a. True
   b. False

10. Post-exposure prophylaxis (PEEP) for HBV is the same for neonates and adults.
    a. True
    b. False

11. In PEEP for HBV, HBIG should be administered immediately and the vaccine series should be started one week later.
    a. True
    b. False

12. Parvovirus B19 causes all of the following, except:
    a. Fifth disease.
    b. Polyarthropathy syndrome.
    c. Transient aplastic crisis.
    d. Acute hepatitis.
    e. Hydrops fetalis.

Chapter numbers refer to "Principles and Practices of Infectious Diseases", sixth edition, edited by Mandell, Bennett, and Dolin, Elsevier/Churchill Livingstone, Philadelphia, PA, 2005.

13. Chronic parvovirus infection causing pure red cell aplasia in AIDS patients is usually treated with which of the following?
    a. Corticosteroids.
    b. Splenectomy.
    c. Ribavirin.
    d. Intravenous IgG.

Answers:

1.	B
2.	C
3.	E
4.	B
5.	A
6.	A
7.	B
8.	A
9.	A
10.	A
11.	B
12.	D
13.	D

Quiz 28
Topic: RNA Viruses 1 (Chapters 144-148)

Chapter numbers refer to "Principles and Practices of Infectious Diseases", sixth edition, edited by Mandell, Bennett, and Dolin, Elsevier/Churchill Livingstone, Philadelphia, PA, 2005.

1. Coltiviruses have a genome consisting of 12 RNA segments.
   a. True
   b. False

2. Colorado Tick Fever (CTF) is transmitted by which of the following arthropods?
   a. *Ixodes dammini.*
   b. *Dermacentor andersoni.*
   c. *Ixodes pacificus.*
   d. *Anpholes mosquitos.*
   e. *Aedes aegypti.*

3. The coltiviruses, which cause CTF, infect the precursors of which blood cell lineage?
   a. RBC.
   b. Granulocytes.
   c. Monocytes/Macrophages.
   d. Platelets.
   e. Lymphocytes.

4. The genome of rotavirus consists of:
   a. Circular dsDNA.
   b. ssRNA 11 segments.
   c. dsRNA 11 segments.
   d. dsRNA 1 segment.

5. Rotavirus seasonal epidemics occur in which of the following seasons?
   a. Summer.
   b. Fall.
   c. Winter.
   d. Spring.

6. Alphaviruses which cause disease in the USA include each of the following, except:
   a. JE.
   b. WEE.
   c. EEE.
   d. VEE.

7. The natural host/reservoir for EEE virus is which of the following?
   a. Humans.
   b. Horses.
   c. Rodents.
   d. Birds.

Questions 8-9: True or False

8. Infants with congenital rubella shed large quantities of virus from body secretions for many months.
   a. True
   b. False

9. The attenuated viral vaccine for rubella can cause congenital rubella syndrome when given to pregnant women.
   a. True
   b. False

10. Which of the following is the most common complication of post-natal rubella infection in women?
    a. Hepatitis.
    b. Thrombocytopenia.
    c. Encephalitis.
    d. Arthritis.

Answers:

1.	A
2.	B
3.	A
4.	C
5.	C
6.	A
7.	D
8.	A
9.	B
10.	D

Quiz 29
Topic: RNA Viruses 2 (Chapters 149-151)

Chapter numbers refer to "Principles and Practices of Infectious Diseases", sixth edition, edited by Mandell, Bennett, and Dolin, Elsevier/Churchill Livingstone, Philadelphia, PA, 2005.

1. Yellow fever occurs in each of the following areas, except:
   a. East Africa.
   b. Asia.
   c. West Africa.
   d. South America.
   e. Central America.

Questions 2-5: True or False

2. Aedes aegypti is primarily found in the woods and forested areas.
   a. True
   b. False

3. >99% of Japanese encephalitis virus infections are subclinical.
   a. True
   b. False

4. European (Central European encephalitis) and Far Eastern (Russia spring-summer encephalitis) tick-borne encephalitis viruses are transmitted vertically in their tick vectors.
   a. True
   b. False

5. Dengue hemorrhagic fever is usually seen in the initial or first infection of children/infants.
   a. True
   b. False

6. The yellow fever vaccine consists of:
   a. An attenuated strain of yellow fever virus.
   b. An inactivated strain form of yellow fever virus.
   c. Viral surface proteins.
   d. Inactivated toxin or toxoid.
   e. Plasmid DNA, which encodes internal viral proteins.

7. The Japanese encephalitis vaccines are which of the following type(s)?
   a. An attenuated strain of yellow fever virus.
   b. An inactivated strain form of yellow fever virus.
   c. Viral surface proteins.
   d. Inactivated toxin or toxoid.
   e. Plasmid DNA, which encodes internal viral proteins.

Questions 8-9: True or False

8. For most travelers, tick-borne encephalitis is best prevented by anti-tick measures.
   a. True
   b. False

9. HCV typically causes a chronic, latent infection.
   a. True
   b. False

10. Which percentage of infected individuals develops chronic HCV infection?
    a. 15%.
    b. 35%.
    c. 50%.
    d. 85%.
    e. >95%.

11. The risk of HCV infection after a needlestick exposure to a health-care worker is approximately:
    a. 0.3%.
    b. 3%.
    c. 30%.
    d. 50%.

12. α-interferon inhibits HCV by which of the following mechanisms?
    a. Protein synthesis inhibition.
    b. Viral polymerase inhibition.
    c. Induction of cellular enzymes, which degrade certain RNAs.
    d. Inhibition of viral entry.
    e. Inhibition of viral uncoating.

Chapter numbers refer to "Principles and Practices of Infectious Diseases", sixth edition, edited by Mandell, Bennett, and Dolin, Elsevier/Churchill Livingstone, Philadelphia, PA, 2005.

Answers:

1.	B
2.	B
3.	A
4.	A
5.	B
6.	A
7.	A, B
8.	B
9.	B
10.	D
11.	B
12.	C

Quiz 30
Topic: RNA Viruses 3 (Chapters 152-156)

Chapter numbers refer to "Principles and Practices of Infectious Diseases", sixth edition, edited by Mandell, Bennett, and Dolin, Elsevier/Churchill Livingstone, Philadelphia, PA, 2005.

1. Which of the following animals is thought to be the host of SARS-CoV?
   a. Gambian rat.
   b. House cat.
   c. Masked palm civet.
   d. Chicken.
   e. Waterfowl.

2. SARS-CoV is thought to be transmitted by all of the following routes, except:
   a. Fomite transmission.
   b. Airborne transmission.
   c. Sexual transmission.
   d. Fecal-oral transmission.

3. The overall mortality rate for SARS is:
   a. 2-5%.
   b. 10-15%.
   c. 40-60%.
   d. 80-90%.

4. Which of the following methods is most commonly used to diagnose SARS?
   a. Acute and convalescent serology.
   b. PCR.
   c. Virus culture.
   d. ELISA for viral proteins.
   e. RT-PCR.

5. Parainfluenza viruses typically cause all of the following syndromes, except:
   a. Pneumonia in transplant patients.
   b. Pneumonia in the elderly.
   c. Croup.
   d. Bronchiolitis.
   e. Otitis media.

Questions 6-9: True or False

6. In mumps meningitis, the CSF findings are often similar to those seen in bacterial meningitis, except that hypoglycorrhacia is rarely seen.
   a. True
   b. False

7. The initial infection with respiratory syncitial virus (RSV) is clinically worse than subsequent infections.
   a. True
   b. False

8. RSV can cause outbreaks in hospital wards.
   a. True
   b. False

9. Metopneumovirus infection typically occurs in early adulthood.
   a. True
   b. False

10. RSV infection is most often diagnosed by which of the following methods?
    a. Acute and convalescent serology.
    b. PCR.
    c. Virus culture.
    d. ELISA for viral proteins.
    e. RT-PCR.

11. Which of the following is the only approved treatment for lower respiratory tract infection of infants?
    a. Palivizumab.
    b. RSV-IGIV.
    c. Pooled, intravenous immunoglobulin.
    d. Oral ribavirin.
    e. Aerosolized ribavirin.

Answers:

1.	C
2.	C
3.	B
4.	E
5.	B
6.	B
7.	A
8.	A
9.	B
10.	D
11.	E

Quiz 31
Topic: RNA Viruses 4 (Chapters 157-161)

Chapter numbers refer to "Principles and Practices of Infectious Diseases", sixth edition, edited by Mandell, Bennett, and Dolin, Elsevier/Churchill Livingstone, Philadelphia, PA, 2005.

1. Measles is spread primarily by which of the following?
   a. Fomites.
   b. Aerosol.
   c. Droplets.
   d. Body fluids.

2. Subacute sclerosing panencephalitis (SSPE) is caused by:
   a. The measles vaccine in immunocompromised hosts.
   b. Re-activation of latent measles virus.
   c. Measles-related virus, agent of canine distemper.
   d. A complex interaction of host factors and viral replicative phenomena.

Questions 3-6: True or False

3. Koplik spots are seen only in measles infection.
   a. True
   b. False

4. The measles rash can be described as morbilliform.
   a. True
   b. False

5. Atypical measles is seen in babies with some degree of passive immunity to the measles virus.
   a. True
   b. False

6. Measles in pregnant women causes fetal abnormalities similar to rubella, but at a decreased frequency.
   a. True
   b. False

7. Adults born in the early 1960s who received the killed version of the measles vaccine should:
   a. Receive a booster with the attenuated measles vaccine.
   b. Have measles virus antibody titers checked, and receive a booster if the titers are low.
   c. Receive a booster with the killed measles vaccine.
   d. Receive no additional vaccine, since the risk of measles is very low.

8. The attenuated measles vaccine is contraindicated in all of the following groups, except:
   a. AIDS patients.
   b. Hypogammaglobulinemia patients.
   c. Pregnant women.
   d. Children with leukemia.
   e. Children with malignancies who received chemotherapy <3 months ago.

9. All of the following are true about Negri bodies, except:
   a. They are most often found in the hippocampal pyramidal cells.
   b. They are round or oval eosinophilic cytoplasmic inclusions.
   c. They are not found in any organ except the brain.

10. If a person is bit by a dog who was provoked, what is the recommended treatment strategy?
    a. Euthanize the dog and perform an autopsy.
    b. Assume the dog is rabid and commence post-exposure prophylaxis.
    c. Observe the dog for 10 days.

Answers:

1.	C
2.	D
3.	A
4.	A
5.	B
6.	B
7.	A
8.	B
9.	C
10.	C

Chapter numbers refer to "Principles and Practices of Infectious Diseases", sixth edition, edited by Mandell, Bennett, and Dolin, Elsevier/Churchill Livingstone, Philadelphia, PA, 2005.

1. Antibodies induced by natural infection have little effect in protecting against influenza infection.
   a. True
   b. False

2. Antigenic drift of influenza viruses occurs secondary to:
   a. Re-assortment of human strains with avian strains.
   b. Immune selection of variants with a few amino acid mutations.
   c. Immune selection of different types of influenza virus.
   d. Evolution within swine populations and then crossover to humans.

3. The most common cause of secondary bacterial pneumonia after influenza infection is which of the following?
   a. *S. pneumoniae*.
   b. *S. aureus*.
   c. *H. influenzae*.
   d. *L. pneumophila*.

4. During an outbreak of influenza A in your community, three of 100 elderly patients in a nursing home develop *Streptococcus pneumoniae* pneumonia approximately one week following a febrile illness accompanied by myalgia and cough. Ten other patients and two nurses in the home also had a nonspecific febrile illness in the past week.
   a. Administer influenza vaccine to patients and staff.
   b. Administer rimantadine to patients and staff.
   c. Administer penicillin prophylaxis to patients and staff.
   d. Administer pneumococcal vaccine to patients.
   e. Isolate patients with known febrile illness.

5. In the setting of an influenza epidemic, hospitalized patients with acute disease should be housed in:
   a. Individual rooms with negative pressure.
   b. Standard rooms with respiratory isolation practices.
   c. Standard rooms with contact isolation practices.
   d. Single rooms or in groups with patients with similar disease.

6. Each of the following is a hantavirus, except:
   a. Sin Nombre virus.
   b. Seuol virus.
   c. Dobrava virus.
   d. Crimean-Congo hemorrhagic fever virus.

7. Hantaviruses are typically transmitted by which of the following?
   a. Tick bite.
   b. Mosquito bite.
   c. Contact with animal blood, carcasses, or hide.
   d. Aerosol from animal excreta.

8. Which arenavirus can spread from human to human?
   a. LCM.
   b. Lassa.
   c. Junin.
   d. Machupo.
   e. Sabia.

9. For which arenavirus infection has a treatment been proven to be effective?
   a. LCM.
   b. Lassa.
   c. Junin.
   d. Machupo.
   e. Sabia.

10. Which drug is effective in the treatment of infection with Question 9's answer?
    a. Cidofovir.
    b. Adefovir.
    c. Lamivudine.
    d. Acyclovir.
    e. Ribavirin.

Quiz 32
Topic: RNA Viruses 5 (Chapters 162-164)

Chapter numbers refer to "Principles and Practices of Infectious Diseases", sixth edition, edited by Mandell, Bennett, and Dolin, Elsevier/Churchill Livingstone, Philadelphia, PA, 2005.

Answers:

1.   B
2.   B
3.   A
4.   B
5.   D
6.   D
7.   D
8.   B
9.   B
10. E

Chapter numbers refer to "Principles and Practices of Infectious Diseases", sixth edition, edited by Mandell, Bennett, and Dolin, Elsevier/Churchill Livingstone, Philadelphia, PA, 2005.

1. HTLV-1 is endemic in all of the following areas, except:
    a. Russia.
    b. Japan.
    c. Indonesia.
    d. Africa.
    e. The Caribbean.

2. Vertical transmission of HTLV-1 occurs predominantly via which of the following routes?
    a. Breast feeding.
    b. Intra-uterine.
    c. Peri-partum.

3. The risk of adult T-cell leukemia (ATL) in HTLV-1 carriers is:
    a. <5%.
    b. 5-10%.
    c. 10-25%.
    d. 30-50%.

4. ATL responds well to chemotherapy.
    a. True
    b. False

5. Which of the following diseases is thought to be secondary to HTLV-1 infection?
    a. Hairy cell leukemia.
    b. Mycosis fungoides.
    c. HAM/TSP.
    d. SLE.

6. Which HTLV-1 protein is thought to be an important transforming agent?
    a. Tax.
    b. Rev.
    c. Rex.
    d. Nef.
    e. Tat.

7. HIV-1 protease is encoded by which of the following genes?
    a. Gag.
    b. Pol.
    c. Vif.
    d. Vpx.
    e. Vpr.

8. The viral genome of HIV-1 consists of:
    a. Negative sense, single strand RNA.
    b. Double-stranded DNA.
    c. Positive sense, single copy RNA.
    d. Positive sense, two copies RNA.

9. Which co-receptor usage is associated with the syncitium-inducing phenotype?
    a. CXCR4.
    b. CCR5.
    c. CCR2b.
    d. CD4.

10. HIV-1 integrase integrates:
    a. RNA into DNA.
    b. DNA genome into the host cell chromosome.
    c. RNA genome into the host cell chromosome.
    d. RT with protease.

Answers:

1.	A
2.	A
3.	A
4.	B
5.	C
6.	A
7.	B
8.	D
9.	A
10.	B

Quiz 34
Topic: Picornaviridae 1 (Chapters 167-169)

Chapter numbers refer to "Principles and Practices of Infectious Diseases", sixth edition, edited by Mandell, Bennett, and Dolin, Elsevier/Churchill Livingstone, Philadelphia, PA, 2005.

1. Throughout the world, enteroviral infections occur throughout the year without seasonal fluctuations.
   a. True
   b. False

2. Of all enteroviral infections, only wild-type poliovirus infections are symptomatic more often than not.
   a. True
   b. False

3. Please explain below the epidemiological theory on why the polio epidemic emerged in the USA in the 20th century. (5 points)

   _____
   _____
   _____
   _____
   _____
   _____
   _____
   _____
   _____
   _____
   _____
   _____
   _____

4. Rhesus macaques are the only other natural host for poliovirus.
   a. True
   b. False

5. Poliovirus (wild-type and attenuated vaccine strains) is most often shed from which of the following?
   a. Feces.
   b. Fomites.
   c. Saliva.
   d. Urine.

6. The major risk factor for chronic, enteroviral meningoencephalitis is which of the following?
   a. DiGeorge's syndrome.
   b. HIV infection.
   c. Severe combined immunodeficiency syndrome.
   d. X-linked agammaglobulinemia.

7. Enteroviruses cause all of the following syndromes, except:
   a. Myopericarditis.
   b. Epidemic keratoconjunctivitis.
   c. Myositis.
   d. Aseptic meningitis.
   e. Acute respiratory tract disease.

8. Which of the following is recommended therapy for enteroviral aseptic meningitis?
   a. Bed rest and NSAID.
   b. Pleconaril.
   c. Ribavirin.
   d. Intravenous IgG.

9. Serum levels of myocardial enzymes are infrequently elevated in enteroviral myopericarditis.
   a. True
   b. False

Answers:

1. B
2. B
3. Improved hygiene created a susceptible, older population. This situation allowed epidemics to occur in older children and young adults. FDR is a classic example. Before the early 20th century, the vast majority of children was infected at a very young age and had mostly unapparent infections.
4. B
5. A
6. D
7. B
8. A
9. B

Chapter numbers refer to "Principles and Practices of Infectious Diseases", sixth edition, edited by Mandell, Bennett, and Dolin, Elsevier/Churchill Livingstone, Philadelphia, PA, 2005.

1. Hepatitis A virus (HAV) is found in many animal species, which are thought to be a major reservoir for human infections.
   a. True
   b. False

2. The major route of HAV transmission is:
   a. Parenteral.
   b. Sexual.
   c. Enteral.
   d. Vertical.

3. HAV food contamination occurs only through water contamination.
   a. True
   b. False

4. Liver inflammation during HAV infection is thought to be:
   a. Secondary to a viral cytopathic effect.
   b. Secondary to viral toxin production.
   c. Immune mediated via CD8+ T-cells.
   d. Immune mediated via anti-HAV antibodies.

5. Travelers going to areas with endemic HAV should receive the HAV vaccine and pooled IG if they are traveling within what period of time before their departure?
   a. 1-2 weeks.
   b. 2-4 weeks.
   c. 6 weeks.
   d. 3 months.

6. People with chronic hepatitis C virus infection are clearly at increased risk of fulminant hepatitis from HAV infection.
   a. True
   b. False

7. Post-exposure prophylaxis with pooled IG can be given up to how much time after the exposure and still be effective?
   a. 48 hours.
   b. 7 days.
   c. 14 days.
   d. 1 month.

8. Pooled IG prophylaxis confers protection for what period of time?
   a. 3 months.
   b. 6 months.
   c. 12 months.

9. Rhinovirus infections are seen most commonly in which of the following two seasons?
   a. Spring.
   b. Summer.
   c. Winter.
   d. Fall.

10. There are approximately how many serotypes of rhinovirus?
    a. 20.
    b. 100.
    c. 1,000.

11. Rhinovirus is typically transmitted by which of the following?
    a. Hand-to-hand contact.
    b. Aerosols.
    c. Droplets.
    d. Fomites.

Answers:

1.	B
2.	C
3.	B
4.	C
5.	A
6.	B
7.	C
8.	A
9.	A, D
10.	B
11.	A

Quiz 36
Topic: Other Viruses (Chapters 172-174)

Chapter numbers refer to "Principles and Practices of Infectious Diseases", sixth edition, edited by Mandell, Bennett, and Dolin, Elsevier/Churchill Livingstone, Philadelphia, PA, 2005.

Questions 1-3: True or False

1. Unlike hepatitis A virus, Norwalk virus is not transmitted by contaminated shellfish.
   a. True
   b. False

2. Norwalk agent-induced diarrhea has white blood cells.
   a. True
   b. False

3. Chronic HEV infection occurs in 5-10% of infected individuals.
   a. True
   b. False

4. Hepatitis E virus (HEV) has a genome consisting of which of the following?
   a. Positive sense RNA.
   b. Negative sense RNA.
   c. Double-stranded DNA.
   d. DNA and RNA.

5. Transmission of HEV is typically by which of the following routes?
   a. Airborne.
   b. Fomites.
   c. Via animals.
   d. Fecal-oral.

6. Which of the following groups has a high mortality with HEV infection?
   a. Cirrhotics.
   b. Diabetics.
   c. CGD patients.
   d. Pregnant women.
   e. Chronic HCV infection.

7. Serum samples for the serologic diagnosis of HEV should be sent to which of the following?
   a. LabCorp.
   b. Specialties Lab.
   c. Quest.
   d. The CDC.

8. People with acute HEV are best treated with:
   a. γ-interferon.
   b. α-interferon.
   c. Ribavirin.
   d. Passive immunotherapy.
   e. Supportive care.

9. HEV infection and transmission is most similar to which of the following?
   a. HAV.
   b. HBV.
   c. HCV.
   d. HGV (GBV-C).

Answers:

1.	B
2.	B
3.	B
4.	A
5.	D
6.	D
7.	D
8.	E
9.	A

Chapter numbers refer to "Principles and Practices of Infectious Diseases", sixth edition, edited by Mandell, Bennett, and Dolin, Elsevier/Churchill Livingstone, Philadelphia, PA, 2005.

1. Prions are:
   a. Closely related to alphaviruses.
   b. Closely related to enteroviruses.
   c. Closely related to pox viruses.
   d. Protein-based infectious pathogens.

2. Prions are inactivated by nucleases and UV radiation.
   a. True
   b. False

3. PrPsc is located in which of the following?
   a. In the cell membrane.
   b. In the cytoplasm.
   c. In the nucleus.
   d. In the endoplasmic reticulum.

4. In theory, PrPsc replicates by which of the following mechanisms?
   a. Causing a mutation in the gene encoding PrPc.
   b. Causing a mutation in another gene which controls PrPc transcription.
   c. Converting PrPc into PrPsc.

5. Kuru is associated with which of the following practices?
   a. Female circumcision.
   b. Male circumcision.
   c. Tattooing.
   d. Cannibalism.

6. Which of the following is characteristic in sCJD?
   a. EEG.
   b. MRI findings.
   c. CSF protein abnormality.
   d. PET scanning.

Questions 7-8: True or False

7. sCJD can be transmitted from person to person via blood transfusion.
   a. True
   b. False

8. Cooking beef inactivates PrPsc found in nvCJD.
   a. True
   b. False

Answers:

1.	D
2.	B
3.	B
4.	C
5.	D
6.	A
7.	B
8.	B

Chapter numbers refer to "Principles and Practices of Infectious Diseases", sixth edition, edited by Mandell, Bennett, and Dolin, Elsevier/Churchill Livingstone, Philadelphia, PA, 2005.

1. Chlamydial inclusion bodies consist of which of the following?
   a. Conglomerates of bacterial protein in the endoplasmic reticulum.
   b. Host cell debris.
   c. Bacterial chromatin.
   d. Reticulate bodies in endocytic vesicles.

2. Chlamydia needs which of the following host cell product(s) for its metabolism?
   a. High energy phosphate compounds.
   b. Phospholipids.
   c. All amino acids.
   d. All of the above.
   e. None of the above.

3. The elementary body is the form of Chlamydia, which infects cells and is stable in an extra cellular environment.
   a. True
   b. False

4. Which group of *Chlamydia trachomatis* serovars causes LGV and severe proctocolitis in homosexual men?
   a. A, B, Ba, and C.
   b. D-K.
   c. L1, L2, and L3.

5. Which group of *C. trachomatis* serovars causes ocular trachoma?
   a. A, B, Ba, and C.
   b. D-K.
   c. L1, L2, and L3.

6. Which group of *C. trachomatis* serovars causes genital tract disease and inclusion conjunctivitis?
   a. A, B, Ba, and C.
   b. D-K.
   c. L1, L2, and L3.

Questions 7-9: True or False

7. The primary lesion of LGV is a painless papule or ulcer which is generally not noticed.
   a. True
   b. False

8. Most adults with inclusion conjunctivitis have concurrent genital tract infections with *C. trachomatis*.
   a. True
   b. False

9. *C. trachomatis* is the cause of >90% of non-gonococcal urethritis.
   a. True
   b. False

10. *C. trachomatis* can infect all of the following tissues in a woman, except:
    a. Cervical epithelium.
    b. Vaginal epithelium.
    c. Urethra.
    d. Bartholin glands.

11. Which of the following types of poultry farmers has the highest attack rate for infection with *Chlamydophila psittaci*?
    a. Chicken farmers.
    b. Goose farmers.
    c. Duck farmers.
    d. Turkey farmers.

12. The rate of *Chlamydophila pneumoniae* infection does not vary with the seasons.
    a. True
    b. False

Quiz 38
Topic: Chlamydia (Chapters 176-179)

Chapter numbers refer to "Principles and Practices of Infectious Diseases", sixth edition, edited by Mandell, Bennett, and Dolin, Elsevier/Churchill Livingstone, Philadelphia, PA, 2005.

Answers:

1.   D
2.   A
3.   A
4.   C
5.   A
6.   B
7.   A
8.   A
9.   B
10. B
11. D
12. A

Chapter numbers refer to "Principles and Practices of Infectious Diseases", sixth edition, edited by Mandell, Bennett, and Dolin, Elsevier/Churchill Livingstone, Philadelphia, PA, 2005.

1. Mycoplasmas are L-forms of bacteria.
   a. True
   b. False

2. Mycoplasmas can grow on cell-free media.
   a. True
   b. False

3. Bullous myringitis is seen in most cases of Mycoplasma pneumonia.
   a. True
   b. False

4. Mycoplasma is a frequent cause of bacterial encephalitis.
   a. True
   b. False

5. Mycoplasmas appear to cause infection as extracellular parasites.
   a. True
   b. False

6. Which of the following dermatologic conditions has the strongest association with mycoplasma infection?
   a. Stevens-Johnson syndrome.
   b. Erythema nodosum.
   c. Erythema marginatum.
   d. Erythema migrans.

7. Which of the following underlying diseases/conditions is associated with severe complications of mycoplasma infection?
   a. Thallasemia.
   b. Paroxysmal nocturnal hemoglobinuria.
   c. Chronic lymphocytic leukemia.
   d. Hereditary spherocytosis.
   e. Sickle cell disease.

8. Cold agglutinins in *M. pneumoniae* infections are which of the following?
   a. IgG antibodies which bind to endothelial cells.
   b. IgG antibodies which bind to IgM antibodies.
   c. IgM antibodies which bind to red blood cells.
   d. IgM antibodies which bind to platelets.

9. Ureaplasmas are not found in normal vaginal flora.
   a. True
   b. False

10. Which of the following organisms is most strongly associated with non-gonococcal urethritis?
    a. *M. hominis.*
    b. *M. genitalium.*
    c. *U. parvum.*
    d. *U. urealyticum.*
    e. *M. fermentans.*

11. Mycoplasmas are not inhibited by which one of the following antibiotics?
    a. Ceftriaxone.
    b. Azithromycin.
    c. Ciprofloxacin.
    d. Doxycycline.

Answers:

1.	B
2.	A
3.	B
4.	B
5.	A
6.	A
7.	E
8.	C
9.	B
10.	B
11.	A

Chapter numbers refer to "Principles and Practices of Infectious Diseases", sixth edition, edited by Mandell, Bennett, and Dolin, Elsevier/Churchill Livingstone, Philadelphia, PA, 2005.

1. Brill-Zinsser is a recrudescence of long latent infection with which of the following organisms?
   a. *R. rickettsii.*
   b. *C. burnetti.*
   c. *R. akari.*
   d. *R. prowazekii.*
   e. *R. typhus.*

2. *Rickettsia rickettsii* is an obligate intracellular parasite.
   a. True
   b. False

3. Which tick is responsible for *R. rickettsii* transmission in the eastern U.S.A.?
   a. *Dermacentor andersoni.*
   b. *Dermacentor variablis.*
   c. *Ixodes scapularis/dammini.*
   d. *Ixodes pacificus.*
   e. *Amblyomma cajennense.*

Questions 4-6: True or False

4. *R. rickettsii* is transmitted trans-stadially.
   a. True
   b. False

5. Most cases of Rocky Mountain spotted fever (RMSF) occur in the fall.
   a. True
   b. False

6. In RMSF patients the CSF usually has increased leukocytes.
   a. True
   b. False

7. *R. rickettsii* infect which of the following cell types?
   a. Macrophages.
   b. Megakaryocytes.
   c. Red blood cells.
   d. Polymorphonuclear cells.
   e. Endothelial cells.

8. The diagnosis of RMSF is made most often and most reliably by which of the following?
   a. Serology.
   b. PCR.
   c. Buffy coat staining.
   d. Culture.

9. The treatment of choice for RMSF in pregnant women is which of the following?
   a. Doxycycline.
   b. Chloramphenicol.
   c. Erythromycin.
   d. Ceftriaxone.
   e. Ciprofloxacin.

10. By which of the following can *R. akari* be differentiated from RMSF?
    a. Type of rash.
    b. Presence of eschar.
    c. Vector.
    d. Absence of headache.
    e. a, b & c.
    f. All of the above.

11. *Coxiella burnetti* infects humans via which of the following routes?
    a. Ingestion of contaminated food products.
    b. Tick bite.
    c. Flea bite.
    d. Inhalation of aerosol.

12. Which of the following tissues has a high concentration of *C. burnetti*?
    a. Milk.
    b. Meat or muscle tissue.
    c. Placenta.
    d. Brain.

13. Q fever is diagnosed by which of the following?
    a. Serology.
    b. PCR.
    c. Buffy coat staining.
    d. Culture.

Chapter numbers refer to "Principles and Practices of Infectious Diseases", sixth edition, edited by Mandell, Bennett, and Dolin, Elsevier/Churchill Livingstone, Philadelphia, PA, 2005.

14. *R. prowazekii* is transmitted by which of the following vectors?
    a. Dog ticks.
    b. Human body louse.
    c. Dog fleas.
    d. Cat fleas.

15. *R. typhus* is transmitted by which of the following vectors?
    a. Dog ticks.
    b. Human body louse.
    c. Dog fleas.
    d. Rat fleas.

Answers:

1. D
2. A
3. B
4. A
5. B
6. B
7. E
8. A
9. B
10. E
11. D
12. C
13. A
14. B
15. D

Quiz 41
Topic: *Staphylococcus aureus* (Chapter 192)

Chapter numbers refer to "Principles and Practices of Infectious Diseases", sixth edition, edited by Mandell, Bennett, and Dolin, Elsevier/Churchill Livingstone, Philadelphia, PA, 2005.

Questions 1-4: True or False:

Differences between Gram-negative bacteria and Gram-positive bacteria.

1. Gram-negative bacteria have a thicker peptido-glycan layer than Gram-positive bacteria.
   a. True
   b. False

2. Only Gram-positive bacteria have an outer membrane.
   a. True
   b. False

3. Only Gram-positive bacteria have techoic acid.
   a. True
   b. False

4. *S. aureus* has a polysaccharide capsule.
   a. True
   b. False

5. All of the following are true about Panton-Valentine toxin-producing *S. aureus* isolates, except:
   a. They cause community-associated MRSA.
   b. They frequently cause osteomyelitis, septicemia, and endocarditis.
   c. They are encoded by a bacteria phage.
   d. They frequently causes furuncles.
   e. They can cause pneumonia.
   f. Their toxin is a hemolysin.

Questions 6-10: True or False:

Toxic Shock Syndrome

6. TSS caused by group A *streptococcus* (GAS) is more often associated with positive cultures from normally sterile sites.
   a. True
   b. False

7. Rash is seen the same percentage of TSS regardless of cause.
   a. True
   b. False

8. Only *S. aureus* TSS is associated with a super-antigen.
   a. True
   b. False

9. GAS TSS has a higher mortality than that caused by *S. aureus*.
   a. True
   b. False

10. TSST-1 gene is rare (<5%) in *S. aureus* from colonizers.
    a. True
    b. False

Questions 11-14: True or False
11. SCCmec is located on a plasmid.
    a. True
    b. False

12. The SCCmec of CA-MRSA isolates is much smaller than the other three types.
    a. True
    b. False

13. The *bla* gene for penicillinase is carried on a plasmid.
    a. True
    b. False

14. GISA strains typically have the Van A resistance phenotype.
    a. True
    b. False

15. The D-test is used to detect *S. aureus* resistance to which of the following?
    a. Cephazolin.
    b. Methicillin.
    c. Tetracycline.
    d. Clarithromycin.
    e. Clindamycin.

Chapter numbers refer to "Principles and Practices of Infectious Diseases", sixth edition, edited by Mandell, Bennett, and Dolin, Elsevier/Churchill Livingstone, Philadelphia, PA, 2005.

16. In adults, *S. aureus* carriage rates range from:
    a. 0-10%.
    b. 10-20%.
    c. 20-40%.
    d. 50-70%

Answers:

1.	B
2.	B
3.	A
4.	A
5.	B
6.	A
7.	B
8.	B
9.	A
10.	B
11.	B
12.	A
13.	A
14.	B
15.	E
16.	C

Quiz 42
Topic: Group A *Streptococcus* (Chapter 195-196)

Chapter numbers refer to "Principles and Practices of Infectious Diseases", sixth edition, edited by Mandell, Bennett, and Dolin, Elsevier/Churchill Livingstone, Philadelphia, PA, 2005.

1. Which of the following has a clear line of demarcation between involved and un-involved skin?
   a. Erysipelas.
   b. Cellulitis.

2. Which of the following is raised above the level of the surrounding skin?
   a. Erysipelas.
   b. Cellulitis.

3. Which of the following is a rare infection caused by Group A streptococci (GAS)?
   a. Lymphangitis.
   b. Pneumonia.
   c. Bacteremia.
   d. Endocarditis.
   e. Pyoderma.

Questions 4-20: True or False:

4. Serogrouping (Lancefield) for streptococci is based on the T-protein.
   a. True
   b. False

5. β-hemolysis refers to incomplete hemolysis.
   a. True
   b. False

6. Group A streptococci (GAS) strains that do not express the M protein are avirulent.
   a. True
   b. False

7. Antibodies against streptolysin S indicate recent infection.
   a. True
   b. False

8. GAS carriage in school aged children is 15-20%.
   a. True
   b. False

9. Children with GAS pharyngitis often complain of nausea, vomiting and abdominal pain.
   a. True
   b. False

10. Bacitracin is used to identify GAS apart from other streptococci, because GAS are exquisitely sensitive to this antibiotic.
    a. True
    b. False

11. 5-10% of GAS strains have increased MIC to penicillin.
    a. True
    b. False

12. Rapid antigen detection tests lack sensitivity and specificity.
    a. True
    b. False

13. Early treatment of GAS pharyngitis is important, because delayed therapy will reduce the efficacy in preventing rheumatic fever.
    a. True
    b. False

14. In the USA, macrolide resistant GAS is steadily increasing and affects the use of this class of antibiotics in empiric therapy of GAS pharyngitis.
    a. True
    b. False

15. The beneficial effects of intravenous immunoglobulin on GAS toxic shock syndrome (TSS) have been proven in a randomized, controlled clinical trial.
    a. True
    b. False

16. Treatment of pyoderma prevents poststreptococcal glomerulonephritis.
    a. True
    b. False

Chapter numbers refer to "Principles and Practices of Infectious Diseases", sixth edition, edited by Mandell, Bennett, and Dolin, Elsevier/Churchill Livingstone, Philadelphia, PA, 2005.

17. In acute rheumatic fever (ARF), arthritis is migratory and polyarticular.
    a. True
    b. False

18. In ARF, the arthritis usually involves the large joints of the extremities.
    a. True
    b. False

19. NSAIDs reduce the progression of ARF chronic carditis.
    a. True
    b. False

20. Penicillin is typically given for many years, sometimes decades, to reduce the likelihood of ARF and acute glomerulonephritis recurrences.
    a. True
    b. False

Answers:

1.	A
2.	A
3.	D
4.	B
5.	B
6.	A
7.	B
8.	A
9.	A
10.	A
11.	B
12.	B
13.	B
14.	B
15.	B
16.	B
17.	A
18.	A
19.	B
20.	B

Quiz 43
Topic: *Brucella* species & *Francisella tularensis* (Chapters 223-224)

Chapter numbers refer to "Principles and Practices of Infectious Diseases", sixth edition, edited by Mandell, Bennett, and Dolin, Elsevier/Churchill Livingstone, Philadelphia, PA, 2005.

1. *Brucellae* are found in high concentrations in the muscle tissue of infected animals.
   a. True
   b. False

2. *Brucellae* replicate primarily within which of the following?
   a. Muscle tissue.
   b. Brain.
   c. Reticuloendothelial system.
   d. Bone marrow.
   e. Bone.

3. The predominant route of transmission of *brucellae* in the southwest USA is now thought to be which of the following?
   a. Ingestion of contaminated goat milk.
   b. Exposure to contaminated placental tissue.
   c. Inhalation of aerosol in meat factories (abattoir).
   d. Contact with infected hares.
   e. Laboratory accidents.

4. Blood cultures are helpful in diagnosing brucellosis.
   a. True
   b. False

5. For the treatment of brucellosis, the World Health Organization recommends the following regimen:
   a. Ceftriaxone 2 gm IV QD for 4-weeks.
   b. Doxycycline 200 mg po QD + Rifampin 600 mg po QD for 6-weeks.
   c. Tetracycline 500 mg po QID for 6-weeks + Streptomycin 1 gm IV QD for the first three weeks.
   d. TMP/SMX DS two tablets po BID for 6-weeks.

Questions 6-12: True or False

6. Tularemia is most common in tropical areas.
   a. True
   b. False

7. Males account for most of the human cases of tularemia.
   a. True
   b. False

8. Human-to-human spread of tularemia, although rare, does occur.
   a. True
   b. False

9. In ulceroglandular tularemia, the skin lesion always precedes the lymphadenopathy.
   a. True
   b. False

10. In tick-borne tularemia, the most common site for the lymphadenopathy is the inguinal region.
    a. True
    b. False

11. *F. tularensis* is routinely seen on Gram-stained smears.
    a. True
    b. False

12. Doxycycline and streptomycin have equivalent efficacy rates in treating tularemia.
    a. True
    b. False

13. The diagnosis of tularemia is usually established by:
    a. Serology.
    b. Blood culture.
    c. Lymph node culture.
    d. Lymph node staining.
    e. Clinical grounds.

Chapter numbers refer to "Principles and Practices of Infectious Diseases", sixth edition, edited by Mandell, Bennett, and Dolin, Elsevier/Churchill Livingstone, Philadelphia, PA, 2005.

Answers:

1.	B
2.	C
3.	A
4.	A
5.	B
6.	B
7.	A
8.	B
9.	B
10.	A
11.	B
12.	B
13.	A

Chapter numbers refer to "Principles and Practices of Infectious Diseases", sixth edition, edited by Mandell, Bennett, and Dolin, Elsevier/Churchill Livingstone, Philadelphia, PA, 2005.

1. Which of the following states/provinces has the highest rate of leptospirosis?
   a. Puerto Rico.
   b. Guam.
   c. Hawaii.
   d. New Jersey.
   e. Brooklyn.

Questions 2-3: True or False

2. Leptospires, excreted in animal urine, can survive for months in the environment.
   a. True
   b. False

3. The main route of infection by leptospires is through ingestion.
   a. True
   b. False

4. Which of the following is prominent during the acute, septicemic phase of leptospirosis?
   a. Aseptic meningitis.
   b. Jaundice.
   c. Acute renal failure.
   d. Increased CPK.
   e. Conjunctival suffusion and muscle tenderness.

5. The preferred method of laboratory diagnosis of leptospirosis is which of the following?
   a. MAT of acute and convalescent sera.
   b. PCR of blood, urine, or CSF.
   c. Blood culture.
   d. Urine culture.

6. Moderate-to-severe leptospirosis should be treated with which of the following?
   a. Doxycycline 200 mg IV q12h.
   b. Penicillin 4 mU IV q6h.
   c. Penicillin 1.5 mU IV q6h.
   d. Chloramphenicol 1 gm IV q6h.

Questions 7-12: True or False:

7. In louse-borne relapsing fever, *B. recurrentis* is transmitted to the human host when the louse defecates while feeding.
   a. True
   b. False

8. Spirochetes are found in 70% of cases when wet blood smears of febrile patients are examined by darkfield microscopy.
   a. True
   b. False

9. Leukocytosis and increased ESR are uncommon in relapsing fever.
   a. True
   b. False

10. Jarisch-Herxheimer reaction is a rare but potentially fatal reaction to treatment of relapsing fever.
    a. True
    b. False

11. Jarsich-Herxheimer reaction only occurs when relapsing fever is treated with a cell wall acting agent, such as penicillin.
    a. True
    b. False

12. Untreated epidemic louse-borne relapsing fever has a mortality of up to 40%.
    a. True
    b. False

Chapter numbers refer to "Principles and Practices of Infectious Diseases", sixth edition, edited by Mandell, Bennett, and Dolin, Elsevier/Churchill Livingstone, Philadelphia, PA, 2005.

Answers:

1.   C
2.   A
3.   B
4.   E
5.   A
6.   C
7.   B
8.   A
9.   B
10.   B
11.   B
12.   A

Quiz 45
Topic: Lyme Disease & *Spirillum minus* (Chapters 239-240)

Chapter numbers refer to "Principles and Practices of Infectious Diseases", sixth edition, edited by Mandell, Bennett, and Dolin, Elsevier/Churchill Livingstone, Philadelphia, PA, 2005.

1. The form of Ixodes ticks which is most responsible for the transmission of Lyme disease to humans is which of the following?
   a. Nymph.
   b. Adult.
   c. Larvae.

Questions 2-7: True or False

2. Deer and white-footed mice are important reservoirs of *B. burgdorferi*.
   a. True
   b. False

3. *I. pacificus* nymphs have a high rate of *B. burgdorferi* carriage.
   a. True
   b. False

4. European Lyme disease is more symptomatic than American disease.
   a. True
   b. False

5. Most patients with EM recall having a tick bite in that area.
   a. True
   b. False

6. The thigh, groin, and axilla are the most common areas for EM.
   a. True
   b. False

7. Typically, patients with EM are seropositive for antibodies against *B. burgdorferi*.
   a. True
   b. False

8. The most common form of cardiac involvement in Lyme disease is which of the following?
   a. Acute myocarditis.
   b. Acute pericarditis.
   c. Chronic pericarditis.
   d. A-V block.
   e. Chronic cardiomyopathy.

9. Lyme disease arthritis usually affects which of the following?
   a. Multiple joints.
   b. Small joints of hands and fingers symmetrically.
   c. Sacral-iliac joint.
   d. Asymmetric large joint(s).

10. Recommended first line therapies for Lyme disease in patients without drug allergies include all of the following, except:
    a. Doxycycline.
    b. Amoxicillin.
    c. Cefuroxime.
    d. Erythromycin.

Questions 11-15: True or False

11. Fluoroquinolones are effective *in vitro* against *B. burgdorferi*.
    a. True
    b. False

12. *Spirillum minus* infections occur after rat bites or oral ingestion.
    a. True
    b. False

13. *S. minus* is more common in Asia than the USA.
    a. True
    b. False

14. The inflamed wound heals just before fever develops in *S. minus* infections.
    a. True
    b. False

15. *S. minus* is typically diagnosed by isolation via blood cultures.
    a. True
    b. False

Chapter numbers refer to "Principles and Practices of Infectious Diseases", sixth edition, edited by Mandell, Bennett, and Dolin, Elsevier/Churchill Livingstone, Philadelphia, PA, 2005.

Answers:

1.	A
2.	B
3.	B
4.	B
5.	B
6.	A
7.	B
8.	D
9.	D
10.	D
11.	B
12.	B
13.	A
14.	B
15.	B

Quiz 46
Topic: *Clostridium tetani* & *Clostridium botulinum* (Chapters 242-243)

Chapter numbers refer to "Principles and Practices of Infectious Diseases", sixth edition, edited by Mandell, Bennett, and Dolin, Elsevier/Churchill Livingstone, Philadelphia, PA, 2005.

1. Tetanus toxin affects which of the following types of neurons?
   a. GABA secreting.
   b. Dopamine secreting.
   c. Acetycholine secreting.
   d. Serotonin secreting.
   e. Glycine secreting.

Questions 2-3: True or False

2. Tetanus toxin is irreversible.
   a. True
   b. False

3. The diagnosis of tetanus is established by culturing of wounds.
   a. True
   b. False

4. When treating tetanus, which of the following should be done within the first hour of presentation?
   a. Reduction of spasms with benzodiazepines.
   b. Antimicrobial therapy.
   c. Passive immunization.
   d. Labetalol therapy to reduce sympathetic hyperactivity.

5. Neonatal tetanus occurs after ingestion of *C. tetani*.
   a. True
   b. False

6. Patients with at-risk wounds should receive passive and active immunization if they have not received active immunization within the past ___ years?
   a. 5.
   b. 10.
   c. 15.
   d. 20.
   e. Not needed if series of immunization has ever been completed.

Questions 7-10: True or False

In classic botulism:
7. Fever is rare.
   a. True
   b. False

8. CNS involvement is uncommon.
   a. True
   b. False

9. The neurologic deficits consist of symmetric motor weakness with corresponding sensory loss.
   a. True
   b. False

10. Weakness begins in the extremities.
    a. True
    b. False

11. Which of the following form(s) of botulism is(are) caused by pre-formed toxin and not endogenous production of the toxin?
    a. Foodborne.
    b. Infant.
    c. Wound.
    d. Undetermined etiology.

12. The diagnosis of botulism is usually made by which of the following?
    a. Anti-toxin antibodies.
    b. EMG.
    c. Edrophonium test.
    d. Toxin assays.
    e. Clinical findings.

13. Which of the following are part of standard botulism therapy?
    a. Administration of anti-toxin.
    b. Active immunization.
    c. Aminoglycoside therapy.
    d. Labetalol therapy.

Chapter numbers refer to "Principles and Practices of Infectious Diseases", sixth edition, edited by Mandell, Bennett, and Dolin, Elsevier/Churchill Livingstone, Philadelphia, PA, 2005.

Answers:

1. A
2. A
3. B
4. A
5. B
6. A
7. A
8. A
9. B
10. B
11. A
12. D
13. A

Quiz 47
Topic: *Mycobacterium tuberculosis* (Chapter 240)

Chapter numbers refer to "Principles and Practices of Infectious Diseases", sixth edition, edited by Mandell, Bennett, and Dolin, Elsevier/Churchill Livingstone, Philadelphia, PA, 2005.

1. Which of the following serve as reservoirs for *M. tuberculosis*?
   a. Chimpanzees.
   b. Macaques.
   c. Guinea pigs.
   d. Deer.
   e. All of the above.
   f. None of the above.

2. Which concentration of organisms is needed before a sputum smear can become positive by acid-fast staining?
   a. 10 organisms/ml.
   b. 100 organisms/ml.
   c. 1,000 organisms/ml.
   d. 10,000 organisms/ml.

Questions 3-4: True or False

3. All body fluids are first treated with decontamination before culturing for *M. tuberculosis*.
   a. True
   b. False

4. DNA PCR is a sensitive and specific way to rule in *M. tuberculosis* infection in smear positive sputum specimens.
   a. True
   b. False

5. *M. bovis* infection usually occurs after which of the following?
   a. Exposure to contaminated placenta.
   b. Exposure to infected person with *M. bovis* cavitary disease.
   c. Exposure to infected cow during veterinary care.
   d. Ingestion of contaminated milk.

6. In the United States, which percentage of household contacts becomes infected with *M. tuberculosis* after they are exposed to smear positive cases?
   a. 5-10%
   b. 20-30%.
   c. 50%.
   d. 80%.
   e. >80%.

Questions 7-9: True or False

7. One possible cause of a false-positive tuberculin 5 TU skin test is repeated tuberculin skin testing within the past year.
   a. True
   b. False

8. False negative tuberculin tests occur in at least 20% of all persons with known active tuberculosis.
   a. True
   b. False

9. Cavitary disease is less common in patients with HIV infection.
   a. True
   b. False

10. If LFTs have become elevated during treatment of tuberculosis, which of the following drugs should be cautiously introduced after discontinuation of INH and RMP and normalization of LFTs?
    a. PZA.
    b. Moxifloxacin.
    c. INH.
    d. RMP.

11. During treatment of pulmonary tuberculosis, the sputum cultures should become negative by which of the following?
    a. 2 weeks.
    b. 4-6 weeks.
    c. 2 months.
    d. 3 months.

Quiz 47
Topic: *Mycobacterium tuberculosis* (Chapter 240)

Chapter numbers refer to "Principles and Practices of Infectious Diseases", sixth edition, edited by Mandell, Bennett, and Dolin, Elsevier/Churchill Livingstone, Philadelphia, PA, 2005.

Questions 12-15: True or False

Answers:

1.	F
2.	D
3.	B
4.	A
5.	D
6.	B
7.	B
8.	A
9.	A
10.	C
11.	C
12.	B
13.	B
14.	B
15.	A
16.	D
17.	B

12. Treatment of contacts of active tuberculosis cases reduces the probability of disease by ~90%.
    a. True
    b. False

13. Contacts should be given INH only after a second skin test at 8 weeks post-exposure is positive.
    a. True
    b. False

14. The BCG reduces the infection rate in children by 60-80%.
    a. True
    b. False

15. Extrapulmonary tuberculosis foci usually respond to treatment more rapidly than pulmonary tuberculosis.
    a. True
    b. False

16. In which of the following forms of tuberculosis has adjunctive corticosteroid therapy been clinically proven to reduce mortality?
    a. Pleural.
    b. Meningeal.
    c. Vertebral osteomyelitis.
    d. Pericardial.

17. People with a history of BCG with a scar should be offered chemoprophylaxis only if their PPD reaction is >= 15 mm.
    a. True
    b. False

Chapter numbers refer to "Principles and Practices of Infectious Diseases", sixth edition, edited by Mandell, Bennett, and Dolin, Elsevier/Churchill Livingstone, Philadelphia, PA, 2005.

Questions 1-8: True or False

1. *C. albicans* has been recovered from soil, animals, hospital environments, inanimate objects, and food.
   a. True
   b. False

2. Thrush patches consist entirely of yeast.
   a. True
   b. False

3. The diagnosis of thrush can be confirmed by culture.
   a. True
   b. False

4. *Candida* esophagitis may occur frequently without thrush.
   a. True
   b. False

5. *Candida* is the most common cause of vaginitis.
   a. True
   b. False

6. Vaginal candidiasis is more common and more refractory to treatment in patients with AIDS.
   a. True
   b. False

7. Most patients with *Candida* endocarditis have positive blood cultures.
   a. True
   b. False

8. Patients with *Candida* endocarditis respond well to treatment with amphotericin B therapy given for 8-10 weeks.
   a. True
   b. False

9. Which of the following is the most common cause of clinical disease?
   a. *A. flavus.*
   b. *A. fumigatus.*
   c. *A. terreus.*
   d. *A. niger.*

10. *Aspergillus* does not colonize humans.
    a. True
    b. False

11. Which one of the following two is an early finding in pulmonary aspergillosis?
    a. Halo sign.
    b. Air-crescent sign.

12. Which of the following is the drug of choice for invasive aspergillosis?
    a. Lipid amphotericin B.
    b. Amphotericin B.
    c. Voriconazole.
    d. Itraconazole.
    e. Caspofungin.

13. Antifungal agents have no proven utility in the treatment of allergic bronchopulmonary aspergillosis.
    a. True
    b. False

Answers:

1.	A
2.	B
3.	B
4.	A
5.	A
6.	B
7.	A
8.	B
9.	B
10.	B
11.	A
12.	C
13.	B

Quiz 49
Topic: Fungi 2 (Chapters 257-261)

Chapter numbers refer to "Principles and Practices of Infectious Diseases", sixth edition, edited by Mandell, Bennett, and Dolin, Elsevier/Churchill Livingstone, Philadelphia, PA, 2005.

Questions 1-2: True or False

1. Medically important Zygomycetes grow in the environment and in tissue as hyphal forms.
   a. True
   b. False

2. Most patients with mucormycosis have rhinocerebral disease.
   a. True
   b. False

3. Which of the following are prominent components of the host response against the Mucorales?
   a. Neutrophils.
   b. T-cells.
   c. B-cells.
   d. NK cells.
   e. Eosinophils.
   f. Mast cells.

4. The most common groups of mucormycosis patients include all of the following, except:
   a. Renal failure patients on deferoxamine.
   b. Patients with prolonged neutropenia.
   c. Patients in DKA.
   d. AIDS patients.

Questions 5-10: True or False

5. The hyphal forms of Mucorales typically appear broader in tissue specimens than that of Aspergillus, Fusarium, and Pseudallescheria.
   a. True
   b. False

6. Voriconazole has excellent activity against the Mucorales fungi.
   a. True
   b. False

7. Patients with lymphocutaneous sporotrichosis typically have fever.
   a. True
   b. False

8. Cigar-shaped yeasts on skin lesion biopsies are characteristic but not diagnostic of sporotrichosis.
   a. True
   b. False

9. For lymphocutaneous sporotrichosis, itraconazole is the treatment of choice.
   a. True
   b. False

10. The diagnosis of chromoblastomycosis is established by the classic triad of painless soft tissue swelling, draining sinus tracts, and extrusion of grains.
    a. True
    b. False

11. In the therapy of cryptococcal meningitis, it has been clearly established that flucytosine, when combined with amphotericin B, leads to:
    a. Improved survival.
    b. Lower relapse rate.
    c. Decreased complications.
    d. Decreased time to sterile CSF cultures.
    e. All of the above.

12. Most complications of cryptococcal meningitis in AIDS patients are secondary to:
    a. Mass effects of cryptococcomas.
    b. Invasion of blood vessels.
    c. Spread to encephalitis.
    d. Increased intracranial pressure.
    e. Fungal toxins.

13. All of the following may be used to treat cryptococcosis, except:
    a. Flucytosine.
    b. Lipid-amphotericin.
    c. Fluconazole.
    d. Caspofungin.
    e. Itraconazole.

Chapter numbers refer to "Principles and Practices of Infectious Diseases", sixth edition, edited by Mandell, Bennett, and Dolin, Elsevier/Churchill Livingstone, Philadelphia, PA, 2005.

14. Which of the following is associated with poor prognosis in cryptococcal meningitis?
    a. Decreased mental status.
    b. CSF WBC count > 20 cells/mm^3.
    c. Strongly positive India ink examination.
    d. High polysaccharide antigen titer (1:1,024).
    e. None of the above.

Answers:

1.	A
2.	A
3.	A
4.	D
5.	A
6.	B
7.	B
8.	B
9.	A
10.	B
11.	D
12.	D
13.	D
14.	B

Quiz 50
Topic: Fungi 3 (Chapters 262-264)

Chapter numbers refer to "Principles and Practices of Infectious Diseases", sixth edition, edited by Mandell, Bennett, and Dolin, Elsevier/Churchill Livingstone, Philadelphia, PA, 2005.

Questions 1-4: True or False

1. Cases of histoplasmosis have been reported on every continent except Antarctica.
   a. True
   b. False

2. There is a strong association between bird and bat guano and the presence of *H. capsulatum*.
   a. True
   b. False

3. Histoplasmosis develops more frequently in females than in males.
   a. True
   b. False

4. The mycelial phase of *H. capsulatum* is present at ambient temperature and the yeast form is present at 37°C or higher.
   a. True
   b. False

5. Which percentage of acute histoplasmosis cases develops acute pericarditis?
   a. 6%.
   b. 16%.
   c. 26%.
   d. 46%.
   e. 66%.

6. The vast majority of progressive disseminated histoplasmosis cases are thought to arise from which of the following?
   a. Acute infection.
   b. Reactivation.
   c. Exuberant immune response against *H. capsulatum* antigens.

7. The mainstay of diagnosis in patients with progressive disseminated histoplasmosis (PDH) is which of the following?
   a. Visualization of the organisms on silver stained buffy coat.
   b. Serology.
   c. Culture of blood, bone marrow, or sputum.
   d. Skin test.
   e. Antigen ELISA of serum or urine.

8. In AIDS patients with PDH, which drug should be used as maintenance therapy?
   a. Itraconazole.
   b. Fluconazole.
   c. Voriconazole.
   d. Ketoconazole.
   e. Weekly amphotericin B.

9. Blastomycosis often occurs as the result of reactivation.
   a. True
   b. False

10. Blastomycosis commonly affects all of the following organs, except:
    a. Prostate.
    b. Bone.
    c. Liver.
    d. Skin.
    e. Lung.

11. Which of the following stains may be used to differentiate *B. dermatitidis* from *C. neoformans*?
    a. Mayer mucicarmine stain.
    b. Gomori methenamine-silver stain.
    c. Periodic acid-Schiff stain.
    d. India ink stain.

12. All of the following shows consistent activity against *B. dermatitidis*, except:
    a. Itraconazole.
    b. Ketoconazole.
    c. Caspofungin.
    d. Amphotericin.
    e. Voriconazole.

Chapter numbers refer to "Principles and Practices of Infectious Diseases", sixth edition, edited by Mandell, Bennett, and Dolin, Elsevier/Churchill Livingstone, Philadelphia, PA, 2005.

13. Patients with coccidioidomycosis frequently develop one or more of the following rashes, except:
   a. Transient, papular rash.
   b. Erythema marginatum.
   c. Erythema multiforme.
   d. Erythema nodosum.

14. Technicians evaluating sputum specimens for the presence of *Coccidioides* spp. should be warned to take precautions against infection.
   a. True
   b. False

15. Patients with coccidioidal meningitis should be treated with which of the following?
   a. Fluconazole.
   b. Itraconazole.
   c. Ketoconazole.
   d. Amphotericin B.

Answers:

1.	A
2.	A
3.	A
4.	D
5.	A
6.	B
7.	B
8.	B
9.	A
10.	B
11.	D
12.	D
13.	D
14.	B
15.	A

Quiz 51
Topic: Protozoa 1 (Chapters 270-272)

Chapter numbers refer to "Principles and Practices of Infectious Diseases", sixth edition, edited by Mandell, Bennett, and Dolin, Elsevier/Churchill Livingstone, Philadelphia, PA, 2005.

Questions 1-2: True or False

1. *E. histolytica* and *E. dispar* trophozoites are morphologically indistinguishable.
   a. True
   b. False

2. *Entamoeba* cysts may remain viable in sewage water for 1 month.
   a. True
   b. False

3. Risk groups for amebiasis include all of the following, except:
   a. Male homosexuals with many sexual contacts.
   b. Institutionalized populations, especially those cognitively impaired.
   c. Residents of southeastern USA.
   d. Immigrants from an endemic area.

4. Both noninvasive and invasive *E. histolytica* infections elicit an IgG response against the lectin protein.
   a. True
   b. False

5. Which of the following is not commonly seen in patients with amebic colitis?
   a. Heme-positive stools.
   b. Normal body temperature (afebrile).
   c. Charcot-Leyden crystals.
   d. Numerous fecal leukocytes.

Questions 6-7: True or False

6. The diagnosis of *E. histolytica* invasive colonic infection is established by simply finding hemophagocytic trophozoites.
   a. True
   b. False

7. Amebic liver abscess is usually diagnosed by fine needle aspiration of the abscess, which reveals the presence of trophozoites.
   a. True
   b. False

8. All of the following are acceptable forms of therapy for patients with amebic liver abscess, except:
   a. Tetracycline plus chloroquine.
   b. Metronidazole plus paromomycin.
   c. Dehydroemetine plus diloxanide furoate.
   d. Dehydroemetine plus paromomycin.

Questions 9-12: True or False

9. Primary amebic meningoencephalitis is caused by *Naegleria fowleri*.
   a. True
   b. False

10. *Acanthamoeba* spp. can be isolated from the human pharynx.
    a. True
    b. False

11. *Acanthamoeba* granulomatous amebic encephalitis occurs predominantly in individuals with no underlying disease.
    a. True
    b. False

12. *Acanthamoeba* keratitis is treated with a combination of surgical debridement and topical antimicrobial agents.
    a. True
    b. False

13. Which form of malaria does not cause some form of chronic infection?
    a. *P. falciparum*.
    b. *P. malariae*.
    c. *P. vivax*.
    d. *P. ovale*.

14. *Plasmodium vivax* preferentially infects reticulocytes.
    a. True
    b. False

Chapter numbers refer to "Principles and Practices of Infectious Diseases", sixth edition, edited by Mandell, Bennett, and Dolin, Elsevier/Churchill Livingstone, Philadelphia, PA, 2005.

15. Chloroquine acts by:
    a. Binding to cytochrome b and inhibiting parasite mitochondrial transport.
    b. Inhibiting dihydrofolate reductase.
    c. Inhibiting protein synthesis by preventing binding of aminacyl-tRNA to the ribosome 30S subunit.
    d. Forming toxic complexes with the heme molecules.

16. First line therapy for *P. malariae* chemoprophylaxis is which of the following?
    a. Chloroquine.
    b. Fansidar.
    c. Doxycycline.
    d. Mefloquine.
    e. Atovaquone/proguanil.

17. All of the following are commonly seen in severe *P. falciparum* infection, except:
    a. Anemia.
    b. Hypoglycemia.
    c. ARDS.
    d. Hepatic failure.
    e. Coma.

18. The Duffy antigen is the erythrocyte receptor for which of the following species of *Plasmodium*?
    a. *P. vivax*.
    b. *P. ovale*.
    c. *P. falciparum*.
    d. *P. malariae*.

19. Chloroquine-resistant *P. falciparum* is not seen in most Caribbean islands.
    a. True
    b. False

Answers:

1.	A
2.	A
3.	C
4.	A
5.	D
6.	A
7.	B
8.	A
9.	A
10.	A
11.	B
12.	A
13.	A
14.	A
15.	D
16.	A
17.	D
18.	A
19.	A

Chapter numbers refer to "Principles and Practices of Infectious Diseases", sixth edition, edited by Mandell, Bennett, and Dolin, Elsevier/Churchill Livingstone, Philadelphia, PA, 2005.

1. *Leishmania donovani* and *L. infantum/chagasi* are responsible for the majority of cases of visceral leishmaniasis.
   a. True
   b. False

2. 90% of the visceral leishmaniasis cases are seen in the following countries, except:
   a. Brazil.
   b. India.
   c. Bangladesh.
   d. Sudan.
   e. El Salvador.

3. Which of the following forms of leishmania occurs in human tissue?
   a. Amastigote.
   b. Merozoite.
   c. Promastigote.
   d. Flagellated.
   e. Sporozoite.

4. Which of the following is the most sensitive way to diagnose visceral leishmaniasis?
   a. Bone marrow biopsies for stain and culture.
   b. Splenic aspirations for stain and culture.
   c. ELISA for anti-leishmania antibodies.
   d. PCR.
   e. Montegro skin test.

5. New World cutaneous leishmaniasis is usually a rural zoonosis.
   a. True
   b. False

6. The treatment of choice for visceral leishmaniasis is which of the following?
   a. Liposomal amphotericin.
   b. Pentavalent antimony.
   c. Pentamidine.
   d. Miltefosine.

7. *T. cruzi* is transmitted by triatomine insect bites when:
   a. Infective forms are carried into the host with saliva.
   b. Infective forms cause the insect to regurgitate into the bite.
   c. Infective forms in the feces penetrate non-intact skin.

8. *T. brucei* complex are transmitted by a tsetse fly bite when:
   a. Infective forms are carried into the host with saliva.
   b. Infective forms cause the insect to regurgitate into the bite.
   c. Infective forms in the feces penetrate non-intact skin.

9. *T. cruzi* causes hypertrophic cardiomyopathy.
   a. True
   b. False

10. Diagnosis of acute Chagas' disease is made by which of the following?
    a. Detecting the organisms in blood smears or buffy coats.
    b. Detecting IgM anti-*T. cruzi* antibodies.
    c. Detecting IgG anti-*T. cruzi* antibodies in the appropriate setting.
    d. PCR for *T. cruzi*.

Questions 11-14: True or False

11. The WHO recommends that all patients with chronic Chagas' disease be treated with nifurtimox or benznidazole.
    a. True
    b. False

12. *T. cruzi* can be transmitted by blood transfusion.
    a. True
    b. False

13. *T. b. gambiense* is found in West Africa.
    a. True
    b. False

Chapter numbers refer to "Principles and Practices of Infectious Diseases", sixth edition, edited by Mandell, Bennett, and Dolin, Elsevier/Churchill Livingstone, Philadelphia, PA, 2005.

14. *T. b. gambiense* causes prominent lymphadenopathy.
    a. True
    b. False

15. CNS East African trypanosomiasis is treated with which of the following?
    a. Pentamidine.
    b. Suramin.
    c. Melarsoprol.
    d. Eflornithine.

Answers:

1.	A
2.	E
3.	A
4.	B
5.	A
6.	A
7.	C
8.	A
9.	B
10.	A
11.	B
12.	A
13.	A
14.	A
15.	C

Quiz 53
Topic: Protozoa 3 (Chapters 276-278)

Chapter numbers refer to "Principles and Practices of Infectious Diseases", sixth edition, edited by Mandell, Bennett, and Dolin, Elsevier/Churchill Livingstone, Philadelphia, PA, 2005.

Questions 1-5: True or False

1. *Toxoplasma gondii* infection is prevalent in game animals, such as bears.
   a. True
   b. False

2. Toxoplasmic encephalitis (TE) in AIDS patients is caused by reactivation.
   a. True
   b. False

3. *T. gondii* can be transmitted through blood transfusion.
   a. True
   b. False

4. TE lesions frequently involve the basal ganglia.
   a. True
   b. False

5. In TE, the CSF typically has a mild mononuclear pleocytosis and a mild-moderately elevated protein level.
   a. True
   b. False

6. The recommended treatment of a pregnant woman acutely infected with *T. gondii* is which of the following?
   a. Atovaquone.
   b. Spiramycin.
   c. Pyrimethamine plus clindamycin.
   d. Pyrimethamine plus sulfadiazine.
   e. Azithromycin.

Questions 7-8: True or False

7. Pregnant women with toxoplasmic retinitis from reactivation do not have a higher risk of vertical transmission of *T. gondii*.
   a. True
   b. False

8. *Giardia lamblia* is flagellated.
   a. True
   b. False

9. Giardiasis outbreaks have been linked to which of the following animals?
   a. Beaver.
   b. Deer.
   c. Bear.
   d. Cats.
   e. Skunks.

10. In patients with giardiasis, diarrhea may last for months.
    a. True
    b. False

11. All of the following may be used to treat giardiasis, except:
    a. Metronidazole.
    b. Albendazole.
    c. Tinidazole.
    d. Clindamycin.
    e. Paromomycin.

Questions 12-15: True or False

12. *Trichomonas vaginalis* is flagellated.
    a. True
    b. False

13. Trichomoniasis is occasionally acquired non-venereally.
    a. True
    b. False

14. Metronidazole blocks the metabolism of alcohol; if they are taken together, flushing, nausea, and vomiting can occur.
    a. True
    b. False

15. *T. vaginalis* is an infrequent cause of urethritis in men.
    a. True
    b. False

Chapter numbers refer to "Principles and Practices of Infectious Diseases", sixth edition, edited by Mandell, Bennett, and Dolin, Elsevier/Churchill Livingstone, Philadelphia, PA, 2005.

16. Vaginal trichomoniasis is most often diagnosed by which of the following techniques?
    a. Wet mount examination of vaginal fluid.
    b. Culture of *T. vaginalis* from vaginal fluid.
    c. DNA probe of vaginal fluid.
    d. PCR of vaginal fluid.

Answers:

1.	A
2.	A
3.	A
4.	A
5.	A
6.	B
7.	A
8.	A
9.	A
10.	A
11.	D
12.	A
13.	A
14.	A
15.	A
16.	A

Quiz 54
Topic: Protozoa 4 (Chapters 279-282)

Chapter numbers refer to "Principles and Practices of Infectious Diseases", sixth edition, edited by Mandell, Bennett, and Dolin, Elsevier/Churchill Livingstone, Philadelphia, PA, 2005.

1. In humans, babesia organisms invade which of the following?
   a. Erythrocytes only.
   b. Erythrocytes and hepatocytes.
   c. Erythrocytes and lymphocytes.
   d. Erythrocytes and monocytes.

2. The predominant cause of human babesiosis in the USA is which of the following?
   a. *B. microti.*
   b. *B. divergens.*
   c. WA1 isolate.
   d. *B. canis.*

3. Patients with babesiosis should be evaluated for simultaneous infection with *Borrelia burgdorferi* and *Ehrlichia chaffeensis*, because:
   a. People who get bitten by ticks often are bitten by many types of ticks.
   b. Co-infection of *B. microti* with either organism is more fulminant.
   c. All three organisms infect the white-tailed deer.
   d. *Ixodes scapularis* can simultaneously carry all three organisms.

4. *B. microti* can cause an asymptomatic, chronic infection.
   a. True
   b. False

5. The recommended treatment for *B. microti* infection is which of the following?
   a. Clindamycin and quinine.
   b. Chloroquine.
   c. Pyrimethamine and sulfadoxine.
   d. Primaquine.

6. All of the following are factors that promote outbreaks of cryptosporidiosis, except:
   a. Cryptosporidium's ability to replicate outside the host.
   b. The oocyst can survive for prolonged periods in the environment.
   c. Chlorination does not kill cryptosporidium.
   d. The oocytes are infectious as soon as they are shed.

7. Cryptosporidiosis in immunocompetent hosts is self-limited and once the diarrhea has resolved, it does not recur.
   a. True
   b. False

8. Which of the following assays on stool specimens is NOT routinely used to diagnose *Cryptosporidium* infection?
   a. Modified acid-fast stain.
   b. Auramine-rhodamine.
   c. Immunofluorescence.
   d. Antigen detection kits.
   e. PCR to detect *Cryptosporidium* DNA.

9. The first treatment option for AIDS patients with chronic cryptosporidiosis should be which of the following
   a. Nitazoxanide.
   b. Paromomycin.
   c. Spiramycin.
   d. Anti-retroviral therapy.

10. Cyclosporiasis can be distinguished from cryptosporidiosis, microsporidosis, and *Isospora* infections based on clinical signs and symptoms.
    a. True
    b. False

11. The first line therapy for cyclosporiasis is which of the following?
    a. Trimethoprim-sulfamethoxazole.
    b. Doxycycline.
    c. Metronidazole.
    d. Spiramycin.

12. The first line therapy for *Isospora* infection is which of the following?
    a. Trimethoprim-sulfamethoxazole.
    b. Doxycycline.
    c. Metronidazole.
    d. Spiramycin.

Chapter numbers refer to "Principles and Practices of Infectious Diseases", sixth edition, edited by Mandell, Bennett, and Dolin, Elsevier/Churchill Livingstone, Philadelphia, PA, 2005.

Questions 13-16: True or False

Answers:

1.	A
2.	A
3.	D
4.	A
5.	A
6.	A
7.	B
8.	E
9.	D
10.	B
11.	A
12.	A
13.	A
14.	A
15.	B
16.	A
17.	D
18.	B

13. Humans are the only host for *Isospora belli*.
    a. True
    b. False

14. *Enterocytozoon bieneusi* is the most frequent cause of microsporidiosis in AIDS patients.
    a. True
    b. False

15. *Enterocytozoon bieneusi* frequently causes disseminated infection in AIDS patients.
    a. True
    b. False

16. *Encephalitozoon intestinalis* causes more inflammation and necrosis than does *Enterocytozoon bieneusi*.
    a. True
    b. False

17. The diagnostic test of choice for intestinal microsporidiosis is which of the following?
    a. Upper GI endoscopy with biopsy.
    b. Colonoscopy.
    c. Electron microscopy of stool samples.
    d. Light microscopy of stool samples treated with chemotrope or chemofluorescent stains.

18. *Enterocytozoon bieneusi* responds well to albendazole therapy.
    a. True
    b. False

Quiz 55
Topic: Helminths 1 (Chapters 285-287)

Chapter numbers refer to "Principles and Practices of Infectious Diseases", sixth edition, edited by Mandell, Bennett, and Dolin, Elsevier/Churchill Livingstone, Philadelphia, PA, 2005.

Questions 1-3: True or False

1. Adult *Ascaris* worms live and mate in the lumen of the small bowel, primarily in the jejunum.
   a. True
   b. False

2. *Ascaris* infection occurs by ingestion of mature eggs.
   a. True
   b. False

3. The *Ascaris* larvae penetrate intact skin and then penetrate the alveoli, before being swallowed and maturing into adult worms.
   a. True
   b. False

4. Which of the following drugs is not recommended for the treatment of Ascariasis?
   a. Piperazine.
   b. Pyrantel pamoate.
   c. Albendazole.
   d. Mebendazole.
   e. Ivermectin.

5. The detection of *T. trichiura* eggs typically requires multiple stool specimens.
   a. True
   b. False

6. Which of the following is the major manifestation of hookworm infection?
   a. Vitamin B12 deficiency.
   b. Hyperinfection syndrome.
   c. Asthma.
   d. Iron deficiency anemia.

7. *Strongyloides stercoralis* infections last for 3-5 years.
   a. True
   b. False

8. The drug of choice for *S. stercoralis* infections is which of the following?
   a. Ivermectin.
   b. Albendazole.
   c. Mebendazole.
   d. Thiabendazole.

9. Periorbital edema is seen in which of the following infections?
   a. Bancroftian filariasis.
   b. Onchocerciasis.
   c. Trichinosis.
   d. Strongloidiasis.
   e. Loiasis.

10. Calabar swellings are seen in which of the following infections?
    a. Bancroftian filariasis.
    b. Onchocerciasis.
    c. Trichinosis.
    d. Strongloidiasis.
    e. Loiasis.

11. Which of the following diseases is established by finding microfilariae in the daytime blood?
    a. Bancroftian filariasis.
    b. Onchocerciasis.
    c. Trichinosis.
    d. Strongloidiasis.
    e. Loiasis.

12. Chronic infection with *S. mansoni* can cause which of the following types of hepatic fibrosis?
    a. Pre-sinusoidal.
    b. Sinusoidal.
    c. Post-sinusoidal.

13. Which organism's egg has a vertical spike?
    a. *S. mansoni*.
    b. *S. japonicum*.
    c. *S. haematobium*.

Chapter numbers refer to "Principles and Practices of Infectious Diseases", sixth edition, edited by Mandell, Bennett, and Dolin, Elsevier/Churchill Livingstone, Philadelphia, PA, 2005.

14. Which of the following infections responds poorly to praziquantel?
    a. *Fasciolopsis buski.*
    b. *Fasciola hepatica.*
    c. *Clonorchis sinensis.*
    d. *Paragonimus westermoni.*

15. Which of the following infections is acquired through the ingestion of undercooked freshwater crustaceans?
    a. *Fasciolopsis buski.*
    b. *Fasciola hepatica.*
    c. *Clonorchis sinensis.*
    d. *Paragonimus westermoni.*

16. Which of the following infections is acquired through the ingestion of undercooked freshwater fish?
    a. *Fasciolopsis buski.*
    b. *Fasciola hepatica.*
    c. *Clonorchis sinensis.*
    d. *Paragonimus westermoni.*

17. Which of the following infections is associated with sheep and cattle?
    a. *Fasciolopsis buski.*
    b. *Fasciola hepatica.*
    c. *Clonorchis sinensis.*
    d. *Paragonimus westermoni.*

18. Which of the following infections is acquired through the ingestion of contaminated water-cress or other aquatic plants?
    a. *Fasciolopsis buski.*
    b. *Fasciola hepatica.*
    c. *Clonorchis sinensis.*
    d. *Paragonimus westermoni.*

Answers:

#	
1.	A
2.	A
3.	B
4.	A
5.	B
6.	D
7.	A
8.	A
9.	C
10.	E
11.	E
12.	A
13.	C
14.	B
15.	D
16.	C
17.	B
18.	B

Chapter numbers refer to "Principles and Practices of Infectious Diseases", sixth edition, edited by Mandell, Bennett, and Dolin, Elsevier/Churchill Livingstone, Philadelphia, PA, 2005.

1. In the cestode lifecycle, eggs are secreted from the _____ host.
   a. Definitive.
   b. Intermediate.

2. For which of the following cestodes are humans either the intermediate or definitive host?
   a. *D. latum.*
   b. *T. saginata.*
   c. *T. solium.*
   d. *E. granulosus*
   e. *E. multilocularis.*

3. Which of the following cestodes can be transmitted from human to human?
   a. *D. latum.*
   b. *E. granulosus.*
   c. *T. saginata.*
   d. *H. nana.*

4. Which of the following two diseases is more aggressive?
   a. Hydatid cyst disease.
   b. Alveolar cyst disease.

Questions 5-6: True or False

5. Therapy for neurocysticercosis is albendazole + dexamethasone.
   a. True
   b. False

6. Negative serology rules out cysticercosis.
   a. True
   b. False

7. Which of the following is the largest tapeworm?
   a. *D. latum.*
   b. *H. nana.*
   c. *T. saginata.*
   d. *T. solium.*

8. Albendazole is the drug of choice for toxocariasis.
   a. True
   b. False

9. Anisakiasis is acquired by which of the following?
   a. Ingestion of contaminated salt-water fish.
   b. Ingestion of contaminated fresh-water fish.
   c. Ingestion of contaminated crustaceans.
   d. Ingestion of food contaminated with eggs.

10. *A. cantonensis* is acquired by which of the following?
    a. Ingestion of food contaminated by rat feces.
    b. Ingestion of contaminated crustaceans.
    c. Ingestion of undercooked rat meat.
    d. Ingestion of eggs.

Questions 11-13: True or False

11. Treatment for *A. cantonensis* meningitis is supportive.
    a. True
    b. False

12. Occasionally, *A. cantonensis* larvae are seen in the CSF.
    a. True
    b. False

13. Swimmer's itch is persistent and refractory to therapy.
    a. True
    b. False

Answers:

1.	A
2.	C
3.	D
4.	B
5.	A
6.	B
7.	A
8.	B
9.	A
10.	B
11.	A
12.	A
13.	B

Quiz 57
Topic: Nosocomial Herpesvirus Infections (Chapter 305)

Chapter numbers refer to "Principles and Practices of Infectious Diseases", sixth edition, edited by Mandell, Bennett, and Dolin, Elsevier/Churchill Livingstone, Philadelphia, PA, 2005.

Questions 1-4: True or False

1. HSV-2 infection of a neonate in an ICU imposes a great risk of infection to other infants in that ICU.
   a. True
   b. False

2. Peripartum pregnant women with herpes simplex virus infection who have secondary genital lesions present and membranes ruptured for more than 4-6 hours should be delivered vaginally.
   a. True
   b. False

3. Peripartum pregnant women with herpes simplex virus infection who have secondary genital lesions present and membranes intact should be delivered by Caesarean section.
   a. True
   b. False

4. Peripartum pregnant women with herpes simplex virus infection who have a history of genital lesions but none currently should be delivered vaginally.
   a. True
   b. False

5. A newborn is considered exposed to VZV if the mother has chickenpox lesions that developed at which of the following?
   a. 1 week before and up to 1 week after delivery.
   b. 5 days before and up to 5 days after delivery.
   c. 5 days before or within 48 hours after delivery.
   d. Within two weeks before delivery.

6. What is the next step if an immunocompromised patient is exposed to VZV?
   a. Draw serology.
   b. Administer VZIG.
   c. Administer varicella vaccine.
   d. Determine history.

7. Which of the following is NOT considered an exposure to VZV?
   a. Patient is examined in an exam room, which had just been used with a patient with varicella.
   b. Playmate contact more than 1 hour of indoor play.
   c. Playmate contact more than 2 hours of outdoor play.
   d. Use of adjacent bed in large ward.

8. The major route of nosocomial CMV transmission is which of the following?
   a. Parenteral route.
   b. Fomites.
   c. Aerosol.
   d. Salvia contamination.

9. The primary means for prevention of CMV infection is which of the following?
   a. Use of blood products treated to remove virus particles.
   b. Use of blood products treated to remove WBCs.
   c. Isolation of patients who are shedding CMV.
   d. Isolation of patients with primary CMV infection.

Questions 10-11; True or False

10. Data support the routine periodic screening for potentially pregnant women whose jobs entail exposure to CMV-infected patients.
    a. True
    b. False

11. Transmission of EBV from patient-to-staff or staff-to-patient has been not been described.
    a. True
    b. False

Quiz 57
Topic: Nosocomial Herpesvirus Infections (Chapter 305)

Chapter numbers refer to "Principles and Practices of Infectious Diseases", sixth edition, edited by Mandell, Bennett, and Dolin, Elsevier/Churchill Livingstone, Philadelphia, PA, 2005.

Answers:

1.	B
2.	A
3.	A
4.	A
5.	C
6.	D
7.	C
8.	A
9.	B
10.	B
11.	A

Quiz 58
Topic: Infections in Transplant Recipients (Chapters 311-312)

Chapter numbers refer to "Principles and Practices of Infectious Diseases", sixth edition, edited by Mandell, Bennett, and Dolin, Elsevier/Churchill Livingstone, Philadelphia, PA, 2005.

Questions 1-2: True or False

1. In hematopoeitic stem-cell transplant (HSCT) patients, diarrhea is usually not secondary to infection.
   a. True
   b. False

2. Primary CMV infection is uncommon in HSCT patients.
   a. True
   b. False

3. CMV screening techniques include which of the following techniques?
   a. Quantitative anti-CMV ELISA.
   b. Quantitative CMV culture.
   c. Quantitative pp65.
   d. Quantitative CMV PCR.

Questions 4-5: True or False

4. HSCT patients who are already seropositive can acquire a second primary VZV infection.
   a. True
   b. False

5. HHV-6 reactivates commonly in HSCT patients but has only rarely been associated with disease.
   a. True
   b. False

6. Which solid organ transplantation is associated with the lowest infection rate?
   a. Kidney.
   b. Heart.
   c. Heart-Lung.
   d. Liver.

7. In solid organ recipients, which of the following is one of the more problematic manifestations of CMV disease?
   a. Mononucleosis syndrome.
   b. Hepatitis.
   c. Pneumonitis.
   d. GI ulcers.

8. Post-transplant lymphoproliferative disorder (PTLD) may be treated with which of the following? More than one answer is correct.
   a. Reduction of immunosuppression.
   b. Intravenous acyclovir.
   c. Monoclonal antibodies against B-cell antigens.
   d. EBV specific CTL.

Questions 9-10: True or False

9. Liver transplant candidates who have HCV viremia before transplantation usually do not re-infect their liver grafts after transplantation.
   a. True
   b. False

10. Patients with chronic graft-versus-host disease should be maintained on antibiotic prophylaxis until immunosuppression is discontinued.
    a. True
    b. False

Answers:

1. A
2. A
3. C,D
4. A
5. A
6. A
7. D
8. A,C,D
9. B
10. A